# CENTRAL REGULATION OF AUTONOMIC FUNCTIONS

# Central Regulation of Autonomic Functions

*Second Edition*

*Edited by*

Ida J. Llewellyn-Smith, PhD

Anthony J. M. Verberne, PhD, DSc

OXFORD
UNIVERSITY PRESS

OXFORD
UNIVERSITY PRESS

Published in the United States of America by Oxford University Press, Inc.,
198 Madison Avenue, New York, NY, 10016
United States of America

Oxford University Press, Inc., publishes works that further Oxford University's objective of excellence in research, scholarship, and education

Oxford is a registered trade mark of Oxford University Press in the UK and in certain other countries


First Edition published in 1990



Library of Congress Cataloging-in-Publication Data
Central regulation of autonomic functions / edited by Ida J. Llewellyn-Smith, Anthony J.M. Verberne. – 2nd ed.
p. ; cm.
Rev. ed. of: Central regulation of autonomic functions. 1990.
Includes bibliographical references and index.
ISBN 978-0-19-530663-7
1. Autonomic nervous system—Physiology. I. Llewellyn-Smith, Ida J. II. Verberne, Anthony J. M.
III. Central regulation of autonomic functions.
[DNLM: 1. Autonomic Nervous System—physiology. WL 600]
QP368.C45 2011
612.8'9—dc22 2010030815

Typeset in Times Roman
Printed on acid-free paper

In Memoriam

Professor David Jordan died unexpectedly while the second edition of *Central Regulation of Autonomic Functions* was in preparation. The chapter that he wrote (Chapter 7, "Parasympathetic Preganglionic Neurons") is an example of the scholarly and thoughtful approach that characterized Dave's research and his teaching. Dave made a significant contribution to our understanding of how neurons in the nucleus of the solitary tract and dorsal motor nucleus of the vagus contribute to central cardiovascular and respiratory control. He is sorely missed by his colleagues and friends.

# Preface

In 1990, Oxford University Press published *Central Regulation of Autonomic Functions*. This seminal volume, edited by Arthur D. Loewy and K. Michael Spyer, was received with wide acclaim. The uniformly high quality of the chapters and an emphasis on identifying gaps in our knowledge about central autonomic control had an immediate impact on research in the field. These features ensured the success of the first volume and have resulted in a continuing high rate of citations, even though the book is now 20 years old.

Since publication of the first edition of *Central Regulation of Autonomic Functions* in 1990, enormous advances have been made in our understanding of how the central nervous system (CNS) controls autonomic function. The sophistication of physiological and anatomical methods used to study central nerve pathways has increased dramatically over the past 20 years and neuroscientists interested in central autonomic control have been quick to adopt these new methods. Thus, the use of *c-fos* expression to identify activated neurons, *in situ* hybridization histochemistry, trans-synaptic viral tracing, juxtacellular neuronal labelling, the increasing refinement of patch clamping techniques, telemetric monitoring, the development of several reduced *in vivo* preparations and, most recently, genetic manipulations that allow neurons to be activated with light have all had an enormous impact on our understanding of how the CNS controls homeostasis. As just one example of how much our knowledge has increased, the idea of a tri-synaptic circuit mediating the arterial baroreceptor reflex was still controversial at the time of publication of the first edition of this book. Now, the medullary pathway that involves the nucleus of the solitary tract (NTS), the caudal ventrolateral medulla and the rostral ventrolateral medulla (RVLM) is accepted as the circuit through which the brain regulates blood pressure on a heartbeat-to-heartbeat basis.

The explosive growth in information about central control of autonomic function and the absence of a recent comprehensive review of the topic convinced us of the need for a second edition of *Central Regulation of Autonomic Functions*. In this volume, we have chosen to focus on areas of central autonomic neuroscience that have experienced significant growth since 1990; and we have selected researchers whom we believe to be acknowledged experts in their respective fields to contribute to this volume. We were also eager for the book to be relevant to physiological problems that are important today. Consequently, the second edition contains chapters that deal with areas not covered in the first edition, including viscerosensory processing in the NTS and central autonomic control of the airways, thermogenesis and energy homeostasis. Capitalizing on the winning format of the first edition, we have asked our authors not only to review knowledge in their areas and highlight recent advances but also to identify key questions that still require investigation. Although the last two decades have seen a substantial increase in information relating to the 20 research areas that are the focus of this book, each area still has a number of important unanswered questions. For example, we know much more about the vasopressor neurons in the RVLM and their roles in blood pressure control than we did in 1990. However, our knowledge about other central autonomic neurons, such as dorsal vagal motor neurons, is still only sketchy.

We have also preserved a number of formatting features from the first edition. All of the chapters in the second edition have a common layout and we have instructed our authors to use a common design for illustrations. In the current edition, some figures have also been reproduced in colour in an insert in the center of the book. As happened for the first edition, we have had each chapter reviewed and the chapters have been revised in response to the reviewers' comments. For the benefit of students and researchers unfamiliar with the field of central autonomic control, we have decided to minimize the number of abbreviations used throughout the book and have insisted that the authors use only abbreviations from the common list that can be found on page xv.

By continuing with the highly successful approach of the first edition, we hope that the second edition of *Central Regulation of Autonomic Functions* will prove as provocative and inspire as much research effort as its predecessor. It will be truly gratifying if the second edition lives up to the exemplary standard set by the first and has a similar impact on the field of central control of autonomic function.

# Acknowledgements

We want to acknowledge the enormous debt we owe to Arthur Loewy and Mike Spyer, the editors of the first edition of *Central Regulation of Autonomic Functions*. Their foresight and dedication led to the development of the concept for the first edition and to its publication. They also have our admiration because the first edition was completed without the assistance of word processors, computer-based artwork, or the internet, which have provided critical underpinning for the second edition.

Our sincere thanks go to our colleagues who contributed chapters to this book. We are enormously grateful for their scholarship, their patience, and their willingness to make all the changes to their chapters that we requested. The success of the second edition of *Central Regulation of Autonomic Functions* rests primarily on their shoulders.

Our authors played another role by acting as reviewers for other chapters, and we also enlisted the services of other reviewers who were not directly involved as contributors to this book. We thank all of these people for helping us ensure that the high scientific standards set by the first edition of *Central Regulation of Autonomic Functions* were maintained in the second edition. We are also indebted to Lee Travis, whose assistance was invaluable in preparing databases of the references for several of the chapters.

Finally, we want to thank all of the people at Oxford University Press (OUP) who have been involved in producing the second edition of *Central Regulation of Autonomic Functions*. Jeffrey House's enthusiastic response to our initial inquiry convinced us of the merits of publishing a second edition. Fiona Stevens was our first editor at OUP. Upon her departure, this role was most ably filled by Craig Panner, who, along with David D'Addona and latterly Kathryn Winder, saw the project through to completion. Craig's enthusiasm for and commitment to the project always remained firm. The editors want to express their immense appreciation for his patience, persistence, and unwavering encouragement.

# Acknowledgements

# Contents

# Contributors

Michael C. Andresen, Ph.D.
*Department of Physiology and Pharmacology*
*Oregon Health and Science University*
*Portland, Oregon*

William W. Blessing, M.B.B.S., Ph.D., F.R.A.C.P.
*Departments of Physiology and Medicine*
*Center for Neuroscience*
*Flinders University*
*Bedford Park, South Australia, Australia*

Kirsteen N. Browning, Ph.D.
*Department of Neural and Behavioral Sciences*
*Penn State College of Medicine*
*Hershey, Pennsylvania*

Brendan J. Canning, Ph.D.
*Johns Hopkins Asthma and Allergy Center*
*Baltimore, Maryland*

J. Patrick Card, Ph.D.
*Department of Neuroscience*
*University of Pittsburgh*
*Pittsburgh, Pennsylvania*

Pascal Carrive, Ph.D.
*School of Medical Sciences*
*University of New South Wales*
*Sydney, New South Wales, Australia*

Roger A. L. Dampney, Ph.D., D.Sc.
*Discipline of Physiology*
*School of Medical Sciences and Bosch Institute*
*University of Sydney*
*Sydney, New South Wales, Australia*

William C. de Groat, Ph.D.
*Department of Pharmacology and Chemical Biology*
*University of Pittsburgh School of Medicine*
*Pittsburgh, Pennsylvania*

Susan A. Deuchars, Ph.D.
*Institute of Membrane and Systems Biology*
*University of Leeds*
*Leeds, West Yorkshire, United Kingdom*

Alastair V. Ferguson, Ph.D.
*Department of Physiology*
*Queen's University, Kingston*
*Ontario, Canada*

Patrice G. Guyenet, Ph.D.
*Department of Pharmacology*
*University of Virginia*
*Charlottesville, Virginia*

Pamela J. Hornby, Ph.D.
*Biologics Research*
*Centocor R&D Biotechnology Center of Excellence*
*Radnor, Pennsylvania*

David Jordan, Ph.D., D.Sc.
*Department of Physiology*
*Royal Free*
*and University College Medical School*
*University College London*
*London, United Kingdom*

Barry E. Levin, M.D.
*Neurology Service*
*Veterans Affairs Medical Center*
*East Orange, New Jersey*

Ida J. Llewellyn-Smith, Ph.D.
*Cardiovascular Medicine, Physiology and Centre for Neuroscience*
*School of Medicine*
*Faculty of Health Sciences*
*Flinders University*
*Bedford Park, South Australia, Australia*

John C. Longhurst, M.D., Ph.D.
*Departments of Medicine, Physiology and Biophysics, Pharmacology and Biomedical Engineering*
*University of California, Irvine*
*Irvine, California*

Lesley Marson, Ph.D.
*Division of Urology*
*Department of Surgery*
*School of Medicine*
*University of North Carolina*
*Chapel Hill, North Carolina*

Shaun F. Morrison, Ph.D.
*Department of Neurological Surgery*
*Oregon Health and Science University*
*Portland, Oregon*

Julian F. R. Paton, Ph.D.
*Department of Physiology and Pharmacology*
*Bristol Heart Institute*
*School of Medical Sciences*
*University of Bristol*
*Bristol, United Kingdom*

Ann M. Schreihofer, Ph.D.
*Department of Integrative Physiology*
*University of North Texas Health Science Center*
*Fort Worth, Texas*

Javier E. Stern, M.D., Ph.D.
*Department of Physiology*
*Medical College of Georgia*
*Augusta, Georgia*

Alison M. Strack, Ph.D.
*Department of Pharmacology*
*Merck Research Laboratories*
*Rahway, New Jersey*

Alan F. Sved, Ph.D.
*Department of Neuroscience*
*University of Pittsburgh*
*Pittsburgh, Pennsylvania*

R. Alberto Travagli, Ph.D.
*Department of Neural and Behavioral Sciences*
*Penn State College of Medicine*
*Hershey, Pennsylvania*

Anthony J. M. Verberne, Ph.D., D.Sc.
*University of Melbourne*
*Clinical Pharmacology and Therapeutics Unit*
*Department of Medicine*
*Austin Health*
*Heidelberg, Victoria, Australia*

Paul R. Wade, Ph.D.
*GI Pharmacology*
*Department of Biosciences*
*Shire Pharmaceuticals*
*Wayne, Pennsylvania*

# List of Abbreviations

| | |
|---|---|
| 5-HT | serotonin |
| ACh | acetylcholine |
| Adr | adrenaline |
| AMP | adenosine monophosphate |
| AMPA | alpha-amino-3-hydroxy-5-methylisoxazole-4-propionate |
| ATP | adenosine triphosphate |
| CART | cocaine and amphetamine regulated transcript |
| CNS | central nervous system |
| CRH | corticotropin-releasing hormone/factor |
| CVLM | caudal ventrolateral medulla |
| DMH | dorsomedial hypothalamic nucleus |
| DVN | dorsal vagal nucleus |
| EPSC | excitatory post-synaptic current |
| EPSP | excitatory post-synaptic potential |
| GABA | gamma amino butyric acid |
| GLUR1-7 | ionotropic glutamate receptors 1-7 |
| IML | intermediolateral cell column |
| IPSC | inhibitory post-synaptic current |
| IPSP | inhibitory post-synaptic potential |
| mRNA | messenger RNA |
| NA | noradrenaline |
| NMDA | *N*-methyl-D-aspartate |
| NTS | nucleus of the solitary tract |
| OVLT | organum vasculosum of the lamina terminalis |
| PAG | periaqueductal grey |
| PNMT | phenylethanolamine *N*-methyltransferase |
| PVN | paraventricular nucleus |
| RVLM | rostral ventrolateral medulla |
| SFO | subfornical organ |
| SON | supraoptic nucleus |
| TRPV | transient receptor potential vanilloid |

# CENTRAL REGULATION OF AUTONOMIC FUNCTIONS

1

# Central Autonomic Pathways

J. PATRICK CARD AND ALAN F. SVED

The central nervous system (CNS) exerts profound regulatory influence over peripheral physiology. This control is essential for homeostasis and for coordinating adaptive changes in physiology and behavior. The CNS influences the physiology of all peripheral organ systems, allowing them to function in concert as well as independently. CNS modulation of many autonomic functions, such as the regulation of arterial blood pressure, also incorporates control mechanisms that allow independent regional control within an organ or tissue. The integrated regulation within and among organs and tissues requires dynamic and responsive neural circuits that can provide the regulatory oversight necessary for proper autonomic function. The CNS meets this challenge by controlling the activity of the autonomic nervous system and through neuroendocrine control over the pituitary gland. The flexibility and precision of central autonomic regulation is coordinated by sensory feedback that the CNS receives from peripheral targets. Although CNS sites that integrate this sensory feedback have been identified, the details regarding the way in which they process sensory input and distribute the processed information to effector systems remain areas for serious investigation.

The purpose of this chapter is to provide an overview of the central circuits that are involved in controlling autonomic function. An extensive literature has identified populations of neurons that modulate the sympathetic and parasympathetic divisions of the autonomic nervous system. Transneuronal tracing using neurotropic viruses, which are retrogradely transported through synaptically connected chains of neurons (see **Box**), has played a critical role in establishing the relationships between groups of neurons involved in controlling various autonomic functions. Viral tracing experiments have been particularly important in identifying "command" neurons that control sympathetic outflow when a "fight-or-flight" response is required. Unfortunately, few studies have examined the synaptic relationships between different central autonomic nuclei or within individual nuclei. These sorts of studies are likely to be vital for understanding the complex interactions that permit the CNS to regulate autonomic function.

In this chapter, we outline the groups of CNS neurons that have been implicated in autonomic control and describe the connections through which they interact. We focus on the circuitry that underlies the ability of central autonomic neurons to respond dynamically to homeostatic and environmental challenges. Most of the chapter deals with the central autonomic neurons that control sympathetic outflow, because this circuitry has been the most extensively studied. To a lesser extent, we discuss central regulation of parasympathetic outflow, emphasizing coordination of sympathetic and parasympathetic activity. (More information about the control of parasympathetic outflow can be found in Chapter 7.) Much of the information relating to autonomic control circuitry that we review here comes from the rat, the species in which this has been the most extensively investigated. However, available data support the conclusion that this organization applies in other species, although little is known about central autonomic neurons in primates.

Box Viral transneuronal tracing

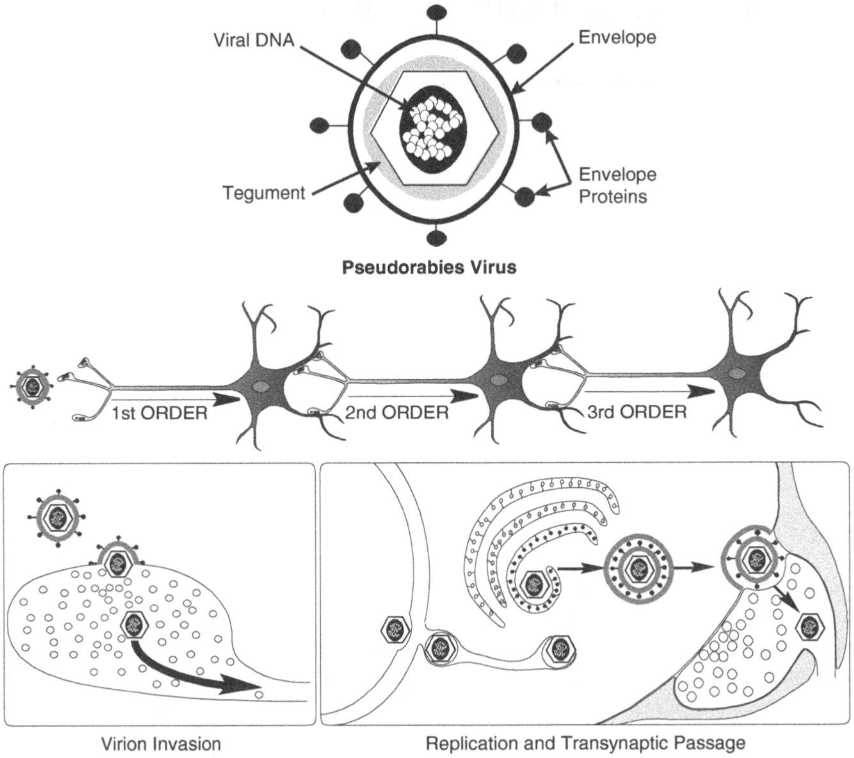


The viral transneuronal tracing method takes advantage of the ability of neurotropic viruses to invade neurons and produce infectious progeny that cross synapses to infect synaptically linked chains of neurons. The main advantage of transneuronal viral tracing is that it reveals polysynaptic circuits that cannot be studied with conventional tracers. Many well-characterized attenuated strains of virus that show directionally selective transport in neurons are now available.

Viral tracers are particularly well suited to analysis of autonomic circuitry and have been applied most extensively to that system. Analysis of viral transport through autonomic circuits has confirmed that the neuron-to-neuron transmission of virus occurs through synapses rather than via spread through the extracellular space after lysis of infected neurons. Studies of central autonomic circuits have also shown that the number of synaptic connections between neurons within a circuit is one of many factors that influence viral replication and transport through the circuit. Hence, the hierarchy of neurons within a circuit labeled by viral transport depends on more than the interval between inoculation and perfusion. These issues highlight the need for careful experimental design, critical analysis of labeling patterns, and conservative interpretation of data from viral tracing studies. A number of reviews provide further details on these issues as they apply to the commonly used alpha herpes viruses[16–19].

There appears to be a hierarchy in central control of autonomic function, which includes three levels of processing: (1) reflex control over individual autonomic targets, (2) integrated control over multiple targets, and (3) matching autonomic adjustments to environmental or homeostatic challenges with behavioral and endocrine responses. In this central processing scheme, sensory feedback is essential at all levels. Sensory information comes from multiple sources and feeds into central autonomic control circuitry at multiple levels. It is important to note that sensory input from a single source often influences several levels of processing. A good example of this organizational principle is the nucleus of the solitary tract (NTS), which receives and distributes information from a variety of different kinds of visceral primary afferents.

## SENSORY INPUT TO CENTRAL SITES INVOLVED IN AUTONOMIC CONTROL

The NTS is the major recipient of the primary sensory information that is essential for precisely regulating autonomic function (see also Chapter 2). This sensory input comes from virtually all autonomically innervated target organs and tissues. The NTS lies in the dorsal caudal brainstem, adjacent to the dorsal vagal motor nucleus and the area postrema. When viewed from a dorsal perspective, the NTS consists of bilateral columns that form a V (Figure 1–1). Each column has usually been separated into three divisions on the basis of location relative to the area postrema. Thus, there is a rostral division anterior to the area postrema, an intermediate division at the level of the area postrema, and a caudal division posterior to the area postrema, where the two columns of the NTS fuse along the midline.

Coronal sections through the NTS reveal a complex cytoarchitecture. Subnuclei within the NTS have been defined on the basis of cell morphology, packing density, and the distribution of sensory afferents. Traditionally, the NTS has been divided into lateral and medial subdivisions, which are separated by the fibers of the solitary tract. Primary sensory afferents travel through the solitary tract to gain access to the NTS (Figure 1–1). Functionally distinct classes of afferents either terminate within NTS subnuclei that are dedicated to organ-specific processing or overlap within a single subnucleus devoted to multi-modal processing. For example, sensory afferents from the esophagus terminate densely within the central subnucleus, where they exert reflex control over parasympathetic preganglionic neurons in the nucleus ambiguus responsible for motor innervation of the esophagus[26]. In contrast, the commissural subnucleus in the posterior NTS receives overlapping projections from functionally diverse primary afferents and distributes sensory information to many brain nuclei involved in central autonomic regulation (see Chapter 2). Neurons that are not confined to cytoarchitecturally distinct subnuclei also project to higher-order central autonomic cell groups. Among these are the A2 catecholamine neurons, which form a long linear column through the NTS and project extensively to areas such as the paraventricular nucleus of the hypothalamus (PVN), the central nucleus of the amygdala, and the bed nucleus of stria terminalis[3,80,103,130]. Thus, pathways originating in the NTS are organized to provide reflex control over individual autonomic targets and to distribute sensory information to other sites that integrate information related to autonomic function.

Although the NTS is often described as a relay for the distribution of sensory information to other regions of the CNS, NTS neurons also serve an important integrative function by processing sensory input. Interneurons in the NTS connect different NTS subnuclei. The time course of viral spread through the NTS after inoculation of autonomic targets in the periphery provides evidence for these local circuits. For example, injection of virus into the esophagus[21] initially produces restricted transneuronal infection of NTS neurons in the central subnucleus; but infection subsequently spreads to other NTS subnuclei at increasing survival times[9]. Similar spread of virus within the NTS occurs from targets such as the stomach and pancreas[70,91]. The extensive intrinsic circuitry in the NTS likely functions to coordinate activity within and among functionally related populations of NTS neurons.

The diversity of CNS afferents terminating within the NTS emphasizes its integrative capacity. The NTS receives afferents from virtually all of the brain sites that participate in regulating autonomic function. These include the rostral ventrolateral medulla (RVLM), the A5 noradrenergic cell group, the parapyramidal region, the lateral hypothalamic area, and the PVN. The area postrema, the parabrachial nucleus, the periaqueductal gray, the dorsomedial hypothalamic nucleus, the central nucleus of amygdala, the insular cortex, and the infralimbic area of the medial prefrontal cortex also provide input to the NTS. Anterograde tracing studies have shown that the majority of these projections are not confined by the boundaries of NTS subnuclei. The fact that dendrites of vagal motor neurons extend into the NTS[92,111] further complicates interpretation of the synaptic targets of these afferents in the NTS. Collectively, these observations suggest that the NTS is a complex integrative center that can influence autonomic outflow either through local brainstem circuits or through projections to other, more distant central autonomic sites. Defining the organizational principles and synaptology through which the NTS exerts its influence remains an important goal of autonomic neuroscience.

Ascending projections from the NTS distribute information about peripheral physiology and organ function through two parallel pathways[98] (Figure 1–2). First, NTS neurons send axons to cell groups in the brainstem, midbrain, diencephalon, limbic forebrain, and restricted regions of the cortex. Some of these efferents go to regions containing neurons that project directly to the sympathetic and parasympathetic preganglionic

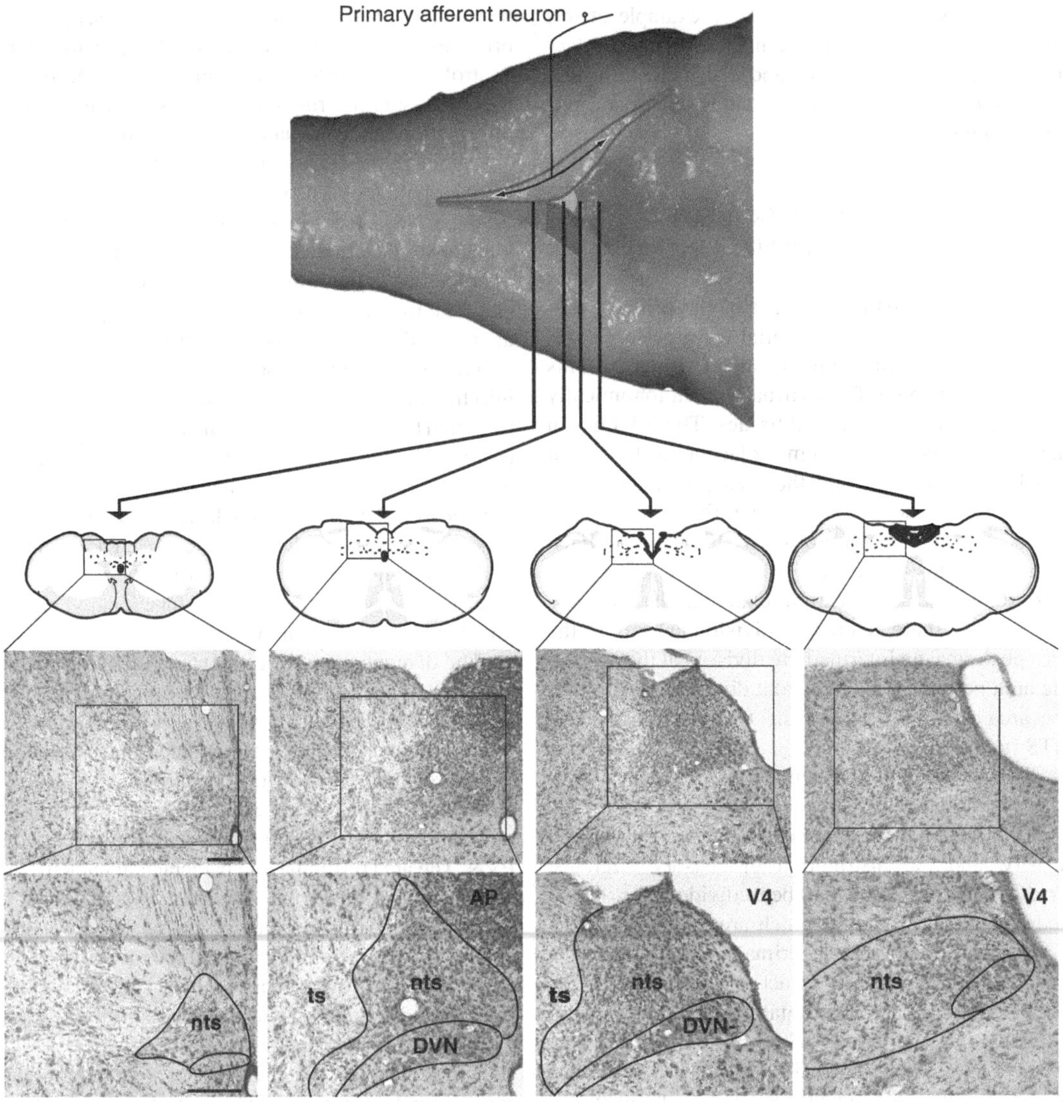


Figure 1–1 Organization of the nucleus of the solitary tract (NTS). For a color version of Figure 1–1, see Color Plate 1–1 between pages 224 and 225. The location of the NTS is mapped onto an image of the dorsal surface of the brainstem. NTS neurons are grouped into two long cell columns that fuse in the midline caudal to the area postrema (AP). The trajectory of primary sensory afferents that enter the NTS via the solitary tract is shown in the top column of the NTS. In the bottom column, the V-shaped structure of the NTS has been divided into three segments based on location relative to AP. The schematics above each column of micrographs show the location of the NTS in four coronal planes. The Nissl-stained photomicrographs below each schematic illustrate the cytoarchitecture of the boxed areas at intermediate and high magnification. AP, area postrema; DVN, dorsal vagal motor nucleus; ts, solitary tract; V4, fourth ventricle.

neurons, including the parapyramidal region, the RVLM, the A5 cell group, the lateral hypothalamic area, and the PVN. Other NTS axons supply areas that influence autonomic outflow indirectly through projections to other central autonomic nuclei. These areas include nuclei in the rostral hypothalamus involved in fluid homeostasis, two nuclei in the limbic forebrain (the central nucleus of amygdala and the bed nucleus of the stria terminalis)[119], and the infralimbic cortex[4]. Information from the NTS reaches these same brain regions and the insular cortex through separate pathways that involve a synapse in the parabrachial nucleus. NTS projections to the

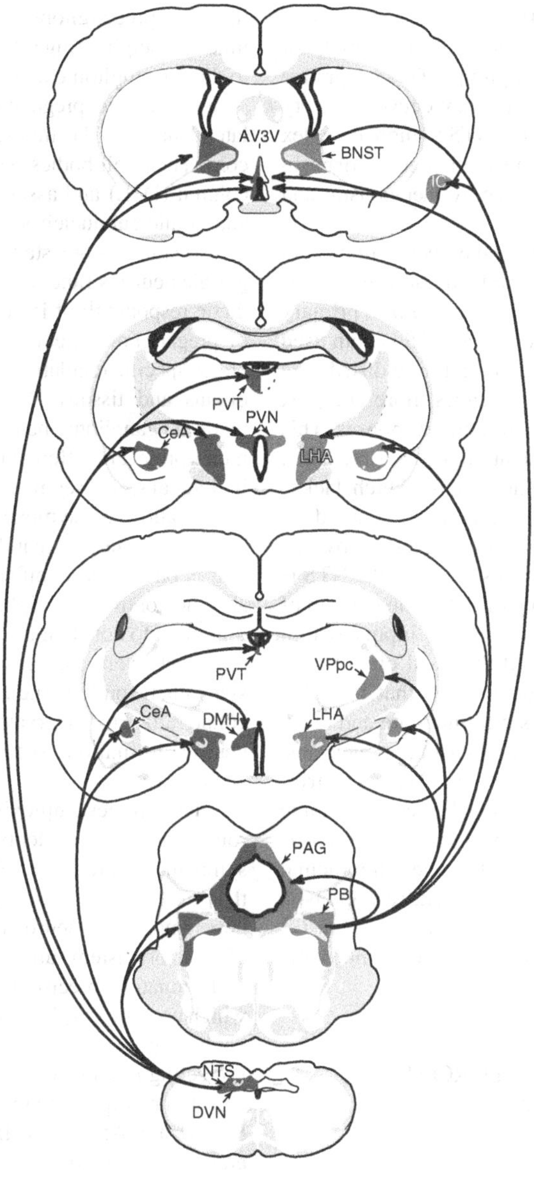


Figure 1–2 Parallel circuits that distribute sensory information received by the NTS. Information from primary sensory afferents synapsing in the NTS is distributed to nuclei in the central autonomic network through two parallel pathways. *Left side*: The NTS distributes information from visceral primary afferents to the parabrachial nucleus and a number of other circumscribed regions of the CNS. *Right side*: Parallel projections from the parabrachial nucleus mirror the projections from the NTS. The parabrachial nucleus also targets the insular cortex both directly and through a thalamic relay. Templates modified from Swanson (1998)[120], with permission. AV3V, anteroventral third ventricle; BNST, bed nucleus of stria terminalis; CeA, central nucleus of amygdala; DMH, dorsomedial hypothalamic nucleus; DVN, dorsal vagal motor nucleus; LHA, lateral hypothalamic area; NTS, nucleus of the solitary tract; PAG, periaqueductal gray; PB, parabrachial nucleus; PVN, paraventricular nucleus of hypothalamus; PVT, paraventricular thalamic nucleus; VPpc, ventroposterior parvocellular thalamic nucleus.

parabrachial nucleus terminate within parabrachial subnuclei that also receive projections from a variety of other non-autonomic CNS cell groups. This integrative relay in the parabrachial nucleus may convert sensory input that is organ-specific in the NTS to more complex regulatory information that affects the entire organism (e.g., to regulate body fluids, energy metabolism, and blood oxygenation)[98].

Taken together, these data make several important points about the way sensory information influences central control of autonomic functions. *First*, primary sensory information received by the NTS is both used for reflex control of autonomic targets and distributed to higher centers where it influences more complex and integrated control over peripheral responses. This neuronal feedback complements hormonal feedback through the circumventricular organs, which lack a blood–brain-barrier and can therefore respond to blood-borne signals. *Second*, as suggested by the relationships and responses of its neurons, the NTS is more than a simple relay. In particular, the overlap of functionally diverse primary afferent inputs within individual NTS subnuclei and the local circuit connections among NTS subnuclei show that the NTS contains circuitry that allows it to integrate and coordinate the activity of various NTS output neurons. *Third*, processed information from the NTS is distributed through parallel pathways. Hence, the same brain regions receive organ-specific information as well as information transformed in the parabrachial nucleus so that it can influence the entire organism. This organization provides an efficient substrate for dynamic and coordinated responses to homeostatic challenges.

## CENTRAL AUTONOMIC NEURONS THAT DIRECTLY CONTROL AUTONOMIC OUTFLOW

The CNS ultimately controls autonomic function by regulating the activity of sympathetic and parasympathetic preganglionic neurons in the brain and spinal cord. These preganglionic neurons provide central regulatory information to neurons in peripheral ganglia ("post-ganglionic neurons"), which, in turn, innervate the organs and tissues that are under autonomic control. Populations of neurons in the brainstem, diencephalon, and limbic forebrain directly control sympathetic and parasympathetic preganglionic neurons. These cell groups are able to function in an integrated manner because of collaterals that feed information forward and recurrent projections that provide feedback. This section outlines the cell groups that regulate autonomic outflow either directly through inputs to preganglionic neurons or indirectly through inputs to neighboring interneurons that are presynaptic to the preganglionic neurons.

Sympathetic preganglionic neurons reside in the lateral horn of the thoracic and upper lumbar spinal cord. Their cell bodies lie in the intermediolateral cell column (IML) and associated cell groups (i.e., spinal autonomic subnuclei; see Chapter 6). Although early investigations suggested that all sympathetic preganglionic neurons functioned as a unit to control sympathetic responses[11], it is now clear that the organization of preganglionic neurons and their inputs allows for target-specific regulation of sympathetically innervated organs and tissues[57,58,79]. Subpopulations of sympathetic preganglionic neurons in the same thoracic segments project to different peripheral targets; and, within individual spinal segments, there also may be a laminar organization of sympathetic preganglionic neurons based on the targets that they innervate. This organization is obviously significant for understanding organ-specific control of peripheral autonomic function. It is important to note that it also implies that the CNS neurons that exert the most widespread influence over sympathetic outflow (i.e., "command control" neurons) collateralize to innervate sympathetic preganglionic neurons in multiple segments in thoracic and lumbar spinal cord.

Many studies employing classical or viral transneuronal tracers have identified neurons that project to sympathetic preganglionic neurons[119]. The neurons that innervate sympathetic preganglionic neurons (i.e., "presympathetic neurons") occur in different regions of the brainstem and diencephalon (Figure 1–3). Unfortunately, precise maps of the spinal segments to which each supraspinal group sends its axons have not yet been published. Prominent populations of spinally projecting neurons occur in the caudal parapyramidal region (i.e., raphé and gigantocellular cell groups), the RVLM, the A5 region, Barrington's nucleus, the lateral hypothalamic area, and the PVN[119]. In addition, direct descending projections have been identified from neurons in the NTS, the Kölliker-Fuse nucleus, the nucleus subcoeruleus, the dorsal and retrochiasmatic hypothalamic areas, the hypothalamic arcuate nucleus, and the infralimbic cortex[4,119]. "Local circuit" interneurons in the spinal cord also innervate sympathetic preganglionic neurons and receive input from at least some of the populations of neurons that provide descending input to the cord (see Chaps. 6 and 8). The sympathetic interneuronal cell bodies occur in the central autonomic area dorsal to the central canal (i.e., dorsal lamina X), among sympathetic preganglionic neurons within the IML, and also diffusely in the cervical and thoracic cord. This interneuronal network within the spinal cord provides an indirect route

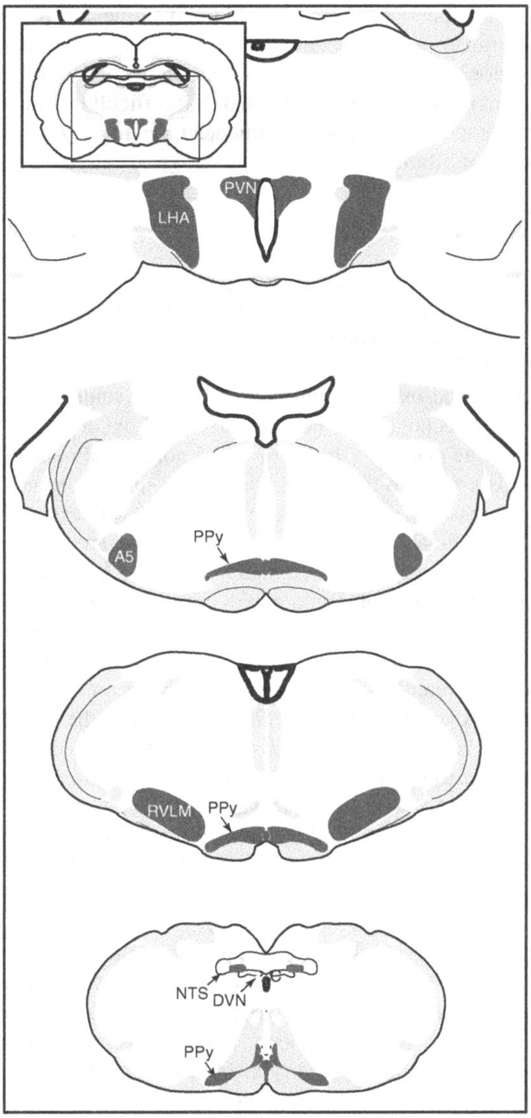


Figure 1–3 Location of cell groups that directly control sympathetic outflow. Diagrams of coronal sections through the rat brain showing preautonomic nuclei, which project directly to the spinal cord to innervate regions containing the cell bodies of sympathetic preganglionic neurons. Templates modified from Swanson (1998)[120], with permission. A5, pontine ventrolateral noradrenergic cell group; DVN, dorsal vagal motor nucleus; LHA, lateral hypothalamic area; NTS, nucleus of the solitary tract; PPy, parapyramidal cell group; PVN, paraventricular nucleus of hypothalamus; RVLM, rostral ventrolateral medulla.

through which descending inputs can influence sympathetic outflow and thereby contribute to the dynamic regulatory capacity of central autonomic circuitry. When interpreting viral transneuronal transport through central autonomic networks, it is critical to remember that spinal interneurons may expand the numbers and locations of neurons in higher centers that are ultimately labeled[15].

Many of the brain regions from which projections to sympathetic preganglionic neurons originate contain a diversity of neurochemically distinct types of neurons. This neurochemical heterogeneity implies that, within any given region, the cell groups that regulate the activity of sympathetic preganglionic neuron are functionally heterogeneous. From this discussion it should be clear that many different central cell groups are involved in controlling even closely related autonomic functions. Thus, regulation of interdependent functions, such as heart rate and arterial pressure, must emerge from the integrated action of the relevant cell groups. Central autonomic circuits must be organized so that they function cooperatively, and they are likely to include input from local interneurons. For many years, we have had only a general understanding of how these complex circuits are "wired" and function. However, studies of the organization and projections of presympathetic cell groups, which directly control the activity of sympathetic preganglionic neurons, are beginning to provide a clearer perspective. The following sections summarize the basic organization of the best-characterized presympathetic cell groups.

## RVLM

The RVLM plays a major role in the regulation of cardiovascular and other autonomic functions (see Chapter 5 and 10). The RVLM gives rise to an extensive projection that terminates throughout the lateral horn but is most dense in rostral thoracic segments. The majority of the bulbospinal RVLM neurons express one of the isoforms of the vesicular glutamate transporter[115] and are therefore likely to be glutamatergic. A subset of the spinally projecting neurons, the C1 cell group, also has a catecholaminergic phenotype[93,94,115]. Interestingly, selective lesions of C1 neurons attenuate, but do not eliminate, the influence of RVLM neurons on tonic and reflex control of cardiovascular function[72,73,106-108]. The majority of RVLM neurons that send axons to the spinal cord appear to be a separate group from RVLM neurons that project to other brain regions[104,114,125,128].

The RVLM is notable in that, unlike the presympathetic cell groups described below, it does not send projections to spinal parasympathetic preganglionic neurons[81,126]. This unique property of the

RVLM suggests that it might have a special role in sympathetic regulation. It is probably relevant that the RVLM predominantly, if not solely, controls sympathetic vasomotor innervation, which has no parasympathetic counterpart.

The data presented above indicate that the RVLM is not just a simple relay. It is also able to coordinate with other cell groups of similar regulatory function to influence the activity of sympathetic preganglionic neurons. The projection-specific topography of neurons within the RVLM also emphasizes the importance of precise anatomical analysis in assessing the functional organization of nuclei involved in central autonomic control.

## Parapyramidal Area

The parapyramidal area, as defined by Helke and colleagues[51], includes the caudal raphé cell groups (raphé pallidus and raphé magnus) as well as the adjacent gigantocellular and paragigantocellular nuclei. Parapyramidal neurons project to other supraspinal nuclei that are involved in central autonomic control. Unfortunately, the organization and extent of these projections are not well defined. However, spinal projections from the parapyramidal area, which influence both sympathetic and parasympathetic outflow, are better characterized[2,53]. As well as innervating spinal autonomic regions, parapyramidal axons target the dorsal horn; and a large body of literature indicates that these neurons are involved in nociception[1,40]. The diversity of its projections suggests that the parapyramidal region may have a complex and multifaceted role in the control of autonomic outflow. In fact, a recent hypothesis proposes that, rather than being dedicated to nociception, parapyramidal neurons play a broad modulatory role in the control of sensory, autonomic, and motor circuits involved in the maintenance of homeostasis[75,76].

Although some studies suggest that parapyramidal nuclei are functionally specialized[76], other data indicate that function is unlikely to be segregated on the basis of individual parapyramidal nuclei . For example, neurons throughout the parapyramidal region are activated when prostaglandin E2 is administered intracerebroventricularly[82,83] or when the $GABA_A$ receptor antagonist bicuculline is microinjected into specific parapyramidal cell groups[84]. Similarly, cold stress activates neurons in raphé pallidus most strongly but also affects neurons throughout the parapyramidal region[14,82]. Furthermore, injection of virus into brown adipose tissue[5,14,82] transneuronally labels neurons across parapyramidal nuclear boundaries. The dendritic arbors of parapyramidal neurons also fail to respect nuclear boundaries defined by cell packing density and neurochemical phenotype[38,46,47,90]. Hence, although some afferents terminate within specific nuclei in the parapyramidal region[39], the presence in any one area of dendrites from many different nuclei makes it difficult to determine which neurons are influenced by any particular type of afferent.

## A5

The A5 noradrenergic cell group in the pons is involved in cardiovascular and cardiorespiratory integration[49,65,74]. It gives rise to one of the most extensive descending projections to the IML, in terms of both density and segmental extent of innervation. Lesion studies with the catecholamine neurotoxin 6-hydroxydopamine indicate that more than 90% of A5 noradrenaline neurons project to the lateral horn of the spinal cord and that these catecholamine neurons account for nearly all of the spinal projection arising from the A5 area[10]. The rapid retrograde transneuronal infection of A5 neurons after injection of pseudorabies virus into peripheral sympathetic targets, such as the kidney, spleen, brown fat, and pineal gland[118], reflects the density and extent of the spinal A5 projection. Like parapyramidal neurons, A5 neurons innervate the dorsal horn of the spinal cord, have been implicated in nociception[25], and also project to other nuclei involved in central autonomic control. A5 neurons are activated by carotid chemoreceptor stimulation and hypercapnia, and their activity displays a respiratory rhythm[49,65]. Injection of excitatory amino acids into the A5 region in anesthetized animals decreases blood pressure[30,37,55,112]. In contrast, electrical stimulation of A5 increases blood pressure[71,129], possibly due to the stimulation of fibers of passage[74]. Like the parapyramidal region, A5 also influences parasympathetic outflow. Although the observations above clearly indicate that the A5 region is involved in the central autonomic control, the full extent of its contributions remains to be established.

## PVN

The PVN is a complex, functionally heterogeneous nucleus that is important in the control of both neuroendocrine and autonomic nervous systems[102,103]. The PVN affects autonomic function through the spinal axons of parvocellular neurons with cell bodies in the dorsal, medial, and lateral subdivisions of the nucleus[121]. PVN axons terminate throughout the lateral horn of thoracic and upper lumbar cord[22] and provide extensive input to parasympathetic preganglionic neurons[88]. It is important to note that PVN neurons also innervate other central autonomic nuclei in the brain[86]. However, surprisingly little is known about how PVN axons segregate or collateralize. Retrograde transport of different tracers from the IML and RVLM has demonstrated that the PVN has the potential to modulate sympathetic outflow directly through projections to the IML, indirectly through projections to the RVLM, and through neurons that innervate both regions[89,110,113]. This organization allows the parvocellular PVN to influence autonomic outflow through direct projections to the preganglionic neurons and indirectly through integrative relays that project to preganglionic neurons. In addition, the PVN receives extensive sensory input, has efferent projections to other central autonomic regions, and has well-defined roles in neuroendocrine and autonomic regulation. All of these features make the PVN one of the most influential nuclei in the central circuitry that controls autonomic function.

### Lateral Hypothalamic Area

The lateral hypothalamic area is similar to the PVN in that it influences autonomic function through direct descending projections to the preganglionic cell groups, as well as indirectly through projections to other central autonomic nuclei[98]. Immunohistochemical and tract-tracing studies have shown that this large region is topographically organized and contains many different neurochemical types of neurons, suggesting considerable functional diversity[67]. Autonomic regions of thoracic and upper lumbar cord receive axons from a number of neurochemically distinct cell groups in the lateral hypothalamic area; and this region also supplies the lower lumbar and sacral cord, where parasympathetic preganglionic neurons are located. The perifornical region of the lateral hypothalamic area is particularly interesting because it contains a number of neurochemically distinct populations of neurons. Prominent among these are hypocretin/orexin neurons that have important roles in controlling behavioral state and autonomic function. The axons of orexin neurons branch to supply other central autonomic nuclei[24], but the extent of branching has not yet been comprehensively analyzed. Classical and viral tracing studies have shown that orexin-containing neurons in the lateral hypothalamic area influence sympathetic outflow though direct descending projections to the lateral horn as well as through polysynaptic circuits that include other central sites involved in autonomic regulation, such as the RVLM[48,127].

### Other Presympathetic Cell Groups

The region of the lumbosacral cord that contains parasympathetic preganglionic neurons is densely innervated by Barrington's nucleus in the dorsal pons as well as receiving input from the parapyramidal region, A5, and hypothalamic cell groups[81,126]. Barrington's nucleus has been classically considered as the pontine micturition center[101], but more recent evidence suggests that it is also involved in the parasympathetic control of other pelvic viscera[126]. Viral labeling from tissues that receive only sympathetic innervation, such as the spleen and brown fat, indicates a role for Barrington's nucleus in controlling sympathetic outflow[12-15]. Collectively, these observations suggest that Barrington's nucleus is involved in coordinating the activity of both the sympathetic and the parasympathetic divisions of the autonomic nervous system.

Other groups of brainstem and hypothalamic neurons are retrogradely labeled after injection of tracers into the region of the thoracic and upper lumbar lateral horn[98,119]. Unfortunately, very little information is available about the organization and possible function of these other presumably presympathetic cell groups. Nevertheless, these additional central sites of retrograde labeling indicate that more groups of neurons are involved in directly controlling sympathetic outflow than just those discussed above.

In summary, a number of basic principles emerge from this discussion of neurons that control autonomic outflow. *First,* circumscribed cell groups in the brainstem and diencephalon provide direct descending control of sympathetic preganglionic neurons. *Second,* the cell groups that give rise to descending inputs to sympathetic preganglionic neurons also innervate, to varying degrees, each other and also brain regions that indirectly control sympathetic outflow. It is unclear the degree to which these projections arise as collaterals of axons projecting to the spinal sympathetic regions. This question requires careful analysis, and its answer will have important implications for understanding the functional organization of the central circuits that control autonomic function. *Third,* spinal axons arising from neurons in the brain can influence sympathetic outflow through interneurons. This spinal cord network (see Chapters 6 and 8) provides a dynamic means of controlling sympathetic outflow and may be the basis for coordinating it with spinal parasympathetic outflow. *Fourth,* many of the cell groups that control sympathetic outflow also influence parasympathetic outflow. This observation highlights the need for detailed characterization of the organization and synaptology of the circuits through which these cell groups coordinate the two branches of the autonomic nervous system.

## CENTRAL AUTONOMIC NEURONS THAT INDIRECTLY CONTROL AUTONOMIC OUTFLOW

The "preautonomic" cell groups discussed above modulate sympathetic and parasympathetic outflow by influencing preganglionic neurons, either directly or through interneurons that synapse on the preganglionic neurons. However, preautonomic nuclei receive input from other cell groups in the brain. Furthermore, autonomic function is modified by stimulation or inhibition of the cell groups that project to preautonomic nuclei, and these cell groups are activated by challenges that require adjustments in autonomic function. In this section, we identify the central regions that participate indirectly in regulating preganglionic neurons and discuss the evidence that supports their involvement in the control of autonomic outflow. The cell groups that fall into this category include relays essential for reflex control, such as the caudal ventrolateral medulla (CVLM); and centers that are involved in more complex integration, such as the periaqueductal gray (PAG) and the parabrachial nucleus (Figure 1–4).

### Caudal Ventrolateral Medulla

The CVLM is an essential component of the brainstem circuitry responsible for reflex control of arterial blood pressure. Baroreceptor afferents synapse on a subpopulation of NTS neurons that excite GABAergic neurons in the CVLM. These CVLM neurons, in turn, project to RVLM and produce a reduction in mean arterial pressure by inhibiting RVLM neurons that innervate sympathetic preganglionic neurons. This well-studied circuit is a good example of the way the CNS exerts reflex control over peripheral autonomic function. However, as with other areas that might be said to serve a relay function, the CVLM is more than a simple relay of baroreceptor reflex function (see Chapter 5).

### A1 Neurons

The location of the A1 noradrenergic neurons partially overlaps with that of the GABAergic CVLM neurons in the caudal brainstem. However, A1 neurons can be distinguished from CVLM neurons because they are catecholaminergic, not GABAergic, and because they innervate different targets. A1 neurons influence cardiovascular function through projections to the hypothalamus, which affect neuroendocrine regulation, and through projections to limbic centers, which coordinate autonomic and behavioral responses. Neuroendocrine effects are achieved, at least in part, through A1 inputs to magnocellular vasopressin neurons[27]. Hemorrhage-induced activation of A1 neurons leads to vasopressin release into the circulation, with the resulting compensatory responses[8]. The A1 neurons also contribute, along with the A2 NTS neurons, to the dense noradrenergic innervation of the median preoptic nucleus in the anteroventral third ventricular region[61,99,100]. The anteroventral third ventricular region also receives sensory information through the organum vasculosum of the lamina terminalis, a circumventricular organ that also regulates vasopressin release due to hormonal signals received directly from the blood[77]. In addition, the A1 cell group heavily innervates preautonomic cell groups that control autonomic outflow, such as the lateral hypothalamic area, PVN, parabrachial nucleus, and NTS[8]. The projections of A1 neurons suggest that they coordinate related autonomic and neuroendocrine functions.

### Parabrachial Nucleus

The parabrachial nucleus is a major target for projections from the NTS, and it heavily innervates preautonomic cell groups[97] (Figure 1–4). Its position in central autonomic circuitry suggests that the parabrachial nucleus distributes sensory information to regulate output from other cell groups involved in central autonomic regulation. The diversity of afferent input received by the parabrachial nucleus suggests that its primary role may be integrative, converting organ-specific sensory input to information that has a more global physiological context[52,98].

The superior cerebellar peduncle divides the parabrachial nucleus into external and internal subdivisions. Projections from the rostral NTS, which is principally related to the sensory processing of taste, are directed to the internal subdivision, while axons from the intermediate and caudal NTS supply almost exclusively the external segment[50,52,60,124]. Cardiovascular afferents from the NTS terminate preferentially in the ventrolateral portion of the external subdivision, and stimulation of this region produces sympathoexcitation and a rise in blood pressure[23].

Reciprocal projections are an important feature of parabrachial circuitry[44]. In many cases, the topographical projections received by individual parabrachial subnuclei are mirrored by reciprocal parabrachial projections to the nucleus that was the source of the afferents. Reciprocal innervation occurs with NTS subnuclei, the medullary reticular formation, the central nucleus of the amygdala, and the bed nucleus of stria terminalis, as well as hypothalamic nuclei implicated in autonomic regulation.

The influence of parabrachial neurons on the compensatory response to hypotensive hemorrhage illustrates how this nucleus contributes to autonomic outflow by working in concert with other central autonomic neurons to produce multifaceted responses. Initially, blood loss reduces arterial blood pressure, unloading baroreceptors and causing a reduction in inhibition of RVLM presympathetic neurons by GABAergic CVLM neurons so that arterial pressure is

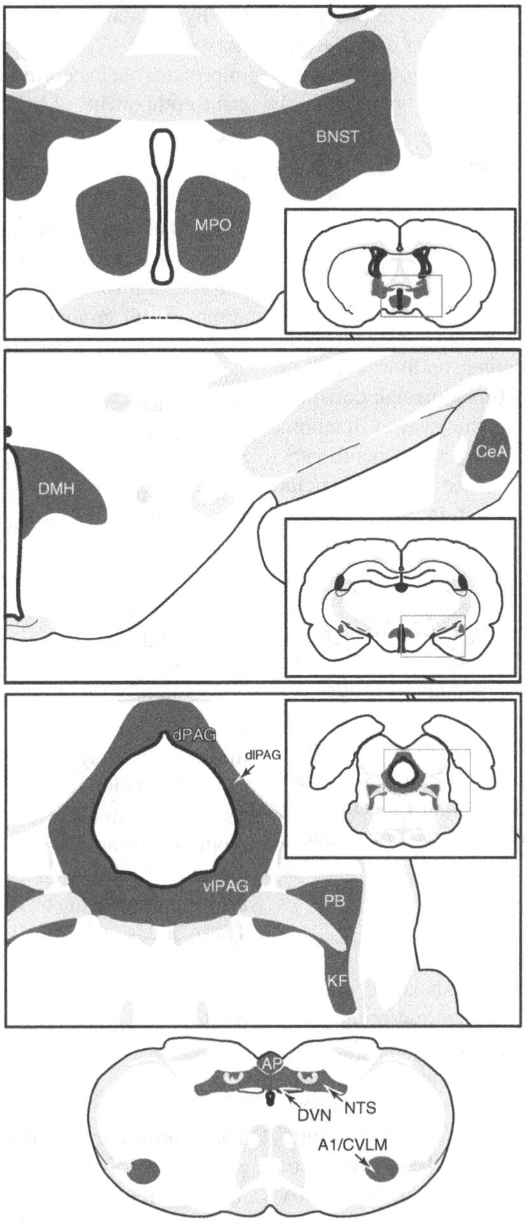


Figure 1–4 Location of cell groups that indirectly control sympathetic outflow. Diagrams of coronal sections through the rat brain showing central autonomic nuclei, which project to preautonomic nuclei to innervate neurons that are involved in the direct control of sympathetic outflow. Templates modified from Swanson (1998)[120], with permission. A1, caudal brainstem ventrolateral noradrenergic cell group; AP, area postrema; BNST, bed nucleus of stria terminalis; CeA, central nucleus of amygdala; CVLM, caudal ventrolateral medulla; DMH, dorsomedial hypothalamic nucleus; Kölliker-Fuse nucleus; MPO, medial preoptic nucleus; NTS, nucleus of the solitary tract; dPAG, dorsal periaqueductal gray; dlPAG, dorsolateral periaqueductal gray; vlPAG, ventrolateral periaqueductal gray; PB, parabrachial nucleus.

increased. If blood loss continues to reduce pressure, the midbrain PAG produces bradycardia and a withdrawal of sympathetic drive[29,105]. Finally, in the third phase of the response, ventrolateral parabrachial neurons restore normal pressure by reinstituting sympathetic vasomotor drive, presumably through projections to the RVLM[6,7].

## Periaqueductal Gray (PAG)

Like the parabrachial nucleus, the PAG consists of a number of functionally distinct subdivisions with well-documented influences on autonomic outflow. The PAG has been divided into columns (dorsomedial, dorsolateral, lateral, and ventrolateral) on the basis of function, cytoarchitecture, projections, and neurochemistry[62]. Stimulation of neurons within these columns elicits complex behavioral responses that include adaptive autonomic adjustments. For example, stimulation of rostral portions of the dorsolateral or lateral columns produces defense responses, whereas stimulation more caudal in these columns produces flight[62]. These behaviors are associated with prototypical "fight or flight" autonomic responses, including changes in heart rate, blood pressure, and perfusion of regional vascular beds. Data such as these indicate that the PAG is an integrative relay through which higher centers orchestrate the autonomic changes that accompany behavioral responses to physiological and environmental challenges.

## Dorsomedial Hypothalamic Nucleus

Activation of the dorsomedial hypothalamic nucleus produces defense behavior with clear and predictable autonomic components (see Chapters 3 and 12). For example, injection of a GABA antagonist or excitatory amino acids into the dorsomedial hypothalamic nucleus produces tachycardia and increased blood pressure, responses that do not occur when these drugs are injected into adjacent sites[31]. Injection of the GABA agonist muscimol into the dorsomedial hypothalamic nucleus abolishes these effects[31]. The pressor effects from dorsomedial hypothalamic stimulation are mediated mainly through RVLM[42,54], whereas raphé pallidus mediates the tachycardia[96]. Axons arising from neurons in the dorsomedial hypothalamic nucleus heavily innervate the PVN[122,123] and functional analyses have revealed that the hypothalamic-pituitary-adrenal axis is activated through the dorsomedial hypothalamic nucleus. Thus, the dense intra-hypothalamic projections of neurons in the dorsomedial hypothalamic nucleus probably provide a means of synchronizing the autonomic responses to stress with activation of the hypothalamic-pituitary-adrenal axis. Overall, the dorsomedial hypothalamic nucleus seems to play an important role in coordinating the autonomic and endocrine components of behavioral responses to stress.

## Bed Nucleus of Stria Terminalis

The bed nucleus of the stria terminalis is one of a group of limbic structures that is involved in organizing behavioral responses to stress, fear, and anxiety[28]. This complex cell group integrates information from cortical, limbic, and subcortical nuclei. It receives a dense noradrenergic input from the A2 neurons in the NTS and A1 neurons in the caudal medulla[3]. Available evidence suggests that these pathways figure prominently in the behavioral, neuroendocrine, and autonomic responses resulting from stress that arises from within the body[43]. The bed nucleus of the stria terminalis also receives significant input from the central nucleus of the amygdala and the medial prefrontal cortex. These projections appear to be important for behavioral, endocrine, and autonomic responses to psychological stressors.

Subregions of the bed nucleus of the stria terminalis project extensively to preautonomic cell groups that influence both sympathetic and parasympathetic outflow[32–36], including the PVN, lateral hypothalamic area, Barrington's nucleus, and the NTS. Areas that modulate the activity of preautonomic cell groups, and therefore indirectly influence autonomic outflow, are also supplied by the bed nucleus of the stria terminalis. These areas include the dorsomedial hypothalamic nucleus and lateral hypothalamic area, both of which have well-established roles in the control of autonomic outflow (see above).

## Central Nucleus of the Amygdala

The central nucleus of the amygdala is an important component of the central circuitry that responds to fear, anxiety, and stress[28,68,95]. Stimulation of this region produces behavioral and autonomic responses classically associated with fear, and lesions of the amygdala prevent fear conditioning[69]. The central nucleus of the amygdala and the bed nucleus of the stria terminalis are highly interconnected, innervate the same regions, and play similar roles in responding to fear, anxiety, and stress, suggesting that these structures work together in a cooperative fashion.

The GABAergic neurons of the central nucleus of the amygdala are grouped into subnuclei. The lateral subnucleus is a major site of termination for afferents to the nucleus. For example, the lateral subnucleus receives an extremely dense input from the cardiovascular subdivision of the parabrachial nucleus[109]. GABAergic neurons in the lateral subnucleus innervate neurons in the adjacent medial subnucleus, which is the major source of output from the central nucleus of the amygdala. Given this organization, feed-forward disinhibitory circuits are probably important in determining the output of the GABAergic projection neurons of the medial subnucleus.

Axons from the medial subnucleus of the central nucleus of the amygdala target many of the central sites involved in autonomic control[95]. The lateral hypothalamic area, PAG, and the dorsal vagal complex receive particularly dense innervations. The extensive output from the central nucleus of the amygdala to other central autonomic areas identifies it as an important component of the central circuitry that regulates autonomic function.

### Cerebral Cortex (See Chapter 11)

The insular cortex contains a topographically organized representation of the viscera and projects to the hypothalamus, the parabrachial nucleus, and the NTS. However, the subregion of the insular cortex that contains the viscerotopic map differs from the area that gives rise to efferent projections that influence autonomic outflow. Stimulation of different regions of the insular cortex evokes autonomic responses as predicted by its viscerotopic representation. For example, bradycardia and depressor responses result from stimulation of caudal agranular insular cortex, while stimulation of more rostral regions of the insular cortex produces the opposite response. These responses are likely to be mediated, at least in part, by a relay in the lateral hypothalamic area[85]. The connections between subregions of the insular cortex suggest that this region is part of the circuitry that regulates responses to challenges that require autonomic adjustments as part of adaptive behavior.

The medial prefrontal cortex is also involved in regulating autonomic function. Its effects are mediated by the infralimbic cortex[45], from which axons innervate the central nucleus of the amygdala, bed nucleus of the stria terminalis, lateral hypothalamic area, PAG, dorsomedial hypothalamic nucleus, RVLM, and NTS. Cortical influences on cardiovascular function probably involve circuits that include the lateral hypothalamic area and PAG. Stimulation of the infralimbic cortex produces hypotension, which is attenuated by injection of lidocaine into the lateral hypothalamic area or PAG[41]. These observations, together with those from studies on the insular cortex, indicate an important role for the lateral hypothalamic area in mediating cortical influences on autonomic function.

## HIERARCHY AND INTEGRATED PROCESSING IN THE CONTROL OF AUTONOMIC OUTFLOW

The information presented above suggests that the central neurons controlling autonomic function are organized into highly interconnected regulatory units. This organization is complex, and the fundamental principles that govern how the behavior of the various units is coordinated and integrated remain to be established. Nevertheless, our understanding has advanced substantially over the past quarter century as technology has become increasingly powerful.

Three levels of integrative processing characterize the central circuitry that controls autonomic function. *First*, there are reflex circuits that control moment-to-moment adjustments in the activity of specific autonomic targets, as occurs, for example, with the baroreceptor reflex. *Second*, there are cell groups, including nuclei in the brainstem and diencephalon, that coordinate activity among autonomic targets. *Finally*, there are cell groups, such as those in cortico-limbic regions, that organize autonomic responses as part of complex behavioral and endocrine responses to environmental and physiological challenges.

The demonstration that peripheral autonomic targets can be regulated independently as well as collectively is one of the most important recent observations in autonomic neuroscience. Sympathetic nerves and their constituent axons have variable responses, depending on the stimuli used to activate them[79]. For example, muscle vasoconstrictor fibers are tonically active and their activity is strongly inhibited by increases in blood pressure, whereas changes in body temperature selectively affect the activity of cutaneous vasoconstrictor fibers[56,58]. Reduction of body temperature increases the activity of nerves innervating brown fat, with little effect on splanchnic nerve activity[78]. Furthermore, stimulating different autonomic areas in the brain produces different sympathetic responses. For example, stimulation of the RVLM increases mean arterial pressure but does not increase the activity of neurons innervating brown fat[78,79]. There are many other examples of this type of segregation of sympathetic function, which have been reviewed elsewhere[79,118]. These different responses of different sympathetic outflows no doubt arise from differences in central processing and connectivity.

Although functionally distinct sympathetic outflows can be activated independently of one another, challenges to homeostasis that require more global reactions can produce a number of simultaneous sympathetic adjustments. This coordinated control over many peripheral targets is a prominent feature of the "fight or flight" response. Viral tracing has been particularly useful in helping us understand how these multifaceted autonomic responses are coordinated. There is a small number of brain regions that are reproducibly labeled when individual sympathetic ganglia or target tissues have been inoculated with virus[116,117] or when viruses with different reporter molecules have been injected into the adrenal medulla and stellate ganglion[59]. The central autonomic regions that show viral labeling from all sympathetic targets are the RVLM, the A5 region, the parapyramidal region (which some studies separate into ventromedial medulla and raphé nuclei), and the PVN. Because these five regions connect directly to sympathetic preganglionic neurons, and because neurons in each show transneuronal virus labeling from multiple sympathetic targets, it has been proposed that these brain regions contain "command" neurons that are responsible for the integrated activation of multiple sympathetic outflows. This hypothesis also implies that other regions with direct projections to sympathetic preganglionic neurons provide more discrete control of autonomic targets.

Since identification of "command" neurons in the brain is based mainly on results of viral tracing studies, it is important to consider both the strengths and limitations of this method. Circuit architecture is particularly important for interpreting the results of experiments that produce transneuronal infection in the brainstem and diencephalon. As discussed above (and see Chapters 6 and 8), a sizeable population of spinal interneurons is presynaptic to sympathetic preganglionic neurons. These neurons collateralize to innervate many spinal segments, and some have cell bodies that lie among sympathetic preganglionic neurons in the IML. Consequently, transneuronal spread of virus through local-circuit interneurons in the spinal cord would expand the segmental distribution of virus that gives rise to retrograde infection of neurons in the brain. Furthermore, density of innervation and the concentration of the injected virus determine the progression of viral infection through a circuit[20]. These factors are particularly important in experiments using two recombinant viruses with unique reporter proteins, where prior infection of a neuron by one virus can render the neuron refractory to infection by the second virus[64]. While neurons in the five regions mentioned above clearly provide important input to sympathetic preganglionic neurons, it is still not clear whether global control over sympathetic outflow is restricted to only these five cell groups.

As well as coordinating different sympathetic outflows, central autonomic circuits are organized to coordinate sympathetic responses with parasympathetic responses. Control over these functionally complementary divisions of the autonomic nervous system often comes from neurons in the same supraspinal regions. Retrograde transport of different tracers from the dorsal motor vagal complex and thoracic spinal cord labels populations of neurons that are separate but overlap in the parvocellular PVN[87,88]. Similarly, areas classically associated with control over parasympathetic function, such as the lateral hypothalamic area and Barrington's nucleus, also contain neurons that project to spinal regions that contain sympathetic preganglionic neurons. Hence, many central autonomic nuclei contribute to both sympathetic and parasympathetic regulation. This makes sense from a regulatory perspective because it is necessary to coordinate the activities of cell groups with complementary functions. Nevertheless, the precise circuitry and synaptic connections involved in coordinating sympathetic and parasympathetic outflow remain to be defined.

In addition to illuminating the circuits that control sympathetic and parasympathetic outflow, transneuronal transport of viruses has provided some unique insights into how autonomic and motor functions are coordinated. Neurons in parapyramidal nuclei are co-infected following injection of one recombinant virus into the adrenal medulla and another into a surgically sympathectomized gastrocnemius muscle[63]. Similarly, dual injection of motor cortex and stellate ganglion has revealed prominent groups of co-infected neurons in the lateral hypothalamic area and pedunculopontine cholinergic cell group[66]. These studies provide further novel information on the identity of CNS cell groups that coordinate autonomic outflow with the contractile state of the peripheral musculature that it serves.

## SUMMARY

Since the publication of the first edition of this book in 1990, considerable progress has been made in defining the organization of the central circuits that regulate autonomic function. Several fundamental principles have emerged. *First*, in addition to preganglionic neurons and interneurons in the spinal cord, central autonomic neurons are concentrated in the brainstem, midbrain, and diencephalon. *Second*, autonomic circuits in the brain include not only neurons that directly control the activity of preganglionic neurons but also higher-order neurons that have the capacity to modify autonomic outflow. *Third*, central cell groups that contribute to the control of autonomic function are hierarchically organized. There are reflex circuits for rapid adjustments of autonomic outflow, cell groups that coordinate autonomic outflows to related targets, and nuclei that integrate multimodal sensory inputs to produce complex behaviors incorporating adaptive autonomic adjustments. *Fourth*, collateralization of axons and reciprocal innervation within and between autonomic cell groups in the brain permits their coordinated activity. *Fifth*, integration of sensory and other inputs at many locations ensures that autonomic responses are appropriate to meet internal and external challenges. Although our knowledge is better than it was in 1990, further detailed characterization of the functional topography and connectivity of central autonomic neurons is necessary if we are to gain greater insight into the way the CNS controls autonomic function.

## References


1. Abols, I. A., and Basbaum, A. I. (1981). Afferent connections of the rostral medulla of the cat: A neural substrate for midbrain-medullary interactions in the modulation of pain. *Journal of Comparative Neurology* 201, 285–297.
2. Allen, G. V., and Cechetto, D. F. (1994). Serotoninergic and nonserotoninergic neurons in the medullary raphe system have axon collateral projections to autonomic and somatic cell groups in the medulla and spinal cord. *Journal of Comparative Neurology* 350, 357–366.
3. Aston-Jones, G., Delfs, J. M., Druhan, J., and Zhu, Y. (1999). The bed nucleus of the stria terminalis: A target site for noradrenergic actions in opiate withdrawal. *Annals of the New York Academy of Sciences* 877, 489–498.
4. Bacon, S. J., and Smith, A. D. (1993). A monosynaptic pathway from an identified vasomotor centre in the medial prefrontal cortex to an autonomic area in the thoracic spinal cord. *Neuroscience* 54, 719–728.
5. Bamshad, M., Song, C. K., and Bartness, T. J. (1999). CNS origins of the sympathetic nervous system outflow to brown adipose tissue. *American Journal of Physiology* 45, R1569–R1578.
6. Blair, M. L., Jaworski, R. L., Want, A., and Piekut, D. T. (2001). Parabrachial nucleus modulates cardiovascular responses to blood loss. *American Journal of Physiology* 280, R1141–R1148.
7. Blair, M. L., and Mickelsen, D. (2006). Activation of lateral parabrachial nucleus neurons restores blood pressure and sympathetic vasomotor drive after hypotensive hemorrhage. *American Journal of Physiology* 291, R742–R750.
8. Blessing, W. W. (1997). *The Lower Brainstem and Bodily Homeostasis*. New York: Oxford University Press.
9. Broussard, D. L., Lynn, R. B., Wiedner, E. B., and Altschuler, S. M. (1998). Solitarial premotor neuron projections to the rat esophagus and pharynx: Implications for control of swallowing. *Gastroenterology* 114, 1268–1275.
10. Byrum, C. E., Stornetta, R., and Guyenet, P. G. (1984). Electrophysiological properties of spinally-projecting A5 noradrenergic neurons. *Brain Research* 303, 15–29.
11. Cannon, W. B., and Rosenblueth, A. (1937). *Autonomic Neuro-Effector Systems*. New York: Macmillan.
12. Cano, G., Card, J. P., Rinaman, L., and Sved, A. F. (1999). Connections of Barrington's nucleus to the sympathetic nervous system. *Journal of the Autonomic Nervous System* 79, 117–128.
13. Cano, G., Card, J. P., and Sved, A. F. (2004). Dual viral transneuronal tracing of central autonomic circuits involved in the innervation of the two kidneys in the rat. *Journal of Comparative Neurology* 471, 462–481.
14. Cano, G., Passerin, A. M., Schiltz, J. C., Card, J. P., Morrison, S. F., and Sved, A. F. (2003). Anatomical substrates for the central control of sympathetic outflow to intercapsular adipose tissue during cold exposure. *Journal of Comparative Neurology* 460, 303–326.
15. Cano, G., Sved, A. F., Rinaman, L., Rabin, B. S., and Card, J. P. (2001). Characterization of the central nervous system innervation of the rat spleen using viral transneuronal tracing. *Journal of Comparative Neurology* 439, 1–18.
16. Card, J. P. (1998). Practical considerations for the use of pseudorabies virus in transneuronal studies of neural circuitry. *Neuroscience and Biobehavioral Reviews* 22, 685–694.
17. Card, J. P. (2001). Pseudorabies virus neuroinvasiveness: A window into the functional organization of the brain. *Advances in Virus Research* 56, 39–71.
18. Card, J. P., and Enquist, L. W. (1995). Neurovirulence of pseudorabies virus. *Critical Reviews in Neurobiology* 9, 137–162.
19. Card, J. P., and Enquist, L. W. (1999). *Transneuronal Circuit Analysis with Pseudorabies Viruses*, pp. 1.5.1–1.5.28. San Diego: John Wiley & Sons.
20. Card, J. P., Enquist, L. W., and Moore, R. Y. (1999). Neuroinvasiveness of pseudorabies virus injected intracerebrally is dependent on viral concentration and terminal field density. *Journal of Comparative Neurology* 407, 438–452.
21. Card, J. P., Rinaman, L., Schwaber, J. S., Miselis, R. R., Whealy, M. E., Robbins, A. K., and Enquist, L. W. (1990). Neurotropic properties of pseudorabies virus: Uptake and transneuronal passage in the rat central nervous system. *Journal of Neuroscience* 10, 1974–1994.

22. Cechetto, D. F., and Saper, C. B. (1988). Neurochemical organization of the hypothalamic projection to the spinal cord in the rat. *Journal of Comparative Neurology* 272, 579–604.
23. Chamberlin, N. L., and Saper, C. B. (1992). Topographic organization of cardiovascular responses to electrical and glutamate microstimulation of the parabrachial nucleus in the rat. *Journal of Comparative Neurology* 326, 245–262.
24. Ciriello, J., McMurray, J. C., Babic, T., and de Oliveira, C. V. (2003). Collateral axonal projections from hypothalamic hypocretin neurons to cardiovascular sites in nucleus ambiguus and nucleus tractus solitarius. *Brain Research* 991, 133–141.
25. Clark, F. M., and Proudfit, H. K. (1993). The projections of noradrenergic neurons in the A5 catecholamine cell group to the spinal cord in the rat: Anatomical evidence that A5 neurons modulate nociception. *Brain Research* 616, 200–210.
26. Cunningham, E. T., and Sawchenko, P. E. (1989). A circumscribed projection from the nucleus of the solitary tract to the nucleus ambiguus in the rat: Anatomical evidence for somatostatin-28-immunoreactive interneurons subserving reflex control of esophageal motility. *Journal of Neuroscience* 9, 1668–1682.
27. Cunningham, E. T., and Sawchenko, P. E. (1991). Reflex control of magnocellular vasopressin and oxytocin secretion. *Trends in Neurosciences* 14, 406–411.
28. Davis, M. (2002). Neural Circuitry of Anxiety and Stress Disorders. In K. L. Davis, D. Charney, J. T. Coyle, and C. Nemeroff, (Eds), *Neuropsychopharmacology: The Fifth Generation of Progress,* pp. 931–951. Philadelphia: Lippincott, Williams & Wilkins.
29. Dean, C. (2004). Hemorrhagic sympathoinhibition mediated through the periaqueductal gray in the rat. *Neuroscience Letters* 354, 79–83.
30. Dickerson, L. W., Panico, W. H., Kuhn, F. E., Willis, A. C., Fitzgerald, J. F., Meyer, E. L., Norman, W. P., and Gillis, R. A. (1997). Stimulation of dog RVLM and A5 area changes sympathetic outflow to vascular beds without effect on the heart. *American Journal of Pathology* 272, R821–R839.
31. DiMicco, J. A., Samuels, B. C., Zaretskaia, M. V., and Zaretsky, D. V. (2002). The dorsomedial hypothalamus and the response to stress: Part renaissance, part revolution. *Pharmacology Biochemistry and Behavior* 71, 469–480.
32. Dong, H.-W., Petrovich, G. D., Watts, A. G., and Swanson, L. W. (2001). Basic organization of projections from the oval and fusiform nuclei of the bed nuclei of the stria terminalis in adult rat brain. *Journal of Comparative Neurology* 436, 430–455.
33. Dong, H.-W., and Swanson, L. W. (2003). Projections from the rhomboid nucleus of the bed nuclei of the stria terminalis: Implications for cerebral hemisphere regulation of ingestive behavior. *Journal of Comparative Neurology* 463, 434–472.
34. Dong, H.-W., and Swanson, L. W. (2006). Projections from bed nuclei of the stria terminalis, anteromedial area: Cerebral hemisphere integration of neuroendocrine, autonomic, and behavioral aspects of energy balance. *Journal of Comparative Neurology* 494, 142–178.
35. Dong, H.-W., and Swanson, L. W. (2006). Projections from bed nuclei of the stria terminalis, magnocellular nucleus: Implications for cerebral hemisphere regulation of micturition, defecation, and penile erection. *Journal of Comparative Neurology* 494, 108–141.
36. Dong, H.-W., and Swanson, L. W. (2006). Projections from the bed nuclei of the stria terminalis, dorsomedial nucleus: Implications for cerebral hemisphere integration of neuroendocrine, autonomic, and drinking responses. *Journal of Comparative Neurology* 494, 75–107.
37. Dyre, R. G., Baisden, R. H., Whittington, D. L., and Woodruff, M. L. (1990). The effects of stimulation of the A5 region on blood pressure and heart rate in rabbits. *Brain Research Bulletin* 24, 33–39.
38. Edward, D. L., Johnston, K. M., Poletti, C. E., and Foote, W. E. (1987). Morphology of pontomedullary raphe and reticular formation neurons in the brainstem of the cat: An intracellular HRP study. *Journal of Comparative Neurology* 256, 257–273.
39. Farkas, E., Jansen, A. S., and Loewy, A. D. (1998). Periaqueductal gray matter input to cardiac-related sympathetic premotor neurons. *Brain Research* 792, 179–192.
40. Fields, H. L., Malick, A., and Burstein, R. (1995). Dorsal horn projection targets of ON and OFF cells in the rostral ventromedial medulla. *Journal of Neurophysiology* 74, 1742–1759.
41. Fisk, G. D., and Wyss, J. M. (2000). Descending projections of infralimbic cortex that mediate stimulation-evoked changes in arterial pressure. *Brain Research* 859, 83–95.
42. Fontes, M. A. P., Tagawa, T., Polson, J. W., Cavanagh, S. J., and Dampney, R. A. (2001). Descending pathways mediating cardiovascular response from dorsomedial hypothalamic nucleus. *American Journal of Physiology* 280, H2891–H2901.

43. Forray, M. I., and Gysling, K. (2004). Role of noradrenergic projections to the bed nucleus of the stria terminalis in the regulation of the hypothalamic-pituitary-adrenal axis. *Brain Research Reviews* 47, 145–160.
44. Fulwiler, C. E., and Saper, C. B. (1984). Subnuclear organization of the efferent connections of the parabrachial nucleus in the rat. *Brain Research* 319, 229–259.
45. Gabbott, P. L. A., Warner, T. A., Jays, P. R. L., Salway, P., and Busby, S. J. (2005). Prefrontal cortex in the rat: Projections to subcortical autonomic, motor, and limbic centers. *Journal of Comparative Neurology* 492, 145–177.
46. Gao, K., and Mason, P. (1997). Somatodendritic and axonal anatomy of intracellularly labeled serotonergic neurons in the rat medulla. *Journal of Comparative Neurology* 389, 309–328.
47. Gao, K., and Mason, P. (2001). Physiological and anatomic evidence for functional subclasses of serotonergic raphe magnus cells. *Journal of Comparative Neurology* 439, 426–439.
48. Geerling, J. G., Mettenleiter, T. C., and Loewy, A. D. (2003). Orexin neurons project to diverse sympathetic outflow systems. *Neuroscience* 122, 541–550.
49. Guyenet, P. G., Koshiya, N., Huangfu, D., Verberne, A. J., and Riley, T. A. (1993). Central respiratory control of A5 and A6 pontine noradrenergic neurons. *American Journal of Physiology* 264, R1035–R1044.
50. Halsell, C. B., and Travers, S. P. (1997). Anterior and posterior oral cavity responsive neurons are differentially distributed among parabrachial subnuclei in rat. *Journal of Neurophysiology* 78, 920–938.
51. Helke, C. J., Thor, K. B., and Sasek, C. A. (1989). Chemical neuroanatomy of the parapyramidal region of the ventral medulla in the rat. *Progress in Brain Research* 81, 17–28.
52. Herbert, H., Moga, M. M., and Saper, C. B. (1990). Connections of the parabrachial nucleus with the nucleus of the solitary tract and the medullary reticular formation in the rat. *Journal of Comparative Neurology* 293, 540–580.
53. Hermann, G. E., Holmes, G. M., Rogers, R. C., Beattie, M. S., and Bresnahan, J. C. (2003). Descending spinal projections from the rostral gigantocellular reticular nuclei complex. *Journal of Comparative Neurology* 455, 210–221.
54. Horiuchi, J., McAllen, R. M., Allen, A. M., Killinger, S., Fontes, M. A. P., and Dampney, R. A. (2004). Descending vasomotor pathways from the dorsomedial hypothalamic nucleus: Role of medullary raphe and RVLM. *American Journal of Physiology* 287, R824–R832.
55. Huangfu, D., Huang, L. J., Riley, T. A., and Guyenet, P. G. (1992). Splanchnic nerve response to A5–area stimulation in rats. *American Journal of Physiology* 263, R437–R446
56. Janig, W. (1988). Pre- and postganglionic vasoconstrictor neurons. *Annual Review of Physiology* 50, 525–539.
57. Janig, W., and Habler, H. J. (2000). Specificity of the organization of the autonomic nervous system: A basis for precise regulation of homeostatic and protective body functions. *Progress in Brain Research* 122, 351–367.
58. Janig, W., and McLachlan, E. M. (1992). Characteristics of function-specific pathways in the sympathetic nervous system. *Trends in Neurosciences* 15, 475–481.
59. Jansen, A. S. P., Van Nguyen, X., Karpitskiy, V., Mettenleiter, T. C., and Loewy, A. D. (1995). Central command neurons of the sympathetic nervous system: Basis of the fight-or-flight response. *Science* 270, 253–260.
60. Karimnamazi. H., Travers, S. P., and Travers, J. B. (2002). Oral and gastric input to the parabrachial nucleus of the rat. *Brain Research* 957, 193–206.
61. Kawano, H., and Muauko, S. (1993). Synaptic inputs of neuropeptide Y-immunoreactive noradrenergic nerve terminals to neurons in the nucleus preopticus medianus which project to the paraventricular nucleus of the hypothalamus of the rat: A combined immunohistochemical and retrograde tracing method. *Brain Research* 600, 74–80.
62. Keay, K. A., and Bandler, R. (2001). Parallel circuits mediating distinct emotional coping reactions to different types of stress. *Neuroscience and Biobehavioral Reviews* 25, 669–678.
63. Kerman, I., Enquist, L. W., Watson, S. J., and Yates, B. J. (2003). Brainstem substrates of sympatho-motor circuitry identified using trans-synaptic tracing with pseudorabies virus recombinants. *Journal of Neuroscience* 23, 4657–4666.
64. Kim, J.-S., Moore, R. Y., Enquist, L. W., and Card, J. P. (1999). Circuit-specific co-infection of neurons in the rat central nervous system with two pseudorabies virus recombinants. *Journal of Virology* 75, 9521–9531.
65. Koshiya, N., and Guyenet, P. G. (1994). A5 noradrenergic neurons and the carotid sympathetic chemoreflex. *American Journal of Physiology* 267, R519–R526.
66. Krout, K. E., Mettenleiter, T. C., and Loewy, A. D. (2003). Single CNS neurons link both central motor and cardiosympathetic

systems: A double-virus tracing study. *Neuroscience* 118, 853–866.

67. Larsen, P. J., Hay-Schmidt, A., and Mikkelsenq, J. D. (1994). Efferent connections from the lateral hypothalamic region and the lateral preoptic area to the hypothalamic paraventricular nucleus in the rat. *Journal of Comparative Neurology* 342, 299–319.
68. LeDoux, J. E. (2000). Emotion circuits in the brain. *Annual Review of Neuroscience* 23, 155–184.
69. LeDoux, J. E. (2003). The emotional brain. fear, and the amygdala. *Cellular and Molecular Neurobiology* 23, 727–738.
70. Loewy, A. D., Franklin, M. F., and Haxhiu, M. A. (1994). CNS monoamine cell groups projecting to pancreatic vagal motor neurons: A transneuronal labeling study using pseudorabies virus. *Brain Research* 638, 248–260.
71. Loewy, A. D., McKellar, S., and Saper, C. B. (1979). Direct projections from the A5 catecholamine cell group to the intermediolateral cell column. *Brain Research* 174, 309–314.
72. Madden, C. J., Ito, S., Rinaman, L., Wiley, R. G., and Sved, A. F. (1999). Lesions of the C1 catecholaminergic neurons of the ventrolateral medulla in rats using anti-DbH-saporin. *American Journal of Physiology* 46, R1063–R1075.
73. Madden, C. J., and Sved, A. F. (2003). Cardiovascular regulation after destruction of the C1 cell group of the rostral ventrolateral medulla in rats. *American Journal of Physiology* 285, 2734–2748.
74. Maiorov, D. N., Malpas, S. C., and Head, G. A. (2000). Influence of pontine A5 region on renal sympathetic nerve activity in conscious rabbits. *American Journal of Physiology* 278, R311–R319.
75. Mason, P. (2005). Deconstructing endogenous pain modulation. *Journal of Neurophysiology* 94, 1659–1663.
76. Mason, P. (2005). Ventromedial medulla: Pain modulation and beyond. *Journal of Comparative Neurology* 493, 2–8.
77. McKinley, M. J., Mathai, M. L., McAllen, R. M., McClear, R. C., Miselis, R. R., Pennington, G. L., Vivas, L., Wade, J. D., and Oldfield, B. J. (2004). Vasopressin secretion: Osmotic and hormonal regulation by the lamina terminalis. *Journal of Neuroendocrinology* 16, 340–347.
78. Morrison, S. F. (1999). RVLM and raphe differentially regulate sympathetic outflows to splanchnic and brown adipose tissue. *American Journal of Physiology* 276, R962–R973.
79. Morrison, S. F. (2001). Differential control of sympathetic outflow. *American Journal of Physiology* 281, R683–R698.
80. Myers, E. A., and Rinaman, L. (2002). Viscerosensory activation of noradrenergic inputs to the amygdala in rats. *Physiology and Behavior* 77, 723–729.
81. Nadelhaft, I., and Vera, P. L. (1996). Neurons in the rat brain and spinal cord labeled after pseudorabies virus injected into the external urethral sphincter. *Journal of Comparative Neurology* 375, 502–517.
82. Nakamura, K., Matsumura, K., Hubschle, T., Nakamura, Y., Hioki, H., Fujiyama, F., Boldogkoi, Z., Konig, M., Thiel, H.-J., Gerstberger, R., Kobayashi, S., and Kaneko, T. (2004). Identification of sympathetic premotor neurons in medullary raphe regions mediated fever and other thermoregulatory functions. *Journal of Neuroscience* 24, 5370–5380.
83. Nakamura, K., Matsumura, K., Kaneko, T., Kobayashi, S., Katoh, H., and Negishi, M. (2002). The rostral raphe pallidus nucleus mediates pyrogenic transmission from the preoptic area. *Journal of Neuroscience* 22, 4600–4610.
84. Nason, M. W., and Mason, P. (2004). Modulation of sympathetic and somatomotor function by the ventromedial medulla. *Journal of Neurophysiology* 92, 510–522.
85. Oppenheimer, T., Saleh, T., and Cechetto, D. F. (1992). Lateral hypothalamic area neurotransmission and neuromodulation of the specific cardiac effects of insular cortex stimulation. *Brain Research* 581, 133–142.
86. Palkovits, M. (1999). Interconnections between the neuroendocrine hypothalamus and the central autonomic system. *Frontiers in Neuroendocrinology* 20, 270–279.
87. Portillo, F., Carrasco, M., and Vallo, J. J. (1996). Hypothalamic neuron projection to autonomic preganglionic levels related with glucose metabolism: A fluorescent labelling study in rat. *Neuroscience Letters* 210, 197–200.
88. Portillo, F., Carrasco, M., and Vallo, J. J. (1998). Separate populations of neurons within the paraventricular hypothalamic nucleus of the rat project to vagal and thoracic autonomic preganglionic levels and express c-Fos protein induced by lithium chloride. *Journal of Chemical Neuroanatomy* 14, 95–102.
89. Pyner, S., and Coote, J. H. (2000). Identification of branching paraventricular neurons of the hypothalamus that project to the rostroventrolateral medulla and spinal cord. *Neuroscience* 100, 549–556.
90. Ramon-Moliner, E., and Nauta, W. J.H. (1966). The isodendritic core of the brain stem. *Journal of Comparative Neurology* 126, 311–335.

91. Rinaman, L., Card, J. P., and Enquist, L. W. (1993). Spatiotemporal responses of astrocytes, ramified microglia, and brain macrophages to central neuronal infection with pseudorabies virus. *Journal of Neuroscience* 13, 685–702.
92. Rinaman, L., and Miselis, R. R. (1987). The organization of vagal innervation of rat pancreas using cholera toxin-horseradish peroxidase conjugate. *Journal of the Autonomic Nervous System* 21, 109–125.
93. Ross, C. A., Armstrong, D. M., Ruggiero, D. A., Pickel, V. M., Joh, T. H., and Reis, D. J. (1981). Adrenaline neurons in the rostral ventrolateral medulla innervate thoracic spinal cord: A combined immunocytochemical and retrograde transport demonstration. *Neuroscience Letters* 25, 257–262.
94. Ross, C. A., Ruggiero, D. A., Park, D. H., Joh, T. H., Sved, A. F., Fernandez-Pardal, J., Saavedra, J. M., and Reis, D. J. (1984). Tonic vasomotor control by the rostral ventrolateral medulla: Effect of electrical or chemical stimulation of the area containing C1 adrenaline neurons on arterial pressure, heart rate, and plasma catecholamines and vasopressin. *Journal of Neuroscience* 4, 474–494.
95. Sah, P., Faber, E. S.L., Lopez de Armentia, M., and Power, J. (2003). The amygdaloid complex: Anatomy and physiology. *Physiology Reviews* 83, 803–834.
96. Samuels, B. C., Zaretsky, D. V., and DiMicco, J. A. (2002). Tachycardia evoked by disinhibition of the dorsomedial hypothalamus in rats is mediated through the medullary raphe. *Journal of Physiology* 538, 941–946.
97. Saper, C. B. (2002). The central autonomic nervous system: Conscious visceral perception and autonomic pattern generation. *Annual Review of Neuroscience* 25, 433–469.
98. Saper, C. B. (2004). Central autonomic system. In: G. Paxinos (Ed.), *The Rat Nervous System,* pp. 761–796. Amsterdam: Elsevier Academic Press,.
99. Saper, C. B., and Levisohn, D. (1983). Afferent connections of the median preoptic nucleus in the rat: Anatomical evidence for a cardiovascular integrative mechanism in the anteroventral third ventricle (AV3V). *region. Brain Research* 288, 21–31.
100. Saper, C. B., Reis, D. J., and Joh, T. H. (1983). Medullary catecholamine inputs to the anteroventral third ventricular cardiovascular region in the rat. *Neuroscience Letters* 42, 285–292.
101. Sasaki, M. (2005). Role of Barrington's nucleus in micturition. *Journal of Comparative Neurology* 493, 21–26.
102. Sawchenko, P. E., Li, H. Y., and Ericsson, A. (2000). Circuits and mechanisms governing hypothalamic responses to stress: A tale of two paradigms. *Progress in Brain Research* 122, 61–87.
103. Sawchenko, P. E., and Swanson, L. W. (1981). Central noradrenergic pathways for the integration of hypothalamic neuroendocrine and autonomic responses. *Science* 214, 685–687.
104. Sawchenko, P. E., Swanson, L. W., Grzanna, R., Howe, P. R. C., Bloom, S. R., and Polak, J. M. (1985). Colocalization of neuropeptide Y immunoreactivity in brainstem catecholamine neurons that project to the paraventricular nucleus of hypothalamus. *Journal of Comparative Neurology* 241, 138–153.
105. Schadt, J. C., Shafford, H. L., and McKnown, M. D. (2005). Neuronal activity within the ventrolateral periaqueductal gray during simulated hemorrhage in conscious rabbits. *American Journal of Physiology* 290, R715–R725.
106. Schreihofer, A. M., and Guyenet, P. G. (2000). Role of presympathetic C1 neurons in the sympatholytic and hypotensive effects of clonidine in rats. *American Journal of Physiology* 279, R1753–R1762.
107. Schreihofer, A. M., and Guyenet, P. G. (2000). Sympathetic reflexes after depletion of bulbospinal catecholaminergic neurons with anti-DbH-saporin. *American Journal of Physiology* 279, R729–R742.
108. Schreihofer, A. M., Stornetta, R., and Guyenet, P. G. (2000). Regulation of sympathetic tone and arterial pressure by rostral ventrolateral medulla after depletion of C1 cells in rats. *Journal of Physiology* 529, 221–236.
109. Schwaber, J. S., Sternini, C., Brecha, N. C., Rogers, W. T., and Card, J. P. (1988). Neurons containing calcitonin gene-related peptide in the parabrachial nucleus project to the central nucleus of the amygdala. *Journal of Comparative Neurology* 270, 416–426.
110. Shafton, A. D., Ryan, A., and Badoer, E. (1998). Neurons in the hypothalamic paraventricular nucleus send collaterals to the spinal cord and to the rostral ventrolateral medulla in the rat. *Brain Research* 801, 239–243.
111. Shapiro, R. E., and Miselis, R. R. (1985). The central organization of the vagus nerve innervating the stomach of the rat. *Journal of Comparative Neurology* 238, 473–488.
112. Stanek, K. A., Neil, J. J., Sawyer, W. B., and Loewy, A. D. (1984). Changes in regional blood flow and cardiac output after L-glutamate stimulation of A5 cell group. *American Journal of Pathology* 246, H44–H51.

113. Stocker, S. D., Cunningham, J. T., and Toney, G. M. (2004). Water deprivation increases Fos immunoreactivity in PVN autonomic neurons with projections to the spinal cord and ventrolateral medulla. *American Journal of Physiology* 287, R1172–R1183.
114. Stornetta, R., Akey, P. J., and Guyenet, P. G. (1999). Location and electrophysiological characterization of rostral medullary adrenergic neurons that contain neuropeptide Y mRNA in rat medulla. *Journal of Comparative Neurology* 415, 482–500.
115. Stornetta, R., Sevigny, C. P., Schreihofer, A. M., Rosin, D. L., and Guyenet, P. G. (2002). Vesicular glutamate transporter DNPI/GLUT2 is expressed by both C1 adrenergic and nonaminergic presympathetic vasomotor neurons of the rat medulla. *Journal of Comparative Neurology* 444, 207–220.
116. Strack, A. M., Sawyer, W. B., Hughes, H. H., Platt, K. B., and Loewy, A. D. (1989). A general pattern of CNS innervation of the sympathetic outflow demonstrated by transneuronal pseudorabies viral infection. *Brain Research* 491, 156–162.
117. Strack, A. M., Sawyer, W. B., Platt, K. B., and Loewy, A. D. (1989). CNS cell groups regulating the sympathetic outflow of the adrenal gland as revealed by transneuronal cell body labeling with pseudorabies virus. *Brain Research* 491, 274–296.
118. Sved, A. F., Cano, G., and Card, J. P. (2001). Neuroanatomical specificity of the circuits controlling sympathetic outflow to different targets. *Clinical and Experimental Pharmacology and Physiology* 28, 115–119.
119. Sved, A. F., and Ruggiero, D. A. (1996). The autonomic nervous system structure and function. In B. J. Yates and A. D. Miller (Eds.), *Vestibular Autonomic Regulation,* pp. 25–51. Boca Raton, FL: CRC Press.
120. Swanson, L. W. (1988). *Brain Maps: Structure of the Rat Brain*, second ed. Amsterdam: Elsevier.
121. Swanson, L. W., and Kuypers, H. G.J. M. (1980). The paraventricular nucleus of the hypothalamus: Cytoarchitectonic subdivision and organization of projections to the pituitary, dorsal vagal complex, and spinal cord as demonstrated by retrograde fluorescence double labeling methods. *Journal of Comparative Neurology* 194, 555–570.
122. ter Horst, G. J., and Luiten, P. G. (1988). The projections of the dorsomedial hypothalamic nucleus in the rat. *Brain Research Bulletin* 16, 231–248.
123. Thompson, R. H., Canteras, N. S., and Swanson, L. W. (1996). Organization of projections from the dorsomedial nucleus of the hypothalamus: A PHA-L study in the rat. *Journal of Comparative Neurology* 376, 143–173.
124. Travers, J. B. (1988). Efferent projections from the anterior nucleus of the solitary tract of the hamster. *Brain Research* 457, 1–11.
125. Tucker, D. C., Saper, C. B., Ruggiero, D. A., and Reis, D. J. (1987). Organization of central adrenergic pathways: I. Relationships of ventrolateral medullary projections to the hypothalamus and spinal cord. *Journal of Comparative Neurology* 259, 591–603.
126. Valentino, R. J., Kosboth, M., Colflesh, M., and Miselis, R. R. (2000). Transneuronal labeling from the rat distal colon: Anatomic evidence for regulation of distal colon function by a pontine corticotropin-releasing factor system. *Journal of Comparative Neurology* 417, 399–414.
127. van den Pol, A. N. (1999). Hypothalamic hypocretin (orexin): Robust innervation of the spinal cord. *Journal of Neuroscience* 19, 3171–3182.
128. Verberne, A. J., Stornetta, R., and Guyenet, P. G. (1999). Properties of C1 and other ventrolateral medullary neurones with hypothalamic projections in the rat. *Journal of Physiology* 517, 477–494.
129. Woodruff, M. L., Baisden, R. H., and Whittington, D. L. (1986). Effects of electrical stimulation on the pontine A5 cell group on blood pressure and heart rate in the rabbit. *Brain Research* 379, 10–23.
130. Zardetto-Smith, A. M., and Gray, T. S. (1995). Catecholamine and NPY efferents from the ventrolateral medulla to the amygdala in the rat. *Brain Research Bulletin* 38, 253–260.

# 2

# The Nucleus of the Solitary Tract: Processing Information from Viscerosensory Afferents

MICHAEL C. ANDRESEN AND JULIAN F. R. PATON

The central nervous system (CNS) is updated continuously on the status of visceral organs by streams of information that directly enter the brainstem at the nucleus of the solitary tract (NTS). This information is carried by the central processes of primary afferent neurons that synapse on second-order neurons in NTS. These viscerosensory afferents provide moment-to-moment updates about the status of respiratory, cardiovascular, gastrointestinal, and other vital organs and initiate adjustments in reflexes that maintain homeostasis. This visceral information also influences neuroendocrine responses and behavior, including exercise, feeding, reward, and stress responses. Excellent recent reviews outline the overall organization of the NTS in relation to key regulatory pathways in the brainstem and also highlight important supramedullary areas that participate in central control of homeostasis[114,142].

This chapter will focus on the intermediate to commissural portions of the caudal NTS and will rely chiefly on evidence from the rat, the most comprehensively studied species. The rostral portion of the NTS mediates gustation and will not be discussed here. Emphasis will be placed on cardiovascular pathways with three aims: (i) to examine the fundamental building blocks of pathways through the NTS with a focus on transmission involving the fast-acting amino acid neurotransmitters, glutamate and γ-amino-butyric acid (GABA), and the baroreceptor reflex; (ii) to outline the mechanisms regulating afferent information transfer to sites beyond the NTS; and (iii) to discuss mechanisms by which afferent information relating to the cardiovascular system is transformed by two major modulators, angiotensin II and nitric oxide.

## CHAOS AT THE GATEWAY

The NTS acts as the gateway to the CNS for sensory information arising from internal organs. Neuroanatomical studies of the NTS have produced a treasure trove of information about the distributions of different types of sensory afferents, the connections of NTS subnuclei with other brain areas, and the neurochemistry of cell bodies and axons within the NTS. The brainstem is heterogeneous in all of these aspects, and the NTS is no exception. NTS neurons express a diverse array of neurotransmitters, neuromodulators, and receptors for transmitters and hormones[25,86,114]. When viewed individually, the subnuclear distributions of these substances and receptors are not strikingly unique or discrete. This heterogeneity is probably responsible for the diverse characteristics of pathways that control different systemic functions. However, placing these various types of NTS neurons into frameworks that clarify central control of autonomic function has proved challenging.

### Visceral Afferent Portal to Reflex Pathways

Despite its heterogeneity, the NTS is commonly represented as a single nucleus in circuitry diagrams (Figure 2–1). A general view of the relationship of the

NTS to other CNS regions has evolved over the last 25 years, and two overarching themes have emerged (see also Chapter 1). First, the NTS has reciprocal connections with a great many CNS structures within and beyond the brainstem. Second, afferents arising from cranial nerves are, in general, viscerotopically distributed within caudal NTS, and these afferent distributions have offered the concept of functional regions; e.g., baroreceptive or respiratory. These two aspects of the anatomy of the NTS remain relatively disconnected; and therefore, precisely how or whether the various afferent inputs to NTS relate to the multiple outputs from NTS are largely unknown. The retrograde spread of trans-synaptic viral tracers from specific peripheral targets follows the same autonomic circuits (Figure 2–1), which were originally assembled from stepwise studies using conventional retrograde neuronal tract tracers[64,138]. However, neither approach can define the afferent identity of the labeled NTS neurons and therefore cannot retrace the complete reflex loop from the initiating afferent to the target.

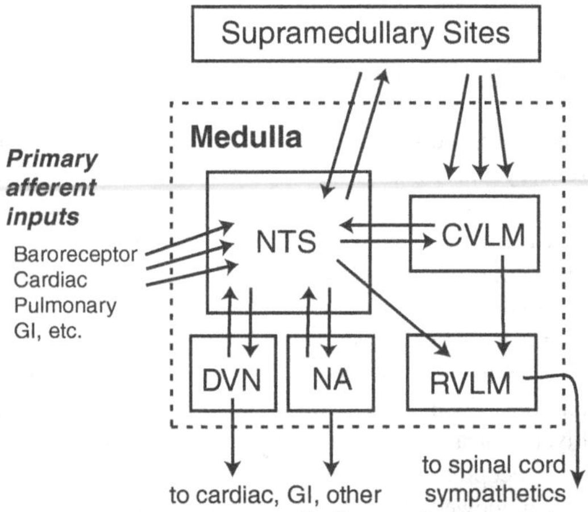


Figure 2–1 Connections between the NTS and other major autonomic brain regions. The caudal ventrolateral medulla (CVLM), dorsal motor nucleus of the vagus (dorsal vagal nucleus, DVN), nucleus ambiguus (NA), and supramedullary sites, including the hypothalamus, are reciprocally connected to the NTS. The rostral ventrolateral medulla (RVLM) receives monosynaptic inputs from the commissural NTS. The DVN, NA, and RVLM are major efferent pathways of the parasympathetic and sympathetic division of the autonomic nervous system.

In one reflex circuit, arterial baroreceptors activate NTS neurons that, in turn, excite cardiac parasympathetic preganglionic neurons in the loose formation of the nucleus ambiguus[149] (see also Chapter 7). The activity of the ambiguual neurons commonly shows a cardiac rhythmicity that is attributed to baroreceptor afferent signals; and the neurons probably receive a direct, monosynaptic input from the NTS[2,69]. The pathway for conveying baroreflex information through the NTS to parasympathetic postganglionic neurons at the heart may include as few as two central neurons and account for loop latencies as short as 26 ms[78]. Similar minimal vago-vagal reflex pathways for parasympathetic regulation of other visceral organs involve the dorsal motor nucleus of the vagus (dorsal vagal nucleus, DVN)[142]. In contrast, the sympathetic portion of the baroreflex engages inhibitory (GABAergic) neurons in the caudal ventrolateral medulla (CVLM), which are activated by NTS neurons that project directly to the CVLM (see Chapter 5). The GABAergic CVLM neurons send axons to the rostral ventrolateral medulla, (RVLM) where they inhibit spinally projecting presympathetic vasomotor neurons. Because of the greater complexity of central sympathetic pathways and their relation to the generation of sympathetic rhythms, it has been much more difficult to determine the role(s) that the NTS and/or visceral afferent inputs play in sympathetic regulation[97], although new insights are emerging.

The brainstem pathways shown in Figure 2–1 outline core circuits that are characteristic of many autonomic reflexes, such as the arterial baroreflex; and these basic reflex responses persist even following decerebration[80,102]. More complicated pathways also exist. Projections from supramedullary sites, such as the hypothalamus, amygdala, and cerebral cortex, modulate the activity of NTS neurons in autonomic pathways and provide integrative control[23]. Whether circuitry within the NTS helps trigger longer loop feedback pathways (e.g., via forebrain structures) is unknown.

## Are there Really Viscerotopic Zones in the NTS?

Visceral information enters the CNS via cranial nerves (mainly IX and X) that form the solitary tract. Visceral primary afferents probably contact most neurons in the NTS directly, and these are called *second-order neurons*. Anterograde tracing from visceral afferent nerve trunks labels broad regions of the intermediate and caudal NTS, suggestive of a general viscerotopic organization (Figure 2–2). The intermediate zone of the caudal NTS may exhibit greater functional segregation of afferents than the commissural region. On the basis of afferent tracing, the NTS has been subdivided into viscerotopic regions that receive cardiovascular, respiratory, and gastrointestinal input (see [85]). Responses to focal electrical stimulation or application of agonists within these viscerotopic regions often mimic reflex responses. For example, microinjection of glutamate into the medial NTS, where arterial baroreceptors terminate[90], evokes hypotension, bradycardia, and respiratory depression, a triad that resembles baroreflex activation[141]. However, activation of other specific subsets of afferents, including pulmonary vagal C-fibers, triggers this triad of responses[68]. Similar microinjection evidence exists for organ-specific changes resembling activation of respiratory[77] and gastrointestinal afferents[142], although NTS injection sites were often quite similar.

In contrast to whole-nerve anatomical data, studies of single NTS neurons or specific subsets of neurons

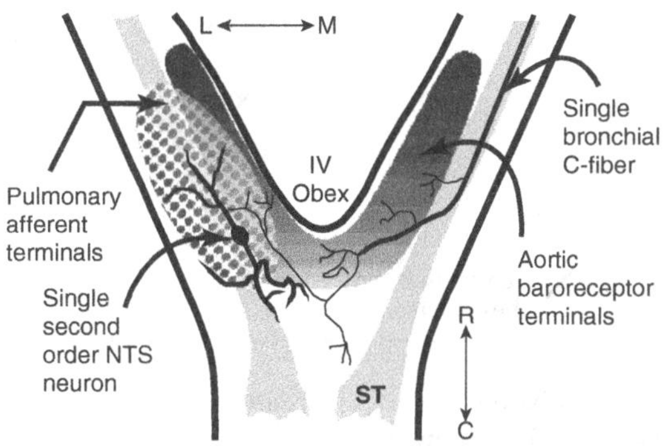


Figure 2–2 Overlap of viscerotopic zones within the NTS. Viscerotopic zones can be defined by mapping subregions that receive input from different classes of cranial visceral afferents (e.g., baroreceptor, gastrointestinal, airway, etc.). This diagram shows two of many such potential zones at the intermediate and commissural levels of the NTS in horizontal section. Aortic baroreceptors terminate in the gray-shaded NTS region medial to the solitary tract (ST). Pulmonary afferents terminate in the stippled zone extending from lateral into medial NTS. Darker stippling indicates greater terminal density, which changes rostrocaudally and mediolaterally. The two termination zones overlap and both extend from intermediate into commissural NTS. Dye-filled second-order NTS neurons (*left side*) may have cell bodies within one zone, but their dendrites extend into other zones and subnuclei. Likewise, single visceral afferent axons (*right side*) reach the NTS via the ST, but may have many branches that extend over great distances, sometimes even crossing the midline to the contralateral side. IV, 4th ventricle.; C, caudal; L, lateral; M, medial; R, rostral.

indicate that, within individual NTS subnuclei, terminations of different functional types of afferent input overlap substantially[6,77,134], and regions feature second-order neurons with various neurochemical phenotypes[10,11]. Such cellular diversity, together with the extensive dendritic arbors of individual second-order NTS neurons, blurs the concept of segregated viscerotopic regions (Figure 2–3)[77,104]. Even in the "*cardiovascular NTS,*" baroreceptive neurons are intermixed with neurons responding to peripheral chemoreceptor or abdominal afferent activation (Figure 2–3[104]).

This blurred viscerotopic representation based on cell body location probably underestimates the functional impact of afferent inputs along distal dendrites. For example, baroreceptive neurons in the dorsal, dorsolateral, and medial NTS extend dendrites medially and laterally into regions many hundreds of micrometers from the cell body, and these processes occasionally cross the midline (Figure 2–3[37]), a pattern also common for respiratory neurons[77]. Little is understood about the functional impact of electrotonic weighting of synaptic inputs at distal compared to proximal sites on NTS neurons, but presumably all contribute to synaptic integration. Even within modalities such as arterial baroreceptors, different sources (aortic nerve and carotid sinus nerve) may be differently distributed.

## Are NTS Zones Defined by Anatomical Criteria Useful?

Cytoarchitectonic approaches, such as Nissl staining, have defined a number of subnuclei within the NTS. However, there is remarkably little correspondence between these subdivisions and zones defined by afferent tracer distributions, functionally defined regions, or neurochemical groups. Neurochemical markers, such as neurotransmitter synthetic enzymes, identify groups of phenotypically similar NTS neurons, but these groups are not confined to the cytoarchitecturally defined subdivisions[70]. In transgenic mice that express green fluorescent protein within neurochemically similar neurons, major neuronal phenotypes, such as GABA- or catecholamine-synthesizing[10,11], or rarer types such as pro-opiomelanocortin subpopulations[9], are distributed across multiple NTS subnuclei. Similarly, retrograde tracing from regions such as the paraventricular nucleus (PVN) in the hypothalamus and the CVLM, identify separate subsets of NTS neurons with distributions that intermingle and cross both viscerotopic zones and histological subregions[60]. Thus, functional subclasses of NTS neurons, whether defined by afferent input, chemical phenotype, or axonal destination, are not confined to well-defined subregions.

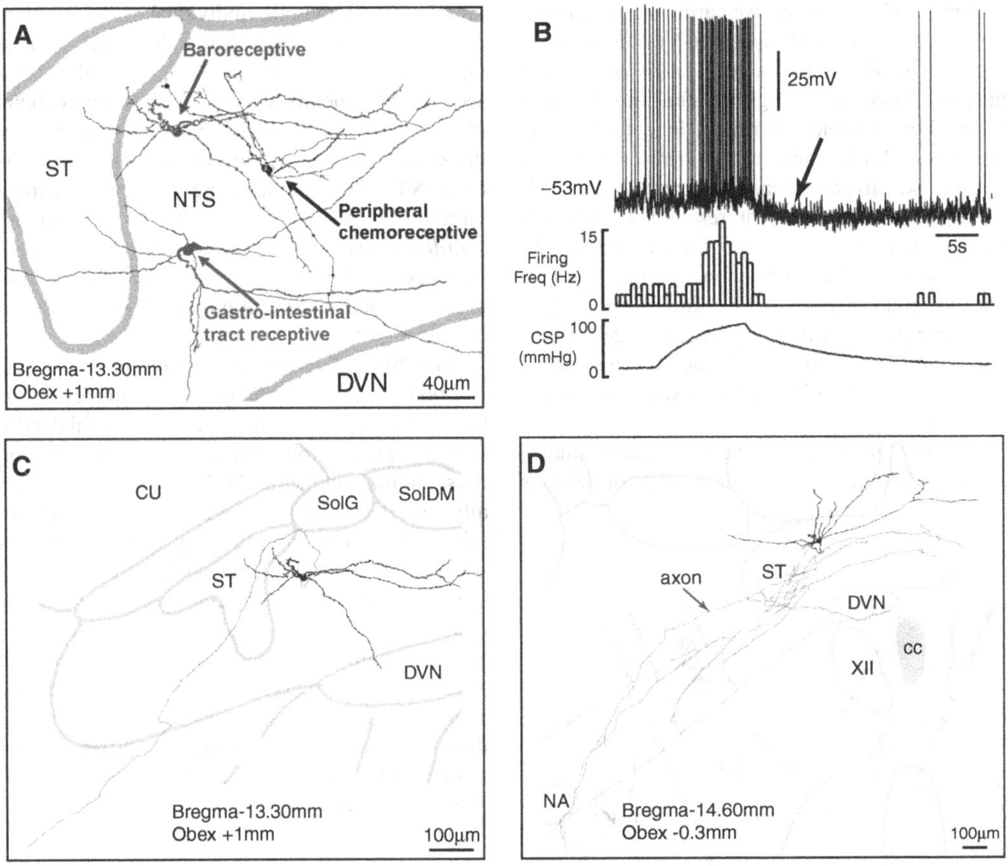


Figure 2–3 Morphological and electrophysiological properties of baroreceptive NTS neurons. For a color version of Figure 2–3, see Color Plate 2–3 between pages 224 and 225. *A*: Individual baroreceptive NTS neurons intermix with neurons belonging to other reflex circuits, suggesting that there is little or no "viscerotopic" organization within the NTS. Microinjection of a drug into the medial NTS would therefore activate many reflex circuits simultaneously, making it very difficult to identify which specific afferent pathway was activated. *B*: Whole-cell recording of a baroreceptive NTS neuron shows the firing frequency (Freq) response to raising carotid sinus pressure (CSP). Note the adaptive nature of the firing, with the peak response occurring before the maximal level of carotid sinus pressure (CSP), and the hyperpolarization following the stimulus (*arrow*). About 30% of baroreceptive NTS neurons exhibited these characteristics, indicating that powerful mechanisms regulate neuronal excitability. *C & D*: Two labeled baroreceptive NTS neurons that received constant short latency inputs after electrical stimulation of the solitary tract (ST). Most putative second-order baroreceptive neurons project out of the NTS towards the ventrolateral medulla (*C & D*), but some also have axons (*D, grey*) that terminate within the NTS. Note the extent to which the dendrites (*black*) arborize ipsi- and contralaterally. CC, central canal; CU, cuneate nucleus; DVN, dorsal vagal nucleus; Gn, gracile nucleus; NA, nucleus ambiguus. Modified from Deuchars et al. (2000)[37] and Paton et al. (2000)[110], with permission.

Anatomical studies often focus on the location of cell bodies, and many labels mark only the cell nuclei without enabling visualization of the dendrites (e.g., Fos). Anterograde tracers often stain axons traversing a region, as well as synaptic terminals. Thus, such tracer-based approaches cannot illustrate functional connections (Figures 2.2 and 2.3). These approaches may overestimate (axons of passage) or underestimate (invisible dendritic arbors) potential structures for interaction. Clearly, combinations of technical approaches will be necessary to establish functionally connected neurons and clarify these uncertainties.

Most visceral organs possess multiple types of afferents (e.g. mechano- and chemo-receptor), and each afferent sends unique information to NTS. The presence within functional groups of myelinated and unmyelinated subtypes of afferents may be one of the most underappreciated aspects of cranial visceral afferent integration. How and where this information is received and combined are major questions for understanding visceral sensory integration. Maps of individual cardiorespiratory afferents based on antidromic activation show that single parent axons commonly branch to reach across multiple subnuclei within the NTS[34]. Intracellular dye-filling of single pulmonary afferent fibers from slowly adapting receptors and second-order NTS neurons has provided anatomical corroboration of the results obtained from extracellular recording studies[4]. Interestingly, the axons of these slowly adapting receptors terminate in dorsomedial sites known to contain arterial baroreceptor terminals. Afferent synapses may be differentially distributed across neurons since, for example, rapidly adapting pulmonary receptor afferents contact dendrites rather than somata[71], whereas aortic baroreceptors tend to be more centralized to the soma and proximal dendrites[46]. Furthermore, individual second-order NTS neurons most often receive input from one type of afferent despite the close proximity of neurons that receive input from other types of afferents (e.g. Figure 2–3A[108]). The morphology of these functionally defined neurons varies[37]. Myelinated and unmyelinated primary afferent inputs appear to be segregated to different second-order neurons in the NTS[6,45]. Thus, modality-specific pathways are intermingled within NTS subregions, although individual neurons may participate in functionally discrete circuits and thus have fewer functional interactions with neighboring neurons than their proximity might imply[88].

## NTS Organization Based on Output Targets

Although afferent inputs are an obvious starting point for pathways within the NTS, NTS neurons send axons to many destinations, offering another feature that identifies organizational themes for NTS viscerosensory processing. (Figure 2–4). The NTS is most likely structured so that neurons are functionally organized based on specific efferent outputs[37,137]. This occurs relatively early in the reflex arc and may reflect visceral afferents' receiving guidance cues that foster appropriate visceral afferent connections during development. Subnuclei within the NTS rapidly differentiate to near-adult topology by embryonic day 19. Symmetric synapses, consistent with GABAergic transmission[155], dominate in the embryo so GABAergic transmission develops first. Maturation of visceral glutamatergic afferents, including myelination, occurs postnatally when there is a rapid shift in synapse distribution toward the soma and proximal dendrites[96] and an increase in synaptic density[79]. Thus, the development of central circuitry probably precedes the establishment of visceral afferent connections within the NTS.

## Where Do Afferents Converge?

Identification of second-order neurons and the source of activation of direct synaptic contacts are essential to answering this question. Second-order NTS neurons are distinguished by direct contacts from afferent terminals that rely on glutamatergic transmission. In the intact brain, activation of peripheral afferents excites second-order neurons and triggers action potentials. Discriminating direct from indirect excitatory responses is critical to such assessments of the pathway of transmission. Intervening neurons produce delays and variation in the response timing that differentiate directly arriving excitation (visceral primary afferent terminals) from that arriving through serial activation of intervening neurons. Physiological activation of peripheral afferents is the most relevant for functional identification of NTS neurons. However, substantial variation in the peripheral transduction process[130] introduces uncertainty in estimates of the central response latency compared to electrical activation, and this makes discrimination of second- from higher-order neurons less certain. Action potentials elicited by closely timed pairs of electrical shocks offer an additional clue, since longer latency responses often fail and are attributed to faulty transmission across multiple synapses in higher-order pathways to NTS neurons. Responses to high-frequency afferent volleys also characteristically undergo substantial frequency-dependent depression[129] as well as increased failures in monosynaptic transmission of C-type fibers[6] at second-order neurons.

Afferent information arrives at second-order neurons via the direct contact of visceral afferent terminals but also indirectly as relayed polysynaptically through excitatory interneurons within the NTS (Figure 2–5). Systematic surveys of individual baroreceptive NTS neurons suggest that less than 15% of NTS neurons receive directly converging inputs from more than one afferent *in vivo*[43,94] or *in vitro*[6,88]. Generally (more than 85% of the time), a single afferent (either A-type, myelinated, or C-type, unmyelinated) provided inputs from either the heart or the lungs to activate individual NTS neurons[43]. Surprisingly few NTS units (<15%) that were activated by aortic depressor nerve stimulation had cardiac rhythms[99]. Similarly, those NTS units that could be activated by chemical stimulation of pulmonary C-fibers and responded at short latency to vagal electrical shocks rarely received baroreceptor inputs. Somewhat higher proportions of NTS neurons

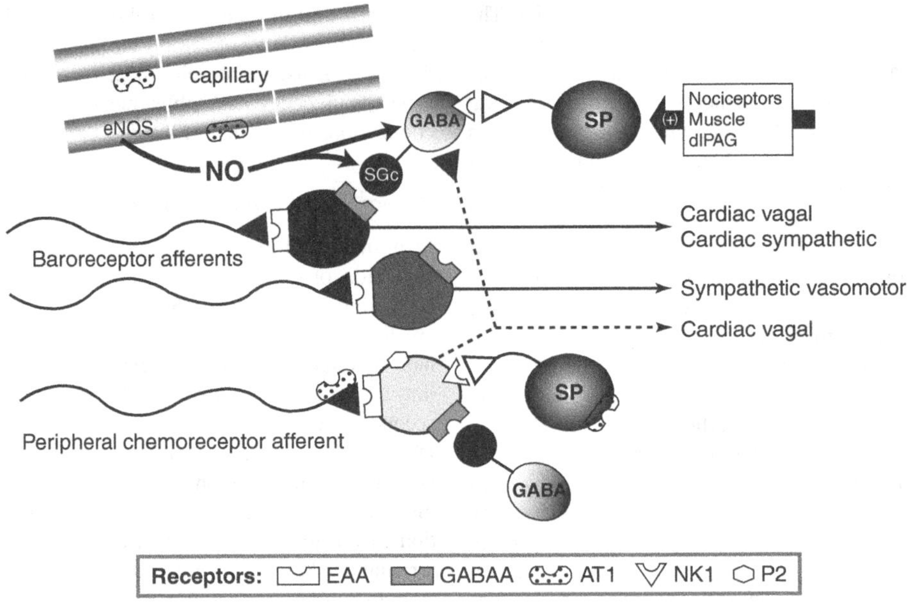


Figure 2–4 Known interactions of angiotensin II, nitric oxide, substance P, soluble guanylate cyclase, and GABA in baroreceptor and peripheral chemoreceptor reflex circuitry in the NTS. NTS neurons that mediate the baroreceptor reflex may be functionally segregated based on their output targets. The excitability of baroreceptive neurons is powerfully regulated by inhibitory transmission, which in turn is modulated by nitric oxide (NO), acting via its receptor soluble guanylate cyclase (sGC), and substance P. Angiotensin II acts on angiotensin type 1 receptors (AT1R) located on blood vessels in the NTS (*see* Figure 2–8A) to activate endothelial nitric oxide synthase (eNOS), thereby triggering nitric oxide release. Nitric oxide increases GABAergic transmission by increasing calcium release from intracellular cyclic adenosine diphosphate ribose regulated ryanodine-sensitive calcium stores. Additionally, substance P acting on neurokinin 1 receptors (NK1R), located on GABAergic interneurons, appears to attenuate the baroreceptor reflex when nociceptors and group III and IV muscle afferents are stimulated. AT1R are also located on visceral afferents and neurons. These receptors increase excitatory transmission and augment the peripheral chemoreceptor reflex, again through substance P acting on NK1R. EAA, excitatory amino acid receptor. See text for references supporting this schema.

(25%–30%) were co-activated by chemoreceptor, cardiac, and cardiopulmonary inputs; but their mono- and polysynaptic character was not tested[103,135]. Thus, most NTS neurons may be dominated by a single afferent modality, but the functions and implications of NTS neurons with multiple convergent afferents are presently unclear.

Surprisingly small proportions of NTS neurons display obvious cardiac rhythmicity[57]. This raises the possibility that cardiac rhythmicity may be encoded by a population of NTS neurons[124]. Despite a near-universal afferent synaptic depression and a general absence of cardiac rhythm within the NTS, pronounced neuronal activity with a cardiac rhythm can be detected at sites further along central cardiovascular pathways, such as the CVLM and RVLM, where neuronal activity positively or negatively correlates with blood pressure, respectively[23,65].

## Autonomic Reflex Pathways May Segregate Early Within the NTS

It is well known that arterial pressure levels can be altered independently of cardiac baroreceptor reflex gain, as during exercise[120]. Thus, the gain of the cardiac baroreflex may be modulated without altering arterial pressure[145]. One obvious site where this differential modulation of the baroreceptor reflex could occur is the NTS.

Baroreceptor reflex control of heart rate but not sympathetic vasomotor activity is highly sensitive to activation of the angiotensin II type 1 receptor[107], the neurokinin type 1 receptor[113], and metabotropic glutamate receptors[137]. These NTS receptors may represent the substrate for selective, differential modulation of vagal versus sympathetic vasomotor reflexes. Hence, separate baroreflex circuits within the NTS

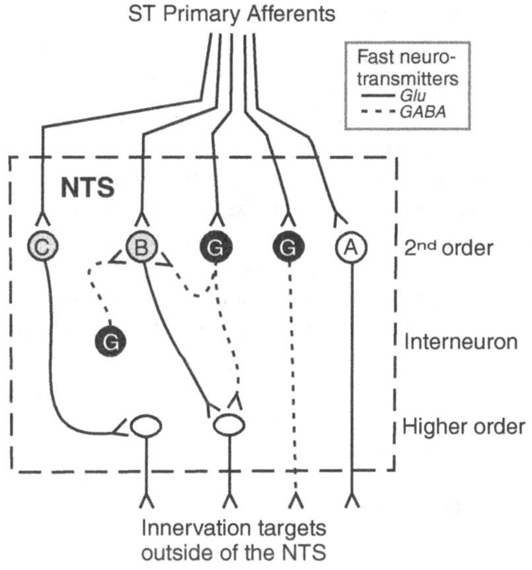


Figure 2–5 Simplest possible organization of autonomic pathways within the NTS. At its simplest, the NTS can be viewed as consisting of solitary tract (ST) afferents contacting and defining second-order neurons (*A, B, C* and *G*). Afferent signals leave the NTS via neurons that send axons outside the NTS. These projection neurons receive synaptic input directly from ST afferents (*A*) or are part of polysynaptic pathways within the NTS (*B, C*). GABAergic neurons (*G*) include interneurons that are generally second-order neurons. Additional neurotransmitters and non-ionotropic receptors also contribute. Evidence supports many of these hypothesized pathways[6,9–11,13,47–49].

may control these distinct autonomic outflows. However, there may be even greater specificity. Activation of angiotensin II receptors in the NTS attenuates both vagal and sympathetic components of the baroreceptor heart rate reflex[21] without affecting baroreflex inhibition of sympathetic vasomotor activity[115]. In other words, NTS baroreceptive neurons may have connections to neurons with distinct functional outputs to different organs (heart, adrenals, kidney). These data suggest a segregation and independence of neuronal function within the NTS analogous to that in the RVLM[33].

Cardiorespiratory afferents that share common output pathways may converge in the NTS. Recordings from physiologically characterized NTS neurons *in vivo* and in the working heart-brainstem preparation, an anesthetized, decerebrate, artificially perfused animal in which connections between visceral afferents and end organs are maintained[102] indicate a degree of convergence of synaptic inputs from cardiorespiratory afferents (see above). Excitatory convergence can occur between cardiac, peripheral chemoreceptor, laryngeal, and pulmonary C-fibers, each modality of which is associated with profound vagal bradycardia. Baroreceptors and peripheral chemoreceptors can have negative interactions, possibly reflecting the opposing actions on sympathetic vasomotor and respiratory responses[61,92–94,103,135]. In support of target-dependent pathways relying on different subsets of NTS neurons, the baroreceptors that mediate vagal reflex bradycardia have significantly higher pressure thresholds for activation than those that evoke reflex sympathoinhibition[136].

It is remains unclear at what stage within a central reflex pathway the neurons gain either functionally defined projections or target their outputs toward sympathetic, parasympathetic, or hypothalamically mediated hormonal control. The destination of the axon of an NTS neuron is a critical determinant of their functional contribution. NTS neurons that receive different types of visceral inputs have been labeled intracellularly[37,106,110]. Second-order baroreceptive NTS neurons receive short, invariant latency excitatory inputs from the solitary tract and have axons that show little branching within the NTS before exiting towards the CVLM, where they form boutons *en passant*[37] (Figure 2–3). Thus, at least some second-order baroreceptive neurons are projection neurons. All NTS neurons retrogradely labeled from CVLM are excited by solitary-tract activation of monosynaptic excitatory postsynaptic currents[13]. Whether such baroreceptive neurons have parasympathetic *versus* sympathetic targets (Figure 2–4) remains to be determined, but a di-synaptic cardiac baroreflex pathway seems required to account for the earliest cardiac vagal efferent volley of action potentials triggered by activation of the carotid sinus nerve[78].

One consequence of intermixed populations of NTS neurons is that interventions like microinjections of drugs will affect multiple pathways with different functions. Interpreting responses to focal activation of neurons must also take into account that reflex responses to chemical stimulation will reflect predominantly actions on the most downstream neurons in a particular pathway. For example, microinjected glutamate may well activate second-order neurons, interneurons, and projection neurons near the injection site, but functional responses will reflect primarily the actions of glutamate at the highest-order neuron within the pathway; i.e., the projection neuron. Thus, evoked responses are unlikely to register actions at upstream neurons, even if they are responsive to glutamate.

The evidence summarized in this section illustrates several important features of NTS organization. Different afferents are unevenly distributed, with a viscerotopic pattern that is stronger rostrally than caudally. Considerable mixing of afferent contacts as well as neurons functionally associated with different visceral organs occurs within NTS. Maps of the distributions of neurochemically distinct classes of NTS neurons show substantial overlap with little clear subnuclear dominance. The functional implications of this intermixing are unclear. A tremendous future challenge is the development of experimental strategies to link specific end organ functions with specific pathways within and beyond the NTS.

## TRANSMISSION OF AFFERENT INFORMATION THROUGH THE NTS

Visceral primary afferents can be categorized by functional modalities and the organ in which their peripheral sensory-transducing endings are located. These were catalogued extensively by their discharge patterns in response to physiological and pharmacological stimuli in the 1950s through to the 1970s[31]. These visceral afferents, in turn, activate various central pathways through connections that begin in the NTS. Perhaps less appreciated are the neurobiological features of cranial visceral afferents that are similar to somatic primary sensory afferents. Two major types of visceral afferent neurons are distinguished on the basis of their myelinated or unmyelinated axons[130]. Individual cranial visceral afferents convey information about local mechanical or chemical conditions within their receptive fields, and afferents are often tuned quite narrowly to transduce one main type of sensory signal. The physiological significance of afferent information arriving at the NTS, and the mechanisms by which this information is processed, are major questions for understanding integrative autonomic control (Figure 2–4). The use of physiological stimuli, such as increases in blood pressure, does not indicate whether the activated pool of NTS neurons is responding primarily to myelinated pathways, where receptors have the lowest pressure thresholds, or to unmyelinated afferents, which represent the overwhelming majority of visceral afferents within a physiological class (e.g., ~90% of rat aortic baroreceptors[5]). Is the information from myelinated and unmyelinated afferents processed, combined, and interpreted differently, and does processing in the NTS yield an output that leads to a physiological response? The answers to these questions remain poorly understood but may be quite important during pathophysiological transformation of these reflexes.

### Pathways Within the NTS

The flow of afferent information clearly depends on the cellular organization within the NTS (Figure 2–5). The frequencies of afferent discharge and activity-dependent mechanisms are important and not uniform, so that the net effects of processing within the NTS will influence the characteristics of the information that reaches particular sites beyond the NTS. *In vivo* studies indicate that neurons at many CNS sites are modulated by visceral afferent information that is processed through the NTS. For example, anatomically separated neurons within the central nucleus of the amygdala respond to either baroreceptor or chemoreceptor activation, suggesting that specific functions are segregated to different parts of the amygdala and rely on specific cardiorespiratory afferent pathways originating in the NTS[28].

### Feedback Inhibition

Excitation is essential for carrying afferent information through the NTS. An overwhelming majority of all NTS neurons are probably second order and directly receive visceral afferent excitatory contacts[88]. Second-order neurons belong to major (GABAergic[11], catecholaminergic[10]) as well as minor (pro-opiomelanocortin[9]) neurochemical groups. Serial, polysynaptic glutamatergic connections from afferents excite higher-order neurons[13] and require a subset of glutamatergic second-order neurons (Figure 2–5). These polysynaptic glutamatergic circuits provide additional excitatory inputs to both second- and higher-order neurons and therefore increase convergence of afferent information onto single neurons[88]. In many cases, the primary synaptic inputs are stronger and more reliable (lower failures) than polysynaptic excitation[13], and this difference in synaptic strength may provide a hierarchy of influences that could impact integrative interactions. GABAergic inhibition is prominent, and initial glutamatergic excitatory postsynaptic potentials (EPSPs) often are followed by inhibitory postsynaptic potentials (IPSPs) with latencies that are consistent with simple di-synaptic pathways[8,11,95]. Multiple mechanisms contribute to depression of viscerosensory afferent drive (Figure 2–6), and these mechanisms, in turn, regulate the levels of NTS activity and the information leaving the NTS. Inhibition derives from both local circuits (i.e., from NTS interneurons[7]) and projections into the NTS[50]. Inhibitory inputs act rapidly enough to contribute to depression of the activity of NTS neurons during repetitive firing of afferents. Presynaptic inhibition probably does not arise from primary afferent depolarization, but rather from more direct mechanisms that include depletion of neurotransmitter vesicles[15] and the

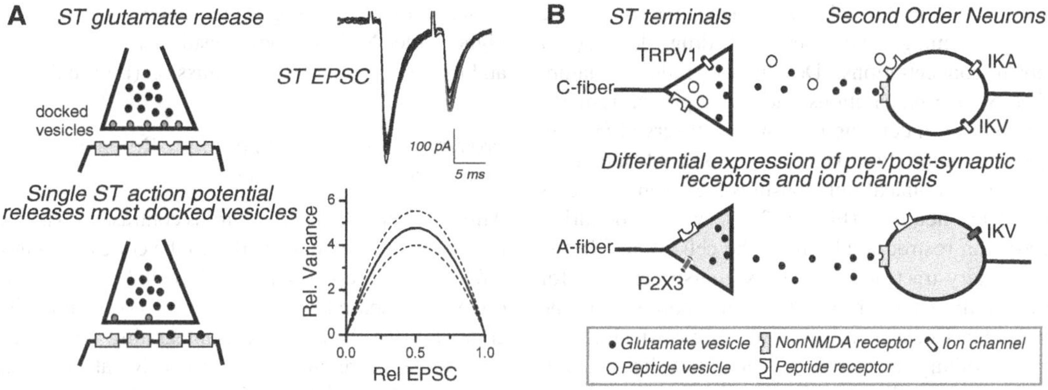


Figure 2–6 Glutamatergic transmission from solitary tract visceral afferents. Visceral afferent transmission in the NTS is highly uniform, with about a 70% release probability at physiological calcium levels. *A*: Solitary tract (ST) synapses release most of their readily releasable (docked) vesicles containing glutamate on the first stimulus. A closely following second stimulus (original traces, *right*) is depressed in amplitude, although the synapse rarely fails to release additional glutamate. A parabola describes the relationship between EPSC amplitude and amplitude variability. This analysis provides an assessment of key factors in synaptic release that result in the evoked EPSC, including the number of functional contacts between the activated afferent axon and the postsynaptic neuron. The shock-to-shock variation in amplitude reflects variations in the probability of release as multiple potential terminals connected to the single afferent axon are activated. Despite the large amount of transmitter that is released, glutamate never saturates the postsynaptic receptors. ST afferent transmission is unusually reliable in its release characteristics compared to most cortical synapses, which fail often. *B*: Synapses from myelinated and unmyelinated ST afferents show key pre- and post-synaptic differences. Unmyelinated C-type terminals express transmembrane proteins, such as TRPV1, that are unique to sensory C-type neurons peripherally. These terminals also release vesicles containing neuropeptides (*large gray circles*) or others containing glutamate (*small black circles*). Purinergic P2X3 receptors are unique to myelinated A-type terminals that also release glutamate. Each neuron has many types of receptors that can be ion channels or receptors that transduce via G-protein coupling. Second-order NTS neurons express voltage-dependent, delayed rectifier potassium channels (IKV), but differentially express the A-type potassium (IKA) channels that mediate delayed excitation[10,12,14].

inhibitory actions of G-protein–coupled receptors, such as metabotropic glutamate receptors, $GABA_B$ receptors, and vasopressin V1a receptors[15,30,66].

The anatomical, physiological, and electrophysiological results reviewed above suggest that the NTS is a complex network (Figure 2–5). The simplest view of NTS organization involves neurons that directly receive (second-order neurons) and transmit (projection neurons) viscerosensory information to distant CNS sites (Figure 2–5). In many cases, a single NTS neuron receives both afferent synaptic input and projects out of the NTS (Figure 2–3)[37]. Interneurons synapse within the NTS and include both GABAergic and glutamatergic neurons. Clearly, axon collaterals from a single NTS neuron may have a local (interneuronal) function, while its projecting axon may also reach targets outside the NTS[37]. The precise sequence of neurons that underlies afferent-activated polysynaptic responses recorded within the NTS is poorly defined. Both pathway structure and modulation of the strength of interactions between neurons will critically influence the translation of primary afferent information into integrated output (Figure 2–6). Patterns in these connections within the NTS (second- or higher-order) are only beginning to emerge[12,13], but the available results suggest that structural organization, together with specific cellular properties, differentially tune or transform (depress or augment) the afferent information that is routed to certain pathways.

## Integration at the Level of the Single Neuron

Thin brainstem slices have offered major improvements in access for studying the mechanisms responsible for excitability and synaptic transmission in NTS neurons. Lengthy, stable intracellular recordings can be obtained, along with direct visualization, precise stimulus timing, and controlled drug delivery at known concentrations. Despite the reduced nature of NTS slice preparations, they have proved remarkably helpful in defining phenomena observed *in vivo*. The horizontal slice preparation takes advantage of the key anatomical relationships between afferents and NTS neurons (Figure 2–2), whose dendritic arbors run rostrocaudally from the cell bodies. In the rat, solitary-tract afferent axons course caudally for many millimeters from their entry points into the brainstem. Consequently, the site of electrical activation of solitary-tract axons in horizontal slices is well separated from the recording site. *In vitro* work has provided important details about the nature of the connections between visceral afferents and NTS neurons.

Electrical shocks delivered to visceral afferent axons in the solitary tract activate afferent axons and, in turn, trigger glutamate release and excitatory postsynaptic currents (EPSCs) under voltage clamp conditions (Figure 2–6). Increases in shock intensity recruit EPSCs in an all-or-none fashion so that EPSC amplitude is unchanged by suprathreshold increments in intensity[15]. This unitary stimulus-response profile for solitary tract–evoked EPSCs, together with variance-mean analysis (Figure 2–6), indicates that a single afferent axon triggers an EPSC through one- to two-dozen active synaptic contacts[6,15,112]. An alternative method of identifying second-order neurons *in vitro* is anterograde transport of fluorescent dyes from a peripheral afferent nerve to central terminals that closely appose second-order cell bodies[44,90]. The NTS neurons apposed by dye-labelled terminals have unitary stimulus recruitment properties identical to second-order neurons identified by solitary tract stimulation[6].

In brainstem slices, solitary tract–evoked EPSCs arrive with nearly invariant latencies on second-order NTS neurons. The standard deviation of the latency is as little as 20 to 30 microseconds (termed "synaptic jitter") and is the electrophysiological signature of a monosynaptic input. These solitary-tract afferents nearly always release some glutamate, but at high frequencies, unmyelinated C-fiber afferents fail substantially more often than lightly myelinated A-fiber afferents[6]. In medial NTS, solitary tract–evoked glutamatergic EPSCs rely predominantly on non–*N*-methyl-D-aspartate (NMDA) receptors [7] (Figure 2.6) and even exogenous NMDA does not activate a current in most second-order NTS neurons[45]. This powerful solitary-tract afferent input has a remarkably high safety factor for generation of action potentials in the second-order neurons that approaches a 100% success rate at low frequencies of stimulation (1–5 Hz)[8,14]. In contrast, activating polysynaptic pathways to higher-order NTS neurons[44] results in variable timing and low success rates of transmission (Figure 2–5).

## Presynaptic Integration at High-Release Viscerosensory Terminals

Afferent contacts on NTS neurons contrast with the pattern in many cortical networks. In the cortex, excitatory afferents often contact primarily distal dendrites, fail often, and release few quanta of neurotransmitter[3]. The cortex is often characterized as integrating weak signals from glutamatergic afferents that arrive at distal dendrites, so that reliable activation of cortical neurons depends on synchronization of multiple, weak, independent inputs[24]. In the NTS, each afferent axon makes multiple close appositions on the somata and proximal dendrites of individual second-order neurons[4], and these contacts rarely fail to release glutamate[6,15,112]. Solitary-tract synapses appear to have quite similar basic vesicular release mechanisms and release substantial amounts of glutamate near the soma of the NTS second-order neurons. The afferent terminal architecture produces large synaptic currents that drive NTS neurons to threshold with single shocks, and this large safety factor means that the multiple presynaptic regulatory mechanisms critically modify afferent release properties.

The unusual strength of visceral afferent synapses has significant ramifications for NTS regulation and integration. Solitary tract–evoked EPSCs in the medial NTS typically range from 200–1000 pA and arise from single solitary-tract axons with multiple contacts onto individual neurons. Analysis of the quantal release of glutamate (Figure 2–6A) reveals that the characteristics of solitary tract–evoked transmission are unusually homogeneous compared to most CNS regions[15]. This uniformity of afferent release properties, both from terminal to terminal and from afferent axon to afferent axon, is surprising in view of the anatomical heterogeneity of the NTS. Differences in the number of contacts or release sites rather than differences in the glutamate-release properties themselves account for variations in synaptic strength across solitary-tract afferents[6,15,112]. On average, each afferent axon makes nearly 20 synapses with a 90% probability of release on each second-order neuron[6,15,112]. In comparison, cortical synapses are highly non-uniform, have markedly lower release probabilities (e.g., 10%–50%), and a cortical EPSC may deliver only a single quantum per afferent axon[125]. The high release properties of viscerosensory inputs to NTS neurons suggest that neurotransmitter depletion accounts for much of use-dependent synaptic depression (Figure 2–6A). These *in vitro* properties also imply that active modulation causes both tonic presynaptic depression of glutamate release and the small synaptic amplitudes recorded in intact brainstem.

## Cranial Visceral Afferents: Presynaptic Differentiation

Cranial afferent neurons with myelinated and unmyelinated axons have distinct discharge properties and pharmacological responsiveness that reflect fundamental differences in their neurobiology[130]. Although the performance of the full baroreflex loop differs between A- and C-fibers, the central bases for these differences remain poorly understood and are seldom tested[48,49].

The vanilloid receptor—transient receptor potential cation channel, subfamily V, member 1 (TRPV1)—binds capsaicin and marks C-fiber afferents from various visceral organs. TRPV1-activation opens a non-selective cation conductance that depolarizes neurons, causing action potentials and triggering synaptic transmission. TRPV1 is present and functional on central C-fiber afferent terminals in the NTS[45,67]. Solitary tract–evoked EPSCs in capsaicin-sensitive neurons are blocked at high concentrations of capsaicin. The actions of capsaicin appear to be accounted for by glutamate release from sensitive afferents, since non-NMDA receptor antagonists block responses measured in NTS neurons. In contrast, capsaicin has no effect on capsaicin-resistant NTS neurons and adenosine triphosphate (ATP) activates presynaptic P2X3 purinergic receptors on capsaicin-resistant solitary-tract afferents to release glutamate[67,83]. TRPV1 and P2X3 receptors in the NTS are rare examples of receptors that facilitate glutamate release from afferents. Presynaptic receptors on afferent terminals more generally suppress glutamate release by activating metabotropic G-protein coupled receptors and their second messengers. Visceral afferent terminals in the NTS also contain neuropeptides, but their functional impacts are largely unknown (Figure 2.4).

Somatic primary afferents include both myelinated and unmyelinated classes, and that field of investigation offers a potentially rich precedent for cranial afferent neurobiology[132]. Unmyelinated cranial visceral afferents may undergo similar chronic, plastic changes in pathophysiological conditions, such as inflammation, hypertension, hypoxia, and environmental insults. Cytokines and peptides may be involved in pathophysiological changes and interactions with other cell types, including vascular endothelium (see Figure 2–4)[109,111,143] and glial cells, may be altered. Another potential contributor might be differences in blood–brain barrier function within different subregions of the NTS. The dorsomedial portions of the caudal NTS show heterogeneous deficits in blood–brain barrier function that resemble those of the area postrema. These deficits are matched by the local absence of critical protein components that maintain barrier patency[87]. In contrast, in hypertension, some barrier proteins are upregulated, suggesting a change in barrier function[146,147]. Thus, neurohumoral signalling in the medial NTS could also importantly alter the processing of information from cranial visceral primary afferents in both health and disease.

## Cranial Nerve Visceral Afferents: Postsynaptic Differentiation

Not only do afferent inputs differ, but the postsynaptic properties of the second-order NTS neurons also show substantial differences. Potassium channels are differentially expressed in second-order NTS neurons[36], leading to selective depression of processing of specific viscerosensory pathways. Differences in potassium channel expression are associated with markedly different excitability, including the presence of delayed excitation in neurons with large A-type potassium currents[10,12,14], and also occur in pathophysiological conditions[19].

All second-order NTS neurons appear to have similar steady-state potassium currents (IKV) that are sensitive to blockade by the potassium channel blocker tetraethylammonium. However, expression of A-type potassium channel (Figure 2–6) differs between subgroups of NTS neurons[14,37], and the presence of these molecules differentiates particular pathways at the earliest stages of processing within the NTS. Potassium channels are pivotal for maintaining fidelity of transmission at high frequency in neuronal pathways. A-type potassium channels are prominent targets for neurotransmitters, including cannabinoids[35] and angiotensin II[148], that can tune afferent transmission. Modulation of A-type potassium channels can fundamentally change the success of transmission through the NTS and therefore substantially alter activity at all subsequent stages of a reflex pathway[26].

## What Shapes the Performance of NTS Pathways?

The interaction between glutamatergic and GABAergic transmission in the NTS involves both ionotropic and metabotropic receptors (Figure 2–7). Metabotropic receptors have much higher affinities for amino acids and are located presynaptically on glutamate- and GABA-containing terminals[66]. On most afferent terminals, metabotropic glutamate receptors provide frequency-dependent, negative feedback to decrease the probability of glutamate release upon subsequent activation[30]. In different NTS neurons, glutamate released from afferent terminals simultaneously either increases or decreases GABA release onto second-order neurons, and this can have functional effects on baroreflex performance[137]. $GABA_B$ receptors are also located presynaptically and inhibit glutamate release from afferent terminals[154]. Thus, within fractions of a second of the arrival of the first action potential, the capacity of the neuron to respond to the next afferent signal will be altered. Such mechanisms can produce a state-dependent change in processing that ultimately changes afferent reflexes at all points beyond the NTS.

Neuronal phenotype differentiates NTS pathways and is partly established by embryonic gene expression. Network activity strongly influences pathway development, with connections between neurons and their activity critically influencing cellular phenotype[20]. Cardiac or baroreceptor afferents, like their reflex pathways, are continuously active. This discharge may shape presynaptic and postsynaptic features of the NTS. Daily engagement of orthostatic reflexes that acutely control blood pressure markedly affects baroreflex gain[52] and may well be a factor in adaptations to hypertension and chronic hypoxia. Most of the details of these basic mechanisms of action remain unresolved for pathways within and beyond the NTS.

One specific NTS neuronal phenotype that has been studied in terms of cardiovascular regulation is the A2 catecholaminergic cell group (for recent review[74]). These neurons receive direct innervation from visceral afferents[10]. Chronic electrical silencing of these neurons was achieved following viral-mediated transgenic expression of a potassium channel targeted specifically to A2 neurons[47], resulting in elevations in arterial pressure that were greater in spontaneously hypertensive rats[47]. Hence, the A2 neurons are active in controlling blood pressure and their role is to chronically suppress arterial pressure, which acts as a compensatory mechanism in the hypertensive rat. Interestingly, these animals also showed changes in respiration, water intake, and urine output, as well as feeding, that emphasized the multi-functional roles of A2 neurons[47].

## MODULATION OF AFFERENT INFORMATION IN THE NTS

### Modulation By Angiotensin II

Of the many transmitters and modulators that occur in the NTS, angiotensin II is particularly interesting because it is involved in regulation of thirst, blood volume, and arterial pressure. Angiotensin II can also increase or decrease the gain of cardiorespiratory reflexes by releasing other transmitters/modulators, such as substance P, GABA, and nitric oxide. Thus, angiotensin II can be viewed as causing "*interactive*" modulation in the NTS.

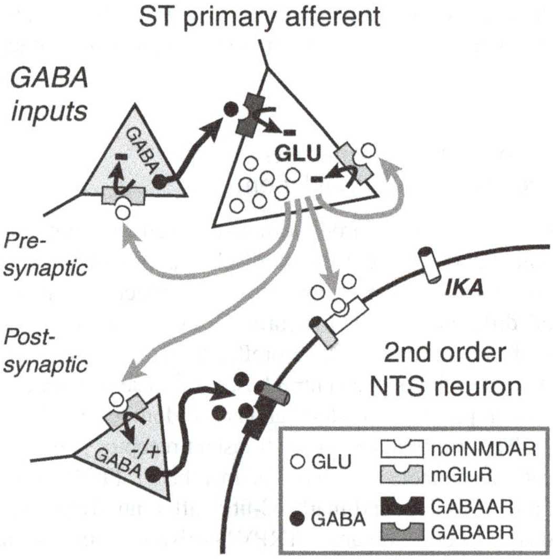


Figure 2–7 Crosstalk between transmitters in the NTS. Second-order NTS neurons receive synapses from afferent terminals that release glutamate (Glu, *white circles*), which primarily excites the neurons through ionotropic (ion channel) non-NMDA receptors (*white*). Glu activates a variety of metabotropic receptors (mGluR, *pale gray*). These provide autofeedback control that reduces Glu release from solitary tract (ST) primary afferent terminals—a form of negative (–) feedback. In addition, second-order NTS neurons commonly receive synaptic contacts from GABA neurons that are themselves second-order NTS neurons and thus activated by ST afferents. Consequently, ST activation can have two actions: an early-arriving EPSP (monosynaptic) from Glu release followed by a later-arriving IPSP (di-synaptic) that then releases GABA (*black circles*) onto $GABA_A$ receptors ($GABA_AR$, *black*) responsible for the IPSP. This IPSP is ST-synchronized and dampens sustained afferent drive by postsynaptic action. GABA release can have a second distinct action presynaptically on ST primary afferent terminals, where GABA strongly inhibits the release of Glu via metabotropic $GABA_B$ receptors ($GABA_BR$, *dark gray*). Note that mGluR receptors can increase or decrease (+/–) the release of GABA and therefore control IPSPs from second-order neurons. Different receptor expression across neurons orchestrates differential synaptic weighting and activity dependence along particular pathways. A-type potassium channels, which are normally substantially inactivated at resting membrane potentials, will become more effective following postsynaptic inhibition by hyperpolarization. Hyperpolarization removes inactivation from these channels and enhances their role of dampening action potential generation. Glu and GABA strongly interact and influence each other's release and efficacy.

### *Angiotensin II-Induced Substance P Release Increases the Gain of Reflexes*

There are several mechanisms by which angiotensin II could enhance excitatory transmission in the NTS. *In vitro*, angiotensin II augments excitatory synaptic transmission either presynaptically or by direct postsynaptic depolarization of NTS neurons[16]. Bradycardia evoked by peripheral chemoreceptor stimulation is facilitated by microinjecting high doses of angiotensin II into the NTS[107]. This effect was prevented by infusing a neurokinin-1 receptor antagonist into the NTS, suggesting that angiotensin II releases substance P, causing an effect that is reflex-specific[17,41] (see Figure 2–4). Furthermore, angiotensin II produced potentiation of electrically evoked EPSPs in some NTS neurons, which was partially blocked by neurokinin-1 receptor antagonism[73].

A role for substance P in the NTS in arterial blood pressure control and baroreceptor reflex modulation is controversial[59]. In otherwise intact, conscious, unrestrained rats after afferent removal, substance P microinjected into the NTS evokes prolonged tachycardia and hypertension[1], consistent with blockade of the baroreceptor reflex. Similarly, NTS microinjections of substance P attenuated the cardiac baroreflex but spared baroreceptor reflex–mediated sympathoinhibition in the working heart brainstem preparation[113].

Substance P can be released in the NTS by afferent stimulation. Blockade of either neurokinin-1 receptors or $GABA_A$ receptors abolished the attenuation of the cardiac baroreflex caused by noxious pinching[22]. Thus, substance P appears to excite local GABAergic neurons via neurokinin-1 receptors, which may, in part, relate to the neurokinin-1 receptor–mediated tachycardia observed during nociception[1,113]. Stimulation of muscle afferents also releases substance P into the NTS, which may contribute to muscle pressor responses[117], and attenuates the cardiac baroreflex via a bicuculline-sensitive mechanism[118]. 5-$HT_3$ receptor activation attenuates baroreceptor reflex bradycardia[68], again through release of substance P onto the neurokinin-1 receptors of GABAergic interneurons[32,91]. Taken together, these data suggest that interactions between substance P, neurokinin-1 receptors, and GABAergic neurons represent a common mechanism of reversibly resetting the cardiac baroreflex gain during acute "stress."

### *Angiotensin II-Induced GABA Release Decreases the Gain of Reflexes*

Circulating[121,109] as well as centrally produced angiotensin II[51] may modulate neuronal signaling within the NTS. Angiotensin type 1 receptors occur on afferents (including carotid sinus and vagal fibers), on the somata and dendrites of NTS neurons, and on blood vessels[89,105]. Most binding sites for angiotensin II are not presynaptic[58]. At relatively low doses, angiotensin II in the NTS evokes hypotension and bradycardia, and, at higher doses, hypertension and tachycardia[98,122]. How these effects relate to those produced by endogenous angiotensin II is unclear, but they suggest multiple functions for angiotensin II in the NTS.

Baro- and chemo-receptor reflexes have been tested in the presence of angiotensin II. Exogenous angiotensin II in the NTS depresses the cardiac component of the baroreceptor reflex[73]. Microinjection of an angiotensin II antagonist into the NTS increased baroreflex gain in anesthetised rats, consistent with a tonic angiotensin II drive[27]. Angiotensin II application in the NTS attenuates baroreflex inhibition of cardiac sympathetic efferent activity[21] but not lumbar sympathetic efferent activity[115], suggesting angiotensin II differentially modulates baroreflex-cardiac sympathetic pathways in the NTS through an inhibitory cellular mechanism. Indeed, angiotensin II does increase the rate of spontaneous IPSPs and facilitates electrically evoked IPSPs. Since these effects are losartan- and bicuculline-sensitive, angiotensin II probably acts presynaptically to increase GABA release, but this action appears to be indirect, via release of nitric oxide (see below and Figure 2–4)[109,111,150].

Modulation of baroreflex function by angiotensin II could be physiological or pathophysiological. Data above indicate that there may be ongoing activation of angiotensin type 1 receptors in the NTS[27], although anesthesia may have dramatically increased renin release[75]. In rats between postnatal days 10 and 20, the cardiac baroreflex undergoes a physiological attenuation that is mediated by angiotensin II acting at the level of the NTS[72] and may be important for switching off the baroreceptor reflex to allow for the maturational rise in arterial blood pressure. A similar mechanism could operate in the development of essential hypertension, where attenuation of the cardiac baroreceptor reflex could allow arterial blood pressure to reach a higher set-point.

### *Angiotensin II-Induced Nitric Oxide Release in the NTS*

Angiotensin II in the NTS potently releases nitric oxide[111] (Figure 2–8), which mediates the angiotensin II-induced depression of the baroreflex[105,152]. Baroreflex depression is also produced by exogenous L-arginine and nitric oxide donors in NTS[105] and prevented by blockade of either nitric oxide synthase or soluble guanylate cyclase, respectively[105]. The source of the nitric oxide released by angiotensin II remains unclear.

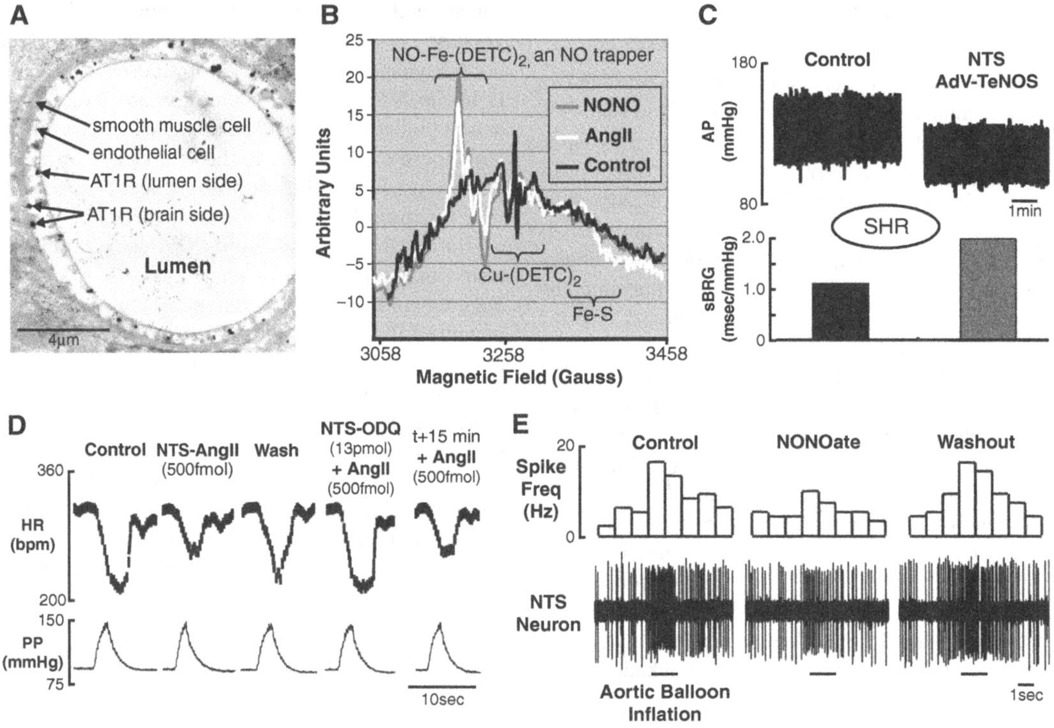


Figure 2–8 Interactive modulation of the baroreflex by angiotensin II and nitric oxide in the NTS. *A*: Angiotensin II type 1 receptors ($AT_1R$) are located on both the luminal and brain side of blood vessels within the NTS. *B*: Microinjection of angiotensin II into the NTS releases nitric oxide that can be trapped and subsequently measured using cryogenic electroparamagnetic resonance. Nitric oxide is trapped using nitric oxide-iron diethyldithiocarbamic acid (NO-Fe-$[DETC]_2$). Signals characteristic of nitric oxide are clearly identified across the 400 Gauss scan following angiotensin II injection into the NTS. A nitric oxide donor (diethylamine NONOate or NONO) was used as a control and shows a similar peak whereas saline injection (control) did not give a response. *C:* Chronic blockade of endothelial nitric oxide synthase in the NTS with an adenovirus (AdV) expressing a dominant negative form of endothelial nitric oxide synthase (truncated eNOS or TeNOS) reduced arterial pressure and increased the cardiac baroreceptor reflex gain in the spontaneously hypertensive rat (SHR). These data indicate that nitric oxide generated by endothelial nitric oxide synthase in NTS plays a major role in the maintenance of hypertension and baroreflex dysfunction in the SHR. *D:* Angiotensin II microinjection into the NTS attenuates the cardiac baroreceptor reflex. This effect is prevented by blocking soluble guanylate cyclase, the receptor for nitric oxide, using 1H-(1,2,4)oxadiazole(4,3-alpha)quinoxaline-1-one (ODQ). *E:* An example showing that nitric oxide (from focal picoejection of diethylamine NONOate) can depress the firing response of an NTS neuron during baroreceptor stimulation. Data modified from Paton et al. (2006)[111] and Waki et al. (2006)[147], with permission.

There is evidence that angiotensin II acting on angiotensin type 1 receptors on the vascular endothelium stimulates endothelial nitric oxide synthase to produce nitric oxide. Increasing evidence supports the notion of vascular-neuronal signaling in the NTS (Figure 2–4). First, the NTS has an extraordinarily dense network of capillaries, and individual capillaries are closely surrounded by neurons and their processes[54]. Thus, the vascular endothelium in the NTS could be a rich source of nitric oxide. Second, blood vessels in the NTS have luminal and extra-luminal angiotensin receptors[111] (Figures 2.4 and 2.8). Finally, angiotensin II-mediated inhibition of the baroreflex is blocked by specific blockade of endothelial but not neuronal nitric oxide synthase[105].

## Modulation by Nitric Oxide

Due to its unique ability to penetrate membranes instantly, nitric oxide is capable of both intra- and inter-cellular signaling and so may act as both an autocrine and paracrine messenger in the NTS. Nitric oxide modulates the activity of many transmitters, including glutamate and GABA (see [119]). Throughout the caudal NTS there are somata, dendrites, and axons that are capable of synthesizing nitric oxide[76]. Some of these neurons respond to increases in arterial pressure, suggesting that neurons mediating the baroreceptor reflex may contain neuronal nitric oxide synthase[29]. *In situ* hybridization[133] or best-practice immunohistochemistry[133] detect endothelial nitric oxide synthase in brain endothelial cells, and this is also likely to be the case in the NTS[147].

Soluble guanylate cyclase, the main intracellular receptor for nitric oxide, generates cyclic guanine monophosphate (cGMP), and cGMP-dependent protein kinase G can phosphorylate many intracellular targets. Nitric oxide can also react with superoxide to produce peroxynitrite ($OONO^-$), which can modulate neurotransmission in both physiological and pathophysiological conditions. These two possible modes of action can be discriminated by using antagonists of soluble guanylate cyclase or by removing peroxynitrite.

### *Nitric Oxide and Excitatory Transmission in the NTS*

In the rat, glutamate has been co-localized immunohistochemically with neuronal nitric oxide synthase in neurons in many NTS subnuclei[82]. Unfortunately, immunoreactivity within cell bodies does not discriminate between metabolic and transmitter pools of glutamate, so it does not confirm that a neuron uses glutamate for transmission. However, in all NTS regions, some terminals of unknown origin contain both neuronal nitric oxide synthase and vesicular glutamate transporter 2, which is a reliable marker for identifying glutamatergic neurons. Almost all NTS neurons immunoreactive for neuronal nitric oxide synthase also contain both the NR-1 subunit of the NMDA glutamate receptor[82] and the alpha-amino-3-hydroxy-5-methylisoxazole-4-propionate (AMPA) glutamate receptor subunit GLUR1. There is also physiological evidence that nitric oxide influences cardiovascular responses to injection of glutamate into the NTS[140]. $Ca^{2+}$ entry via NMDA receptors could be one of the mechanisms through which neuronal nitric oxide synthase is activated.

Nitric oxide and glutamate act in the NTS at both neuronal and systems levels. Inhibition of nitric oxide synthase in the NTS decreased the firing response to stimulation of AMPA but not NMDA receptors[39], without affecting either spontaneous or vagus nerve–evoked potentials. Furthermore, a nitric oxide donor enhanced AMPA- but not NMDA-mediated firing,. *In vitro,* nitric oxide potentiates EPSPs evoked by electrical stimulation of the solitary tract[150]. Thus, nitric oxide facilitates AMPA receptor–mediated transmission in the NTS. At the level of the cardiovascular system, antagonizing the activity of either neuronal nitric oxide synthase or soluble guanylate cyclase in the NTS attenuated the hypotension and bradycardia induced by application of glutamate or NMDA[81]. Conversely, antagonism of NMDA and non-NMDA receptors in the NTS reduced the depressor/bradycardic response induced by NTS microinjection of L-arginine[81]. Thus, nitric oxide and glutamate receptors interact reciprocally within the NTS to affect cardiovascular variables.

### *Nitric Oxide Modulation of NTS Circuitry Regulating Arterial Pressure*

Nitric oxide in the NTS appears to play a major role in the control of arterial blood pressure and heart rate. Many studies have shown that the precursor for nitric oxide, L-arginine, and various nitric oxide donors injected into the NTS produce bradycardia and a depressor response[55,147]. These responses can be prevented by blockade of soluble guanylate cyclase[153], suggesting that the response is due to nitric oxide rather than peroxynitrite. Overexpression of endothelial nitric oxide synthase in the NTS, which chronically elevates levels of nitric oxide, also results in bradycardia and depressor responses[127]. These are also prevented by soluble guanylate cyclase inhibitors[139]. Nitric oxide synthase inhibitors injected into the NTS, as well as expression of antisense oligonucleotides for neuronal nitric oxide synthase, produce tachycardia and hypertension[55].

The role of nitric oxide in the baroreceptor reflex is less clear. Some authors report that either blockade of nitric oxide synthase in the NTS or microinjection of nitric oxide donors failed to affect the baroreceptor reflex gain in anesthetized[55] and awake animals[116]. Blocking nitric oxide synthase in the NTS attenuated baroreceptor reflex bradycardia and suppressed the inhibition of renal sympathetic nerve activity evoked by intravenous phenylephrine in anesthetised rats[84]. However, others have described an increase in the reflex heart rate range following baroreceptor stimulation when an inhibitor of all nitric oxide synthase isoforms was microinjected into the NTS, suggesting an inhibitory role for nitric oxide on baroreflex function[116]. Furthermore, L-arginine, sodium nitroprusside, and a nitric oxide donor all attenuated baroreceptor reflex-mediated bradycardia, and a soluble guanylate cyclase inhibitor blocked nitric oxide–induced baroreflex inhibition, indicating that these effects are mediated by nitric oxide[111]. Nitric oxide mediation of baroreflex inhibition was supported by studies in which endothelial nitric oxide synthase in the NTS has been chronically blocked. The result is enhanced spontaneous baroreflex gain in both normotensive and spontaneously hypertensive rats[147] (Figure 2–8), with a maintained bradycardia and depressor response in the spontaneously hypertensive rats. Furthermore, in this rat strain, endothelial nitric oxide synthase mRNA is upregulated in the NTS compared to normotensive rats[147]. Hence, nitric oxide generated by endothelial nitric oxide synthase may make a major contribution to maintaining hypertension and depressing baroreflex gain in spontaneously hypertensive rats.

### *Nitric Oxide Modulation of GABA Transmission in the NTS*

Aortic distension during focal application of a nitric oxide donor to barosensitive NTS neurons reduces their firing response (Figure 2–8), an effect that is prevented by pre-exposure to bicuculline. In contrast, application of a nitric oxide donor to non-barosensitive neurons produces no response or excitation or inhibition (J. W. Polson and J. F. R. Paton, unpublished observations). Therefore, nitric oxide appears to selectively increase GABAergic drive to neurons mediating the baroreceptor reflex. Low nanomolar concentrations of nitric oxide increase intracellular calcium levels in GABAergic NTS neurons[150] (Figure 2–9), with the largest responses found from the putative axons of GABAergic interneurons. Moreover, nitric oxide potentiated the electrically evoked IPSPs and EPSPs in NTS neurons in the presence of non-NMDA receptor blockade with a lower-threshold nitric oxide concentration for EPSPs than IPSPs (Figure 2–9)[150].

Nitric oxide is a highly indiscriminate signaling molecule, affecting targets up to 150 μm from its source[63]. Given the tight packing of NTS neurons and the intermixing of different types of reflex-specific neurons and circuits, how could nitric oxide modulate reflexes selectively, and what roles could nitric oxide from endothelial versus neuronal sources play? Possible mechanisms by which nitric oxide could exert selective actions in the NTS include:

- Putting the source of nitric oxide next to the target, restricting effective spread
- Nitric oxide scavenging by buffers and hemoglobin to reduce spread
- Inactivation of nitric oxide to restrict both its half-life (~100 ms) and the maximal distance traveled (see [53])
- Interaction between the nitric oxide synthase isoform involved and the transmitter system modulated. The transmitter system affected could depend on nitric oxide concentration, or the amounts of nitric oxide produced could depend on the isoform of nitric oxide synthase involved[109]
- Regulating the responsiveness of soluble guanylate cyclase to nitric oxide in the target cell. This process may be dynamic because soluble guanylate cyclase is negatively regulated by cytosolic $Ca^{2+}$ [101]
- Desensitizing soluble guanylate cyclase to influence the duration of nitric oxide's actions via the cGMP pathway[18]. In cells maintaining normal ATP concentrations, soluble guanylate cyclase activity is inhibited by more than 50%[126]. Decreases in ATP levels due to metabolic stress or hypoxia could potentiate responses[126], and a response to nitric oxide could depend on brainstem oxygenation
- Regulating soluble guanylate cyclase, the rate of cGMP breakdown, and phosphodiesterase activity to regulate nitric oxide signaling[18]
- Modulating excitatory and inhibitory synapses via differential sensitivity of biochemical pathways to nitric oxide in different neuronal populations

Clearly, more precise experimental interventions that better respect the subtleties of nitric oxide release and signaling are needed to determine how nitric oxide exerts it effects. If, for example, endogenous nitric oxide signaling does occur in microdomains, then the use of nitric oxide donors, which release unknown amounts of nitric oxide, becomes questionable because spatial accuracy and concentration-dependent effects will be lost. Such factors could help explain inconsistent results about the role of nitric oxide in the NTS on cardiovascular variables and baroreflex gain described above.

## LOOKING TO THE FUTURE

Considerably more is now known about the encoding of sensory afferent information, integration, neuromodulation, and circuit wiring in the NTS than in 1990. Diversity, heterogeneity, and pathway specificity are all obvious features of the NTS, and these are reflected in the information that reaches distant destinations within the CNS. However, because of the number and diversity of NTS inputs and outputs, as well as the lack of clear visceral topography and intermixing of neurons, there remains a great need to define the phenotypes of neurons within specific reflex circuits and to develop more sophisticated tools, such as cell-type–specific transgenic models, to selectively target them. However, NTS neurons contain multiple transmitters, so there may be no single phenotype that identifies a

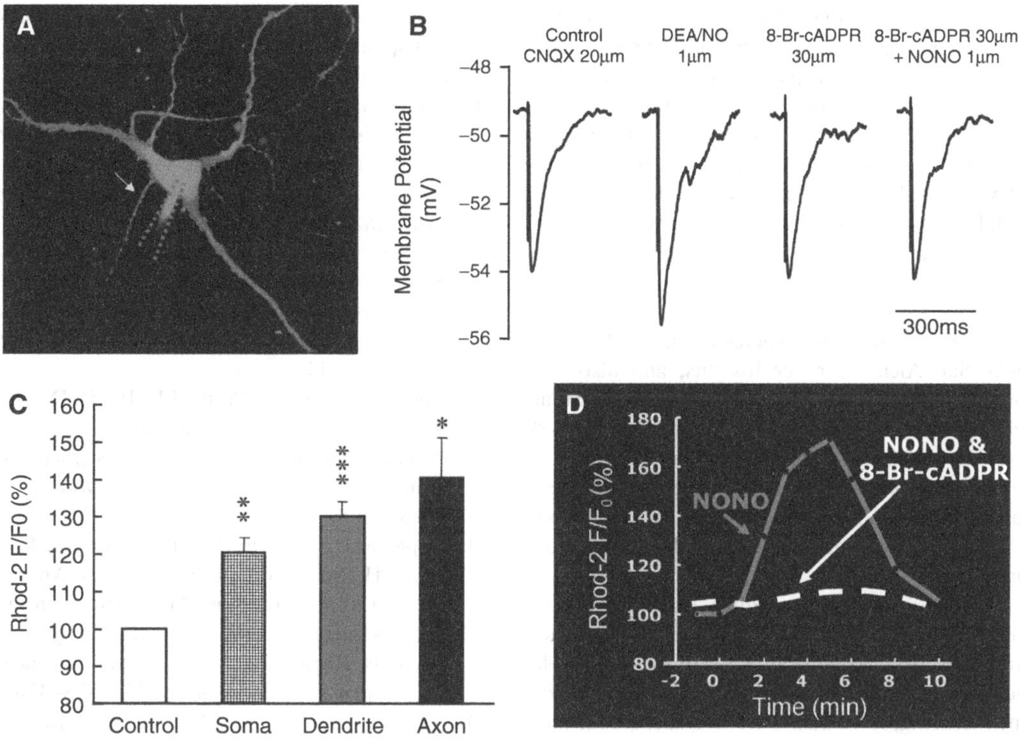


Figure 2–9 Nitric oxide effects on GABAergic transmission in the NTS. For a color version of Figure 2–9, see Color Plate 2–9 between pages 224 and 225. *A:* GABA-containing neuron in the NTS revealed using an adenovirus-expressing enhanced green fluorescent protein under the control of the GAD67 promoter. The dotted line indicates the position of the patch pipette. *B:* Electrically evoked monosynaptic IPSPs are augmented by the nitric oxide donor, diethylamine NONOate. This augmentation is prevented by selective antagonism of cyclic adenosine diphosphate ribose regulated ryanodine-sensitive intracellular calcium stores (cADPR) using 8-Br-cADPR. *C:* Measurements of intracellular calcium from different cellular compartments of GABAergic interneurons in the NTS when exposed to a nitric oxide donor. Neurons were loaded with a calcium-sensitive dye (Rhod-2) from the patch pipette. The most sensitive compartment was axonal. *D:* The rise in intracellular calcium recorded from a GABAergic interneuron when exposed to nitric oxide. Note that the response is abolished when 8-Br-cADPR blocks calcium release from cADPR-ryanodine sensitive intracellular stores. Data modified from Wang et al. (2006)[151], with permission.

specific pathway. Activity affects phenotype in other CNS systems. Is there a different role for activity in shaping and maintaining the characteristics of tonically active afferent pathways (e.g., cardiovascular or respiratory), compared to pathways with lower periodicities (e.g., gastrointestinal or C-fiber afferent)? Functional roles of neurons with certain phenotypes, such as those expressing neurokinin 1 receptors, can be assessed by destroying them with saporin toxins[123]. However, ablation may cause unpredictable plasticity, including neuronal sprouting and changes in connectivity and/or transmitters. Future studies might refine this approach by inactivating specific phenotypes through silencing without destroying them[47] or genetically deleting receptors on specific types of neurons[38].

The neurobiology of primary afferents in the spinal cord predicts that there could be dynamic competition among myelinated and unmyelinated afferents for stable synaptic contacts within the NTS. In the spinal cord, central connections change when stable contacts are lost; for instance, after injury. Does an injury such as sinoaortic denervation affect NTS and brainstem circuits? Attention also needs to focus on the mechanisms of activation and involvement of non-neuronal cells, such as glia[56], pericytes[62] and endothelium[111], and of signaling molecules other than neurotransmitters/neuromodulators, such as cytokines[144] and prostaglandins[131], in sensory afferent processing and modulation.

Regarding cardiovascular control, the NTS is a possible site for determining the set-point of arterial pressure[42]. What is the substrate for this? Does it depend on baroreceptor inputs or not? The rejuvenated idea of a central baroreceptor is an attractive proposition for regulating set-point independently of arterial baroreceptors[100]. Chemosensitive neurons in the commissural NTS with sympathoexcitatory outputs to the RVLM[128] would make plausible candidates, if, for example, they can detect blood flow by changes in blood gases or pH[40].

ACKNOWLEDGEMENTS Michael C. Andresen thanks Sue Aicher for her insights, and also Tim Bailey, Young-Ho Jin, Suzanne Appleyard, Stuart McDougall, Jim Peters, Luciano Fernandes, and Mark Doyle for countless discussions about the world of neurobiology and their own discoveries. Financial support from the National Heart, Lung and Blood Institute of the National Institutes of Health made our work possible.

The ideas expressed by Julian F. R. Paton have evolved through experimentation as well as discussion with colleagues and collaborators. In this regard, he would like to thank Michael Spyer, Sergey Kasparov, Tony Pickering, Jeff Potts, and Jim Deuchars for their insights. The financial support of the British Heart Foundation, Biotechnology and Biological Sciences Research Council and The Royal Society are fully appreciated. Paton holds a Royal Society–Wolfson Research Merit Award.

## References

1. Abdala, A. P., Haibara, A. S., and Colombari, E. (2003). Cardiovascular responses to substance P in the nucleus tractus solitarii: Microinjection study in conscious rats. *American Journal of Physiology. Heart and Circulatory Physiology* 285, H891–H898.
2. Agarwal, S. K., and Calaresu, F. R. (1992). Electrical stimulation of nucleus tractus solitarius excites vagal preganglionic cardiomotor neurons of the nucleus ambiguus in rats. *Brain Research* 574, 320–324.
3. Allen, C., and Stevens, C. F. (1994). An evaluation of causes for unreliability of synaptic transmission. *Proceedings of the National Academy of Science USA* 91, 10380–10383.
4. Anders, K., Ohndorf, W., Dermietzel, R., and Richter, D. W. (1993). Synapses between slowly adapting lung stretch receptor afferents and inspiratory beta-neurons in the nucleus of the solitary tract of cats: A light and electron microscopic analysis. *Journal of Comparative Neurology* 335, 163–172.
5. Andresen, M. C., Krauhs, J. M., and Brown, A. M. (1978). Relationship of aortic wall baroreceptor properties during development in normotensive and spontaneously hypertensive rats. *Circulation Research* 43, 728–738.
6. Andresen, M. C., and Peters, J. H. (2008). Comparison of baroreceptive to other afferent synaptic transmission to the solitary tract nucleus. *American Journal of Physiology. Heart and Circulatory Physiology* 295, H2032–H2042.
7. Andresen, M. C., and Yang, M. (1990). Non-NMDA receptors mediate sensory afferent synaptic transmission in medial nucleus tractus solitarius. *American Journal of Physiology* 259, H1307–H1311.
8. Andresen, M. C., and Yang, M. (1995). Dynamics of sensory afferent synaptic transmission in aortic baroreceptor regions of nucleus tractus solitarius. *Journal of Neurophysiology* 74, 1518–1528.
9. Appleyard, S. M., Bailey, T. W., Doyle, M. W., Jin, Y.-H., Smart, J. L., Low, M. J., and Andresen, M. C. (2005). Proopiomelanocortin neurons in nucleus tractus solitarius are activated by visceral afferents: Regulation by cholecystokinin and opioids. *Journal of Neuroscience* 25, 3578–3585.
10. Appleyard, S. M., Marks, D., Kobayashi, K., Okano, H., Low, M. J., and Andresen, M. C. (2007). Visceral afferents directly activate catecholamine neurons in the solitary tract nucleus. *Journal of Neuroscience* 27, 13292–13302.
11. Bailey, T. W., Appleyard, S. M., Jin, Y. H., and Andresen, M. C. (2008). Organization and proportion of GABAergic neurons in solitary tract nucleus (NTS). *Journal of Neurophysiology* 99, 1712–1722.
12. Bailey, T. W., Hermes, S. M., Aicher, S. A., and Andresen, M. C. (2007). Target-specific, dynamic pathway tuning by A-type potassium channels in solitary tract nucleus: Cranial visceral afferent pathways to caudal ventrolateral medulla or paraventricular hypothalamus. *Journal of Physiology* 582, 613–628.
13. Bailey, T. W., Hermes, S. M., Andresen, M. C., and Aicher, S. A. (2006). Cranial visceral afferent pathways through the nucleus of the solitary tract to caudal ventrolateral medulla or paraventricular hypothalamus: Target-specific synaptic reliability and convergence patterns. *Journal of Neuroscience* 26, 11893–11902.
14. Bailey, T. W., Jin, Y.-H., Doyle, M. W., and Andresen, M. C. (2002). Vanilloid sensitive afferents activate neurons with prominent A-type potassium currents in nucleus tractus solitarius. *Journal of Neuroscience* 22, 8230–8237.
15. Bailey, T. W., Jin, Y.-H., Doyle, M. W., Smith, S. M., and Andresen, M. C. (2006). Vasopressin inhibits

glutamate release via two distinct modes in the brainstem. *Journal of Neuroscience* 26, 6131–6142.

16. Barnes, K. L., Deweese, D. M., and Andresen, M. C. (2003). Angiotensin potentiates excitatory synaptic transmission to medial solitary tract nucleus neurons. *American Journal of Physiology. Regulatory, Integrative and Comparative Physiology* 284, R1340–R1353.
17. Barnes, K. L., Diz, D. I., and Ferrario, C. M. (1991). Functional interactions between angiotensin II and substance P in the dorsal medulla. *Hypertension* 17, 1121–1126.
18. Bellamy, T. C., Wood, J., Goodwin, D. A., and Garthwaite, J. (2000). Rapid desensitization of the nitric oxide receptor, soluble guanylyl cyclase, underlies diversity of cellular cGMP responses. *Proceedings of the National Academy of Science USA* 97, 2928–2933.
19. Belugin, S., and Mifflin, S. W. (2005). Transient voltage-dependent potassium currents are reduced in NTS neurons isolated from renal wrap hypertensive rats. *Journal of Neurophysiology* 94, 3849–3859.
20. Borodinsky, L. N., Root, C. M., Cronin, J. A., Sann, S. B., Gu, X., and Spitzer, N. C. (2004). Activity-dependent homeostatic specification of transmitter expression in embryonic neurons. *Nature* 429, 523–530.
21. Boscan, P., Allen, A. M., and Paton, J. F. R. (2001). Baroreflex inhibition of cardiac sympathetic outflow is attenuated by angiotensin II in the nucleus of the solitary tract. *Neuroscience* 103, 153–160.
22. Boscan, P., Kasparov, S., and Paton, J. F. R. (2002). Somatic nociception activates NK1 receptors in the nucleus tractus solitarii to attenuate the baroreceptor cardiac reflex. *European Journal of Neuroscience* 16, 907–920.
23. Brown, D. L., and Guyenet, P. G. (1985). Electrophysiological study of cardiovascular neurons in the rostral ventrolateral medulla in rats. *Circulation Research* 56, 359–369.
24. Bruno, R. M., and Sakmann, B. (2006). Cortex is driven by weak but synchronously active thalamocortical synapses. *Science* 312, 1622–1627.
25. Burton, M. D., and Kazemi, H. (2000). Neurotransmitters in central respiratory control. *Respiration Physiology* 122, 111–121.
26. Butcher, J. W., and Paton, J. F. R. (1998). $K^+$ channel blockade in the NTS alters efficacy of two cardiorespiratory reflexes in vivo. *American Journal of Physiology* 274, R677–R685.
27. Campagnole-Santos, M. J., Diz, D. I., and Ferrario, C. M. (1988). Baroreceptor reflex modulation by angiotensin II at the nucleus tractus solitarii. *Hypertension* 11 (Supplement I), 167–171.
28. Cechetto, D. F., and Calaresu, F. R. (1984). Units in the amygdala responding to activation of carotid baro- and chemoreceptors. *American Journal of Physiology* 246, R832–R836.
29. Chan, R. K., Jarvina, E. V., and Sawchenko, P. E. (2000). Effects of selective sinoaortic denervations on phenylephrine-induced activational responses in the nucleus of the solitary tract. *Neuroscience* 101, 165–178.
30. Chen, C. Y., Ling Eh, E. H., Horowitz, J. M., and Bonham, A. C. (2002). Synaptic transmission in nucleus tractus solitarius is depressed by group II and III but not group I presynaptic metabotropic glutamate receptors in rats. *Journal of Physiology* 538, 773–786.
31. Coleridge, H. M., and Coleridge, J. C. G. (1980). Cardiovascular afferents involved in regulation of peripheral vessels. *Annual Review of Physiology* 42, 413–427.
32. Comet, M. A., Laguzzi, R., Hamon, M., and Sevoz-Couche, C. (2005). Functional interaction between nucleus tractus solitarius NK(1) and 5-HT(3) receptors in the inhibition of baroreflex in rats. *Cardiovascular Research* 65, 930–939.
33. Dampney, R. A., and McAllen, R. M. (1988). Differential control of sympathetic fibres supplying hindlimb skin and muscle by subretrofacial neurones in the cat. *Journal of Physiology* 395, 41–56.
34. Davies, R. O., and Kubin, L. (1986). Projection of pulmonary rapidly adapting receptors to the medulla of the cat: An antidromic mapping study. *Journal of Physiology* 373, 63–86.
35. Deadwyler, S. A., Hampson, R. E., Mu, J., Whyte, A., and Childers, S. (1995). Cannabinoids modulate voltage sensitive potassium A-current in hippocampal neurons via a CAMP-dependent process. *Journal of Pharmacology and Experimental Therapeutics* 273, 734–743.
36. Dekin, M. S., Getting, P. A., and Johnson, S. M. (1987). In vitro characterization of neurons in the ventral part of the nucleus tractus solitarius. I. Identification of neuronal types and repetitive firing properties. *Journal of Neurophysiology* 58, 195–196.
37. Deuchars, J., Li, Y. W., Kasparov, S., and Paton, J. F. R. (2000). Morphological and electrophysiological properties of neurones in the dorsal vagal complex of the rat activated by arterial baroreceptors. *Journal of Comparative Neurology* 417, 233–249.
38. Dhillon, H., Zigman, J. M., Ye, C., Lee, C. E., McGovern, R. A., Tang, V., Kenny, C. D.,

Christiansen, L. M., White, R. D., Edelstein, E. A., Coppari, R., Balthasar, N., Cowley, M. A., Chua, S., Jr., Elmquist, J. K., and Lowell, B. B. (2006). Leptin directly activates SF1 neurons in the VMH and this action by leptin is required for normal body-weight homeostasis. *Neuron* 49, 191–203.

39. Dias, A. C., Colombari, E., and Mifflin, S. W. (2003). Effect of nitric oxide on excitatory amino acid-evoked discharge of neurons in NTS. *American Journal of Physiology. Heart and Circulatory Physiology* 284, H234–H240.
40. Dickinson, C. J. (1991). Neurogenic hypertension, a synthesis and review, pp. 107–117. London: Chapman and Hall Medical.
41. Diz, D. I., Fantz, D. L., Benter, I. F., and Bosch, S. M. (1997). Acute depressor actions of angiotensin II in the nucleus of the solitary tract are mediated by substance P. *American Journal of Physiology* 273, R28–R34.
42. Doba, N., and Reis, D. J. (1973). Acute fulminating neurogenic hypertension produced by brainstem lesions in the rat. *Circulation Research* 32, 584–593.
43. Donoghue, S., Felder, R. B., Gilbey, M. P., Jordan, D., and Spyer, K. M. (1985). Post-synaptic activity evoked in the nucleus tractus solitarius by carotid sinus and aortic nerve afferents in the cat. *Journal of Physiology* 360, 261–273.
44. Doyle, M. W., and Andresen, M. C. (2001). Reliability of monosynaptic transmission in brain stem neurons in vitro. *Journal of Neurophysiology* 85, 2213–2223.
45. Doyle, M. W., Bailey, T. W., Jin, Y.-H., and Andresen, M. C. (2002). Vanilloid receptors presynaptically modulate visceral afferent synaptic transmission in nucleus tractus solitarius. *Journal of Neuroscience* 22, 8222–8229.
46. Doyle, M. W., Bailey, T. W., Jin, Y.-H., Appleyard, S. M., Low, M. J., and Andresen, M. C. (2004). Strategies for cellular identification in nucleus tractus solitarius slices. *Journal of Neuroscience Methods* 37, 37–48.
47. Duale, H., Waki, H., Howorth, P., Kasparov, S., Teschemacher, A. G., and Paton, J. F. (2007). Restraining influence of A2 neurons in chronic control of arterial pressure in spontaneously hypertensive rats. *Cardiovascular Research* 76, 184–193.
48. Fan, W., and Andresen, M. C. (1998). Differential frequency-dependent reflex integration of myelinated and nonmyelinated rat aortic baroreceptors. *American Journal of Physiology* 275, H632–H640.
49. Fan, W., Schild, J. H., and Andresen, M. C. (1999). Graded and dynamic reflex summation of myelinated and unmyelinated rat aortic baroreceptors. *American Journal of Physiology* 277, R748–R756.
50. Felder, R. B., and Mifflin, S. W. (1988). Modulation of carotid sinus afferent input to nucleus tractus solitarius by parabrachial nucleus stimulation. *Circulation Research* 63, 35–49.
51. Ferguson, A. V., and Washburn, D. L. (1998). Angiotensin II: A peptidergic neurotransmitter in central autonomic pathways. *Progress in Neurobiology* 54, 169–192.
52. Fritsch, J. M., Charles, J. B., Bennett, B. S., Jones, M. M., and Eckberg, D. L. (1992). Short-duration spaceflight impairs human carotid baroreceptor-cardiac reflex responses. *Journal of Applied Physiology* 73, 664–671.
53. Griffiths, C., and Garthwaite, J. (2001). The shaping of nitric oxide signals by a cellular sink. *Journal of Physiology* 536, 855–862.
54. Gross, P. M. (1991). Morphology and physiology of capillary systems in subregions of the subfornical organ and area postrema. *Canadian Journal of Physiology and Pharmacology* 69, 1010–1025.
55. Harada, S., Tokunaga, S., Momohara, M., Masaki, H., Tagawa, T., Imaizumi, T., and Takeshita, A. (1993). Inhibition of nitric oxide formation in the nucleus tractus solitarius increases renal sympathetic nerve activity in rabbits. *Circulation Research* 72, 511–516.
56. Haydon, P. G., and Carmignoto, G. (2006). Astrocyte control of synaptic transmission and neurovascular coupling. *Physiological Reviews* 86, 1009–1031.
57. Hayward, L. F., and Felder, R. B. (1995). Cardiac rhythmicity among NTS neurons and its relationship to sympathetic outflow in rabbits. *American Journal of Physiology* 269, H923–H933.
58. Healy, D. P., Rettig, R., Nguyen, T., and Printz, M. P. (1989). Quantitative autoradiography of angiotensin II receptors in the rat solitary-vagal area: Effects of nodose ganglionectomy or sino-aortic denervation. *Brain Research* 484, 1–12.
59. Helke, C. J., and Seagard, J. L. (2004). Substance P in the baroreceptor reflex: 25 years. *Peptides* 25, 413–423.
60. Hermes, S. M., Mitchell, J. L., and Aicher, S. A. (2006). Most neurons in the nucleus tractus solitarii do not send collateral projections to multiple autonomic targets in the rat brain. *Experimental Neurology* 198, 539–551.
61. Hines, T., Toney, G. M., and Mifflin, S. W. (1994). Responses of neurons in the nucleus tractus solitarius to stimulation of heart and lung receptors in the rat. *Circulation Research* 74, 1188–1196.

62. Hirase, H., Creso, J., Singleton, M., Bartho, P., and Buzsaki, G. (2004). Two-photon imaging of brain pericytes in vivo using dextran-conjugated dyes. *Glia* 46, 95–100.
63. Jacoby, S., Sims, R. E., and Hartell, N. A. (2001). Nitric oxide is required for the induction and heterosynaptic spread of long-term potentiation in rat cerebellar slices. *Journal of Physiology* 535, 825–839.
64. Jansen, A. S., and Loewy, A. D. (1994). Viral tracing of innervation. *Science* 265, 121–122.
65. Jeske, I., Morrison, S. F., Cravo, S. L., and Reis, D. J. (1993). Identification of baroreceptor reflex interneurons in the caudal ventrolateral medulla. *American Journal of Physiology* 264, R169–R178.
66. Jin, Y.-H., Bailey, T. W., and Andresen, M. C. (2004). Cranial afferent glutamate heterosynaptically modulates GABA release onto second-order neurons via distinctly segregated MGLURS. *Journal of Neuroscience* 24, 9332–9340.
67. Jin, Y.-H., Bailey, T. W., Li, B. Y., Schild, J. H., and Andresen, M. C. (2004). Purinergic and vanilloid receptor activation releases glutamate from separate cranial afferent terminals. *Journal of Neuroscience* 24, 4709–4717.
68. Jordan, D. (2005). Vagal control of the heart: Central serotonergic (5–HT) mechanisms. *Experimental Physiology* 90, 175–181.
69. Jordan, D., Khalid, M. E., Schneiderman, N., and Spyer, K. M. (1982). The location and properties of preganglionic vagal cardiomotor neurones in the rabbit. *Pflugers Archives* 395, 244–250.
70. Kalia, M., Fuxe, K., and Goldstein, M. (1985). Rat medulla oblongata. *II.* Dopaminergic, noradrenergic (A1 and A2) and adrenergic neurons, nerve fibers and presumptive terminal processes. *Journal of Comparative Neurology* 233, 308–332.
71. Kalia, M., and Richter, D. W. (1988). Rapidly adapting pulmonary receptor afferents: II. Fine structure and synaptic organization of central terminal processes in the nucleus of the tractus solitarius. *Journal of Comparative Neurology* 274, 574–594.
72. Kasparov, S., Butcher, J. W., and Paton, J. F. R. (1998). Angiotensin II receptors within the nucleus of the solitary tract mediate the developmental attenuation of the baroreceptor vagal reflex in pre-weaned rats. *Journal of the Autonomic Nervous System* 74, 160–168.
73. Kasparov, S., and Paton, J. F. R. (1999). Differential effects of angiotensin II in the nucleus tractus solitarii of the rat—plausible neuronal mechanisms. *Journal of Physiology* 521, 227–238.
74. Kasparov, S., and Teschemacher, A. G. (2008). Altered central catecholaminergic transmission and cardiovascular disease. *Experimental Physiology* 93, 725–740.
75. Keeton, T. K., and Campbell, W. B. (1980). The pharmacologic alteration of renin release. *Pharmacological Reviews* 32, 81–227.
76. Krowicki, Z. K., Sharkey, K. A., Serron, S. C., Nathan, N. A., and Hornby, P. J. (1997). Distribution of nitric oxide synthase in rat dorsal vagal complex and effects of microinjection of nitric oxide compounds upon gastric motor function. *Journal of Comparative Neurology* 377, 49–69.
77. Kubin, L., Alheid, G. F., Zuperku, E. J., and McCrimmon, D. R. (2006). Central pathways of pulmonary and lower airway vagal afferents. *Journal of Applied Physiology* 101, 618–627.
78. Kunze, D. L. (1972). Reflex discharge patterns of cardiac vagal efferent fibres. *Journal of Physiology* 222, 1–15.
79. Lachamp, P., Tell, F., and Kessler, J. P. (2002). Successive episodes of synapses production in the developing rat nucleus tractus solitarii. *Journal of Neurobiology* 52, 336–342.
80. Lee, J. S., Andresen, M. C., Morrow, D., and Chang, K. S. K. (2002). Isoflurane depresses baroreflex control of heart rate in decerebrate rats. *Anesthesiology* 96, 1214–1222.
81. Lin, H. C., Wan, F. J., and Tseng, C. J. (1999). Modulation of cardiovascular effects produced by nitric oxide and ionotropic glutamate receptor interaction in the nucleus tractus solitarii of rats. *Neuropharmacology* 38, 935–941.
82. Lin, L. H., Emson, P. C., and Talman, W. T. (2000). Apposition of neuronal elements containing nitric oxide synthase and glutamate in the nucleus tractus solitarii of rat: A confocal microscopic analysis. *Neuroscience* 96, 341–350.
83. Llewellyn-Smith, I. J., and Burnstock, G. (1998). Ultrastructural localization of $P2x_3$ receptors in rat sensory neurons. *Neuroreport* 9, 2545–2550.
84. Lo, W. J., Liu, H. W., Lin, H. C., Ger, L. P., Tung, C. S., and Tseng, C. J. (1996). Modulatory effects of nitric oxide on baroreflex activation in the brainstem nuclei of rats. *Chinese Journal of Physiology* 39, 57–62.
85. Loewy, A. D. (1990). Central autonomic pathways. In A. D. Loewy and K. M. Spyer (Eds.), *Central Regulation of Autonomic Functions*, pp. 88–103. New York: Oxford.
86. Luckman, S. M., and Lawrence, C. B. (2003). Anorectic brainstem peptides: More pieces to the puzzle. *Trends in Endocrinology and Metabolism* 14, 60–65.

87. Maolood, N., and Meister, B. (2009). Protein components of the blood–brain barrier (BBB) in the brainstem area postrema-nucleus tractus solitarius region. *Journal of Chemical Neuroanatomy* 37, 182–195.
88. McDougall, S. J., Peters, J. H., and Andresen, M. C. (2009). Convergence of cranial visceral afferents within the solitary tract nucleus. *Journal of Neuroscience* 29, 12886–12895.
89. McKinley, M. J., Albiston, A. L., Allen, A. M., Mathai, M. L., May, C. N., McAllen, R. M., Oldfield, B. J., Mendelsohn, F. A., and Chai, S. Y. (2003). The brain renin-angiotensin system: Location and physiological roles. *International Journal of Biochemistry and Cell Biology* 35, 901–918.
90. Mendelowitz, D., Yang, M,. Andresen, M. C., and Kunze, D. L. (1992). Localization and retention in vitro of fluorescently labeled aortic baroreceptor terminals on neurons from the nucleus tractus solitarius. *Brain Research* 581, 339–343.
91. Merahi, N., Orer, H. S., Laporte, A.-M., Gozlan, H., Hamon, M., and Laguzzi, R. (1992). Baroreceptor reflex inhibition induced by the stimulation of serotonin$_3$ receptors in the nucleus tractus solitarius of the rat. *Neuroscience* 46, 91–100.
92. Mifflin, S. W. (1992). Arterial chemoreceptor input to nucleus tractus solitarius. *American Journal of Physiology* 263, R368–R375.
93. Mifflin, S. W. (1993). Laryngeal afferent inputs to the nucleus of the solitary tract. *American Journal of Physiology* 265, R269–R276.
94. Mifflin, S. W. (1996). Convergent carotid sinus nerve and superior laryngeal nerve afferent inputs to neurons in the NTS. *American Journal of Physiology* 271, R870–R880.
95. Mifflin, S. W., and Felder, R. B. (1988). An intracellular study of time-dependent cardiovascular afferent interactions in nucleus tractus solitarius. *Journal of Neurophysiology* 59, 1798–1813.
96. Miller, A. J., McKoon, M., Pinneau, M., and Silverstein, R. (1983). Postnatal synaptic development of the nucleus tractus solitarius (NTS) of the rat. *Developmental Brain Research* 8, 205–213.
97. Morrison, S. F. (2001). Differential control of sympathetic outflow. *American Journal of Physiology. Regulatory, Integrative and Comparative Physiology* 281, R683–R698.
98. Mosqueda-Garcia, R., Tseng, C.-J., Appalsamy, M., and Robertson, D. (1990). Cardiovascular effects of microinjection of angiotensin II in the brainstem of renal hypertensive rats. *Journal of Pharmacology and Experimental Therapeutics* 255, 374–381.
99. Nosaka, S., Murase, S., Murata, K., and Inui, K. (1995). "Aortic baroreceptor" neurons in the nucleus tractus solitarius in rats: Convergence of cardiovascular inputs as revealed by heartbeat-locked activity. *Journal of the Autonomic Nervous System* 55, 69–80.
100. Osborn, J. W. (2005). Hypothesis: Set-points and long term control of arterial pressure. A theoretical argument for a long term arterial pressure control system in the brain rather than the kidney. *Clinical and Experimental Pharmacology and Physiology* 32, 384–393.
101. Parkinson, S. J., Jovanovic, A., Jovanovic, S., Wagner, F., Terzic, A., and Waldman, S. A. (1999). Regulation of nitric oxide-responsive recombinant soluble guanylyl cyclase by calcium. *Biochemistry* 38, 6441–6448.
102. Paton, J. F. R. (1996). A working heart-brainstem preparation of the mouse. *Journal of Neuroscience Methods* 65, 63–68.
103. Paton, J. F. R. (1998). Convergence properties of solitary tract neurones driven synaptically by cardiac vagal afferents in the mouse. *Journal of Physiology* 508, 237–252.
104. Paton, J. F. R. (1999). The Sharpey-Schafer Prize lecture: Nucleus tractus solitarii: Integrating structures. *Experimental Physiology* 84, 815–833.
105. Paton, J. F. R., Boscan, P., Murphy, D., and Kasparov, S. (2001). Unravelling mechanisms of action of angiotensin II on cardiorespiratory function using in vivo gene transfer. *Acta Physiologica Scandinavica* 173, 127–137.
106. Paton, J. F. R., Deuchars, J., Li, Y. W., and Kasparov, S. (2001). Properties of solitary tract neurones responding to peripheral arterial chemoreceptors. *Neuroscience* 105, 231–248.
107. Paton, J. F. R., and Kasparov, S. (1999). Differential effects of angiotensin II on cardiorespiratory reflexes mediated by nucleus tractus solitarii—a microinjection study in the rat. *Journal of Physiology* 521, 213–225.
108. Paton, J. F. R., and Kasparov, S. (2000). Sensory channel specific modulation in the nucleus of the solitary tract. *Journal of the Autonomic Nervous System* 80, 117–129.
109. Paton, J. F. R., Kasparov, S., and Paterson, D. J. (2002). Nitric oxide and autonomic control of heart rate: A question of specificity. *Trends in Neurosciences* 25, 626–631.
110. Paton, J. F. R., Li, Y. W., Deuchars, J., and Kasparov, S. (2000). Properties of solitary tract neurons receiving inputs from the sub-diaphragmatic vagus nerve. *Neuroscience* 95, 141–153.
111. Paton, J. F. R., Lonergan, T., Deuchars, J., James, P. E., and Kasparov, S. (2006). Detection of angiotensin II mediated nitric oxide release within the nucleus of the solitary tract using

electron-paramagnetic resonance (EPR) spectroscopy. *Autonomic Neuroscience* 126, 193–201.
112. Peters, J. H., McDougall, S. J., Kellett, D. O., Jordan, D., Llewellyn-Smith, I. J., and Andresen, M. C. (2008). Oxytocin enhances cranial visceral afferent synaptic transmission to the solitary tract nucleus. *Journal of Neuroscience* 28, 11731–11740.
113. Pickering, A. E., Boscan, P., and Paton, J. F. R. (2003). Nociception attenuates parasympathetic but not sympathetic baroreflex via NK1 receptors in the rat nucleus tractus solitarii. *Journal of Physiology* 551, 589–599.
114. Pilowsky, P. M., and Goodchild, A. K. (2002). Baroreceptor reflex pathways and neurotransmitters: 10 years on. *Journal of Hypertension* 20, 1675–1688.
115. Polson, J. W., Dampney, R. A., Boscan, P., Pickering, A. E., and Paton, J. F. (2007). Differential baroreflex control of sympathetic drive by angiotensin II in the nucleus tractus solitarii. *American Journal of Physiology. Regulatory, Integrative and Comparative Physiology* 293, R1954–R1960.
116. Pontieri, V., Venezuela, M. K., Scavone, C., and Michelini, L. C. (1998). Role of endogenous nitric oxide in the nucleus tractus solitarii on baroreflex control of heart rate in spontaneously hypertensive rats. *Journal of Hypertension* 16, 1993–1999.
117. Potts, J. T., Fuchs, I. E., Li, J. H., Leshnower, B., and Mitchell, J. H. (1999). Skeletal muscle afferent fibres release substance P in the nucleus tractus solitarii of anaesthetized cats. *Journal of Physiology* 514, 829–841.
118. Potts, J. T., Paton, J. F. R., Mitchell, J. H., Garry, M. G., Kline, G., Anguelov, P. T., and Lee, S. M. (2003). Contraction-sensitive skeletal muscle afferents inhibit arterial baroreceptor signalling in the nucleus of the solitary tract: Role of intrinsic GABA interneurons. *Neuroscience* 119, 201–214.
119. Prast, H., and Philippu, A. (2001). Nitric oxide as modulator of neuronal function. *Progress in Neurobiology* 64, 51–68.
120. Raven, P. B., Fadel, P. J., and Ogoh, S. (2005). Arterial baroreflex resetting during exercise: A current perspective. *Experimental Physiology* 91, 37–49.
121. Reid, I. A. (1992). Interactions between Ang II, sympathetic nervous system and baroreceptor reflexes in regulation of blood pressure. *American Journal of Physiology* 262, E763–E778.
122. Rettig, R., Healy, D. P., and Printz, M. P. (1986). Cardiovascular effects of microinjections of angiotensin II into the nucleus tractus solitarii. *Brain Research* 364, 233–240.
123. Riley, J., Lin, L. H., Chianca, D. A., Jr., and Talman, W. T. (2002). Ablation of NK1 receptors in rat nucleus tractus solitarii blocks baroreflexes. *Hypertension* 40, 823–826.
124. Rogers, R. F., Paton, J. F. R., and Schwaber, J. S. (1993). NTS neuronal responses to arterial pressure and pressure changes in the rat. *American Journal of Physiology* 265, R1355–R1368.
125. Rosenmund, C., Clements, J. D., and Westbrook, G. L. (1993). Nonuniform probability of glutamate release at a hippocampal synapse. *Science* 262, 754–757.
126. Ruiz-Stewart, I., Tiyyagura, S. R., Lin, J. E., Kazerounian, S., Pitari, G. M., Schulz, S., Martin, E., Murad, F., and Waldman, S. A. (2004). Guanylyl cyclase is an ATP sensor coupling nitric oxide signaling to cell metabolism. *Proceedings of the National Academy of Science USA* 101, 37–42.
127. Sakai, K., Hirooka, Y., Matsuo, I., Eshima, K., Shigematsu, H., Shimokawa, H., and Takeshita, A. (2000). Overexpression of ENOS in NTS causes hypotension and bradycardia in vivo. *Hypertension* 36, 1023–1028.
128. Sato, M. A., Colombari, E., and Morrison, S. F. (2002). Inhibition of neurons in commissural nucleus of solitary tract reduces sympathetic nerve activity in SHR. *American Journal of Physiology. Heart And Circulatory Physiology* 282, H1679–H1684.
129. Scheuer, D. A., Zhang, J., Toney, G. M., and Mifflin, S. W. (1996). Temporal processing of aortic nerve evoked activity in the nucleus of the solitary tract. *Journal of Neurophysiology* 76, 3750–3757.
130. Schild, J. H., Clark, J. W., Hay, M., Mendelowitz, D., Andresen, M. C., and Kunze, D. L. (1994). A- and C-Type nodose sensory neurons: Model interpretations of dynamic discharge characteristics. *Journal of Neurophysiology* 71, 2338–2358.
131. Schiltz, J. C., and Sawchenko, P. E. (2003). Signaling the brain in systemic inflammation: The role of perivascular cells. *Frontiers in Bioscience* 8, S1321–S1329.
132. Scholz, J., and Woolf, C. J. (2007). The neuropathic pain triad: Neurons, immune cells and glia. *Nature Neuroscience* 10, 1361–1368.
133. Seidel, B., Stanarius, A., and Wolf, G. (1997). Differential expression of neuronal and endothelial nitric oxide synthase in blood vessels of the rat brain. *Neuroscience Letters* 239, 109–112.
134. Sekizawa, S., Joad, J. P., and Bonham, A. C. (2003). Substance P presynaptically depresses the transmission of sensory input to bronchopulmonary neurons in the guinea pig

nucleus tractus solitarii. *Journal of Physiology* 552, 547–559.

135. Silva-Carvalho, L., Paton, J. F. R., Rocha, I., Goldsmith, G. E., and Spyer, K. M. (1998). Convergence properties of solitary tract neurons responsive to cardiac receptor stimulation in the anesthetized cat. *Journal of Neurophysiology* 79, 2374–2382.
136. Simms, A. E., Paton, J. F., and Pickering, A. E. (2007). Hierarchical recruitment of the sympathetic and parasympathetic limbs of the baroreflex in normotensive and spontaneously hypertensive rats. *Journal of Physiology* 579, 473–486.
137. Simms, A. E., Paton, J. F. R., and Pickering, A. E. (2006). Disinhibition of the cardiac limb of the arterial baroreflex in rat: A role for metabotropic glutamate receptors in the nucleus tractus solitarii. *Journal of Physiology* 575, 727–738.
138. Standish, A., Enquist, L. W., and Schwaber, J. S. (1994). Innervation of the heart and its central medullary origin defined by viral tracing. *Science* 263, 232–234.
139. Tai, M. H., Hsiao, M., Chan, J. Y., Lo, W. C., Wang, F. S., Liu, G. S., Howng, S. L., and Tseng, C. J. (2004). Gene delivery of endothelial nitric oxide synthase into nucleus tractus solitarii induces biphasic response in cardiovascular functions of hypertensive rats. *American Journal of Hypertension* 17, 63–70.
140. Talman, W. T., Dragon, D. N., Ohta, H., and Lin, L. H. (2001). Nitroxidergic influences on cardiovascular control by NTS: A link with glutamate. *Annals of the New York Academy of Science* 940, 169–178.
141. Talman, W. T., Perrone, M. H., and Reis, D. J. (1980). Evidence for L-glutamate as the neurotransmitter of baroreceptor afferent nerve fibers. *Science* 209, 813–815.
142. Travagli, R. A., Hermann, G. E., Browning, K. N., and Rogers, R. C. (2006). Brainstem circuits regulating gastric function. *Annual Review of Physiology* 68, 279–305.
143. Waki, H., Gouraud, S. S., Maeda, M., and Paton, J. F. R. (2008). Gene expression profiles of major cytokines in the nucleus tractus solitarii of the spontaneously hypertensive rat. *Autonomic Neuroscience* 142, 40–44.
144. Waki, H., Gouraud, S. S., Maeda, M., and Paton, J. F. R. (2008). Specific inflammatory condition in nucleus tractus solitarii of the SHR: Novel insight for neurogenic hypertension? *Autonomic Neuroscience* 142, 25–31.
145. Waki, H., Kasparov, S., Katahira, K., Shimizu, T., Murphy, D., and Paton, J. F. R. (2003). Dynamic exercise attenuates spontaneous baroreceptor reflex sensitivity in conscious rats. *Experimental Physiology* 88, 517–526.
146. Waki, H., Liu, B., Miyake, M., Katahira, K., Murphy, D., Kasparov, S., and Paton, J. F. R. (2007). Junctional adhesion molecule-1 is upregulated in spontaneously hypertensive rats: Evidence for a prohypertensive role within the brain stem. *Hypertension* 49, 1321–1327.
147. Waki, H., Murphy, D., Yao, S. T., Kasparov, S., and Paton, J. F. R. (2006). Endothelial nitric oxide synthase in the nucleus tractus solitarii contributes to the hypertension in the spontaneously hypertensive rat. *Hypertension* 48, 644–650.
148. Wang, D. S., Sumners, C., Posner, P., and Gelband, C. H. (1997). A-type $K^+$ current in neurons cultured from neonatal rat hypothalamus and brain stem: Modulation by angiotensin II. *Journal of Neurophysiology* 78, 1021–1029.
149. Wang, J., Irnaten, M., Neff, R. A., Venkatesan, P., Evans, C., Loewy, A. D., Mettenleiter, T. C., and Mendelowitz, D. (2001). Synaptic and neurotransmitter activation of cardiac vagal neurons in the nucleus ambiguus. *Annals of the New York Academy of Science* 940, 237–246.
150. Wang, S., Paton, J. F.R., and Kasparov, S. (2007). Differential sensitivity of excitatory and inhibitory synaptic transmission to modulation by nitric oxide in rat nucleus tractus solitarii. *Experimental Physiology* 92, 371–382.
151. Wang, S., Teschemacher, A. G., Paton, J. F. R., and Kasparov, S. (2006). Mechanism of nitric oxide action on inhibitory GABAergic signaling within the nucleus tractus solitarii. *The FASEB Journal* 20, 1537–1539.
152. Wong, L. F., Polson, J. W., Murphy, D., Paton, J. F. R., and Kasparov, S. (2002). Genetic and pharmacological dissection of pathways involved in the angiotensin II-mediated depression of baroreflex function. *The FASEB Journal* 16, 1595–1601.
153. Wu, W. C., Wang, Y., Kao, L. S., Tang, F. I., and Chai, C. Y. (2002). Nitric oxide reduces blood pressure in the nucleus tractus solitarius: A real-time electrochemical study. *Brain Research Bulletin* 57, 171–177.
154. Zhang, J., and Mifflin, S. W. (1998). Receptor subtype specific effects of GABA agonists on neurons receiving aortic depressor nerve inputs within the nucleus of the solitary tract. *Journal of the Autonomic Nervous System* 73, 170–181.
155. Zhang, L. L., and Ashwell, K. W. (2001). Development of the cyto- and chemoarchitectural organization of the rat nucleus of the solitary tract. *Anatomy and Embryology (Berlin)* 203, 265–282.

3

# The Hypothalamus and Autonomic Regulation: An Overview

ROGER A. L. DAMPNEY

The hypothalamus was first identified as a distinct region within the diencephalon by His in 1893 (for review, see [19]). Later, during the 1920s and 1930s, Ranson and Hess and their colleagues demonstrated that lesions or localized electrical stimulation of sites within the hypothalamus had profound effects on a range of behaviors that included autonomic functions, such as feeding and drinking, reproductive behavior, thermoregulatory responses, and responses to stress. At that time, it was thought that these effects were due to actions on neuronal cell bodies within the hypothalamus; but it is now recognized that the effects of lesions or electrical stimulation may also be due in part to effects on ascending or descending axons of passage within the hypothalamus. Nevertheless, even with the advent of new methods that have allowed the effects of specific inhibition or excitation of neuronal cell bodies within the hypothalamus to be studied, it is still clear that hypothalamic nuclei are essential components of the central circuitry that subserves the integrated behavioral responses referred to above.

This chapter will briefly review the structure of the hypothalamus and its main connections and functions. Although particular attention will be paid to the regulation of autonomic functions, these are virtually always components of more generalized, often quite stereotyped, behavioral responses. Thus, a major challenge is to understand how the connections and properties of hypothalamic neurons can produce these responses. This chapter will not attempt to describe these properties in detail but will instead discuss our current understanding of the general principles of the relationship between structure and function in the hypothalamus and will also attempt to define key unanswered questions.

## OVERVIEW OF HYPOTHALAMIC STRUCTURE

The hypothalamus can be subdivided both rostrocaudally and mediolaterally. Rostrocaudally, it is most commonly divided into three parts (anterior, middle, and posterior parts). As shown in Figure 3–1, the rostral boundary is the lamina terminalis, which extends from the optic chiasm to the anterior commissure and also forms part of the rostral wall of the third ventricle. The caudal limits of the hypothalamus are the mamillary nuclei. The anterior part of the hypothalamus is also referred to as the *preoptic area*, the middle as the *tuberal part*, and the posterior as the *mammillary part*.

In the mediolateral direction, the hypothalamus is traditionally divided into three longitudinal cell columns, as first described by Gurdijian[42] and Krieg[60]. These are referred to as the *periventricular*, *medial* and *lateral* zones. Most of the major nuclei of the hypothalamus are within the medial zone and usually have a distinct cytoarchitecture. In contrast, neurons within the lateral zone are more diffusely distributed and do not form anatomically distinct nuclei. The lateral hypothalamus also contains the medial forebrain bundle, which connects the hypothalamus with brainstem nuclei via descending axons, and with neurons in the forebrain, including the basal forebrain, amygdala, and cerebral cortex, by ascending axons.

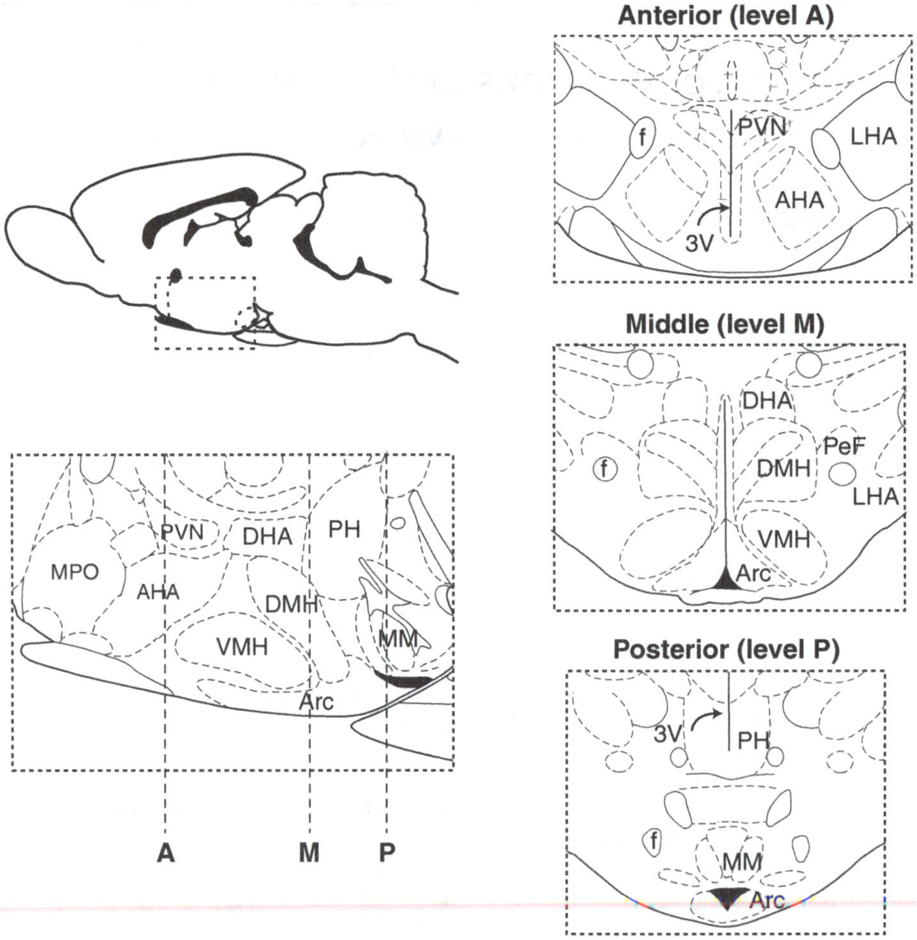


Figure 3–1 Hypothalamic regions in the rat that influence autonomic functions. The lower left panel shows a sagittal section 0.4 mm lateral to the midline, in the region indicated by the hatched rectangle in the drawing of the rat brain (upper left panel). The three panels on the right show coronal sections at anterior, middle and posterior levels of the hypothalamus. 3V, third ventricle; AHA, anterior hypothalamic area; Arc, arcuate nucleus; DHA, dorsal hypothalamic area; DMH, dorsomedial hypothalamic nucleus; f, fornix; LHA, lateral hypothalamic area; MM, medial mammillary nucleus; MPO, median preoptic nucleus; PeF, perifornical area; PH, posterior hypothalamic nucleus; PVN, paraventricular nucleus; VMH, ventromedial hypothalamic nucleus.

The medial forebrain bundle also contains axons that pass through the hypothalamus without making synaptic connections.

As summarized by Card et al.[19], during embryogenesis the hypothalamus develops from the diencephalic vesicle of the neural tube. Differentiation of the germinal epithelium in the ventral diencephalon occurs in stages. The cells that ultimately are located within the lateral hypothalamus form first and then migrate laterally. Then, the cells that ultimately are part of the medial subdivision differentiate and migrate to a position medial to the lateral group. The periventricular cell groups are also formed from the germinal epithelium and are located adjacent to the wall of the third ventricle.

As discussed in more detail below, the relationship between structure and function in the hypothalamus is complex. At the same time, it is possible to make some generalizations concerning the overall functions of different parts of the hypothalamus. In particular, the anterior area contains neurons that respond directly to signals indicating deviations from physiological set-points. This includes neurons sensitive to increases in body temperature, to circulating cytokines that are released in response to inflammatory stimuli, to an increased level of blood osmolality, to alterations in blood glucose level, or to the levels of circulating hormones, such as angiotensin II. Second, neurons controlling the release of hormones from the pituitary gland (vasopressin and oxytocin from its posterior part, and adrenocorticotropic hormone, thyroid-stimulating hormone, growth hormone, luteinizing hormone, follicle-stimulating hormone, and prolactin) are largely located within the periventricular zone of the hypothalamus, including the paraventricular, anterior periventricular, and arcuate nuclei (Figure 3–1).

A feature of hypothalamic structure is the large degree of interconnection between different nuclei and regions, particularly within the periventricular and medial zones. For example, the dorsomedial hypothalamus has major projections to other hypothalamic nuclei, including all nuclei in the periventricular zone except the arcuate nucleus[104]. The dorsomedial hypothalamus also receives inputs from a wide range of other hypothalamic nuclei, including nearly all the major nuclei in the anterior, middle, and posterior parts of the hypothalamus[103]. Other nuclei within the medial or periventricular zone (e.g., the median preoptic nucleus or ventromedial hypothalamic nucleus) also have extensive interconnections with other hypothalamic nuclei[104].

## OUTPUTS: CONNECTIONS WITH SYMPATHETIC AND PARASYMPATHETIC PREGANGLIONIC NEURONS

### Direct Connections

Neurons within the hypothalamus can regulate autonomic outflow via either direct or indirect connections with sympathetic or parasympathetic preganglionic neurons. Neurons that make direct monosynaptic connections with preganglionic neurons (so-called sympathetic or parasympathetic premotor neurons) have been identified using the method of trans-synaptic transport of viruses, such as pseudorabies virus or herpes simplex virus. In studies using this method, virus is injected into either the target organ (e.g., heart or kidney), a nerve, or a ganglion. One of the problems with this method is that it can be difficult to determine whether an infected central neuron is one or more than one synapse removed from the preganglionic neuron to which it projects[55,98]. A second possible problem is that not all neurons may transport viruses, so that some neurons with appropriate connections may not be labeled. Nevertheless, when the results of such studies are considered together with those of studies using conventional retrograde tracers, which do not cross synapses, a relatively clear picture emerges (Figure 3–2).

First, the paraventricular nucleus (PVN) is the major location of both sympathetic and parasympathetic premotor neurons in the hypothalamus[16,18,56,87,94,98,101]. This nucleus contains neurons that project to all levels of the sympathetic outflow to innervate sympathetic preganglionic neurons, which regulate all, or nearly all, target organs that receive a sympathetic innervation. Parasympathetic premotor neurons regulating the vagal outflow to the heart, pancreas, and liver are also located within the PVN[15,16,99,101], suggesting that this nucleus may also regulate the vagal outflow to all organs that receive a vagal innervation.

Second, apart from the PVN, the dorsal hypothalamic area, lateral hypothalamic area, perifornical area, and retrochiasmatic nucleus also contain spinally projecting neurons[16,21,50,86,108]. Studies using anterograde axonal tracing indicate that neurons in all of these regions terminate in areas of the spinal cord that contain preganglionic neurons[81,86,106]. Consistent with this, studies using trans-synaptically transported viruses also indicate that neurons in all of these regions project to the sympathetic outflows that innervate a variety of organs, including the spleen, heart, adrenal

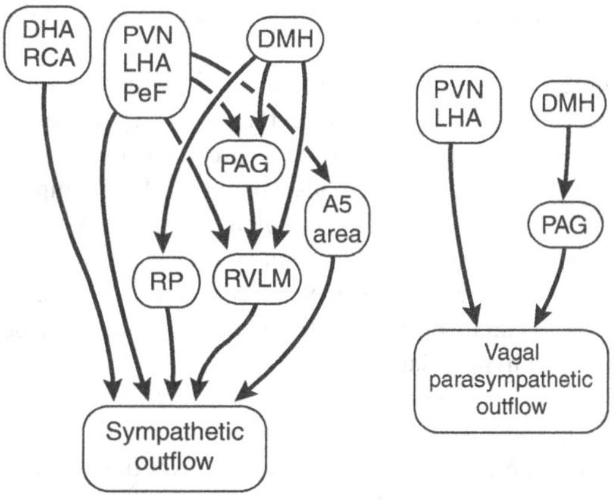


Figure 3–2 Main direct and indirect hypothalamic projections that control autonomic outflow. Diagrams showing the projections from hypothalamic nuclei to the sympathetic outflow (*left*) and vagal parasympathetic outflow (*right*). DHA, dorsal hypothalamic area; DMH, dorsomedial hypothalamic nucleus; LHA, lateral hypothalamic area; RP, raphe pallidus; PAG, periaqueductal gray; PeF, perifornical area; PVN, paraventricular nucleus; RCA, retrochiasmatic area; RVLM, rostral ventrolateral medulla.

gland, kidney, urethra, and white adipose tissue[16,18,56,94,101,107]. Neurons in the lateral hypothalamic area project directly to the dorsal vagal nucleus[49], indicating that this region, like the PVN, contains parasympathetic as well as sympathetic premotor neurons.

## Indirect Connections

Hypothalamic neurons can also make connections with sympathetic preganglionic neurons via synapses with premotor sympathetic neurons, such as those in the rostral ventrolateral medulla (RVLM), medullary raphé nuclei, or A5 area in the pons. Connections also occur via more complex polysynaptic pathways that include synapses with neurons in other regions, such as the midbrain periaqueductal gray (PAG), parabrachial complex, or nucleus of the solitary tract (NTS), all of which project to sympathetic premotor nuclei. For example, as shown in Figure 3–2, neurons in the PVN, dorsomedial hypothalamus, and lateral hypothalamic area project to the RVLM[27,28,37,41] and also to other supramedullary regions, such as the midbrain PAG and Kölliker-Fuse nucleus in the pons[49,102], which in turn project to the RVLM[27,28,37].

Apart from the RVLM, other sympathetic premotor neurons also receive both direct and indirect inputs from hypothalamic nuclei. For example, there is a direct input from a discrete group of neurons in the dorsomedial hypothalamic area to the raphé nuclei in the midline medulla, which contains sympathetic premotor neurons[83]. Sympathetic premotor neurons in the raphé also receive a significant afferent input from subregions within the midbrain PAG[35], which, in turn, receive inputs from a wide range of hypothalamic nuclei[10]. Similarly, sympathetic premotor neurons in the A5 area in the pons also receive afferent inputs from the midbrain PAG[35], as well as from the PVN and perifornical area in the hypothalamus[17,51]. Thus, there are multiple routes by which premotor sympathetic neurons can receive inputs from neurons within a wide range of hypothalamic nuclei.

Less is known about indirect connections between the hypothalamus and parasympathetic preganglionic neurons. Neurons in the dorsomedial hypothalamus do not appear to project directly to vagal preganglionic nuclei; but studies using retrograde trans-synaptic transport of viruses indicates that they project indirectly to these nuclei, perhaps via the midbrain PAG[15,101].

## Are there Command Neurons or Specific Sub-Groups of Autonomic Neurons?

As discussed by Blessing[11], Cannon first proposed that the sympathetic nervous system is activated in a generalized fashion in response to challenges, such as hemorrhage or hypoxia and during exercise or emotional arousal. There is now a very large body of evidence demonstrating that different sympathetic outflows, and also parasympathetic outflows, can be regulated in a highly specific and differentiated fashion (for review see [54]). There is also physiological evidence that, within the RVLM, subsets of sympathetic premotor neurons preferentially, or even exclusively, regulate the sympathetic outflow to the heart or to blood vessels in specific vascular beds[29,64,68]. Trans-synaptic transport of viruses has indicated that sympathetic premotor neurons in the PVN are topographically organized so that subgroups project specifically to particular sympathetic outflows[98], (Figure 3–3). Furthermore, parasympathetic premotor neurons in the PVN appear to be a separate population from the sympathetic premotor neurons in the same nucleus[16].

The evidence that there are subgroups of autonomic neurons within the hypothalamus, each of which regulates a particular component of the autonomic outflow, does not rule out the possibility that other subsets of neurons within the hypothalamus have parallel outputs to more than one type of sympathetic preganglionic neuron. Such "command neurons" (i.e., neurons with projections to more than one type of sympathetic outflow) are likely to exist within the hypothalamus. Jansen et al.[55], using trans-synaptic labeling with two different viruses, identified neurons in the PVN, lateral hypothalamic area, and perifornical area that make connections with both the sympathetic outflow to the heart and the outflow to the adrenal gland. These neurons may be activated under circumstances when there is a generalized increase in the sympathetic outflow to the heart, adrenal glands, blood vessels, and other effectors; for example, during exercise or acute psychological stress. There is also evidence for the existence of hypothalamic neurons with outputs to both the somatomotor and autonomic systems (see "Relationship between hypothalamic structure and function: general principles" below).

Thus, at the level of the hypothalamus, there are subgroups of neurons that preferentially, or possibly even exclusively, project to particular components of the autonomic outflow. There is also evidence for hypothalamic neurons with collateralized projections to sympathetic premotor neurons that drive the sympathetic outflow to quite different target organs, and/or other neurons regulating the somatomotor outflow. Such putative "command neurons" could help coordinate autonomic and somatomotor responses during exercise or other types of stress (see below).

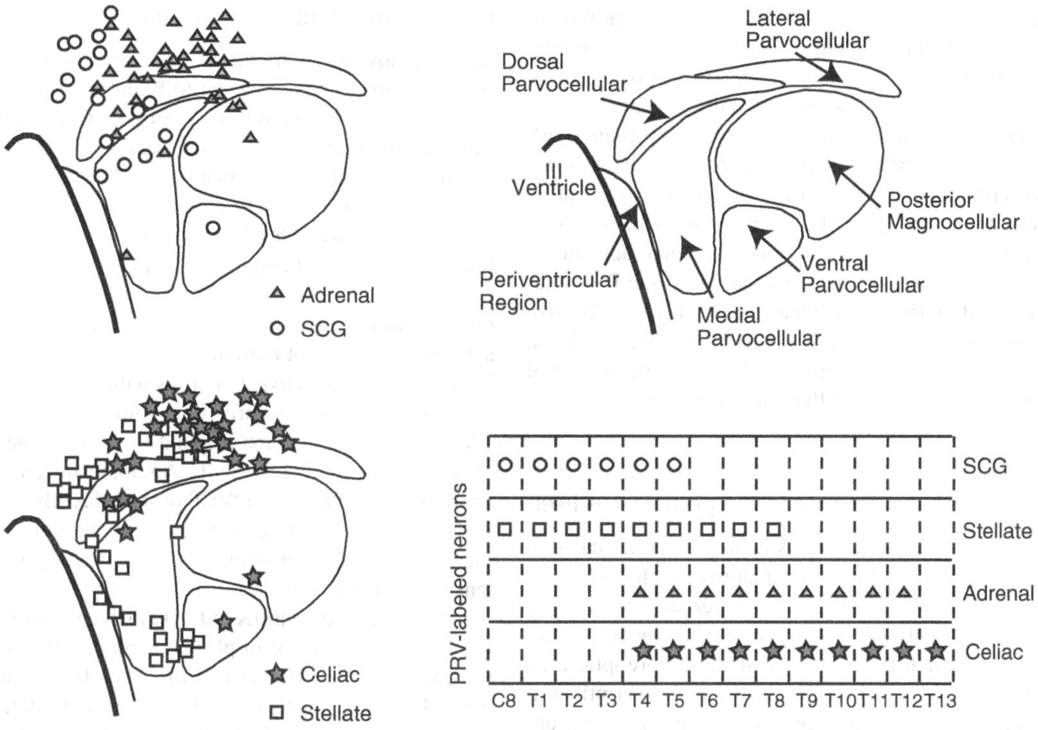


Figure 3–3 Distribution of neurons within and surrounding the PVN that are trans-synaptically labeled from different sympathetically innervated targets. Pseudorabies virus (PRV) was injected into either the adrenal medulla, the superior cervical ganglion (SCG), the stellate ganglion or celiac ganglion. The distribution of PRV-labeled neurons within each of the spinal cord segments is also shown. Note the different topographical distribution of the neurons in the hypothalamus that were labeled from the different targets. Modified from Strack et al.[98], with permission.

## INPUTS TO HYPOTHALAMIC NEURONS CONTROLLING AUTONOMIC FUNCTION

### Inputs from Visceral Receptors and Pain Receptors

Signals arising from visceral receptors (e.g., baroreceptors, chemoreceptors, cardiopulmonary receptors, etc.) and somatic pain receptors are known to regulate the release of vasopressin and of adrenocorticotropic hormone. This occurs via inputs to vasopressin-synthesizing neurons in the magnocellular PVN and supraoptic nucleus (SON) and inputs to neurons containing corticotropin-releasing factor in the parvicellular PVN. Afferent axons from these visceral receptors terminate in the NTS. From there, sensory information is transmitted to the PVN and SON both directly and via the ventrolateral medulla. Most, but not all, of the neurons in the NTS and ventrolateral medulla that project to the PVN and SON are noradrenaline-synthesizing neurons of the A2 and A1 groups, respectively[25]. Neurons in the A1 and A2 groups also convey signals to the PVN in response to an immune challenge and psychological stressors[30].

There are other indirect routes connecting the NTS and ventrolateral medulla with hypothalamic nuclei. For example, there are major topographically organized projections from NTS subnuclei to subregions of the parabrachial complex in the pons and to the PAG in the midbrain[45,46]. These nuclei, in turn, are major sources of input to hypothalamic nuclei that regulate autonomic activity, including the PVN and lateral hypothalamic area[1,8,57,58,72,78,112]. Whether these inputs specifically regulate autonomic neurons in these hypothalamic regions and what particular signals they convey are unknown.

Although it is well established that the ascending signals relayed via the NTS and ventrolateral medulla regulate magnocellular neuroendocrine neurons in the PVN, their role in the regulation of autonomic neurons in this nucleus is less clear. For example, challenges such as hemorrhage or hypoxia (which unloads baroreceptors and activates chemoreceptors, respectively), result in Fos expression in many neurons in the PVN and other hypothalamic regions. Nevertheless, very few of the activated neurons project to the spinal sympathetic outflow or to the RVLM[26]. On the other hand, an immune challenge activates a subset of neurons in the dorsal parvicellular PVN that project directly to the spinal cord[114]. It is not known, however, whether these neurons are activated via ascending signals from the NTS or ventrolateral medulla, or via other pathways activated by circulating pyrogens (see below).

## Inputs from Neurons in the Hypothalamus Itself

The hypothalamus contains neurons that are capable of sensing and signaling changes in physiological variables, particularly core temperature and blood glucose levels. Temperature-sensing neurons are located primarily in the hypothalamic preoptic area and include neurons that sense both warmth and cold[2,14]. Hypothalamic thermosensitive neurons are crucial for maintaining body temperature. Small alterations in hypothalamic temperature evoke thermoregulatory responses of much greater magnitude than those evoked by equivalent temperature changes detected by receptors elsewhere in the body[14]. The firing rate of these thermosensitive hypothalamic neurons is also influenced by pyrogens, and this appears to be the mechanism by which fever can cause alterations in the set-point for body temperature. As discussed in Chapter 18, activation of thermosensitive hypothalamic neurons elicits highly patterned and coordinated somatomotor and autonomic responses.

It was first demonstrated over 50 years ago that neurons that sense changes in extracellular glucose concentration are located in the hypothalamus (see [62] for a review, and Chapter 17). Such glucose-sensitive neurons are activated by hypoglycemia and trigger the secretion of adrenaline from the adrenal medulla, leading to a compensatory increase in the level of blood glucose[62]. The neurons that sense glucoprivation and trigger this response are located in the ventromedial hypothalamic nucleus as well as the arcuate nucleus and the lateral hypothalamic area[13,62]. Recently, it has been shown that glucoprivation activates neurons in the ventromedial hypothalamic nucleus via local release of noradrenaline[31]. Neurons that are activated by hyperglycemia have also been described, and these may play a role in regulation of energy balance[62].

## Inputs from Circulating Substances

The circumventricular organs are specialized structures that are located adjacent to brain ventricles and have a reduced blood–brain barrier (see Chapter 16). Three of the circumventricular organs—the subfornical organ (SFO), the organum vasculosum of the lamina terminalis (OVLT), and the area postrema—contain neuronal cell bodies that project to a variety of brain regions, including the hypothalamus. Because of the reduced blood–brain barrier in circumventricular organs, various circulating hormones and other substances, which do not normally affect neurons in other brain regions, can activate neurons within the circumventricular organs[70]. In particular, neurons in the SFO, OVLT, and area postrema respond to increased levels of circulating angiotensin II. Angiotensin-sensitive neurons in the SFO and OVLT project directly to the PVN and SON[5,77]. These connections are thought to be major routes by which an increase in circulating angiotensin II can lead to increased release of vasopressin[70].

There are also neurons in the OVLT and SFO that respond to an increase in plasma osmolality[69]. These osmosensitive neurons also project to the hypothalamic PVN and SON, but they appear to be largely separate populations from the angiotensin-sensitive neurons[69]. Like angiotensin-sensitive neurons, osmosensitive neurons in the OVLT and SFO activate vasopressin-synthesising neurons in the PVN and SON[70].

Trans-synaptic viral tracing studies have shown that there are polysynaptic connections from neurons in the OVLT and SFO to the sympathetic outflow[38,110]. Some of these OVLT and SFO neurons also express the angiotensin type 1 receptor and are thus presumably angiotensin-sensitive. Activation of both angiotensin-sensitive and osmosensitive neurons in the forebrain circumventricular organs can excite sympathetic activity via their connections with PVN neurons that project to the spinal cord or RVLM[6,96,97,105].

Apart from their inputs to the PVN, neurons in the OVLT and SFO also project to several other hypothalamic regions known to have an autonomic function, including the lateral hypothalamic area, perifornical area, and dorsomedial hypothalamus[70]. The functions of these connections are unknown, but potentially they are other routes by which signals transmitted via circumventricular organs can influence autonomic function by actions in the hypothalamus.

## Inputs from Other Brain Regions

Afferent inputs to the hypothalamus arise from a wide variety of nuclei and are too complex to be described in detail here. Nevertheless, some general points can be made. First, the parabrachial complex in the pons and the PAG in the midbrain are the main sources of ascending inputs to the hypothalamus; and they project to all, or nearly all, hypothalamic regions[1,8,20,57,58,71,78,103,112]. Some of the hypothalamus-projecting neurons in the PAG and parabrachial complex may transmit signals originating from peripheral receptors (see "Inputs from visceral receptors and pain receptors" above). However, they may also relay information from higher centers of the brain, since both the PAG and parabrachial complex receive major inputs from the cortex and basal forebrain[71,74].

Secondly, brain regions subserving autonomic responses to emotional stimuli, such as the amygdala, provide a relatively small amount of direct input to the PVN, which is the main location of sympathetic premotor neurons in the hypothalamus[48]. Instead, information from the amygdala and other limbic regions may reach the PVN via two routes. One is through interneurons, including GABAergic inhibitory interneurons, which surround and send axons into the PVN[47,48,82]. Another route is through other hypothalamic nuclei, such as the dorsomedial hypothalamus, medial preoptic area, or lateral hypothalamic area, which send axons directly to the PVN[47]. The functional significance of the presence of an intervening synapse between the amygdala and other limbic regions and the output neurons of the PVN is unclear. However, it has been suggested that emotional stimuli may or may not require activation of sympathetic premotor or neuroendocrine neurons, depending on the context of the emotional stimulus[48]. Thus, the additional connections provide the opportunity for further processing of signals associated with emotional stimuli antecedent to the PVN. In contrast, other challenges such as hemorrhage, which require an immediate emergency response, are signaled via direct inputs to the PVN from the NTS and other nuclei (see "Inputs from visceral receptors and pain receptors" above).

### Inputs from the External World

The hypothalamus receives information about the external environment, particularly in regard to temperature, light and, odor. Information about ambient external temperature reaches the hypothalamus via skin thermoreceptors and, together with inputs from thermoreceptors in the hypothalamus itself, triggers behavioral and autonomic thermoregulatory responses (see Chapter 18). Information about the ambient light level is transmitted to the hypothalamus by direct inputs from retinal ganglion cells, mainly to the suprachiasmatic nucleus[39,76]. These signals then synchronize the intrinsic rhythm of neurons in the suprachiasmatic nucleus to the normal light–dark cycle[85]. The suprachiasmatic nucleus, via its projections to other hypothalamic nuclei (principally the subparaventricular zone and the dorsomedial hypothalamus) regulates the circadian rhythms of temperature, sleep and waking, locomotor activity, feeding, and corticosteroid production[85]. Because circadian rhythms of locomotor activity are also closely correlated with similar variations in blood pressure and heart rate[65], it seems likely that the diurnal variations in these variables are also generated by neurons within the same hypothalamic nuclei.

It has long been known that pheromones—species-specific chemical signals that trigger mating and reproductive behavior—exert their effects by activating neurons in the hypothalamic preoptic area that synthesize gonadotropin-releasing hormone[93]. Until recently, specialized sensors in the vomeronasal organ were generally believed to detect pheromones, whereas the olfactory epithelium within the nasal cavity detects common odors (for a review see [92]). However, recent studies have shown that both common odors and pheromones activate the main olfactory pathway to the gonadotropin-releasing hormone neurons in the hypothalamus, which includes synapses in the olfactory cortex and olfactory bulb[111]. Pheromones also activate an accessory pathway that projects to gonadotropin-releasing hormone neurons via the amygdala[12]. Nevertheless, the main olfactory pathway seems to be essential for normal mating because specific lesions of this pathway result in deficiencies in mating behavior[66].

## RELATIONSHIP BETWEEN HYPOTHALAMIC STRUCTURE AND FUNCTION: GENERAL PRINCIPLES

Since the work of Ranson and Hess, the hypothalamus has been acknowledged to contain the neural mechanisms that subserve somatomotor, autonomic, and neuroendocrine responses associated with different behaviors, such as feeding, drinking, reproductive behavior, thermoregulation, and defensive behavior. Each behavior can be quite stereotyped, even if it is species-specific. Thus, there must be different sets of neurons in the hypothalamus, each of which can generate coordinated patterns of autonomic and other components of these behavioral responses.

There is a general acceptance that pattern generators exist in the hypothalamus, as well as possibly in other brain regions[7,11,84,104]. Nevertheless, the precise neural substrates that are capable of producing coordinated behavior patterns are unknown. The simplest model that can explain these coordinated patterns of behavior is a set of "command" neurons with collateralized projections directly or indirectly innervating autonomic, somatomotor, and hormone-synthesizing neurons that are activated as part of a specific behavioral response (Figure 3–4). These command neurons would presumably also receive inputs from a variety of sources that are known to trigger the particular pattern of response. Experimental evidence to support the existence of putative command neurons includes studies using trans-synaptic tracing with two viruses. Krout et al.[61] identified neurons within the lateral hypothalamus with projections to both the stellate ganglion and the motor cortex. These neurons could conceivably control both the sympathetic outflow to the heart as well as simultaneously regulate somatomotor function. Interestingly, about half of neurons in the lateral hypothalamus that connect with both the sympathetic outflow and motor cortex contain orexin[61]. Orexin-containing neurons are confined to the lateral hypothalamus and are particularly active during periods of arousal and activity[73], when blood pressure and heart rate are also increased[65]. Hence, orexin neurons that project to both sympathetic preganglionic neurons in the spinal cord and the motor cortex may be putative command neurons controlling coordinated autonomic and somatomotor responses.

Another set of hypothalamic neurons with properties suggestive of command neurons are neurons in the medial preoptic nucleus that receive direct inputs from gonadotropin-releasing hormone neurons[12]. The medial preoptic nucleus innervates both autonomic nuclei and somatomotor regions in the brain and is essential for the expression of male sexual behavior, which includes stereotyped autonomic, somatomotor, and hormonal components[79]. Furthermore, injections of gonadotropin-releasing hormone into the cerebral ventricles activate neurons in medial preoptic nucleus and also evoke sexual behavior[109]. Taken together, these observations suggest that these medial preoptic neurons could be command neurons regulating stereotyped sexual behavior, including its autonomic and non-autonomic components.

The examples above support the view that the hypothalamus contains command neurons that are

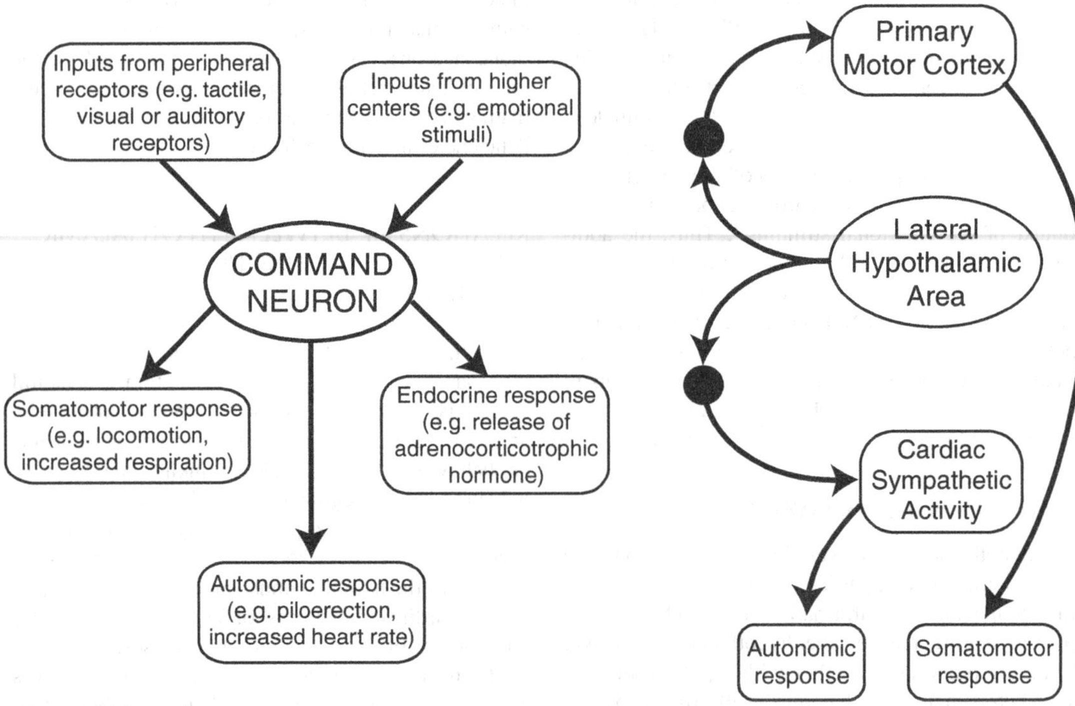


Figure 3–4 "Command neurons" in the hypothalamus and how they might control coordinated autonomic, hormonal, and behavioral responses. *Left*, Diagram illustrating the concept of a "command neuron" in the hypothalamus that regulates the autonomic, hormonal, and somatomotor components of a coordinated response that may be triggered by either external stimuli or inputs from higher centers. *Right*, Diagram showing the organization of pathways originating from putative "command neurons" within the lateral hypothalamus, which have been shown to have collateral projections to both the primary motor cortex and to the cardiac sympathetic outflow. Modified from Krout et al.[61], with permission.

specific for certain coordinated responses. Neurons with similar properties are likely to exist outside the hypothalamus. For example, the midbrain PAG is known to contain columns of neurons, each of which integrates a different pattern of defensive behavior with stereotyped somatomotor and autonomic components[7]. Activation of neurons in the lateral column of the PAG trigger fight-or-flight behavior accompanied by increased blood pressure and heart rate, responses that are characteristic of an active coping strategy. In contrast, neurons in the ventrolateral column of the PAG trigger hypoactivity accompanied by decreases in blood pressure and heart rate, characteristic of a passive coping strategy[7]. Neurons in both the lateral and ventrolateral columns of the PAG have strong reciprocal connections with hypothalamic neurons[10,72] so that the full expression of these stereotyped responses may depend upon the connections between the hypothalamus and midbrain PAG.

## HYPOTHALAMIC CONTROL OF THE AUTONOMIC NERVOUS SYSTEM IN DISEASE

The hypothalamus is thought to play an important role in generating abnormal patterns of autonomic activity in various cardiovascular disorders. In particular, overactivity of neurons in the PVN is believed to contribute to the increased sympathetic activity in neurogenic hypertension and heart failure. Furthermore, neurons in the dorsomedial hypothalamus are thought to be part of the central circuitry activated during panic attacks, which are characterized by increases in blood pressure, heart rate, and respiratory activity. In this section, the evidence supporting these views will be briefly reviewed.

### Neurogenic Hypertension

Early studies showed that lesions of the anteroventral boundary of the third ventricle attenuated or prevented various types of experimental hypertension, including renal hypertension, deoxycorticosterone acetate–salt induced hypertension, and Dahl salt-sensitive hypertension[9,40,44]. However, these studies did not clarify whether the lesions attenuated the hypertension by reducing sympathetic activity or by reducing the level of circulating vasopressin or other pressor substances. More recently, in the spontaneously hypertensive rat, inhibition of neurons within the PVN has been shown to greatly reduce lumbar sympathetic activity[4], indicating that, at least in this model, hypertension depends upon the tonic activity of the PVN-sympathetic pathway. This pathway includes a synapse with sympathetic premotor neurons in the RVLM. Angiotensin II type 1 receptors in the RVLM are also required for the increased sympathetic activity[3,52,53,100].

Sympathetic activity is also increased in obesity-related hypertension. Levels of the hormone, leptin, are increased in obesity; and it has been proposed that the sympathetic activation in obesity-related hypertension is leptin-dependent[43,80]. This suggestion is not counter-intuitive, because in obesity there is thought to be selective leptin resistance; the anorexic and weight-reducing effects of leptin are prevented, while the sympathoexcitatory and pressor actions are preserved[43]. Leptin exerts its effects by actions on hypothalamic nuclei. In particular, it can increase sympathetic vasomotor activity by an action on neurons in the ventromedial hypothalamus[67,75].

The data summarized above show that neurons in the hypothalamus can generate sustained increases in sympathetic activity, at least in some models of hypertension. Whether this is also the case in other models of neurogenic hypertension remains to be determined.

### Heart Failure

Severe congestive heart failure is associated with a marked increase in sympathetic activity, particularly cardiac and renal sympathetic activity[34]. Recent studies indicate that neurons in the hypothalamic PVN play a key role in generating this sympathetic overactivity[36,63]. PVN neurons that control sympathetic activity (PVN-sympathetic neurons) have an increased activity in heart failure[113], at least in part as a result of a reduced tonic GABAergic inhibition[63]. This reduced inhibition is associated with reduced expression of the neuronal isoform of nitric oxide synthase in the PVN[63]. Nitric oxide may normally facilitate the release of GABA in the PVN. Consequently, when neuronal nitric oxide synthase is downregulated, less GABA is released; and the PVN-sympathetic neurons are disinhibited[63,95]. The activity of sympathoexcitatory neurons in the PVN depends upon the balance between tonic excitatory effects mediated by excitatory amino acid and angiotensin type 1 receptors and tonic inhibitory effects mediated by GABA receptors[22,23]. In heart failure, blockade of glutamate or angiotensin II receptors in the PVN reduces sympathetic activity[63,113]. Thus, a shift in the balance between the inhibitory effects of GABA/nitric oxide and the excitatory effects of glutamate/angiotensin II on PVN-sympathetic neurons could lead to the sympathetic overactivity characteristic of heart failure[63].

The links between heart failure and the increased activity of PVN-sympathetic neurons are not absolutely clear, but there is evidence that circulating cytokines may play a role. An increase in the level of circulating tumor necrosis factor-alpha results in increased activity of both PVN and RVLM neurons, which is associated with increased sympathetic activity, arterial pressure and heart rate[115]. The levels of circulating tumor necrosis factor-alpha and other cytokines are increased in heart failure[24]. Hence, the cytokines may act on neurons in the hypothalamus to trigger the release of prostaglandins, which then excite PVN-sympathetic neurons[36].

### Panic Disorder

Panic disorder is characterized by increased anxiety and sympathetic activity[33]. In patients with this disorder, panic attacks can be triggered by intravenous sodium lactate injections[89]. Neurons in the dorsomedial hypothalamus are an essential component of the central circuitry mediating this response. In rats, disinhibition of neurons in the dorsomedial hypothalamus evokes a cardiovascular response, together with increased anxiety[32,88]. In rats with chronic impairment of GABAergic neurotransmission in the dorsomedial hypothalamus, intravenous injection of lactate results in the generation of a panic-like response, which is characterized by marked increases in anxiety-like behavior, blood pressure, and heart rate[90]. In contrast, chronic impairment of GABAergic neurotransmission in the PVN does not have this effect[90]. The inputs to the dorsomedial hypothalamus that trigger panic attacks are not fully defined but most likely include inputs from neurons in the basolateral nucleus of the amygdala[91].

## CONCLUDING REMARKS AND UNANSWERED QUESTIONS

Despite the progress that has been made in recent years in elucidating the connections and functions of hypothalamic neurons that regulate autonomic outflow, many fundamental questions remain unanswered. First, relatively little information is available about the organization of descending pathways from the hypothalamus that regulate autonomic changes associated with naturally evoked behaviors in conscious animals, such as thermoregulatory responses or defensive behavior. Second, the mechanisms by which hypothalamic neurons are able to act as "pattern generators," triggering coordinated autonomic, endocrine, and somatomotor components of stereotyped responses, are still unclear. Third, although synaptic transmission in the hypothalamus is profoundly affected by neurotransmitters, such as noradrenaline, serotonin, angiotensin II, and nitric oxide, very little is known about the factors and mechanisms that regulate their release. Finally, plasticity obviously occurs in autonomic circuitry within the hypothalamus, including altered properties after exercise training and in disease states such as heart failure[59,116]; but the cellular mechanisms that lead to these plastic changes are poorly understand. Nevertheless, the great progress that has been made since the publication of the previous edition of this book in 1990 indicates that at least some of these important questions are likely to be answered within the next decade.

ACKNOWLEDGEMENTS The work from my laboratory referred to here was supported by the National Health and Medical Research Council of Australia, the Australian Research Council and the National Heart Foundation of Australia.

## References

1. Abrahamson, E. E., and Moore, R. Y. (2001). The posterior hypothalamic area: Chemoarchitecture and afferent connections. *Brain Research* 889, 1–22.
2. Alam, N., Szymusiak, R., and McGinty, D. (1995). Local preoptic/anterior hypothalamic warming alters spontaneous and evoked neuronal activity in the magno-cellular basal forebrain. *Brain Research* 696, 221–230.
3. Allen, A. M. (2001) Blockade of angiotensin AT1-receptors in the rostral ventrolateral medulla of spontaneously hypertensive rats reduces blood pressure and sympathetic nerve discharge. *Journal of the Renin-Angiotensin-Aldosterone System* 2 Suppl 1, S120–S124.
4. Allen, A. M. (2002). Inhibition of the hypothalamic paraventricular nucleus in spontaneously hypertensive rats dramatically reduces sympathetic vasomotor tone. *Hypertension* 39, 275–280.
5. Anderson, J. W., Smith, P. M., and Ferguson, A. V. (2001). Subfornical organ neurons projecting to paraventricular nucleus: Whole-cell properties. *Brain Research* 921, 78–85.
6. Bains, J. S., and Ferguson, A. V. (1995). Paraventricular nucleus neurons projecting to the spinal cord receive excitatory input from the subfornical organ. *American Journal of Physiology* 268, R625–R633.
7. Bandler, R., Keay, K. A., Floyd, N., and Price, J. (2000). Central circuits mediating patterned autonomic activity during active vs. passive emotional coping. *Brain Research Bulletin* 53, 95–104.
8. Barone, F. C., Wayner, M. J., Scharoun, S. L., Guevara-Aguilar, R., and Aguilar-Baturoni, H. U. (1981). Afferent connections to the lateral hypothalamus: A horseradish peroxidase study in the rat. *Brain Research Bulletin* 7, 75–88.

9. Bealer, S. L. (1984). Hypothalamic knife cuts attenuate maintenance of deoxycorticosterone acetate-salt induced hypertension. *Brain Research* 309, 192–195.
10. Beitz, A. J. (1982). The organization of afferent projections to the midbrain periaqueductal gray of the rat. *Neuroscience* 7, 133–159.
11. Blessing, W. W. (1997). *The Lower Brainstem and Bodily Homeostasis*. New York: Oxford University Press.
12. Boehm, U., Zou, Z., and Buck, L. B. (2005). Feedback loops link odor and pheromone signaling with reproduction. *Cell* 123, 683–695.
13. Borg, M. A., Sherwin, R. S., Borg, W. P., Tamborlane, W. V., and Shulman, G. I. (1997). Local ventromedial hypothalamus glucose perfusion blocks counterregulation during systemic hypoglycemia in awake rats. *Journal of Clinical Investigation* 99, 361–365.
14. Boulant, J. A. (2000). Role of the preoptic-anterior hypothalamus in thermoregulation and fever. *Clinical Infectious Diseases* 31 Suppl 5, S157–S161.
15. Buijs, R. M., and Kalsbeek, A. (2001). Hypothalamic integration of central and peripheral clocks. *Nature Reviews Neuroscience* 2, 521–526.
16. Buijs, R. M., la Fleur, S. E., Wortel, J., Van Heyningen, C., Zuiddam, L., Mettenleiter, T. C., Kalsbeek, A., Nagai, K., and Niijima, A. (2003). The suprachiasmatic nucleus balances sympathetic and parasympathetic output to peripheral organs through separate preautonomic neurons. *Journal of Comparative Neurology* 464, 36–48.
17. Byrum, C. E., and Guyenet, P. G. (1987). Afferent and efferent connections of the A5 noradrenergic cell group in the rat. *Journal of Comparative Neurology* 261, 529–542.
18. Cano, G., Sved, A. F., Rinaman, L., Rabin, B. S., and Card, J. P. (2001). Characterization of the central nervous system innervation of the rat spleen using viral transneuronal tracing. *Journal of Comparative Neurology* 439, 1–18.
19. Card, J. P., Swanson, L. W., and Moore, R. Y. (1999). The hypothalamus: an overview of regulatory systems. In M. J. Zigmond, F. E. Bloom, S. C. Landis, J. L. Roberts, and L. R. Squire (Eds.), *Fundamental Neuroscience*, pp. 1013–1026. San Diego: Academic Press.
20. Carstens, E., Leah, J., Lechner, J., and Zimmermann, M. (1990). Demonstration of extensive brainstem projections to medial and lateral thalamus and hypothalamus in the rat. *Neuroscience* 35, 609–626.
21. Cechetto, D. F., and Saper, C. B. (1988). Neurochemical organization of the hypothalamic projection to the spinal cord in the rat. *Journal of Comparative Neurology* 272, 579–604.
22. Chen, Q. H., Haywood, J. R., and Toney G. M. (2003). Sympathoexcitation by PVN-injected bicuculline requires activation of excitatory amino acid receptors. *Hypertension* 42, 725–731.
23. Chen, Q. H., and Toney, G. M. (2003). Responses to GABA-A receptor blockade in the hypothalamic PVN are attenuated by local AT1 receptor antagonism. *American Journal of Physiology. Regulatory, Integrative and Comparative Physiology* 285, R1231–R1239.
24. Chrousos, G. P. (2000). The stress response and immune function: Clinical implications. The 1999 Novera H. Spector Lecture. *Annals of the New York Academy of Sciences* 937, 38–67.
25. Cunningham, E. T., and Sawchenko, P. E. (1988). Anatomical specificity of noradrenergic inputs to the paraventricular and supraoptic nuclei of the rat hypothalamus. *Journal of Comparative Neurology* 274, 60–76.
26. Dampney, R. A. L., and Horiuchi, J. (2003). Functional organisation of central cardiovascular pathways: Studies using c-Fos gene expression. *Progress in Neurobiology* 71, 359–384.
27. Dampney, R. A. L. (1994). Functional organization of central pathways regulating the cardiovascular system. *Physiological Reviews* 74, 323–364.
28. Dampney, R. A. L., Czachurski, J., Dembowsky, K., Goodchild, A. K., and Seller, H. (1987). Afferent connections and spinal projections of the pressor region in the rostral ventrolateral medulla of the cat. *Journal of the Autonomic Nervous System* 20, 73–86.
29. Dampney, R. A. L., and McAllen, R. M. (1988). Differential control of sympathetic fibres supplying hindlimb skin and muscle by subretrofacial neurones in the cat. *Journal of Physiology* 395, 41–56.
30. Dayas, C. V., Buller, K. M., Crane, J. W., Xu, Y., and Day, T. A. (2001). Stressor categorization: Acute physical and psychological stressors elicit distinctive recruitment patterns in the amygdala and in medullary noradrenergic cell groups. *European Journal of Neuroscience* 14, 1143–1152.
31. de Vries, M. G., Lawson, M. A., and Beverly, J. L. (2005). Hypoglycemia-induced noradrenergic activation in the VMH is a result of decreased ambient glucose. *American Journal of Physiology. Regulatory, Integrative and Comparative Physiology* 289, R977–R981.
32. DiMicco, J. A., Samuels, B. C., Zaretskaia, M. V., and Zaretsky, D. V. (2002). The dorsomedial hypothalamus and the response to stress: Part

renaissance, part revolution. *Pharmacology, Biochemistry & Behavior* 71, 469–480.
33. Esler, M., Alvarenga, M., Lambert, G., Kaye, D., Hastings, J., Jennings, G., Morris, M., Schwarz, R., and Richards, J. (2004). Cardiac sympathetic nerve biology and brain monoamine turnover in panic disorder. *Annals of the New York Academy of Sciences* 1018, 505–514.
34. Esler, M., and Kaye, D. (1998). Increased sympathetic nervous system activity and its therapeutic reduction in arterial hypertension, portal hypertension and heart failure. *Journal of the Autonomic Nervous System* 72, 210–219.
35. Farkas, E., Jansen, A. S., and Loewy, A. D. (1998). Periaqueductal gray matter input to cardiac-related sympathetic premotor neurons. *Brain Research* 792, 179–192.
36. Felder, R. B., Francis, J., Zhang, Z. H., Wei, S. G., Weiss, R. M., and Johnson, A. K. (2003). Heart failure and the brain: New perspectives. *American Journal of Physiology. Regulatory, Integrative and Comparative Physiology* 284, R259–R276.
37. Fontes, M. A., Tagawa, T., Polson, J. W., Cavanagh, S. J., and Dampney, R. A. L. (2001). Descending pathways mediating cardiovascular response from dorsomedial hypothalamic nucleus. *American Journal of Physiology. Heart and Circulatory Physiology* 280, H2893–H2901.
38. Giles, M. E., Sly, D. J., McKinley, M. J., and Oldfield, B. J. (2001). Neurons in the lamina terminalis which project polysynaptically to the kidney express angiotensin AT1A receptor. *Brain Research* 898, 9–12.
39. Gooley, J. J., Lu, J., Fischer, D., and Saper, C. B. (2003). A broad role for melanopsin in nonvisual photoreception. *Journal of Neuroscience* 23, 7093–7106.
40. Goto, A., Ganguli, M., Tobian, L., Johnson, M. A., and Iwai, J. (1982). Effect of an anteroventral third ventricle lesion on NaCl hypertension in Dahl salt-sensitive rats. *American Journal of Physiology* 243, H614–H618.
41. Granata, A. R., and Chang, H. T. (1994). Relationship of calbindin D-28k with afferent neurons to the rostral ventrolateral medulla in the rat. *Brain Research* 645, 265–277.
42. Gurdijian, E. S. (1927). The diencephalon of the albino rat. *Journal of Comparative Neurology* 43, 1–114.
43. Haynes, W. G. (2005). Role of leptin in obesity-related hypertension. *Experimental Physiology* 90, 683–688.
44. Haywood, J. R., Fink, G. D., Buggy, J., Boutelle, S., Johnson, A. K., and Brody, M. J. (1983). Prevention of two-kidney, one-clip renal hypertension in rat by ablation of AV3V tissue. *American Journal of Physiology* 245, H683–H689.
45. Herbert, H., Moga, M. M., and Saper, C. B. (1990). Connections of the parabrachial nucleus with the nucleus of the solitary tract and the medullary reticular formation in the rat. *Journal of Comparative Neurology* 293, 540–580.
46. Herbert, H., and Saper, C. B. (1992). Organization of medullary adrenergic and noradrenergic projections to the periaqueductal gray matter in the rat. *Journal of Comparative Neurology* 315, 34–52.
47. Herman, J. P., Cullinan, W. E., Ziegler, D. R., and Tasker, J. G. (2002). Role of the paraventricular nucleus microenvironment in stress integration. *European Journal of Neuroscience* 16, 381–385.
48. Herman, J. P., Tasker, J. G., Ziegler, D. R., and Cullinan, W. E. (2002). Local circuit regulation of paraventricular nucleus stress integration: Glutamate-GABA connections. *Pharmacology, Biochemistry and Behavior* 71, 457–468.
49. Holstege, G. (1987). Some anatomical observations on the projections from the hypothalamus to brainstem and spinal cord: An HRP and autoradiographic tracing study in the cat. *Journal of Comparative Neurology* 260, 98–126.
50. Hosoya, Y. (1980). The distribution of spinal projection neurons in the hypothalamus of the rat, studied with the HRP method. *Experimental Brain Research* 40, 79–87.
51. Hosoya, Y., Sugiura, Y., Ito, R., and Kohno, K. (1990). Descending projections from the hypothalamic paraventricular nucleus to the A5 area, including the superior salivatory nucleus, in the rat. *Experimental Brain Research* 82, 513–518.
52. Ito, S., Hiratsuka, M., Komatsu, K., Tsukamoto, K., Kanmatsuse, K., and Sved, A. F. (2003). Ventrolateral medulla AT1 receptors support arterial pressure in Dahl salt-sensitive rats. *Hypertension* 41, 744–750.
53. Ito, S., Komatsu, K., Tsukamoto, K., Kanmatsuse, K., and Sved, A. F. (2002). Ventrolateral medulla AT1 receptors support blood pressure in hypertensive rats. *Hypertension* 40, 552–559.
54. Janig, W., and Habler, H. J. (2000). Specificity in the organization of the autonomic nervous system: A basis for precise neural regulation of homeostatic and protective body functions. *Progress in Brain Research* 122, 351–367.
55. Jansen, A. S., Nguyen, X. V., Karpitskiy, V., Mettenleiter, T. C., and Loewy, A. D. (1995). Central command neurons of the sympathetic nervous system. Basis of the fight-or-flight response. *Science* 270, 644–646.

56. Jansen, A. S., Wessendorf, M. W., and Loewy, A. D. (1995). Transneuronal labeling of CNS neuropeptide and monoamine neurons after pseudorabies virus injections into the stellate ganglion. *Brain Research* 683, 1–24.
57. Kita, H., and Oomura, Y. (1982a). An HRP study of the afferent connections to rat lateral hypothalamic region. *Brain Research Bulletin* 8, 63–71.
58. Kita, H., and Oomura, Y. (1982b). An anterograde HRP study of retinal projections to the hypothalamus in the rat. *Brain Research Bulletin* 8, 249–253.
59. Kramer, J. M., Beatty, J. A., Plowey, E. D., and Waldrop, T. G. (2002). Exercise and hypertension: A model for central neural plasticity. *Clinical and Experimental Pharmacology and Physiology* 29, 122–126.
60. Krieg, W. J. (1932). The hypothalamus of the albino rat. *Journal of Comparative Neurology* 55, 19–89.
61. Krout, K. E., Mettenleiter, T. C., and Loewy, A. D. (2003). Single CNS neurons link both central motor and cardiosympathetic systems: A double-virus tracing study. *Neuroscience* 118, 853–866.
62. Levin, B. E., Routh, V. H., Kang, L., Sanders, N. M., and Dunn-Meynell, A. A. (2004). Neuronal glucosensing: What do we know after 50 years? *Diabetes* 53, 2521–2528.
63. Li, Y. F., and Patel, K. P. (2003). Paraventricular nucleus of the hypothalamus and elevated sympathetic activity in heart failure: The altered inhibitory mechanisms. *Acta Physiologica Scandinavica* 177, 17–26.
64. Lovick, T. A. (1987). Differential control of cardiac and vasomotor activity by neurones in nucleus paragigantocellularis lateralis in the cat. *Journal of Physiology* 389, 23–35.
65. Makino, M., Hayashi, H., Takezawa, H., Hirai, M., Saito, H., and Ebihara, S. (1997). Circadian rhythms of cardiovascular functions are modulated by the baroreflex and the autonomic nervous system in the rat. *Circulation* 96, 1667–1674.
66. Mandiyan, V. S., Coats, J. K., and Shah, N. M. (2005). Deficits in sexual and aggressive behaviors in Cnga2 mutant mice. *Nature Neuroscience* 8, 1660–1662.
67. Marsh, A. J., Fontes, M. A. P., Killinger, S., Pawlak, D. B., Polson, J. W., and Dampney, R. A. L. (2003). Cardiovascular responses evoked by leptin acting on neurons in the ventromedial and dorsomedial hypothalamus. *Hypertension* 42, 488–493.
68. McAllen, R. M., May, C. N., and Campos, R. R. (1997). The supply of vasomotor drive to individual classes of sympathetic neuron. *Clinical and Experimental Hypertension* 19, 607–618.
69. McKinley, M. J., Allen, A. M., Burns, P., Colvill, L. M., and Oldfield, B. J. (1998). Interaction of circulating hormones with the brain: The roles of the subfornical organ and the organum vasculosum of the lamina terminalis. *Clinical and Experimental Pharmacology and Physiology* 25, S61–S67.
70. McKinley, M. J., McAllen, R. M., Davern, P., Giles, M. E., Penschow, J., Sunn, N., Uschakov, A., and Oldfield, B. J. (2003). The sensory circumventricular organs of the mammalian brain. *Advances in Anatomy, Embryology and Cell Biology* 172, 1–122.
71. Meller, S. T., and Dennis, B. J. (1986). Afferent projections to the periaqueductal gray in the rabbit. *Neuroscience* 19, 927–964.
72. Meller, S. T., and Dennis, B. J. (1993). Efferent projections of the periaqueductal gray in the rabbit. *Neuroscience* 40, 193–216.
73. Mileykovskiy, B. Y., Kiyashchenko, L. I., and Siegel, J. M. (2005). Behavioral correlates of activity in identified hypocretin/orexin neurons. *Neuron* 46, 787–798.
74. Moga, M. M., Herbert, H., Hurley, K. M., Yasui, Y., Gray, T. S., and Saper, C. B. (1990). Organization of cortical, basal forebrain, and hypothalamic afferents to the parabrachial nucleus in the rat. *Journal of Comparative Neurology* 295, 624–661.
75. Montanaro, M. S., Allen, A. M., and Oldfield, B. J. (2005). Structural and functional evidence supporting a role for leptin in central neural pathways influencing blood pressure in rats. *Experimental Physiology* 90, 689–696.
76. Moore, R. Y., and Lenn, N. J. (1972). A retinohypothalamic projection in the rat. *Journal of Comparative Neurology* 146, 1–14.
77. Oldfield, B. J., Badoer, E., Hards, D. K., and McKinley, M. J. (1994). Fos production in retrogradely labelled neurons of the lamina terminalis following intravenous infusion of either hypertonic saline or angiotensin II. *Neuroscience* 60, 255–262.
78. Pan, B., Castro-Lopes, J. M., and Coimbra, A. (1999). Central afferent pathways conveying nociceptive input to the hypothalamic paraventricular nucleus as revealed by a combination of retrograde labeling and c-Fos activation. *Journal of Comparative Neurology* 413, 129–145.
79. Panzica, G. C., Viglietti-Panzica, C., and Balthazart, J. (1996). The sexually dimorphic medial preoptic nucleus of quail: A key brain area mediating steroid action on male sexual behavior. *Frontiers in Neuroendocrinology* 17, 51–125.
80. Rahmouni, K., Correia, M. L., Haynes, W. G., and Mark, A. L. (2005). Obesity-associated

hypertension: New insights into mechanisms. *Hypertension* 45, 9–14.
81. Ribeiro-Barbosa, E. R., Skorupa, A. L., Cipolla-Neto, J., and Canteras, N. S. (1999). Projections of the basal retrochiasmatic area: A neural site involved in the photic control of pineal metabolism. *Brain Research* 839, 35–40.
82. Roland, B. L., and Sawchenko, P. E. (1993). Local origins of some GABAergic projections to the paraventricular and supraoptic nuclei of the hypothalamus in the rat. *Journal of Comparative Neurology* 332, 123–143.
83. Samuels, B. C., Zaretsky, D. V., and DiMicco, J. A. (2004). Dorsomedial hypothalamic sites where disinhibition evokes tachycardia correlate with location of raphe-projecting neurons. *American Journal of Physiology. Regulatory, Integrative and Comparative Physiology* 287, R472–R478.
84. Saper, C. B. (2002). The central autonomic nervous system: Conscious visceral perception and autonomic pattern generation. *Annual Review of Neuroscience* 25, 433–469.
85. Saper, C. B., Lu, J., Chou, T. C., and Gooley, J. (2005). The hypothalamic integrator for circadian rhythms. *Trends in Neurosciences* 28, 152–157.
86. Saper, C. B., Loewy, A. D., Swanson, L. W., and Cowan, W. M. (1976). Direct hypothalamo-autonomic connections. *Brain Research* 117, 305–312.
87. Schramm, L. P., Strack, A. M., Platt, K. B., and Loewy, A. D. (1993). Peripheral and central pathways regulating the kidney: A study using pseudorabies virus. *Brain Research* 616, 251–262.
88. Shekhar, A., and Katner, J. S. (1995). Dorsomedial hypothalamic GABA regulates anxiety in the social interaction test. *Pharmacology, Biochemistry and Behavior* 50, 253–258.
89. Shekhar, A., and Keim, S. R. (1997). The circumventricular organs form a potential neural pathway for lactate sensitivity: Implications for panic disorder. *Journal of Neuroscience* 17, 9726–9735.
90. Shekhar, A., Keim, S. R., Simon, J. R., and McBride, W. J. (1996). Dorsomedial hypothalamic GABA dysfunction produces physiological arousal following sodium lactate infusions. *Pharmacology, Biochemistry and Behavior* 55, 249–256.
91. Shekhar, A., Sajdyk, T. J., Gehlert, D. R., and Rainnie, D. G. (2003). The amygdala, panic disorder, and cardiovascular responses. *Annals of the New York Academy of Sciences* 985,308–325.
92. Shepherd, G. M. (2006). Behavior, smells, brains and hormones. *Nature* 439, 149–151.
93. Simerly, R. B. (2002). Wired for reproduction: Organization and development of sexually dimorphic circuits in the mammalian forebrain. *Annual Review of Neuroscience* 25, 507–536.
94. Sly, D. J., Colvill, L., McKinley, M. J., and Oldfield, B. J. (1999). Identification of neural projections from the forebrain to the kidney, using the virus pseudorabies. *Journal of the Autonomic Nervous System* 77, 73–82.
95. Stern, J. E. (2004). Nitric oxide and homeostatic control: an intercellular signalling molecule contributing to autonomic and neuroendocrine integration? *Progress in Biophysics and Molecular Biology* 84, 197–215.
96. Stocker, S. D., Cunningham, J. T., and Toney, G. M. (2004). Water deprivation increases Fos immunoreactivity in PVN autonomic neurons with projections to the spinal cord and rostral ventrolateral medulla. *American Journal of Physiology. Regulatory, Integrative and Comparative Physiology* 287, R1172–R1183.
97. Stocker, S. D., and Toney, G. M. (2005). Median preoptic neurones projecting to the hypothalamic paraventricular nucleus respond to osmotic, circulating Ang II and baroreceptor input in the rat. *Journal of Physiology* 568, 599–615.
98. Strack, A. M., Sawyer, W. B., Hughes, J. H., Platt, K. B., and Loewy, A. D. (1989). A general pattern of CNS innervation of the sympathetic outflow demonstrated by transneuronal pseudorabies viral infections. *Brain Research* 491, 156–162.
99. Stuesse, S. L., and Fish, S. E. (1984). Projections to the cardioinhibitory region of the nucleus ambiguus of rat. *Journal of Comparative Neurology* 229, 271–278.
100. Tagawa, T., and Dampney, R. A. L. (1999). AT receptors mediate excitatory inputs to rostral ventrolateral medulla pressor neurons from hypothalamus. *Hypertension* 34, 1301–1307.
101. Ter Horst, G. J., Hautvast, R. W., De Jongste, M. J., and Korf, J. (1996). Neuroanatomy of cardiac activity-regulating circuitry: A transneuronal retrograde viral labelling study in the rat. *European Journal of Neuroscience* 8, 2029–2041.
102. Thompson, R. H., Canteras, N. S., and Swanson, L. W. (1996). Organization of projections from the dorsomedial nucleus of the hypothalamus: A PHA-L study in the rat. *Journal of Comparative Neurology* 376, 143–173.
103. Thompson, R. H., and Swanson, L. W. (1998). Organization of inputs to the dorsomedial nucleus of the hypothalamus: A reexamination with Fluorogold and PHAL in the rat. *Brain Research Reviews* 27, 89–118.
104. Thompson, R. H., and Swanson, L. W. (2003). Structural characterization of a hypothalamic

visceromotor pattern generator network. *Brain Research Reviews* 41, 153–202.

105. Toney, G. M., Chen, Q. H., Cato, M. J., and Stocker, S. D. (2003). Central osmotic regulation of sympathetic nerve activity. *Acta Physiologica Scandinavica* 177, 43–55.
106. van den Pol, A. N. (1999). Hypothalamic hypocretin (orexin): Robust innervation of the spinal cord. *Journal of Neuroscience* 19, 3171–3182.
107. Vizzard, M. A., Erickson, V. L., Card, J. P., Roppolo, J. R., and de Groat, W. C. (1995). Transneuronal labeling of neurons in the adult rat brainstem and spinal cord after injection of pseudorabies virus into the urethra. *Journal of Comparative Neurology* 355, 629–640.
108. Vrang, N., Mikkelsen, J. D., and Larsen, P. J. (1997). Direct link from the suprachiasmatic nucleus to hypothalamic neurons projecting to the spinal cord: A combined tracing study using cholera toxin subunit B and *Phaseolus vulgaris*-leucoagglutinin. *Brain Research Bulletin* 44, 671–680.
109. Westberry, J., and Meredith, M. (2003). The influence of chemosensory input and gonadotropin releasing hormone on mating behavior circuits in male hamsters. *Brain Research* 974, 1–16.
110. Westerhaus, M. J., and Loewy, A. D. (1999). Sympathetic-related neurons in the preoptic region of the rat identified by viral transneuronal labeling. *Journal of Comparative Neurology* 414, 361–378.
111. Yoon, H., Enquist, L. W., and Dulac, C. (2005). Olfactory inputs to hypothalamic neurons controlling reproduction and fertility. *Cell* 123, 669–682.
112. Yoshida, K., McCormack, S., Espana, R. A., Crocker, A., and Scammell, T. E. (2006). Afferents to the orexin neurons of the rat brain. *Journal of Comparative Neurology* 494, 845–861.
113. Zhang, Z. H., Francis, J., Weiss, R. M., and Felder, R. B. (2002). The renin-angiotensin-aldosterone system excites hypothalamic paraventricular nucleus neurons in heart failure. *American Journal of Physiology. Heart and Circulatory Physiology* 283, H423–H433.
114. Zhang, Y. H., Lu, J., Elmquist, J. K., and Saper, C. B. (2000). Lipopolysaccharide activates specific populations of hypothalamic and brainstem neurons that project to the spinal cord. *Journal of Neuroscience* 20, 6578–6586.
115. Zhang, Z. H., Wei, S. G., Francis, J., and Felder, R. B. (2003). Cardiovascular and renal sympathetic activation by blood-borne TNF-alpha in rat: The role of central prostaglandins. *American Journal of Physiology. Regulatory, Integrative and Comparative Physiology* 284, R916–R927.
116. Zucker, I. H., Wang, W., Pliquett, R. U., Liu, J. L., and Patel, K. P. (2001). The regulation of sympathetic outflow in heart failure. The roles of angiotensin II, nitric oxide, and exercise training. *Annals of the New York Academy of Sciences* 940, 431–443.

# 4

# Autonomic and Neuroendocrine Roles of the Paraventricular Nucleus

JAVIER E. STERN

## THE PVN: A CENTER FOR AUTONOMIC AND NEUROENDOCRINE INTEGRATION

Maintenance of bodily homeostasis involves complex interactions between three major information-processing systems within the brain and spinal cord, namely the *endocrine*, the *neuroendocrine*, and the *autonomic nervous systems*. Concerted actions among these systems are generally required for proper adaptive cardiovascular, fluid, and energy balance responses. It is important to note that an unbalanced interaction amongst these systems may result in maladaptive responses characteristic of various disease conditions, such as stress[29], heart failure[136], and the metabolic syndrome[47,85].

Despite the importance of balanced and coordinated autonomic-neuroendocrine outputs, relatively little is known about the mechanisms underlying the generation and integration of complex patterns of homeostatic responses, particularly at the cellular and/or network levels.

Evidence accumulated over more than 20 years supports the view that the paraventricular nucleus of the hypothalamus (PVN) is a key neuronal substrate in homeostatic control[116,117]. To subserve this complex function, the PVN must be able to monitor and integrate information about the body's internal environment. In concert with other central autonomic nuclei, the PVN also needs to generate appropriate efferent autonomic and neuroendocrine signals so that a constant internal environment is maintained.

Information about the status of the internal environment reaches the PVN by means of viscerosensory afferents as well as through blood-borne signals[77] (see Figure 4–1). For example, key sensory information regarding fluid-balance homeostasis and cardiovascular control arises primarily from aortic baroreceptors[43], atrial volume receptors[93], and peripheral chemoreceptors[96], as well as central osmoreceptors located in the circumventricular organs[70]. These include the subfornical organ (SFO) and the organum vasculosum of the lamina terminalis (OVLT), which are known to mediate the actions of circulating angiotensin II on drinking behavior, vasopressin release, and sympathetic outflow [65]. Other critical afferent pathways/signals within the PVN that influence fluid balance and cardiovascular homeostasis include projections from the suprachiasmatic nucleus, which provide cues for the day/night rhythmic control of autonomic/neuroendocrine patterns[16] and circulating steroids[31].

Efferent projections from the PVN can be largely segregated into three main groups, including (a) axons that target the posterior pituitary, which secrete the neurohormones oxytocin and vasopressin and play a role in fluid balance and reproductive homeostasis; (b) axons that supply the median eminence, which secretes a variety of hypophysiotropic hormones and participates in the control of the major hypothalamic-pituitary axes; and (c) long, descending projections to autonomic centers in the brainstem and spinal cord, including the rostral ventrolateral medulla (RVLM), the nucleus of the solitary tract (NTS), the dorsal motor nucleus of the vagus (dorsal vagal nucleus [DVN]) and sympathetic preganglionic neurons located in the lateral horn of the thoracic and upper lumbar spinal cord[115] (see Figure 4–1).

The autonomic-related projections from the PVN play important roles in control of the cardiovascular system and fluid balance[20,23]. For example, activation of PVN neurons induces sympathoexcitatory and pressor responses via excitatory connections with the RVLM[118,130], and PVN-RVLM projections contribute to elevated sympathoexcitatory activity during hypertension[1,2]. Projections from the PVN to the NTS have been shown to modulate the firing activity of NTS neurons[11,27] and glutamatergic visceral afferent transmission within the NTS[8,86]. These actions are thought to play a role in baroreflex suppression mediated by the PVN[19,28,68] and in autonomic and circulatory adjustments to exercise in trained rats[69]. Thus, through modulatory actions on the baroreceptor reflex and on the activities of sympathetic and parasympathetic neurons, the PVN is in a pivotal position to contribute to the short- and long-term control of the cardiovascular system.

Taken together, these data indicate that, in response to afferent signals carrying information about the status of the internal environment, the PVN is capable of generating complex patterns of neuroendocrine and autonomic output by means of reciprocal interconnections with autonomic centers in the brainstem and spinal cord, as well as through projections to the median eminence and posterior pituitary. These homeostatic responses include a *humoral component,*

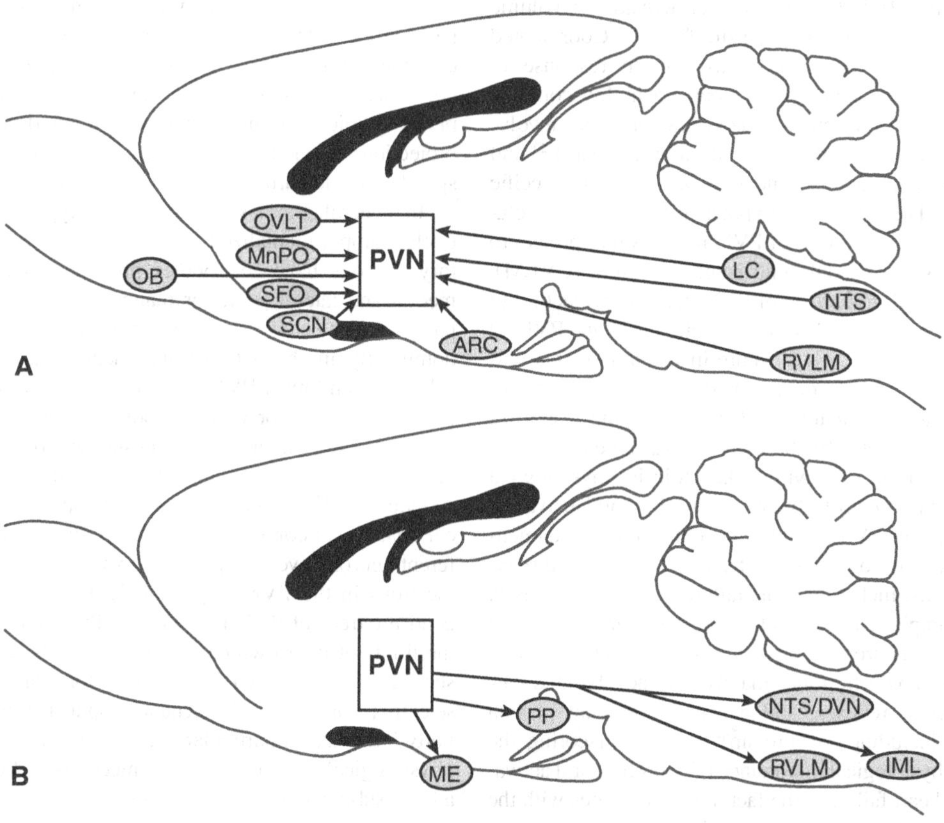


Figure 4–1 Afferent and efferent pathways of the paraventricular nucleus (PVN). Schematic diagram summarizing the major afferents (*A*) and efferent (*B*) pathways of the PVN. ARC, arcuate nucleus; DVN, dorsal motor nucleus of the vagus; IML, intermediolateral column of the spinal cord; LC, locus coeruleus; ME, median eminence; MnPO, median preoptic nucleus; NTS, nucleus of the solitary tract; OB, olfactory bulb; OVLT, organum vasculosum of the lamina terminalis; PP, posterior pituitary; RVLM; rostral ventrolateral medulla; SCN, suprachiasmatic nucleus; SFO, subfornical organ. Modified from Burbach et al. (2001)[17], with permission.

in the form of neurosecretion of vasopressin, oxytocin and hypophysiotropic factors; and a *neuronal component*, which modulates sympathetic and parasympathetic outflows.

Challenges to fluid-balance homeostasis provide a good example of the coordinated nature of homeostatic responses involving the PVN. During dehydration, both neurosecretory and autonomic neurons in the PVN are activated, as shown by the expression of the early-gene *c-fos*[66,111], resulting in increased vasopressin secretion[113] and sympathoexcitation[109,110]. A role for the PVN in the modulation of drinking responses is also well established[40,67] These coordinated autonomic, neuroendocrine, and behavioral responses result ultimately in the proper restoration and maintenance of blood pressure and blood volume.

In addition to dehydration, other cardiovascular-related challenges also modulate the activity, and/or increase *c-fos* expression in, both neurosecretory and autonomic PVN neurons. These include circulating angiotensin II[9,18,56,71], baroreceptor activation[43], volume loading[6,21,58,94], and hypotension[49,55,88,99]. Coordinated neurosecretory/autonomic activation in response to these various challenges is clearly a highly complex and incompletely characterized phenomenon, involving the activation of distinct afferent pathways [22] and selective populations of neurons, according to specific stimuli. Thus, whereas hypotension activates a relatively large proportion of PVN neurons that project to the NTS and caudal ventrolateral medulla (CVLM), only a small proportion of PVN neurons projecting to sympathetic related areas (e.g., spinal cord and RVLM) are activated[7,14,22]. Thus, future investigations that elucidate the mechanisms and pathways underlying specific patterns of autonomic/neuroendocrine responses that are integrated by the PVN are warranted.

In addition to playing a key role in physiological homeostatic control, abnormal neurohumoral activation driven by the PVN is believed to constitute a fundamental pathophysiological mechanism in various disease conditions, including heart failure[79,136] and diabetes[135]. For example, a hallmark of congestive heart failure is an increased neurohumoral drive, characterized by elevated sympathetic tone (mainly cardiac), blunted cardiovascular reflexes, and elevated hormonal plasma levels, including vasopressin[64,76,136]. Underscoring the pathophysiological importance of neurohumoral activation in heart failure is the fact that it correlates with the severity of the disease, determining to a large extent the risk, prognosis, and mortality of heart failure patients[30].

A growing body of evidence supports an important contribution of the PVN to increased neurohumoral drive during heart failure; and changes in various neurotransmitter systems, including glutamate, nitric oxide, and GABA[76,79,80,81,82,123,132], as well as proinflammatory cytokines[42,131], have been identified as key underlying mechanisms. Moreover, manipulations that improve neurohumoral drive during heart failure, including exercise[45,134], modify the efficacy of these neurotransmitter systems, alleviating the elevated neurohumoral drive in this condition. This example underpins both the physiological and pathological relevance of understanding the precise mechanisms underlying autonomic/neuroendocrine integration by the PVN.

## Cellular Organization of Neuroendocrine and Autonomic Regions of the PVN

Discrete populations of anatomically and functionally differentiated neurons control the three principal modalities by which the PVN influences homeostasis[115,124]. These include: a) magnocellular neurosecretory neurons, which synthesize oxytocin and vasopressin, project to the posterior pituitary, and participate in the control of reproduction and fluid balance; b) parvocellular neuroendocrine neurons, which project to the median eminence and secrete hypophysiotropic hormones, including corticotropin-releasing factor, thyrotropin-releasing hormone, and somatostatin; and c) parvocellular preautonomic neurons, which send long descending projections to autonomic centers in the brainstem and spinal cord and participate in autonomic control[62].

In general, these various neuronal types are relatively compartmentalized. Magnocellular neurosecretory neurons have cell bodies predominantly in the medial and lateral posterior magnocellular subnuclei; parvocellular neuroendocrine neurons are located predominantly in the anterior and medial parvocellular subnuclei, and most PVN-preautonomic neurons lie in the ventromedial (or ventral subdivision of the medial parvocellular subnucleus), posterior (or lateral parvocellular), and dorsal cap (or dorsal parvocellular) subnuclei[5,115,117,124] (see Figure 4–2). Despite this apparent anatomical compartmentalization, functionally different neurons overlap spatially at various rostrocaudal locations in the PVN (Figure 4–3). Furthermore, the dendritic trees of PVN neurons usually extend beyond the limits of their own compartments[103]. Thus, caution should be taken when considering, for example, the selectivity of a particular synaptic input that preferentially innervates a particular region of the PVN, or the physiological responses to microinjections of drugs into a PVN subnucleus.

Neuroanatomical studies have shown that largely segregated populations of PVN-preautonomic neurons project to parasympathetic- and sympathetic-related autonomic targets in the spinal cord and brainstem areas, including the dorsal vagal complex, the RVLM, and the spinal cord[87,91,95,101]. Interestingly, a small proportion of neurons have been shown to project to both

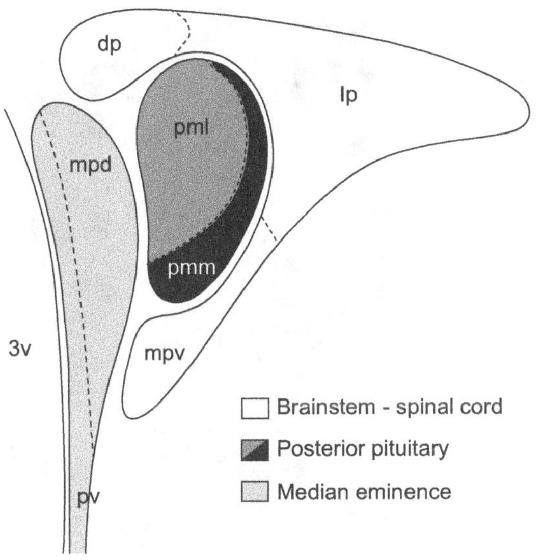


Figure 4–2 Functional and anatomical subdivisions of the PVN. dp, dorsal parvocellular subnucleus; lp, lateral parvocellular subnucleus; mpd, v, dorsal and ventral subdivisions of the medial parvocellular subnucleus; pml, pmm, lateral (vasopressinergic, *dark grey*) and medial (oxytocinergic, *black*) subdivisions of the posterior magnocellular subnucleus; pv, periventricular nucleus; 3V, third ventricle. Modified from Swanson and Sawchenko (1983)[117], with permission.

the RVLM and the spinal cord[92,101]. Whether the latter constitute an anatomically and functionally distinct subgroup within the population of PVN-preautonomic neurons is at present unknown. Studies using transneuronal viral tracing support a segregation between PVN-preautonomic neurons in sympathetic versus parasympathetic circuits and suggest that PVN preautonomic neurons are topographically organized according to the innervated tissue[16,112,114].

Cellular heterogeneity within the PVN is not only reflected in the presence of functionally different neurons (e.g., endocrine, neuroendocrine, and autonomic) but also by the wide array of neuroactive substances expressed by these neurons. For example, in addition to oxytocin and vasopressin, various other neuropeptides are co-expressed in magnocellular neurosecretory neurons[33]. Of particular interest is the co-localization and co-release of vasopressin and dynorphin from the same neurosecretory vesicles in vasopressin neurons. This co-release modulates the rhythmical electrical activity of secreting neurons in an autocrine fashion[15,100]. Finally, activity-dependent changes in the peptidergic phenotype of neurons in the PVN and supraoptic nucleus (SON)[12] add another layer of complexity to the cellular heterogeneity associated with these structures.

Although they are studied to a much lesser extent, evidence indicates that preautonomic neurons in the PVN are also neurochemically heterogeneous[98]. For example, various peptides, most predominantly oxytocin and vasopressin, are expressed in PVN-preautonomic neurons. Similarly to their magnocellular neurosecretory counterparts, PVN-preautonomic neurons show highly complex patterns of expression of peptides. For example, while some evidence supports the idea that specific neurochemical types of PVN neurons occur in specific PVN subnuclei[36,98], neurons projecting to a single target may express different peptides. Besides the well-established occurrence of peptides in descending pathways from the PVN, it is becoming increasingly clear that the excitatory amino acid glutamate is also a key neurotransmitter in these neurons[111,129]. Furthermore, the specific activation during water deprivation of neurons expressing vesicular glutamate transporter 2, but not oxytocin- or vasopressin-containing PVN-preautonomic neurons[111], supports a link between neurochemical and functional heterogeneity within the PVN. Clearly, more studies are needed to determine the functional significance of neurochemical heterogeneity within the PVN.

In addition to the main output neurons, inhibitory GABAergic and excitatory glutamatergic interneurons are found within the PVN and in regions surrounding the PVN [119]. Furthermore, PVN neurons are intimately associated with local astroglial cells and the microvasculature. While glial cells are known to play a key role in the modulation of magnocellular neurosecretory neurons[37,122,34], their potential roles in the control of autonomic function in health and disease are at present unknown.

## ANATOMICAL AND FUNCTIONAL DISTINCTIONS BETWEEN NEUROENDOCRINE AND AUTONOMIC PVN NEURONS

In the early 1990s, elegant work combining intracellular recordings, intracellular labeling, and immunohistochemistry established some basic electrophysiological criteria that enabled the distinction of PVN neurons into two major groups: type I (putative magnocellular neurosecretory neurons), and type II (putative parvocellular neurons)[38,120]. The most prominent difference between type I (putative magnocellular) and type II (putative parvocellular) neurons is their ability to generate either a pronounced transient outward rectifying current (present in type I but not type II neurons) or a $Ca^{2+}$-dependent low-threshold spike (present in some type II but not in

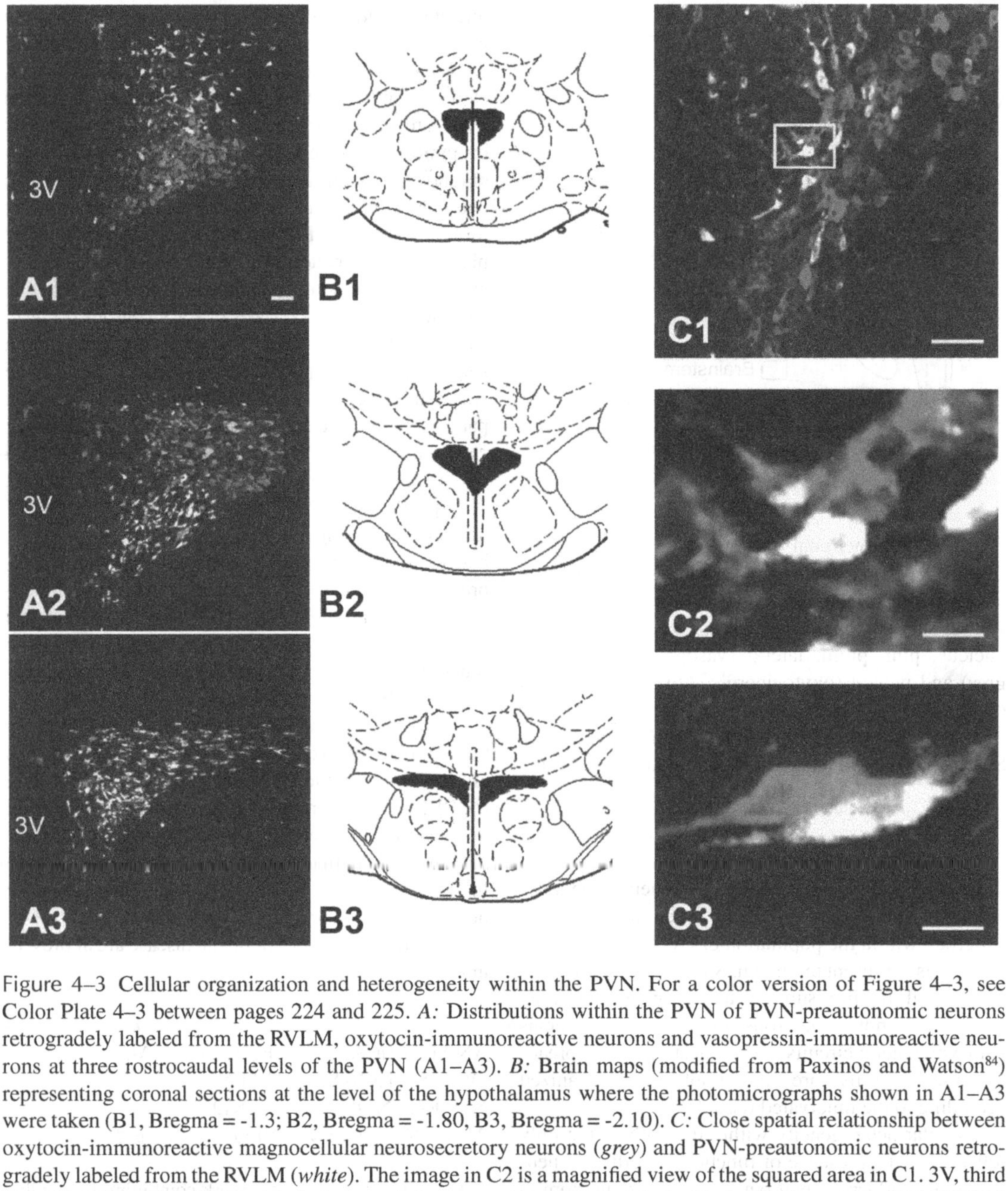


Figure 4–3 Cellular organization and heterogeneity within the PVN. For a color version of Figure 4–3, see Color Plate 4–3 between pages 224 and 225. *A:* Distributions within the PVN of PVN-preautonomic neurons retrogradely labeled from the RVLM, oxytocin-immunoreactive neurons and vasopressin-immunoreactive neurons at three rostrocaudal levels of the PVN (A1–A3). *B:* Brain maps (modified from Paxinos and Watson[84]) representing coronal sections at the level of the hypothalamus where the photomicrographs shown in A1–A3 were taken (B1, Bregma = -1.3; B2, Bregma = -1.80, B3, Bregma = -2.10). *C:* Close spatial relationship between oxytocin-immunoreactive magnocellular neurosecretory neurons (*grey*) and PVN-preautonomic neurons retrogradely labeled from the RVLM (*white*). The image in C2 is a magnified view of the squared area in C1. 3V, third ventricle. There are double-labeled oxytocin/vasopressin neurons and double-labeled oxytocin/PVN-RVLM neurons. Bars: A, 100 μm; C1, 80 μm; C2–C3, 20 μm.

type I neurons). Differences in the balance between two main subthreshold conductances, namely the A-type $K^+$ current IA, (found predominantly in type I cells) and the T-type $Ca^{2+}$ current $I_T$ (found predominantly in type II neurons) have subsequently been shown to underlie these two different electrophysiological responses[63]. Although this approach continues to be used to differentiate magnocellular from parvocellular neurons, it does not distinguish between functionally different subtypes of parvocellular neurons, such as parvocellular neuroendocrine and PVN-preautonomic neurons.

Using a multidisciplinary approach as described above, we have recently obtained a detailed morphological and electrophysiological characterization of different subsets of PVN-preautonomic neurons[54,103] and have further expanded the available knowledge on the cellular mechanisms underlying neuronal excitability and plasticity in PVN and SON neurons[4,39,105,13,78,102]. Morphologically, PVN-preautonomic neurons have longer dendrites with more branching than their neuroendocrine counterparts[97,103] (Figure 4–4).

Some distinctive structural features of PVN-preautonomic neurons include the presence of dendrites ending in close apposition to the walls of the third ventricle, with dendritic branches crossing to the contralateral PVN. In addition, in a large proportion of neurons, axons were found to originate from proximal dendrites[103]. Electrophysiologically, PVN-preautonomic neurons are characterized by the presence of $Ca^{2+}$-dependent low-threshold spikes and a robust $I_T$[103] and display either continuous irregular firing or firing in spontaneous, brief bursts[54,103] (Figure 4–4).

Despite these characteristic features, there is still a high degree of structural and functional heterogeneity within PVN-preautonomic neurons, which appears to be, at least in part, dependent on the targets that they innervate. While PVN-preautonomic neurons that project to the RVLM and PVN-preautonomic neurons that project to the NTS are similarly inhibited by nitric oxide[54], we found that noradrenaline inhibits more PVN neurons that project to the NTS than PVN neurons that project to the RVLM (Figure 4–4). Since noradrenaline potently excites magnocellular neurosecretory neurons[3,24], these results suggest that noradrenaline may have a gating role within the PVN, increasing neurosecretory output while inhibiting autonomic output. However, the specific condition/s under which this mechanism would become functionally relevant are at present unknown.

## PARACRINE SIGNALING MECHANISMS UNDERLYING TRANSFER OF INFORMATION WITHIN AND BETWEEN AUTONOMIC AND NEUROENDOCRINE CIRCUITS IN THE PVN

Homeostatic responses coordinated by the PVN involve concomitant changes in autonomic and endocrine/neuroendocrine outputs. Consequently, local integrative processes, as well as information transfer across the functionally diverse circuits within the PVN, are thought to contribute to generation of the various output patterns from the PVN that affect homeostasis[104,116,124].

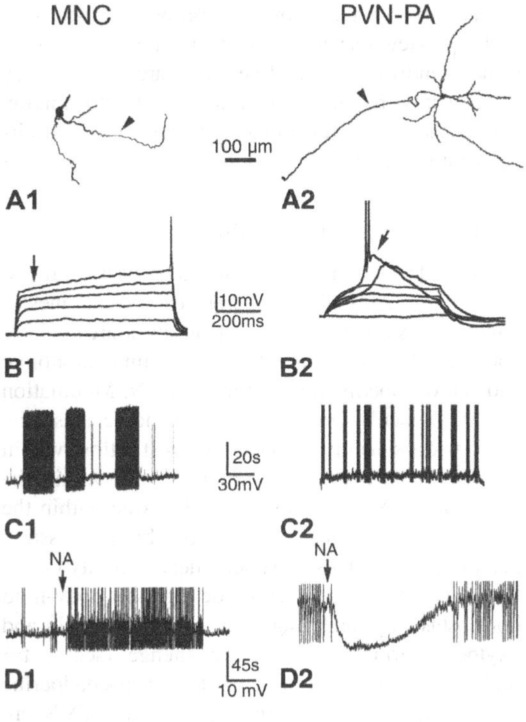


Figure 4–4 Morphological and functional distinctions between magnocellular neuroendocrine (magnocellular neurosecretory neuron) and preautonomic (PVN-preautonomic) PVN neurons. *A:* Representative examples of an intracellularly filled and reconstructed magnocellular neurosecretory neuron (*A1*) and a PVN neuron that projects to the nucleus of the solitary tract (*B1*). Note that the NTS-projecting PVN neuron has a more complex and extensive dendritic arbor. Arrowheads, axons. *B:* In response to membrane depolarization, magnocellular neurosecretory neurons display a strong transient outward rectification (*B1, arrow*), which delays the occurrence of an action potential. On the other hand, PVN-preautonomic neurons respond with a low-threshold depolarization (*B2, LTD, arrow*), which usually triggers a few overriding action potentials. *C:* Bursting firing pattern obtained from a vasopressin-immunoreactive magnocellular neurosecretory neuron (*C1*) and from an NTS-projecting PVN-preautonomic neuron (*C2*). The magnocellular neurosecretory neuron has longer-lasting bursts than the PVN-preautonomic neuron. *D:* Changes in the membrane potential and discharge of a magnocellular neurosecretory neuron (*D1*) and an NTS-projecting PVN-preautonomic neuron in response to application of noradrenaline (NA, 200 μM) (*D2*). NA induces membrane depolarization and increased firing in the magnocellular neurosecretory neuron but the opposite occurs in the PVN-preautonomic neuron.

As summarized below, emerging evidence supports the view that nitric oxide signaling, as well as somatodendritic release of peptides, are potential key mechanisms required for transfer of information within and across functionally distinct neuronal circuits within the PVN.

## Nitric Oxide Signaling within the PVN

Nitric oxide is a non-conventional gaseous neurotransmitter that readily diffuses across cell membranes to affect targets relatively distant from its source of production[128]. It is a key molecule controlling autonomic and neuroendocrine function in the PVN. Modulation of cardiovascular and fluid-balance homeostasis by nitric oxide is mainly mediated by direct actions within the central nervous system, in particular within the SON and PVN. For example, nitric oxide within the PVN induces a reduction in arterial blood pressure, heart rate, and renal sympathetic nerve activity (see [48] for review). Likewise, nitric oxide regulates body-fluid homeostasis by inhibiting release of vasopressin and oxytocin during an osmotic challenge (see [41] for review). The effects of nitric oxide on neuroendocrine and autonomic output from the SON and PVN are mediated by inhibition of the activity of both magnocellular neurosecretory neurons[10,57,106,108] and PVN-preautonomic neurons[52,54]. It is important to note that inhibition of both PVN cell types by nitric oxide is mediated indirectly by activation of local GABAergic interneurons (see [104] for review), supporting nitric oxide–GABA interactions as a key signaling mechanism within the PVN, which probably contributes to the coordination of neuroendocrine and autonomic responses (Figure 4–5).

Important factors influencing the efficacy of nitric oxide as a signaling molecule include (a) the nitric oxide synthase isoforms involved in its synthesis, (b) the cell type producing nitric oxide, and (c) how close the site of nitric oxide synthesis is to its cellular targets (see [83] for review). Neuronal nitric oxide synthase is the most abundant isoform in the brain. This isoform is highly expressed in the SON and PVN[126], where its expression is non-uniformly distributed among functionally different neuronal populations. While both oxytocin- and vasopressin-containing magnocellular neurosecretory neurons express abundant levels of neuronal nitric oxide synthase[75], only a relatively small proportion of PVN-preautonomic neurons express detectable levels of the protein[44,54,127]. Since nitric oxide efficiently modulates autonomic function, as well as the discharge of most PVN-preautonomic neurons, the low abundance of neuronal nitric oxide synthase protein expression in PVN-preautonomic neurons suggests that nitric oxide produced by and diffusing from an alternative source, such as the magnocellular neurosecretory neurons, contributes to the nitric oxide–mediated modulation of autonomic outflow from the PVN[104]. In this scenario, nitric oxide could act as a bridging molecule, facilitating communication between cells and circuits in the neuroendocrine and autonomic compartments of the PVN. This intercellular and inter-network communication would be particularly important under conditions in which synchronized neuroendocrine and autonomic responses are required.

In addition to neuronal nitric oxide synthase, other isoforms also contribute to nitric oxide availability and actions within the SON and PVN. For example, endothelial nitric oxide synthase protein is expressed both by endothelial[32] and glial cells in the PVN and contributes to constitutive nitric oxide availability and to the modulation of neuronal activity in the SON and PVN[104] (Figure 4–5). Moreover, expression of endothelial nitric oxide synthase in the PVN is modulated by activation of β-type estrogen receptors[32], which are mainly expressed in PVN-preautonomic neurons[107]. Thus, nitric oxide produced by both endothelial and glial cells can efficiently modulate neurohumoral output from the PVN by regulating the activity of magnocellular neurosecretory and PVN-preautonomic neurons. Since the activity of endothelial nitric oxide synthase can also be stimulated by neurotransmitters, including glutamate and ATP[53], it is likely that nitric oxide signaling among neurons, glial cells, and the local microvasculature contributes to communication within and across neuroendocrine and autonomic circuits in the PVN. A similar mechanism has been recently proposed to control secretion of gonadotropin-releasing hormone from the median eminence[90].

## Somatodendritic Release of Peptides as an Autocrine/Paracrine Signal within the SON and PVN

It has become increasingly clear in recent years that in addition to secretion from their terminals in the posterior pituitary, vasopressin and oxytocin are also released from somata and dendrites of magnocellular neurosecretory neurons within the SON and PVN[60]. Large dense-core vesicles contain neuropeptides, and ultrastructural studies have revealed the presence of many large dense-core vesicles in the dendrites of magnocellular neurosecretory neurons. Furthermore, these dendrites also show exocytotic profiles, which are the ultrastructural signatures for the release of the contents of a synaptic vesicle. These observations provide evidence for release of peptides from the dendrites of magnocellular neurosecretory neurons[89] (see also Figure 4–6). It is important to note that dendritic and axonal release of peptides can be modulated independently, depending upon the nature of the physiological stimulus[60]. Release of peptides from dendrites requires an elevation in intracellular $Ca^{2+}$.

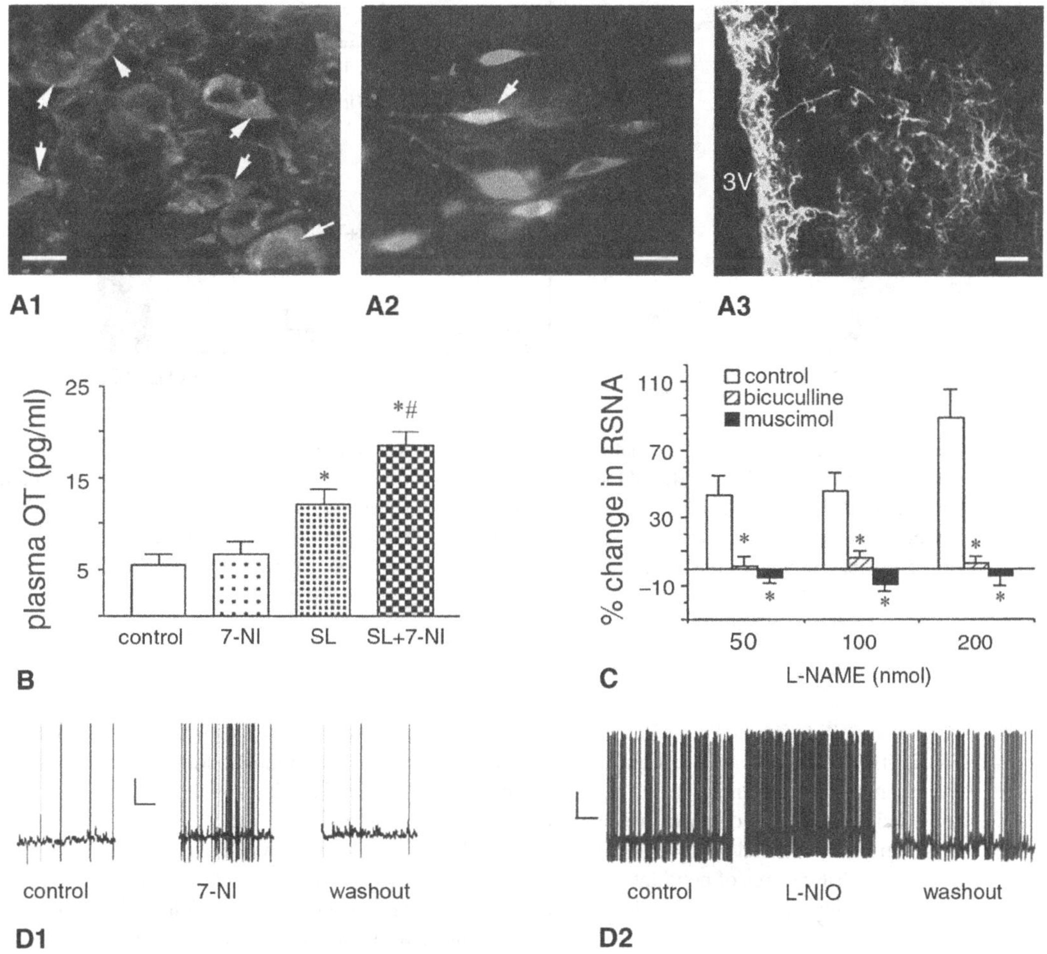


Figure 4–5 Nitric oxide modulatory actions on the autonomic and neuroendocrine PVN. For a color version of Figure 4–5, see Color Plate 4–5 between pages 224 and 225. *A:* Neuronal nitric oxide synthase immunoreactivity in vasopressin-immunoreactive magnocellular neurosecretory neurons and in PVN-preautonomic neurons retrogradely labeled from the NTS. Arrows, double-labeled neurons. *A3*: Double staining for glial fibrillary acidic protein (GFAP) and endothelial nitric oxide synthase (eNOS) in the PVN. There is a high degree of co-localization of the two immunoreactivities. *B:* Effects of 7-nitroindazole (7-NI; 50 mg/kg), which blocks the activity of neuronal nitric oxide synthase, on plasma levels of oxytocin 24 hours after salt loading (SL). The increase in plasma oxytocin induced by SL is potentiated in the presence of 7-NI. *P< 0.05 compared with control; # P< 0.05 compared with SL group. *C:* Change in renal sympathetic nerve activity (RSNA) following microinjections of L-nitroarginine methyl ester (L-NAME), a non-specific antagonist of nitric oxide synthase, into the PVN in the absence or presence of the GABAA receptor antagonist, bicuculline, or agonist, muscimol, respectively. *P< 0.05 compared with control. *D:* Blockade of neuronal nitric oxide synthase (7-NI, 100 μM, *D1*) or endothelial nitric oxide synthase with *N*-iminoethyl-L-ornithine (L-NIO, 10 μM, *D2*), increases the firing of PVN-preautonomic neurons that project to the RVLM. Scale bars in *A1* and *A2:* 25 μm, Bar in A3: 70 μm. Vertical and horizontal bars in *D1* and *D2:* 20 mV and 2 s, and 20 mV and 10 s, respectively. *B1* reproduced from Ventura et al. (2005)[125], with permission. *C* reproduced from Zhang and Patel (1998)[133], with permission. *D1* modified from Li et al. (2003)[54], with permission.

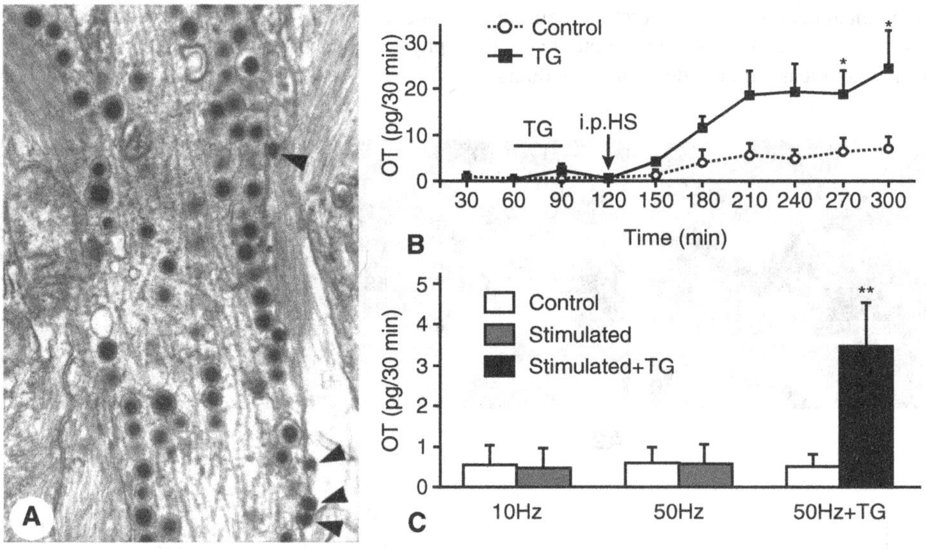


Figure 4–6 Release of peptides from somata and dendrites in the magnocellular neurosecretory system. *A:* Electron micrograph of a dendrite in the SON showing exocytosed vesicle cores (arrowheads) detected using tannic acid treatment. *B:* Thapsigargin (TG), an agent that mobilizes intracellular $Ca^{2+}$ stores, promotes dendritic release of oxytocin in response to an osmotic stimulus, intraperitoneal injection of hypertonic saline (i.p. HS), or *C:* in response to antidromic stimulation of the neural stalk. Modified from Morris and Ludwig (2004)[73], with permission.

Thus, signals that mobilize intracellular $Ca^{2+}$ stores, such as oxytocin itself[50], or induce an influx of $Ca^{2+}$ through voltage-gated $Ca^{2+}$ channels, such as vasopressin[25], can efficiently trigger dendritic release of peptides. In addition, mobilization of intracellular $Ca^{2+}$ stores primes dendritic stores of peptides, making them available for subsequent activity-dependent release[60] (see Figure 4–6).

Activity-dependent somatodendritic release of neuropeptides plays an important role in neuroendocrine control, mostly by modulating the discharge of vasopressin and oxytocin neurons. For example, blockade of the V1a subtype of vasopressin receptors in the SON increased the discharge rate of vasopressin neurons, suggesting that endogenous vasopressin is auto-inhibitory[59]. However, another study showed that modulatory effects of vasopressin depend on the initial level of activity in vasopressin neurons. This observation supports the idea that the release of vasopressin within the PVN may serve as a feedback mechanism by which the activity of the entire population of vasopressin neurons is equalized to an average level[35]. Similarly, locally released oxytocin facilitates the activity of oxytocin neurons and pituitary hormone–release in an autocrine/paracrine manner[46,72,74]. Thus, somatodendritic release of oxytocin and vasopressin provides autocrine/paracrine signals by which magnocellular neurosecretory neurons can modulate their own electrical activity as well as hormone-release.

In addition to this well-established modality of cell-type specific auto-modulation, recent evidence suggests that somatodendritic release of oxytocin and vasopressin by magnocellular neurosecretory neurons may affect other cell types within the PVN (e.g., PVN-preautonomic neurons and astrocytes), contributing to inter-network communication within the PVN. For instance, activation of oxytocin receptors on hypothalamic astrocytes in culture increases intracellular $Ca^{2+}$ in these cells[26]. Furthermore, activation of oxytocin receptors in hypothalamic slices rapidly induces glial plasticity in the SON, including retraction of glial processes and reduction of the coverage of neurons by astrocytic processes[51], similar to that observed *in vivo*[121]. It is important to note that the increase in astroglial $Ca^{2+}$ induced by neuropeptides could in turn lead to the activation of endothelial nitric oxide synthase, the subsequent release of nitric oxide, and modulation of distant targets. Thus, enhanced release of vasopressin with the PVN during dehydration[61] may contribute to the increase in sympathoexcitation driven by the PVN during this state[110]. Taken together, these data suggest that activity-dependent, somatodendritic release of PVN peptides, acting either in a nitric oxide–dependent or independent manner, may be an important signaling mechanism contributing to cell–cell communication and autonomic and neuroendocrine integration within the PVN.

## SUMMARY AND CONCLUSIONS

Homeostatic control involves intricate interactions among peripheral humoral signals and afferent neuronal pathways, along with complex integrative properties that result from extensive bidirectional connections between the endocrine/neuroendocrine and autonomic systems[77]. Based on its complex pattern of inputs and outputs, its neurochemical heterogeneity, and the presence of functionally discrete neuronal circuits, the PVN is capable of orchestrating complex and coordinated patterns of endocrine, neuroendocrine, and autonomic responses, making it a pivotal structure for the maintenance of homeostasis.

Despite the importance of the PVN in homeostatic control, little is yet known about the detailed mechanisms underlying its ability to coordinate neurohumoral output in response to specific challenges. Insights into this functionally relevant problem will emerge from further studies on the mechanisms controlling neuronal activity within each of the functionally discrete PVN circuits, as well as those mediating cell–cell communication among these circuits.

### References

1. Akine, A., Montanaro, M., and Allen, A. M. (2003). Hypothalamic paraventricular nucleus inhibition decreases renal sympathetic nerve activity in hypertensive and normotensive rats. *Autonomic Neuroscience* 108, 17–21.
2. Allen, A. M. (2002). Inhibition of the hypothalamic paraventricular nucleus in spontaneously hypertensive rats dramatically reduces sympathetic vasomotor tone. *Hypertension* 39, 275–280.
3. Armstrong, W. E., Gallagher, M. J., and Sladek, C. D. (1986). Noradrenergic stimulation of supraoptic neuronal activity and vasopressin release *in vitro*: Mediation by an alpha 1-receptor. *Brain Research* 365, 192–197.
4. Armstrong, W. E., and Stern, J. E. (1998). Phenotypic and state-dependent expression of the electrical and morphological properties of oxytocin and vasopressin neurones. *Progress in Brain Research* 119, 101–113.
5. Armstrong, W. E., Warach, S., Hatton, G. I., and McNeill, T. H. (1980). Subnuclei in the rat hypothalamic paraventricular nucleus: A cytoarchitectural, horseradish peroxidase and immunocytochemical analysis. *Neuroscience* 5, 1931–1958.
6. Badoer, E., McKinlay, D., Trigg, L., and McGrath, B. P. (1997). Distribution of activated neurons in the rabbit brain following a volume load. *Neuroscience* 81, 1065–1077.
7. Badoer, E., and Merolli, J. (1998). Neurons in the hypothalamic paraventricular nucleus that project to the rostral ventrolateral medulla are activated by haemorrhage. *Brain Research* 791, 317–320.
8. Bailey, T. W., Jin, Y. H., Doyle, M. W., Smith, S. M., and Andresen, M. C. (2006). Vasopressin inhibits glutamate release via two distinct modes in the brainstem. *Journal of Neuroscience* 26, 6131–6142.
9. Bains, J. S., and Ferguson, A. V. (1995). Paraventricular nucleus neurons projecting to the spinal cord receive excitatory input from the subfornical organ. *American Journal of Physiology* 268, R625–R633.
10. Bains, J. S., and Ferguson, A. V. (1997). Nitric oxide regulates NMDA-driven GABAergic inputs to type I neurones of the rat paraventricular nucleus. *Journal of Physiology* 499, 733–746.
11. Banks, D., and Harris, M. C. (1987). Activation within dorsal medullary nuclei following stimulation in the hypothalamic paraventricular nucleus in rats. *Pflügers Archiv* 408, 619–627.
12. Bertini, L. T., and Kiss, J. Z. (1991). Hypophysiotrophic neurons are capable of altering the ratio of co-packaged neurohormones. *Neuroscience* 42, 237–244.
13. Biancardi, V. C., Campos, R. R., and Stern, J. E. (2010). Altered balance of gamma-aminobutyric acidergic and glutamatergic afferent inputs in rostral ventrolateral medulla-projecting neurons in the paraventricular nucleus of the hypothalamus of renovascular hypertensive rats. *Journal of Comparative Neurology* 518, 567–585.
14. Blair, M. L., Piekut, D., Want, A., and Olschowka, J. A. (1996). Role of the hypothalamic paraventricular nucleus in cardiovascular regulation. *Clinical and Experimental Pharmacology and Physiology* 23, 161–165.
15. Brown, C. H. (2004). Rhythmogenesis in vasopressin cells. *Journal of Neuroendocrinology* 16, 727–739.
16. Buijs, R. M., la Fleur, S. E., Wortel, J., Van Heyningen, C., Zuiddam, L., Mettenleiter, T. C., Kalsbeek, A., Nagai, K., and Niijima, A. (2003). The suprachiasmatic nucleus balances sympathetic and parasympathetic output to peripheral

organs through separate preautonomic neurons. *Journal of Comparative Neurology* 464, 36–48.

17. Burbach, J. P., Luckman, S. M., Murphy, D., and Gainer, H. (2001). Gene regulation in the magnocellular hypothalamo-neurohypophysial system. *Physiological Reviews* 81, 1197–1267.
18. Cato, M. J., and Toney, G. M. (2005). Angiotensin II excites paraventricular nucleus neurons that innervate the rostral ventrolateral medulla: An *in vitro* patch-clamp study in brain slices. *Journal of Neurophysiology* 93, 403–413.
19. Chen, Y. L., Chan, S. H., and Chan, J. Y. (1996). Participation of galanin in baroreflex inhibition of heart rate by hypothalamic PVN in rat. *American Journal of Physiology* 271, H1823–H1828.
20. Coote, J. H. (2005). A role for the paraventricular nucleus of the hypothalamus in the autonomic control of heart and kidney. *Experimental Physiology* 90, 169–173.
21. Cunningham, J. T., Bruno, S. B., Higgs, K. A., and Sullivan, M. J. (2002). Intrapericardial procaine affects volume expansion-induced fos immunoreactivity in unanesthetized rats. *Experimental Neurology* 174, 181–192.
22. Dampney, R. A., and Horiuchi, J. (2003). Functional organisation of central cardiovascular pathways: Studies using c-fos gene expression. *Progress in Neurobiology* 71, 359–384.
23. Dampney, R. A., Polson, J. W., Potts, P. D., Hirooka, Y., and Horiuchi, J. (2003). Functional organization of brain pathways subserving the baroreceptor reflex: Studies in conscious animals using immediate early gene expression. *Cellular and Molecular Neurobiology* 23, 597–616.
24. Day, T. A., and Renaud, L. P. (1984). Electrophysiological evidence that noradrenergic afferents selectively facilitate the activity of supraoptic vasopressin neurons. *Brain Research* 303, 233–240.
25. Dayanithi, G., Widmer, H., and Richard, P. (1996). Vasopressin-induced intracellular $Ca^{2+}$ increase in isolated rat supraoptic cells. *Journal of Physiology* 490, 713–727.
26. Di Scala-Guenot, D., Mouginot, D., and Strosser, M. T. (1994). Increase of intracellular calcium induced by oxytocin in hypothalamic cultured astrocytes. *Glia* 11, 269–276.
27. Duan, Y. F., Kopin, I. J., and Goldstein, D. S. (1999). Stimulation of the paraventricular nucleus modulates firing of neurons in the nucleus of the solitary tract. *American Journal of Physiology* 277, R403–R411.
28. Duan, Y. F., Winters, R., McCabe, P. M., Green, E. J., Huang, Y., and Schneiderman, N. (1997). Cardiorespiratory components of defense reaction elicited from paraventricular nucleus. *Physiology and Behavior* 61, 325–330.
29. Engelmann, M., Landgraf, R., and Wotjak, C. T. (2004). The hypothalamic-neurohypophysial system regulates the hypothalamic-pituitary-adrenal axis under stress: an old concept revisited. *Frontiers in Neuroendocrinology* 25, 132–149.
30. Esler, M. D., Lambert, G. W., Ferrier, C., Kaye, D. M., Wallin, B. G., Kalff, V., Kelly, M. J., and Jennings, G. L. (1995). Central nervous system noradrenergic control of sympathetic outflow in normotensive and hypertensive humans. *Clinical and Experimental Hypertension* 17, 409–423.
31. Fink, G., Rosie, R., Sheward, W. J., Thomson, E., and Wilson, H. (1991). Steroid control of central neuronal interactions and function. *Journal of Steroid Biochemistry and Molecular Biology* 40, 123–132.
32. Gingerich, S., and Krukoff, T. L. (2005). Estrogen modulates endothelial and neuronal nitric oxide synthase expression via an estrogen receptor beta-dependent mechanism in hypothalamic slice cultures. *Endocrinology* 146, 2933–2941.
33. Glasgow, E., Kusano, K., Chin, H., Mezey, E., Young, W. S., III, and Gainer, H. (1999). Single cell reverse transcription-polymerase chain reaction analysis of rat supraoptic magnocellular neurons: Neuropeptide phenotypes and high voltage-gated calcium channel subtypes. *Endocrinology* 140, 5391–5401.
34. Gordon, G. R., Iremonger, K. J., Kantevari, S., Ellis-Davies, G. C., MacVicar, B. A., and Bains, J. S. (2009). Astrocyte-mediated distributed plasticity at hypothalamic glutamate synapses. *Neuron* 64, 391–403.
35. Gouzenes, L., Desarmenien, M. G., Hussy, N., Richard, P., and Moos, F. C. (1998). Vasopressin regularizes the phasic firing pattern of rat hypothalamic magnocellular vasopressin neurons. *Journal of Neuroscience* 18, 1879–1885.
36. Hallbeck, M., Larhammar, D., and Blomqvist, A. (2001). Neuropeptide expression in rat paraventricular hypothalamic neurons that project to the spinal cord. *Journal of Comparative Neurology* 433, 222–238.
37. Hatton, G. I. (2004). Dynamic neuronal-glial interactions: An overview 20 years later. *Peptides* 25, 403–411.
38. Hoffman, N. W., Tasker, J. G., and Dudek, F. E. (1991). Immunohistochemical differentiation of electrophysiologically defined neuronal populations in the region of the rat hypothalamic paraventricular nucleus. *Journal of Comparative Neurology* 307, 405–416.

39. Jackson, K., Silva, H. M., Zhang, W., Michelini, L. C., and Stern, J. E. (2005). Exercise training differentially affects intrinsic excitability of autonomic and neuroendocrine neurons in the hypothalamic paraventricular nucleus. *Journal of Neurophysiology* 94, 3211–3220.
40. Johnson, A. K., and Thunhorst, R. L. (1997). The neuroendocrinology of thirst and salt appetite: Visceral sensory signals and mechanisms of central integration. *Frontiers in Neuroendocrinology* 18, 292–353.
41. Kadekaro, M. (2004). Nitric oxide modulation of the hypothalamo-neurohypophyseal system. *Brazilian Journal of Medical and Biological Research* 37, 441–450.
42. Kang, Y. M., He, R. L., Yang, L. M., Qin, D. N., Guggilam, A., Elks, C., Yan, N., Guo, Z., and Francis, J. (2009). Brain tumour necrosis factor-alpha modulates neurotransmitters in hypothalamic paraventricular nucleus in heart failure. *Cardiovascular Research* 83, 737–746.
43. Kannan, H., and Yamashita, H. (1983). Electrophysiological study of paraventricular nucleus neurons projecting to the dorsomedial medulla and their response to baroreceptor stimulation in rats. *Brain Research* 279, 31–40.
44. Kantzides, A., and Badoer, E. (2005). nNOS-containing neurons in the hypothalamus and medulla project to the RVLM. *Brain Research* 1037, 25–34.
45. Kleiber, A. C., Zheng, H., Schultz, H. D., Peuler, J. D., and Patel, K. P. (2008). Exercise training normalizes enhanced glutamate-mediated sympathetic activation from the PVN in heart failure. *American Journal of Physiology. Regulatory, Integrative and Comparative Physiology.* 294, R1863–R1872.
46. Kombian, S. B., Hirasawa, M., Mouginot, D., and Pittman, Q. J. (2002). Modulation of synaptic transmission by oxytocin and vasopressin in the supraoptic nucleus. *Progress in Brain Research* 139, 235–246.
47. Kreier, F., Kap, Y. S., Mettenleiter, T. C., van Heijningen, C., van der Vliet, J., Kalsbeek, A., Sauerwein, H. P., Fliers, E., Romijn, J. A., and Buijs, R. M. (2006). Tracing from fat tissue, liver, and pancreas: A neuroanatomical framework for the role of the brain in type 2 diabetes. *Endocrinology* 147, 1140–1147.
48. Krukoff, T. L. (1999). Central actions of nitric oxide in regulation of autonomic functions. *Brain Research Reviews* 30, 52–65.
49. Krukoff, T. L., Mactavish, D., and Jhamandas, J. H. (1997). Activation by hypotension of neurons in the hypothalamic paraventricular nucleus that project to the brainstem. *Journal of Comparative Neurology* 385, 285–296.
50. Lambert, R. C., Dayanithi, G., Moos, F. C., and Richard, P. (1994). A rise in the intracellular $Ca^{2+}$ concentration of isolated rat supraoptic cells in response to oxytocin. *Journal of Physiology* 478, 275–287.
51. Langle, S. L., Poulain, D. A., and Theodosis, D. T. (2003). Induction of rapid, activity-dependent neuronal-glial remodelling in the adult rat hypothalamus in vitro. *European Journal of Neuroscience* 18, 206–214.
52. Li, D. P., Chen, S. R., and Pan, H. L. (2002). Nitric oxide inhibits spinally projecting paraventricular neurons through potentiation of presynaptic GABA release. *Journal of Neurophysiology* 88, 2664–2674.
53. Li, N., Sul, J. Y., and Haydon, P. G. (2003). A calcium-induced calcium influx factor, nitric oxide, modulates the refilling of calcium stores in astrocytes. *Journal of Neuroscience* 23, 10302–10310.
54. Li, Y., Zhang, W., and Stern, J. E. (2003). Nitric oxide inhibits the firing activity of hypothalamic paraventricular neurons that innervate the medulla oblongata: Role of GABA. *Neuroscience* 118, 585–601.
55. Li, Y. W., and Dampney, R. A. (1994). Expression of Fos-like protein in brain following sustained hypertension and hypotension in conscious rabbits. *Neuroscience* 61, 613–634.
56. Li, Z., and Ferguson, A. V. (1993). Angiotensin II responsiveness of rat paraventricular and subfornical organ neurons *in vitro*. *Neuroscience* 55, 197–207.
57. Liu, Q. S., Jia, Y. S., and Ju, G. (1997). Nitric oxide inhibits neuronal activity in the supraoptic nucleus of the rat hypothalamic slices. *Brain Research Bulletin* 43, 121–125.
58. Lovick, T. A., and Coote, J. H. (1988). Effects of volume loading on paraventriculo-spinal neurones in the rat. *Journal of the Autonomic Nervous System* 25, 135–140.
59. Ludwig, M., and Leng, G. (1997). Autoinhibition of supraoptic nucleus vasopressin neurons *in vivo*: A combined retrodialysis/electrophysiological study in rats. *European Journal of Neuroscience* 9, 2532–2540.
60. Ludwig, M., and Leng, G. (2006). Dendritic peptide release and peptide-dependent behaviours. *Nature Reviews Neuroscience* 7, 126–136.
61. Ludwig, M., and Pittman, Q. J. (2003). Talking back: Dendritic neurotransmitter release. *Trends in Neurosciences* 26, 255–261.
62. Luiten, P. G., ter Horst, G. J., Karst, H., and Steffens, A. B. (1985). The course of paraventricular

hypothalamic efferents to autonomic structures in medulla and spinal cord. *Brain Research* 329, 374–378.

63. Luther, J. A., and Tasker, J. G. (2000). Voltage-gated currents distinguish parvocellular from magnocellular neurones in the rat hypothalamic paraventricular nucleus. *Journal of Physiology* 523, 193–209.
64. Mancia, G. (1990). Sympathetic activation in congestive heart failure. *European Heart Journal* 11 Suppl A, 3–11.
65. McKinley, M. J., Allen, A. M., Burns, P., Colvill, L. M., and Oldfield, B. J. (1998). Interaction of circulating hormones with the brain: The roles of the subfornical organ and the organum vasculosum of the lamina terminalis. *Clinical and Experimental Pharmacology and Physiology* 25, S61–S67.
66. McKinley, M. J., Hards, D. K., and Oldfield, B. J. (1994). Identification of neural pathways activated in dehydrated rats by means of Fos-immunohistochemistry and neural tracing. *Brain Research* 653, 305–314.
67. McKinley, M. J., and Johnson, A. K. (2004). The physiological regulation of thirst and fluid intake. *News in Physiological Sciences* 19, 1–6.
68. Michelini, L. C. (1994). Vasopressin in the nucleus tractus solitarius: A modulator of baroreceptor reflex control of heart rate. *Brazilian Journal of Medical and Biological Research* 27, 1017–1032.
69. Michelini, L. C. (2001). Oxytocin in the NTS. A new modulator of cardiovascular control during exercise. *Annals of the New York Academy of Sciences* 940, 206–220.
70. Miselis, R. R. (1981). The efferent projections of the subfornical organ of the rat: A circumventricular organ within a neural network subserving water balance. *Brain Research* 230, 1–23.
71. Mitchell, L. D., Callahan, M. F., Wilkin, L. D., Bellin, S. I., and Johnson, A. K. (1985). Systemic angiotensin II, blood pressure and supraoptic neuronal activity. *Peptides* 6 Suppl 1, 153–158.
72. Moos, F. C. (1994). [Positive control of oxytocin on its secretory system]. *Pathologie-biologie (Paris)* 42, 133–137.
73. Morris, J. F., and Ludwig, M. (2004). Magnocellular dendrites: Prototypic receiver/transmitters. *Journal of Neuroendocrinology* 16, 403–408.
74. Neumann, I., Douglas, A. J., Pittman, Q. J., Russell, J. A., and Landgraf, R. (1996). Oxytocin released within the supraoptic nucleus of the rat brain by positive feedback action is involved in parturition-related events. *Journal of Neuroendocrinology* 8, 227–233.
75. Nylen, A., Skagerberg, G., Alm, P., Larsson, B., Holmqvist, B. I., and Andersson, K. E. (2001). Detailed organization of nitric oxide synthase, vasopressin and oxytocin immunoreactive cell bodies in the supraoptic nucleus of the female rat. *Anatomy and Embryology* 203, 309–321.
76. Packer, M. (1988). Neurohormonal interactions and adaptations in congestive heart failure. *Circulation* 77, 721–730.
77. Palkovits, M. (1999). Interconnections between the neuroendocrine hypothalamus and the central autonomic system. Geoffrey Harris Memorial Lecture, Kitakyushu, Japan, October 1998. *Frontiers in Neuroendocrinology* 20, 270–295.
78. Park, J. B., Jo, J. Y., Zheng, H., Patel, K. P., and Stern, J. E. (2009). Regulation of tonic GABA inhibitory function, presympathetic neuronal activity and sympathetic outflow from the paraventricular nucleus by astroglial GABA transporters. *Journal of Physiology* 587, 4645–4660.
79. Patel, K. P., and Zhang, K. (1996). Neurohumoral activation in heart failure: Role of paraventricular nucleus. *Clinical and Experimental Pharmacology and Physiology* 23, 722–726.
80. Patel, K. P., Zhang, K., Kenney, M. J., Weiss, M., and Mayhan, W. G. (2000). Neuronal expression of Fos protein in the hypothalamus of rats with heart failure. *Brain Research* 865, 27–34.
81. Patel, K. P., Zhang, K., Zucker, I. H., and Krukoff, T. L. (1996). Decreased gene expression of neuronal nitric oxide synthase in hypothalamus and brainstem of rats in heart failure. *Brain Research* 734, 109–115.
82. Patel, K. P., Zhang, P. L., and Krukoff, T. L. (1993). Alterations in brain hexokinase activity associated with heart failure in rats. *American Journal of Physiology* 265, R923–R928.
83. Paton, J. F., Kasparov, S., and Paterson, D. J. (2002). Nitric oxide and autonomic control of heart rate: A question of specificity. *Trends in Neurosciences* 25, 626–631.
84. Paxinos, G., and Watson, C. (1986). *The rat brain in stereotaxic coordinates*, Second Edition. Sydney: Academic Press.
85. Perez-Tilve, D., Stern, J. E., and Tschop, M. (2006). The brain and the metabolic syndrome: Not a wireless connection. *Endocrinology* 147, 1136–1139.
86. Peters, J. H., McDougall, S. J., Kellett, D. O., Jordan, D., Llewellyn-Smith, I. J., and Andresen, M. C. (2008). Oxytocin enhances cranial visceral afferent synaptic transmission to the solitary tract nucleus. *Journal of Neuroscience* 28, 11731–11740.
87. Portillo, F., Carrasco, M., and Vallo, J. J. (1998). Separate populations of neurons within the

paraventricular hypothalamic nucleus of the rat project to vagal and thoracic autonomic preganglionic levels and express c-Fos protein induced by lithium chloride. *Journal of Chemical Neuroanatomy* 14, 95–102.

88. Potts, P. D., Polson, J. W., Hirooka, Y., and Dampney, R. A. (1997). Effects of sinoaortic denervation on Fos expression in the brain evoked by hypertension and hypotension in conscious rabbits. *Neuroscience* 77, 503–520.
89. Pow, D. V., and Morris, J. F. (1989). Dendrites of hypothalamic magnocellular neurons release neurohypophysial peptides by exocytosis. *Neuroscience* 32, 435–439.
90. Prevot, V. (2002). Glial-neuronal-endothelial interactions are involved in the control of GnRH secretion. *Journal of Neuroendocrinology* 14, 247–255.
91. Pyner, S., and Coote, J. H. (1999). Identification of an efferent projection from the paraventricular nucleus of the hypothalamus terminating close to spinally projecting rostral ventrolateral medullary neurons. *Neuroscience* 88, 949–957.
92. Pyner, S., and Coote, J. H. (2000). Identification of branching paraventricular neurons of the hypothalamus that project to the rostroventrolateral medulla and spinal cord. *Neuroscience* 100, 549–556.
93. Pyner, S., Deering, J., and Coote, J. H. (2002). Right atrial stretch induces renal nerve inhibition and c-fos expression in parvocellular neurones of the paraventricular nucleus in rats. *Experimental Physiology* 87, 25–32.
94. Randolph, R. R., Li, Q., Curtis, K. S., Sullivan, M. J., and Cunningham, J. T. (1998). Fos expression following isotonic volume expansion of the unanesthetized male rat. *American Journal of Physiology* 274, R1345–R1352.
95. Ranson, R. N., Motawei, K., Pyner, S., and Coote, J. H. (1998). The paraventricular nucleus of the hypothalamus sends efferents to the spinal cord of the rat that closely appose sympathetic preganglionic neurones projecting to the stellate ganglion. *Experimental Brain Research* 120, 164–172.
96. Reddy, M. K., Patel, K. P., and Schultz, H. D. (2005). Differential role of the paraventricular nucleus of the hypothalamus in modulating the sympathoexcitatory component of peripheral and central chemoreflexes. *American Journal of Physiology. Regulatory, Integrative and Comparative Physiology* 289, R789–R797.
97. Rho, J. H., and Swanson, L. W. (1989). A morphometric analysis of functionally defined subpopulations of neurons in the paraventricular nucleus of the rat with observations on the effects of colchicine. *Journal of Neuroscience* 9, 1375–1388.
98. Sawchenko, P. E., and Swanson, L. W. (1982). Immunohistochemical identification of neurons in the paraventricular nucleus of the hypothalamus that project to the medulla or to the spinal cord in the rat. *Journal of Comparative Neurology* 205, 260–272.
99. Schiltz, J. C., Hoffman, G. E., Stricker, E. M., and Sved, A. F. (1997). Decreases in arterial pressure activate oxytocin neurons in conscious rats. *American Journal of Physiology* 273, R1474–R1483.
100. Scott, V., Bishop, V. R., Leng, G., and Brown, C. H. (2009). Dehydration-induced modulation of kappa-opioid inhibition of vasopressin neurone activity. *Journal of Physiology* 587, 5679–5689.
101. Shafton, A. D., Ryan, A., and Badoer, E. (1998). Neurons in the hypothalamic paraventricular nucleus send collaterals to the spinal cord and to the rostral ventrolateral medulla in the rat. *Brain Research* 801, 239–243.
102. Sonner, P. M., Filosa, J. A., and Stern, J. E. (2008). Diminished A-type potassium current and altered firing properties in presympathetic PVN neurones in renovascular hypertensive rats. *Journal of Physiology* 586, 1605–1622.
103. Stern, J. E. (2001). Electrophysiological and morphological properties of pre-autonomic neurones in the rat hypothalamic paraventricular nucleus. *Journal of Physiology* 537, 161–177.
104. Stern, J. E. (2004). Nitric oxide and homeostatic control: An intercellular signalling molecule contributing to autonomic and neuroendocrine integration? *Progress in Biophysics and Molecular Biology* 84, 197–215.
105. Stern, J. E., and Armstrong, W. E. (1996). Changes in the electrical properties of supraoptic nucleus oxytocin and vasopressin neurons during lactation. *Journal of Neuroscience* 16, 4861–4871.
106. Stern, J. E., and Ludwig, M. (2001). NO inhibits supraoptic oxytocin and vasopressin neurons via activation of GABAergic synaptic inputs. *American Journal of Physiology. Regulatory, Integrative and Comparative Physiology* 280, R1815–R1822.
107. Stern, J. E., and Zhang, W. (2003). Preautonomic neurons in the paraventricular nucleus of the hypothalamus contain estrogen receptor beta. *Brain Research* 975, 99–109.
108. Stern, J. E., and Zhang, W. (2005). Cellular sources, targets and actions of constitutive nitric oxide in the magnocellular neurosecretory

system of the rat. *Journal of Physiology* 562, 725–744.

109. Stocker, S. D., Hunwick, K. J., and Toney, G. M. (2005). Hypothalamic paraventricular nucleus differentially supports lumbar and renal sympathetic outflow in water-deprived rats. *Journal of Physiology* 563, 249–263.
110. Stocker, S. D., Keith, K. J., and Toney, G. M. (2004). Acute inhibition of the hypothalamic paraventricular nucleus decreases renal sympathetic nerve activity and arterial blood pressure in water-deprived rats. *American Journal of Physiology. Regulatory, Integrative and Comparative Physiology* 286, R719–R725.
111. Stocker, S. D., Simmons, J. R., Stornetta, R. L., Toney, G. M., and Guyenet, P. G. (2006). Water deprivation activates a glutamatergic projection from the hypothalamic paraventricular nucleus to the rostral ventrolateral medulla. *Journal of Comparative Neurology* 494, 673–685.
112. Strack, A. M., Sawyer, W. B., Hughes, J. H., Platt, K. B., and Loewy, A. D. (1989). A general pattern of CNS innervation of the sympathetic outflow demonstrated by transneuronal pseudorabies viral infections. *Brain Research* 491, 156–162.
113. Stricker, E. M., Callahan, J. B., Huang, W., and Sved, A. F. (2002). Early osmoregulatory stimulation of neurohypophyseal hormone secretion and thirst after gastric NaCl loads. *American Journal of Physiology. Regulatory, Integrative and Comparative Physiology* 282, R1710–R1717.
114. Sved, A. F., Cano, G., and Card, J. P. (2001). Neuroanatomical specificity of the circuits controlling sympathetic outflow to different targets. *Clinical and Experimental Pharmacology and Physiology* 28, 115–119.
115. Swanson, L. W., and Kuypers, H. G. (1980). The paraventricular nucleus of the hypothalamus: Cytoarchitectonic subdivisions and organization of projections to the pituitary, dorsal vagal complex, and spinal cord as demonstrated by retrograde fluorescence double-labeling methods. *Journal of Comparative Neurology* 194, 555–570.
116. Swanson, L. W., and Sawchenko, P. E. (1980). Paraventricular nucleus: A site for the integration of neuroendocrine and autonomic mechanisms. *Neuroendocrinology* 31, 410–417.
117. Swanson, L. W., and Sawchenko, P. E. (1983). Hypothalamic integration: Organization of the paraventricular and supraoptic nuclei. *Annual Review of Neuroscience* 6, 269–324.
118. Tagawa, T., and Dampney, R. A. (1999). AT(1) receptors mediate excitatory inputs to rostral ventrolateral medulla pressor neurons from hypothalamus. *Hypertension* 34, 1301–1307.
119. Tasker, J. G., Boudaba, C., and Schrader, L. A. (1998). Local glutamatergic and GABAergic synaptic circuits and metabotropic glutamate receptors in the hypothalamic paraventricular and supraoptic nuclei. *Advances in Experimental Medicine and Biology* 449, 117–121.
120. Tasker, J. G., and Dudek, F. E. (1991). Electrophysiological properties of neurones in the region of the paraventricular nucleus in slices of rat hypothalamus. *Journal of Physiology* 434, 271–293.
121. Theodosis, D. T., Montagnese, C., Rodriguez, F., Vincent, J. D., and Poulain, D. A. (1986). Oxytocin induces morphological plasticity in the adult hypothalamo-neurohypophysial system. *Nature* 322, 738–740.
122. Theodosis, D. T., and Poulain, D. A. (1999). Contribution of astrocytes to activity-dependent structural plasticity in the adult brain. *Advances in Experimental Medicine and Biology* 468, 175–182.
123. Vahid-Ansari, F., and Leenen, F. H. (1998). Pattern of neuronal activation in rats with CHF after myocardial infarction. *American Journal of Physiology* 275, H2140–H2146.
124. Van Den Pol, A. N. (1982). The magnocellular and parvocellular paraventricular nucleus of rat: Intrinsic organization. *Journal of Comparative Neurology* 206, 317–345.
125. Ventura, R. R., Giusti-Paiva, A., Gomes, D. A., Elias, L. L., and Antunes-Rodrigues, J. (2005). Neuronal nitric oxide synthase inhibition differentially affects oxytocin and vasopressin secretion in salt loaded rats. *Neuroscience Letters* 379, 75–80.
126. Vincent, S. R. (1994). Nitric oxide: A radical neurotransmitter in the central nervous system. *Progress in Neurobiology* 42, 129–160.
127. Weiss, M. L., Chowdhury, S. I., Patel, K. P., Kenney, M. J., and Huang, J. (2001). Neural circuitry of the kidney: NO-containing neurons. *Brain Research* 919, 269–282.
128. Wood, J., and Garthwaite, J. (1994). Models of the diffusional spread of nitric oxide: Implications for neural nitric oxide signalling and its pharmacological properties. *Neuropharmacology* 33, 1235–1244.
129. Yang, Z., Bertram, D., and Coote, J. H. (2001). The role of glutamate and vasopressin in the excitation of RVL neurones by paraventricular neurones. *Brain Research* 908, 99–103.
130. Yang, Z., and Coote, J. H. (1998). Influence of the hypothalamic paraventricular nucleus on

cardiovascular neurones in the rostral ventrolateral medulla of the rat. *Journal of Physiology* 513, 521–530.

131. Yu, Y., Zhang, Z. H., Wei, S. G., Serrats, J., Weiss, R. M., and Felder, R. B. (2010). Brain perivascular macrophages and the sympathetic response to inflammation in rats after myocardial infarction. *Hypertension* 55, 652–659.
132. Zhang, K., Li, Y. F., and Patel, K. P. (2002). Reduced endogenous GABA-mediated inhibition in the PVN on renal nerve discharge in rats with heart failure. *American Journal of Physiology. Regulatory, Integrative and Comparative Physiology* 282, R1006–R1015.
133. Zhang, K., and Patel, K. P. (1998). Effect of nitric oxide within the paraventricular nucleus on renal sympathetic nerve discharge: Role of GABA. *American Journal of Physiology* 275, R728–R734.
134. Zheng, H., Li, Y. F., Cornish, K. G., Zucker, I. H., and Patel, K. P. (2005). Exercise training improves endogenous nitric oxide mechanisms within the paraventricular nucleus in rats with heart failure. *American Journal of Physiology. Heart and Circulatory Physiology* 288, H2332–H2341.
135. Zheng, H., Mayhan, W. G., Bidasee, K. R., and Patel, K. P. (2006). Blunted nitric oxide-mediated inhibition of sympathetic nerve activity within the paraventricular nucleus in diabetic rats. *American Journal of Physiology. Regulatory, Integrative and Comparative Physiology* 290, R992–R1002.
136. Zucker, I. H., Schultz, H. D., Li, Y. F., Wang, Y., Wang, W., and Patel, K. P. (2004). The origin of sympathetic outflow in heart failure: The roles of angiotensin II and nitric oxide. *Progress in Biophysics and Molecular Biology* 84, 217–232.

# 5

# The Ventrolateral Medulla and Sympathetic Regulation of Arterial Pressure

ANN M. SCHREIHOFER AND ALAN F. SVED

The ventrolateral medulla oblongata is essential for the normal regulation of cardiovascular function by the autonomic nervous system. Historically, the ventrolateral medulla has been divided into functional regions defined by their ability to alter arterial pressure when activated or inhibited. Pressor and depressor regions were named by their relative rostral or caudal positions (Figure 5–1), generating some confusion regarding precise anatomical location and promoting the simplistic notion that these heterogeneous regions of the reticular formation each serve a singular and unique function within distinct boundaries. Although the traditional nomenclature persists, recent advances have yielded important insights into these highly interconnected, complex medullary regions in both normal and pathophysiological cardiovascular regulation. This chapter briefly reviews the role of the ventrolateral medulla in sympathetic control of cardiovascular function from a historical perspective and focuses on new observations gained since the first edition of this book. For a more detailed historical account, see the chapter in the earlier edition[35] and others on the subject[10].

## THE VENTROLATERAL MEDULLA: A SERIES OF LONGITUDINAL COLUMNS THAT REGULATE ARTERIAL PRESSURE

The ventrolateral medulla contains columns of neurons involved in sympathetic cardiovascular regulation that extend rostrally to the ponto-medullary junction and caudally to the junction with the cervical spinal cord (Figure 5–1). The organization appears roughly similar in all species examined. This chapter will focus on data from the rat, and differences with other species will be noted. Although there is an underlying assumption that the human medulla oblongata has a similar anatomical and functional organization, only limited data are available for primates[4].

The anatomical location of regions will be described using schematics from a rat atlas of Paxinos and Watson[82], although the exact placement of neurons important for cardiovascular regulation does not precisely coincide with the illustrated nuclei. Regions of the ventrolateral medulla will be described in relation to ventral landmarks to improve accuracy (Figures 5–1 and 5–2). Generally, the functional zones do not fit strict anatomical boundaries, a factor that has contributed to confusion in nomenclature when neuroanatomical terms are used synonymously with functional classifications. The functional zones have been mapped by: (1) observing physiological responses to localized neuronal excitation or inhibition, (2) identifying neurons affected by cardiovascular perturbations with electrophysiological recordings or expression of the early response gene *c-fos*, and (3) establishing connections electrophysiologically or neuroanatomically to other regions considered important in cardiovascular regulation.

The most thoroughly examined region of the ventrolateral medulla is the pressor region within the rostral ventrolateral medulla (RVLM), which tonically activates sympathetic nerve activity to increase arterial pressure and heart rate. For this discussion, "sympathetic nerve activity" broadly refers to the

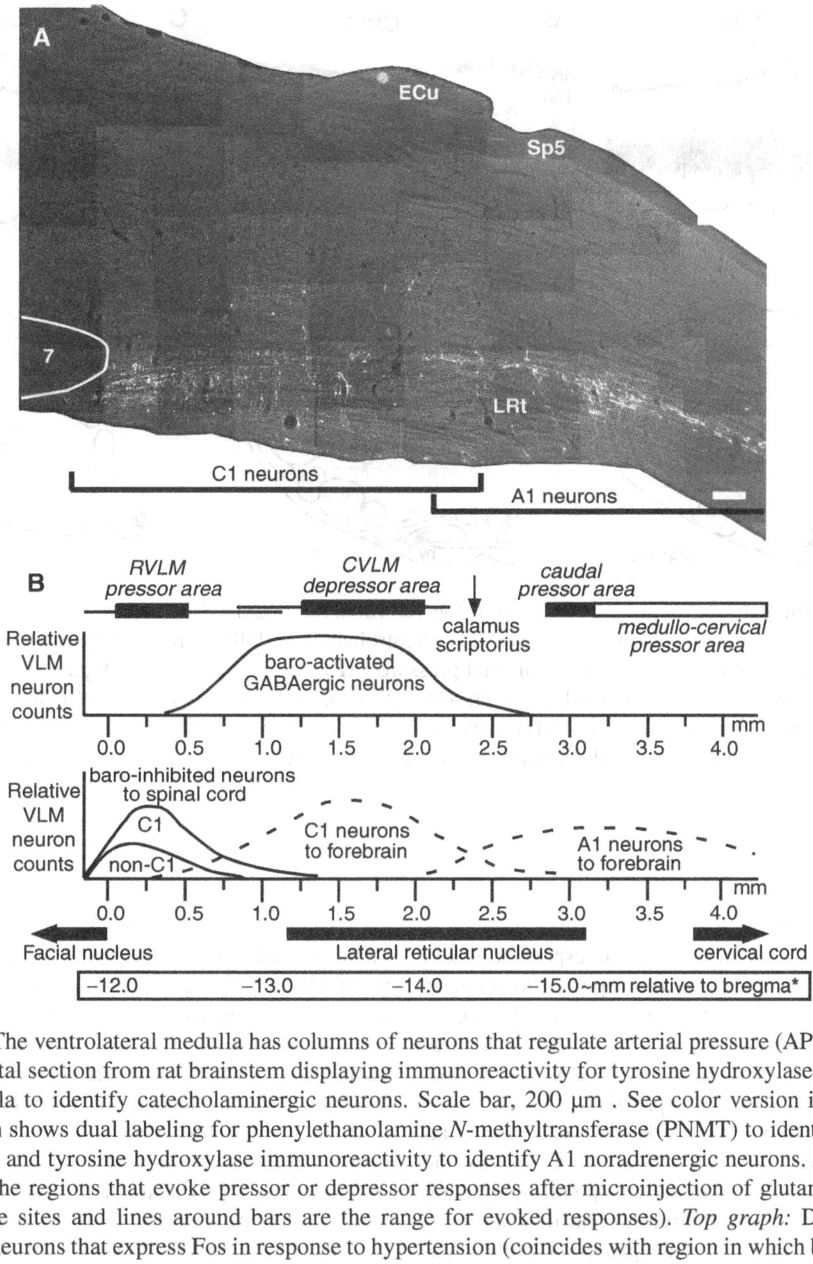


Figure 5–1 The ventrolateral medulla has columns of neurons that regulate arterial pressure (AP). *A:* Montage of a parasagittal section from rat brainstem displaying immunoreactivity for tyrosine hydroxylase in the ventrolateral medulla to identify catecholaminergic neurons. Scale bar, 200 μm . See color version in Card et al., 2006[18], which shows dual labeling for phenylethanolamine *N*-methyltransferase (PNMT) to identify C1 adrenergic neurons and tyrosine hydroxylase immunoreactivity to identify A1 noradrenergic neurons. *B:* Bars at the top indicate the regions that evoke pressor or depressor responses after microinjection of glutamate (bars are most effective sites and lines around bars are the range for evoked responses). *Top graph:* Distribution of GABAergic neurons that express Fos in response to hypertension (coincides with region in which baro-activated GABAergic neurons can be recorded) that most likely contribute to the depressor responses evoked from the caudal ventrolateral medulla (CVLM). *Bottom graph:* Solid lines show distribution of C1 adrenergic and non-catecholaminergic neurons that lie within 500 micrometers caudal to the facial nucleus, project to the thoracic spinal cord and likely contribute to pressor responses of evoked from the rostral ventrolateral medulla (RVLM). Dotted lines depict caudal C1 neurons that project to the forebrain. The caudal C1 neurons are interspersed with baro-activated GABAergic CVLM neurons and overlap caudally with forebrain-projecting A1 neurons that are adjacent to the unidentified neurons of the caudal pressor area. For reference to ventral landmarks, the facial nucleus and lateral reticular nucleus are depicted on the rostrocaudal axis. The approximate bregma levels according to Paxinos and Watson[82] are also listed in relation to these ventral landmarks. ECu, external cuneate nucleus; Lrt, Lateral reticular nucleus; Sp5, spinal trigeminal nucleus; VLM, ventrolateral medulla; 7, facial nucleus. *These levels vary slightly in different versions of atlases by Paxinos and Watson. Adapted from Schreihofer and Guyenet, 2002, with permission[97].

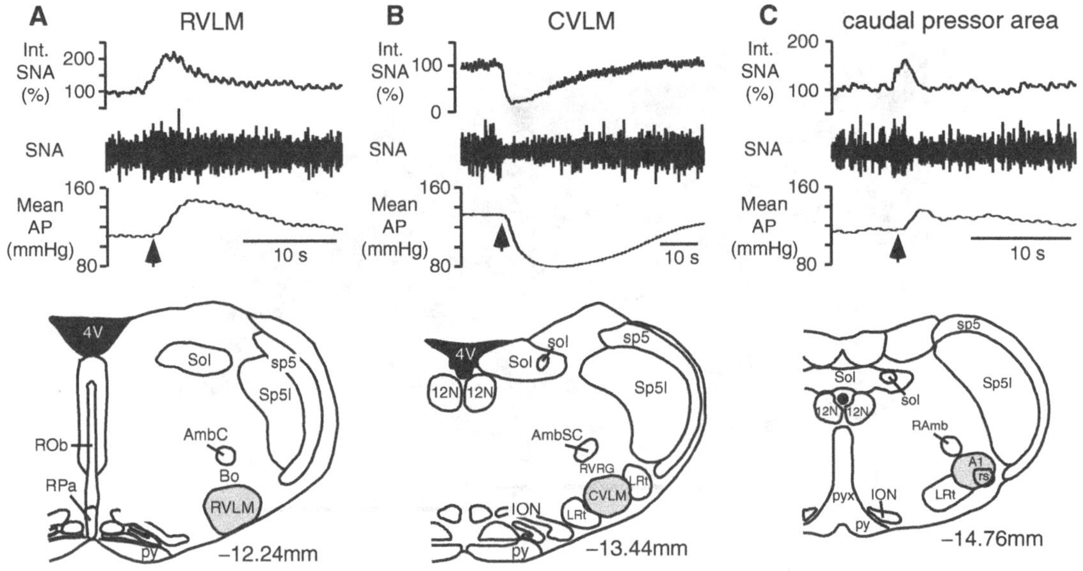


Figure 5–2 Stimulation of vasoactive regions of the ventrolateral medulla. The effects of stimulation (1 nmol glutamate in 100 nl vehicle) of vasoactive sites in the ventrolateral medulla on raw and integrated (Int) splanchnic sympathetic nerve activity (SNA) and arterial pressure (AP). At the bottom of each panel, the approximate site of the injection is shown as a shaded region on schematics adapted from Paxinos and Watson[82] *A:* Stimulation of the rostral ventrolateral medulla (RVLM) increases SNA and AP in a urethane-anesthetized rat. *B:* Stimulation of the depressor region of the CVLM decreases SNA and AP. *C:* Stimulation of the caudal pressor area increases SNA and AP.

activity of sympathetic nerves that serve cardiac or vasomotor functions. In rats, pressor responses evoked from RVLM coincide with the reported location of neurons that are inhibited by increases in arterial pressure (i.e., baro-inhibited) and project to the thoracic spinal cord (Figures 5–1B, 5–2A, and 5–3A). Hypotension-induced Fos expression in spinally projecting neurons reveals a similar distribution of putative pre-sympathetic RVLM neurons[114]. (We use the term "pre-sympathetic" to denote spinally projecting neurons that directly or indirectly control sympathetic preganglionic neurons). This group of pre-sympathetic neurons is often collectively referred to as the RVLM, though pre-sympathetic neurons only account for a small percentage of total neurons in the RVLM. In the rat, pre-sympathetic RVLM neurons are on average 1.8 mm from the midline, and their mediolateral extent is approximately 1 mm at the core of the RVLM (Figure 5–2A). The pre-sympathetic RVLM neurons are ventral and slightly medial to the nucleus ambiguus, with some neurons located near the ventral surface and the majority lying within 300 micrometers of it[58,94]. Most pre-sympathetic RVLM neurons are glutamatergic[106] and 50% to 70% of baro-inhibited, bulbospinal RVLM neurons are in the rostral portion of the C1 adrenergic cell group (Figures 5–1B and 5–3B–D)[94,114,118]. Non-catecholaminergic pre-sympathetic RVLM neurons are located slightly more rostrally (Figure 5–1B), interspersed with the catecholaminergic pre-sympathetic neurons[94]. Single-unit recording experiments place the baro-inhibited RVLM neurons immediately ventral to respiratory-related neurons of the Bötzinger complex[94,100].

Immediately caudal to the RVLM is a depressor region commonly referred to as the caudal ventrolateral medulla (CVLM; Figures 5–1B, and 5–2B). In early studies, the depressor neurons were thought to coincide with the A1 noradrenergic cell group; and there was speculation about a role for these catecholaminergic neurons in the observed depressor response[11]. Instead, the A1 neurons play an important role in hypovolemia-induced release of vasopressin from the posterior pituitary[104]. More recent studies have identified the critical depressor neurons as GABAergic and projecting toward the RVLM to presumably innervate pre-sympathetic RVLM neurons (see details below). These GABAergic neurons are rostral to the A1 neurons and are intermingled with the

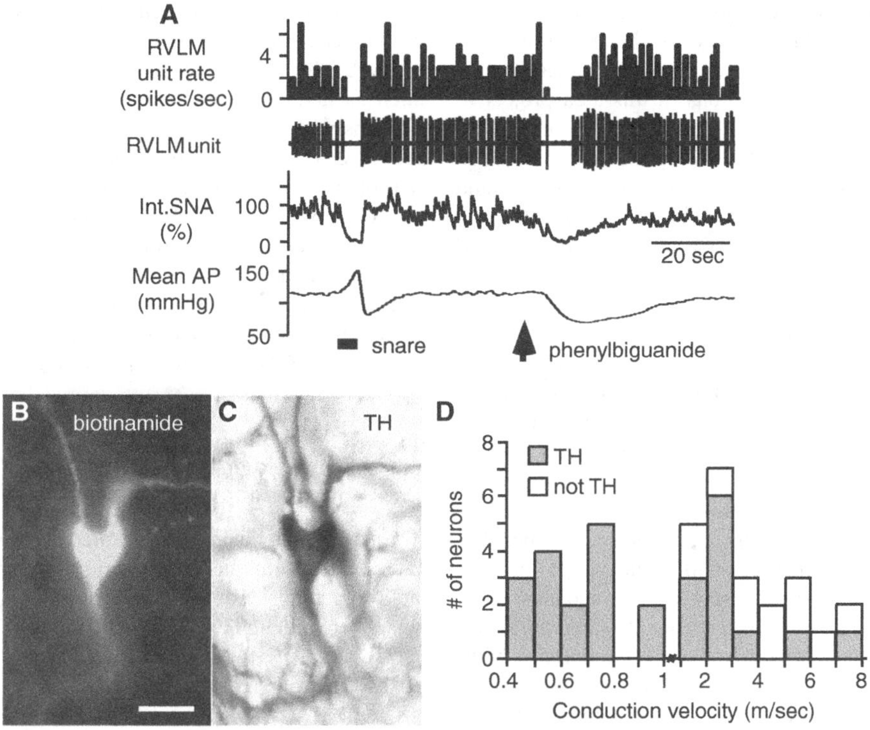


Figure 5–3 Characteristics of bulbospinal neurons of the RVLM. *A:* In a chloralose-anesthetized rat, a spinally projecting neuron in the RVLM is silenced by increasing AP due to constriction of an abdominal aortic snare or stimulation of the von Bezold-Jarisch reflex by phenylbiguanide (20 μg/kg, iv) coincident with inhibition of splanchnic SNA. Raw and integrated (Int) SNA are shown. A spinally projecting baro-inhibited RVLM neuron filled with biotinamide (B) by juxtacellular labeling and revealed with streptavidin-Cy3 is immunoreactive for tyrosine hydroxylase (C). Reproduced from Schreihofer and Guyenet (2000)[95], with permission. *D:* Slowly conducting baro-inhibited bulbospinal RVLM neurons are catecholaminergic, as indicated by tyrosine hydroxylase (TH) immunoreactivity; and faster conducting RVLM neurons are more likely to be non-catecholaminergic. Reproduced from Schreihofer and Guyenet (1997)[94], with permission.

forebrain-projecting caudal portion of the C1 cell group (Figure 5–1B)[98,118]. In rats, depressor responses to microinjections of glutamate place the CVLM approximately 1.5 mm caudal to the facial nucleus[89] or 1 mm rostral to calamus scriptorius (Figures 5–1B and 5.2B). At their rostral extent, the critical GABAergic neurons are located ventral to the nucleus ambiguus and between the lateral wings of the rostral lateral reticular nucleus (Figure 5–2B), and at their caudal extent they are immediately dorsal to the lateral reticular nucleus. Recordings of individual baro-activated GABAergic CVLM neurons place them immediately ventral to respiratory-related neurons of the pre-Bötzinger complex and the rostral portion of the ventral respiratory group. The GABAergic CVLM neurons that express Fos in response to hypertension and project to the RVLM span approximately 2 mm rostrocaudally, with some encroachment into the region containing pre-sympathetic RVLM neurons[19] (Figure 5–1). To distinguish it from the A1 region more caudally, Dampney and colleagues[23] proposed that the CVLM be renamed the intermediate ventrolateral medulla; however, the traditional nomenclature is still typically used.

Caudal to the depressor region of the CVLM lies another pressor region in the ventrolateral medulla referred to as the caudal pressor area to distinguish it from the pressor region in the RVLM. First described in rats by Gordon and McCann[34], microinjections of glutamate increase arterial pressure when centered in the ventrolateral medulla 1 mm to 2 mm caudal to the depressor area of the CVLM (Figures 5–1B and 5–2C). The most responsive region is dorsolateral to the caudal end of the lateral reticular nucleus and ventromedial to the medullary dorsal horn at the level of the pyramidal decussation[81,108]. In contrast to the RVLM and CVLM, properties of the critical neurons that evoke pressor responses from the caudal pressor area are not known. Neurons in this area project to several medullary regions associated with autonomic control but not directly to the spinal cord[108]. Evoked pressor responses are sympathetically mediated and appear to require activation of pre-sympathetic RVLM neurons[15]. The caudal pressor area is medial to, and distinct from, the caudal A1 cell group[108]. A pressor region in this part of the ventrolateral medulla has also been described in cats[30].

Recently, a pressor region located caudal to the caudal pressor area at the junction of the medulla and the cervical spinal cord was described in rat[102]. Stimulation of this region of the ventrolateral medulla increases arterial pressure; but, unlike the caudal pressor area, the pressor response does not require connections rostral to the CVLM. This region, named the medullo-cervical pressor area, contains glutamatergic neurons that project to the thoracic spinal cord[102] and most likely corresponds to the neurons retrogradely and trans-synaptically labeled after injection of pseudorabies virus into sympathetic ganglia[44]. These neurons do not contribute to basal sympathetic vasomotor tone in anesthetized rats, and their function remains to be elucidated. Given the paucity of information on this region, it will not be discussed further here.

## THE ROSTRAL VENTROLATERAL MEDULLA

The RVLM provides the major tonic excitatory drive for basal sympathetic vasomotor tone and functions as a key site for integration of numerous reflexively mediated changes in sympathetic nerve activity and arterial pressure. Excitation of the RVLM markedly increases sympathetic nerve activity, arterial pressure, and heart rate. Conversely, in anesthetized animals, acute inhibition of the RVLM reduces these parameters to the same extent as cervical spinal cord transection, suggesting that neurons in the RVLM provide the primary drive for basal sympathetic nerve activity to the cardiovascular system under these conditions. Interestingly, in conscious rats, acute inhibition of the RVLM reduces arterial pressure but increases heart rate by activation of β-adrenoceptors. This observation suggests that the RVLM is critical for maintaining sympathetic vasomotor tone, but other regions of the CNS may regulate sympathoadrenal control of the heart rate independently of the RVLM[71]. During the past decade, our knowledge of the anatomy and physiology of pre-sympathetic RVLM neurons has advanced greatly. Yet the original electrophysiological criteria for identification of pre-sympathetic RVLM neurons originally outlined by Guyenet and colleagues are still the standard today[35]. The recent development of new methods, such as juxtacellular labeling of individual RVLM neurons with extracellular recording[94] and immunotoxins that can selectively target C1 adrenergic neurons[63,96], have greatly advanced our understanding of how the RVLM modulates cardiovascular function. Nevertheless, some key questions remain unanswered, perhaps awaiting the development of other tools or new insights into how the brainstem regulates the autonomic function of targets important for control of the cardiovascular system.

### Electrophysiological Properties of Pre-Sympathetic RVLM Neurons

The RVLM can be precisely located using stereotaxic coordinates combined with antidromic mapping of field potentials from the adjacent facial nucleus, which are elicited by electrical stimulation of the facial nerve[35,79,94]. Identification of pre-sympathetic RVLM neurons requires demonstration of an axonal projection to the spinal cord. Within the RVLM immediately caudal to the facial nucleus, more than 90% of baro-inhibited neurons project to the spinal cord[94]. The baro-inhibited RVLM neurons have a wide range of conduction velocities (Figure 5–3D)[35,79,94], suggesting that the population contains neurons with unmyelinated and lightly myelinated axons. Firing rates also appear to be related to conduction velocity, with faster-conducting neurons having the highest firing rates and patterns of activity that resemble patterns observed in sympathetic nerve activity[35,94] With anesthetics that elevate sympathetic nerve activity, such as halothane or intraperitoneally administered urethane, the firing rates of pre-sympathetic RVLM neurons are also higher, along with reduced sensitivity to baroreceptor and respiratory inputs[35]. Pre-sympathetic RVLM neurons are exquisitely sensitive to changes in arterial pressure and are readily silenced by increases in arterial pressure coincident with an abolition of sympathetic nerve activity (Figure 5–3A). As observed in sympathetic nerve recordings, these neurons display activity that is related to the cardiac cycle if arterial pressure is high enough to produce sufficient arterial baroreceptor tone[35,79]. Within the cardiac cycle, RVLM neuronal activity peaks when arterial pressure is lowest during diastole and immediately preceding the cardiac-related peaks in sympathetic nerve activity[79], as would be expected if they are driving that activity. Neurons in the RVLM of rabbits and cats with similar electrophysiological properties have been reported[6,116].

## Neurochemistry of Pre-Sympathetic RVLM Neurons

Pre-sympathetic RVLM neurons are excitatory to sympathetic preganglionic neurons innervating cardiac and vasoconstrictor targets. The activity of pre-sympathetic RVLM neurons is directly correlated with sympathetic nerve activity[79], and stimulation of neuronal cell bodies in the RVLM with glutamate produces dose-dependent increases in arterial pressure[88] that are sympathetically mediated. In contrast, acute inhibition of neuronal cell bodies in the RVLM can virtually abolish the activity of sympathetic vasomotor nerves[101], reducing arterial pressure to levels observed after spinal transection[88,99]. The majority of pre-sympathetic RVLM neurons express vesicular glutamate transporter 2 mRNA[106], suggesting that they use glutamate as a neurotransmitter. In agreement, at least half of all axon profiles making contact with sympathetic preganglionic neurons in the thoracic spinal cord of the rat contain glutamate, with most of the remaining contacts containing GABA[60] (see Chapter 6). These data suggest that all other neurotransmitters released onto sympathetic preganglionic neurons are co-released with either glutamate or GABA. Therefore, as pre-sympathetic RVLM neurons are not GABAergic, the primary neurotransmitter of these neurons is likely to be glutamate. Although some of the influence of pre-sympathetic RVLM neurons may not be through direct synaptic contacts onto sympathetic preganglionic neurons, anterogradely labeled terminals from RVLM neurons contain glutamate and make synaptic contacts onto dendrites in the intermediolateral cell column, the thoracolumbar spinal nucleus that contains the cell bodies of sympathetic preganglionic neurons[78]. Spinally projecting C1 neurons also make synaptic contacts on sympathetic preganglionic neurons[73], but the majority of bulbospinal C1 neurons in the RVLM are also glutamatergic[102].

Physiological evidence indicates that bulbospinal RVLM neurons use the neurotransmitter glutamate to excite sympathetic preganglionic neurons. Injection of kynurenate, a broad-spectrum ionotropic glutamate receptor antagonist, into the subarachnoid space of the thoracic spinal cord dramatically reduces arterial pressure and inhibits sympathoexcitatory and pressor responses produced by stimulation of the RVLM[7]. Similarly, injection of glutamate receptor antagonists at discrete levels of the thoracic sympathetic column blocks RVLM-evoked increases in sympathetic outflow from that level[64,110]. Kynurenate also decreases the spontaneous activity of individually recorded sympathetic preganglionic neurons and prevents RVLM-evoked excitatory responses in anesthetized rats[78]. Although these data do not prove glutamate is acting at the synapse between RVLM neurons and sympathetic preganglionic neurons, the timing of the RVLM-evoked excitatory responses in sympathetic preganglionic neurons is suggestive of a fast neurotransmitter, such as an excitatory amino acid[78].

In contrast, the precise role of catecholamines in the regulation of sympathetic vasomotor tone by the RVLM is still not well understood. Approximately 50% to 70% of pre-sympathetic RVLM are C1 catecholaminergic neurons (Figures 5–1A, 5–3B, and 5–3C)[94,114,118]. Juxtacellular labeling of individually recorded pre-sympathetic RVLM neurons reveals that the slowly conducting neurons are catecholaminergic, and the faster-conducting neurons are catecholaminergic and non-catecholaminergic neurons (Figure 5–3D)[94]. However, vesicular glutamate transporter 2 mRNA is expressed in at least 80% of catecholaminergic pre-sympathetic RVLM neurons, suggesting they also use glutamate as a neurotransmitter[38]. The presence of noradrenaline and absence of detectable adrenaline in the intermediolateral region of thoracic spinal cord[111] indicates that C1 neurons may use noradrenaline as a neurotransmitter when catecholamines are released. The modulatory effects of catecholamines upon the activity of sympathetic preganglionic neurons are complex and depend upon the type of adrenoceptor that is activated and the state of the inputs to the target neuron[21]. *In vivo* studies have shown that iontophoretic application of noradrenaline or adrenaline inhibits the activity of sympathetic preganglionic neurons, contrary to the proposed sympathoexcitatory role of pre-sympathetic C1 neurons in the RVLM. However, the inhibitory influence of noradrenaline can be reversed to excitation by increasing the local concentration of a glutamate analogue, DL-homocysteic acid. *In vitro* studies have also shown both inhibitory and excitatory effects of catecholamines on the activity of sympathetic preganglionic neurons, which are probably mediated by $\alpha_2$- and $\alpha_1$-adrenoceptors, respectively. Thus, catecholamines may serve multiple purposes, including amplification of excitatory inputs or buffering to limit over-excitation of sympathetic preganglionic neurons by setting their level of excitability to other inputs.

The selective lesion of C1 pre-sympathetic RVLM neurons slightly decreases baseline arterial pressure[62,63] and impairs the ability of the RVLM to increase sympathetic nerve activity and arterial pressure[62,63,96,101], suggesting that the lesions may remove an excitatory influence of catecholamines on sympathetic preganglionic neurons. Alternatively, the elimination of C1 neurons may reduce the number of RVLM neurons that release glutamate to stimulate sympathetic nerve activity. Although glutamate appears to be essential for the ability of the RVLM to alter sympathetic nerve activity, blockade of adrenoceptors intrathecally does not affect tachycardic or pressor responses evoked by stimulation of the RVLM[20,64,72]. The conditions under which the pre-sympathetic RVLM neurons release catecholamines and the physiological effects of this neurotransmitter on the activity of sympathetic preganglionic neurons require further investigation.

The pre-sympathetic RVLM neurons also synthesize neuropeptides and other neuroactive substances that may play important roles in modulating sympathetic nerve activity. Trans-synaptic labeling of RVLM neurons by injection of pseudorabies virus into sympathetic targets reveals that pre-sympathetic RVLM neurons also contain neuropeptide Y, somatostatin, VIP, substance P, and met-enkephalin, suggesting that neuropeptides modulate RVLM-mediated regulation of sympathetic preganglionic neurons[45]. Pituitary adenylate cyclase-activating polypeptide is also found in bulbospinal catecholaminergic RVLM neurons, and administration of this peptide into the spinal cord increases splanchnic sympathetic nerve activity[29]. In addition, bulbospinal RVLM neurons also contain superoxides and cocaine- and amphetamine-related transcript[14,68]. The conditions under which these neuromodulators may be released from RVLM neurons and their effects upon sympathetic vasomotor tone are not well understood.

## The Generation of Sympathetic Vasomotor Tone by Tonic Activation of the RVLM

The mechanisms underlying the generation of tonic activity in pre-sympathetic RVLM neurons and sympathetic nerves is one of the most important, yet least understood, concepts in central neural control of the circulation. Even without the benefit of sensory inputs communicated through the NTS, the contribution of the RVLM to sympathetic nerve activity and arterial pressure remains at a normal set-point[99]. Historically, two views regarding the generation of tonic activity in pre-sympathetic RVLM neurons have been proposed. As initially described by Guyenet and colleagues[35], under certain conditions, pre-sympathetic RVLM neurons can display pacemaker-like activity and generate action potentials that are independent of synaptic inputs. In contrast, others have argued for a network-driven control of RVLM neurons that requires synaptic inputs to generate tonic activity. Based on intracellular recording *in vivo* and *in vitro*, Lipski and co-workers[59] concluded that all action potentials in RVLM neurons are preceded by excitatory post-synaptic potentials produced by synaptic input, and that these cells lack known pacemaker currents. Thus, while RVLM neurons may have pacemaker properties under some unusual conditions (*in vitro* slices from neonatal rats or intracisternal injection of kynurenic acid), under normal physiological conditions the activity of RVLM neurons seems to be produced by the balance of a multitude of excitatory and inhibitory inputs received by these neurons. Although a few key inputs will be described in the following sections, at present how the critical excitatory inputs generate the tonic activity of the RVLM pre-sympathetic neurons is unclear.

## Inputs to Pre-Sympathetic RVLM Neurons

The RVLM receives numerous projections from other regions of the CNS associated with autonomic control, many of which are reciprocal. Inputs to the RVLM include, but are not limited to, the NTS, CVLM (see below), contralateral RVLM, medullary respiratory neurons, medullary lateral tegmental field, midline raphé nuclei, A5 cell group, parabrachial nuclei, cerebellar nuclei, midbrain periaqueductal gray, lateral and periventricular nuclei of the hypothalamus, and prefrontal cortex (see Chapter 1). Details regarding the anatomical and physiological properties of most of these inputs are beyond the scope of this chapter, and the reader is referred to an excellent review by Dampney[25]. Whereas these afferent inputs to RVLM have been mapped in elegant neuroanatomical studies, most investigators have not ascertained whether these inputs are directed to pre-sympathetic neurons or to other neurons in this heterogeneous region. Studies conducted at the electron microscopic level have documented excitatory and inhibitory inputs, but sources and physiological roles are not certain in many cases. Both glutamate and angiotensin peptides clearly play important excitatory roles in regulating the activity of pre-sympathetic RVLM neurons (see below), and GABA is the major inhibitory influence (see section on CVLM). In addition, other neuroactive substances such as catecholamines, acetylcholine, opioids, estrogen, nitric oxide, substance P, corticotropin-releasing factor, superoxide, serotonin, and vasopressin clearly affect the activity of the RVLM, but are beyond the scope of this chapter.

## Glutamate as a Tonic Excitatory Input to the RVLM

Because glutamate is a major excitatory neurotransmitter in the CNS, it would be logical to assume that this excitatory amino acid would play an important role in generating the tonic activity of pre-sympathetic RVLM neurons. However, reports that bilateral blockade of glutamate receptors in the RVLM with kynurenic acid produces no detectable effects on resting arterial pressure suggested that glutamate does not provide a significant tonic activation of pre-sympathetic RVLM neurons[37,48]. Ito and Sved[42] challenged this notion with their observation that if the CVLM is first inhibited, subsequent blockade of glutamate receptors in the RVLM markedly reduces arterial pressure. In their model, glutamatergic inputs to the RVLM directly excite pre-sympathetic neurons and indirectly excite GABAergic inhibition of the RVLM, and the lack of change in arterial pressure with kynurenic acid in the RVLM reflects the balance of these two actions. However, this concept was challenged by Dampney and colleagues[41], who were unable to replicate the key observation of changes in arterial pressure or in renal sympathetic nerve activity. In contrast, Miyawaki and colleagues[74] found that after blockade of GABAergic inputs within the RVLM, injection of kynurenic acid produced some inhibition of splanchnic and lumbar sympathetic nerve activity. These observations suggested a tonic glutamatergic input to RVLM neurons under their experimental conditions, but also the existence of additional sources of drive to these neurons. Insights into the apparent differences in the outcomes of these studies may be gained from animal models that have elevated basal sympathetic nerve activity, such as hypertension or water deprivation, where inhibition of glutamate receptors in the RVLM consistently lowers sympathetic nerve activity and arterial pressure[13,113]. In these instances, the balance between glutamatergic drives and inhibitory influences appears shifted toward excitation. Although the level of glutamatergic excitation in relative balance with other inputs seems to vary with the physiological state of the animal, it is clear that, in the absence of both glutamatergic and GABAergic inputs to pre-sympathetic RVLM neurons, significant activity remains to drive sympathetic nerve activity and maintain arterial pressure.

## Angiotensins as Tonic Excitatory Inputs to the RVLM

Microinjection of angiotensin peptides into RVLM increases arterial pressure and sympathetic nerve activity; and angiotensin II activates pre-sympathetic RVLM neurons (see [113]), consistent with the presence of angiotensin type 1 receptors in this region (see [12]) and an excitatory action of the peptides. Likewise, blockade of angiotensin type 1 receptors in RVLM reduces the increase in arterial pressure and sympathetic nerve activity evoked by disinhibition of the paraventricular nucleus of the hypothalamus (PVN), suggesting that PVN-evoked excitation of the RVLM is mediated by angiotensin[115]. In contrast, the existence of a tonic contribution of angiotensins to the basal activity of RVLM neurons has been more controversial. The observation that bilateral injection into the RVLM of sarcosine-containing peptide antagonists of angiotensin receptors (e.g., Sarthran) markedly decreases arterial pressure has been replicated in several laboratories with multiple analogues, but more recent studies show this response is not due to an action on any known type of angiotensin receptor[43,85]. In particular, local injection of selective antagonists of type 1 or type 2 angiotensin receptors has no effect on baseline arterial pressure in anesthetized rats, suggesting there is little tonic contribution to the maintenance of sympathetic nerve activity and arterial pressure. As with glutamate, the contribution of angiotensins to the tonic activity of pre-sympathetic RVLM neurons is likely to vary with the state of the animal, as selective blockade of angiotensin type 1 receptors decreases arterial pressure in several rat models of hypertension[113]. The cellular mechanisms underlying the production and utilization of angiotensin peptides as neurotransmitters in the RVLM are also not fully understood. The notion of an angiotensinergic neuron is equivocal and it is more likely that glia release angiotensinogen that is converted to active angiotensin peptides in the interstitial fluid. Furthermore, Allen and colleagues[3] observed an increase in arterial pressure after using an adenoviral vector to express a constitutively active form of the angiotensin type 1 receptor in rat RVLM, but here the expression of the active angiotensin type 1 receptor occurred in astrocytes rather than neurons. Further study is clearly needed to elucidate the role of angiotensin peptides in the tonic regulation of the activity of pre-sympathetic RVLM neurons and the mechanisms underlying the synthesis and utilization of angiotensins in the RVLM.

## The RVLM and Generation of Sympathetic Reflexes and Centrally Mediated Changes in Sympathetic Nerve Activity

The RVLM is a major site of integration for phasic changes in sympathetic vasomotor tone initiated by peripheral inputs or by neurons in central autonomic-related nuclei. Sympathoinhibitory reflexes initiated by peripheral afferent nerves to the NTS, such as the arterial baroreflex and von Bezold-Jarisch reflex, are produced by GABAergic inhibition of pre-sympathetic RVLM neurons via activation of the CVLM (see next section). In contrast, for many sympathoexcitatory reflexes, glutamate plays a clear, essential role in the activation of pre-sympathetic RVLM neurons to increase sympathetic nerve activity. For example, stimulation of the peripheral chemoreflex activates many pre-sympathetic RVLM neurons and increases sympathetic nerve activity. This sympathoexcitatory response is greatly reduced by blockade of glutamate receptors in the RVLM[52]. Analogous observations have been reported for other sympathoexcitatory responses, including those elicited by the somatic pressor reflex[48], the nasopharyngeal reflex[70], and stimulation of the gall bladder[124]. Although the source of the glutamatergic input to the RVLM for the chemoreflex is believed to be the NTS[52], for these other reflexes the source of glutamate is not known.

In addition to integrating signals from the periphery, the RVLM is also a site of integration for centrally mediated increases in sympathetic nerve activity. Most autonomic-related nuclei do not directly influence sympathetic nerves by projections to the spinal cord but instead project to the RVLM. Many centrally evoked pressor responses are produced, at least in part, by excitation of the RVLM, including those elicited from the nuclei in the hypothalamus (see Chapter 3), dorsolateral PAG[61], central nucleus of the amygdala[90], or cuneiform nucleus[117]. In contrast, serotonergic inputs to the RVLM from the midline raphé nuclei appear to provide an inhibitory influence upon RVLM neurons, and this input may be activated during painful stimuli and under conditions of stress[5].

## THE CAUDAL VENTROLATERAL MEDULLA

The depressor region of the CVLM provides tonic and phasic inhibitory control of pre-sympathetic RVLM neurons. Stimulation of the CVLM reduces sympathetic nerve activity and arterial pressure via inhibition of the RVLM in rats and other species examined[2,27,55,122], probably due to activation of $GABA_A$ receptors on pre-sympathetic RVLM neurons[9]. The magnitude of increases in arterial pressure, sympathetic nerve activity, and plasma noradrenaline produced by blockade of $GABA_A$ receptors in the RVLM is mimicked by inhibition of the CVLM[80,99], suggesting that the CVLM is the major source of tonic inhibition to pre-sympathetic RVLM neurons. GABAergic neurons in the CVLM provide a crucial restraint to the activity of the RVLM and sympathetic nerves to maintain a normal arterial pressure. In addition, most sympathoinhibitory reflexes that occur by inhibition of the RVLM appear to be produced through activation of GABAergic CVLM neurons.

Before considering these GABAergic CVLM neurons in more detail, we must acknowledge that these neurons exist in a heterogeneous region of the medullary reticular formation and are intermixed with neurons utilizing different neurotransmitters that serve a variety of functions. One such group of neurons within the CVLM region is the caudal portion of the C1 cell group. These baro-inhibited neurons, which innervate forebrain structures[118], mimic the activity observed in the spinally projecting rostral C1 neurons, providing a mechanism for coordination of forebrain systems with control of sympathetic preganglionic neurons. Although the detailed function of the caudal C1 neurons has not been the focus of much study, these neurons may play a role in the response to deficits in blood glucose[87] and possibly other stressful conditions[93].

### Identification of Putative CVLM Inhibitory Neurons Regulating RVLM

Studies in the 1980s characterizing the CVLM depressor area also highlighted its critical role in baroreceptor reflex control of sympathetic nerve activity and arterial pressure. The essential role of CVLM neurons in relaying baroreceptor-related signals from the NTS to the RVLM, and providing the required inhibitory link in this reflex pathway, has now been fully documented[112]. Extracellular recordings within the depressor region of the CVLM reveal a population of neurons with attributes suggesting that they are the critical interneurons in the baroreflex pathway. In contrast to pre-sympathetic RVLM neurons, CVLM neuronal activity is briskly activated by slight increases in arterial pressure (baro-activated) and is inversely related to sympathetic nerve activity (Figures 5–4A and 5–4B)[97,98]. The activity of CVLM neurons is tightly coupled to mean arterial pressure (Figures 5–4C and 5–4D). Especially with elevated arterial pressure, these neurons are prominently modulated in relation to the cardiac cycle (pulse-modulated), with most of their activity occurring during the rising phase of systole (Figure 5–4C). Baro-activated CVLM neurons are also activated by other stimuli that produce sympathoinhibition. For example, systemic cholecystokinin or stimulation of the von Bezold-Jarisch reflex with the $5HT_3$ agonist phenylbiguanide excite baro-activated CVLM neurons immediately preceding the inhibition of sympathetic nerve activity (Figures 5–4A and 5–4B)[98]. In addition, baro-activated CVLM neurons display patterns of central respiratory modulation that appear to be inversely related to patterns observed in pre-sympathetic RVLM neurons (see Chapter 10)[39,65]. Juxtacellular labeling of baro-activated, pulse-modulated CVLM neurons paired with *in situ* hybridization histochemistry for GAD67 mRNA demonstrates these neurons are GABAergic (Figures 5–4E and 5–4F)[97,98]. This phenotypic identification is needed to identify the inhibitory interneurons, because adjacent cholinergic vagal motor neurons in the nucleus ambiguus are also activated by baroreceptors and phenylbiguanide and display respiratory-related activity[32,47,86]. Lastly, baro-activated, pulse-modulated CVLM neurons have been antidromically activated from the pressor region of the RVLM[1,31,46]. Although this observation does not prove a synaptic connection,

CVLM neurons with this combination of properties are prime candidates for the inhibitory neurons that regulate pre-sympathetic RVLM neurons.

## The CVLM and the Production of Sympathetic Reflexes

The stimulation of numerous reflexes requiring activation of vagal afferent nerves evokes inhibition of sympathetic nerve activity that is mediated by GABAergic inhibition of the pre-sympathetic RVLM neurons[107,119]. In each of these cases, the GABAergic inhibition appears to arise from the CVLM[112]. The most-studied of these reflexes, the arterial baroreflex, is initiated by raising arterial pressure to stimulate baroreceptors in the aortic arch and carotid sinus, the axons of which travel via vagal and glossopharyngeal afferent nerves, respectively. The baroreceptor afferents activate second-order neurons in the NTS, which in turn excite GABAergic interneurons in the CVLM via a glutamatergic input[112]. These baro-activated GABAergic CVLM neurons most likely inhibit pre-sympathetic RVLM neurons, thereby inhibiting sympathetic nerve activity and returning arterial pressure to normal levels. Disruption or impairment of this reflex is linked with impaired short-term control of arterial pressure and hypertension (see below).

The stimulation of chemosensitive cardiac vagal afferent nerves by activation of $5HT_3$ receptors to elicit the von Bezold-Jarisch reflex evokes profound inhibition of sympathetic nerve activity and hypotension by the same tri-synaptic medullary pathway (Figures 5–3A and 5–4B)[119]. Recently, activation of gastrointestinal vagal afferents by cholecystokinin has been shown to inhibit pre-sympathetic RVLM neurons coincident with inhibition of splanchnic sympathetic nerve activity[92]. This effect also requires activation of the CVLM neurons[76]. Interestingly, this stimulus produces opposing effects on other sympathetic nerves, and differential effects are reflected in recordings of individual barosensitive CVLM and RVLM neurons (see below)[76,92]. Analogous to stimulation of vagal afferent nerves, stimulation of some sympathetic afferents, such as the greater splanchnic nerve, also evokes sympathoinhibition requiring the CVLM[83].

The inhibition CVLM neuronal activity also appears to contribute to sympathoexcitatory responses via disinhibition of pre-sympathetic RVLM neurons. Hypotension reduces the drive to baroreceptor

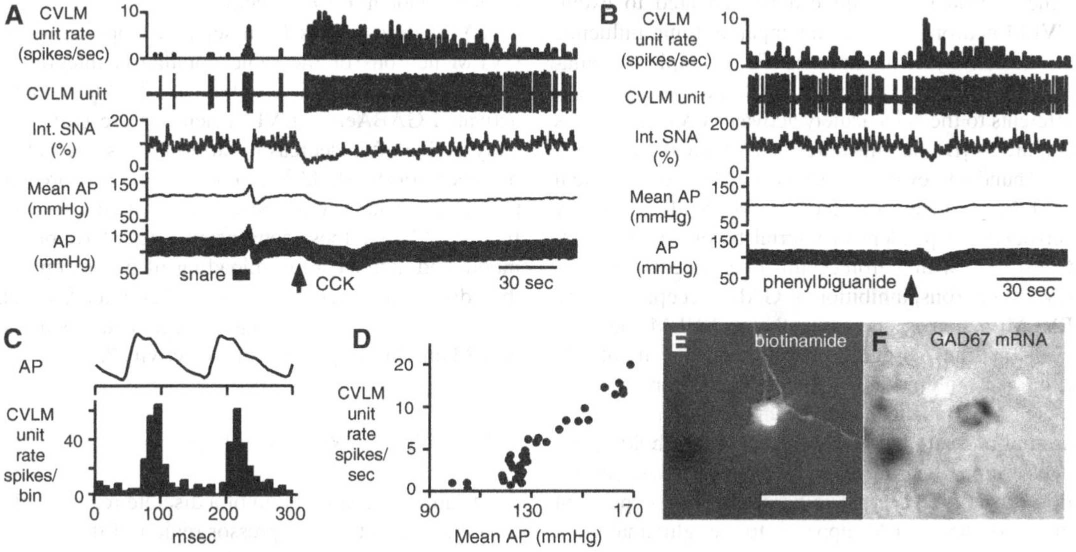


Figure 5–4 Characteristics of baro-activated neurons in the CVLM. In a chloralose-anesthetized rat, a neuron in the CVLM is activated by either (*A*) raising AP with a snare and injection of cholecystokinin (CCK, 10 μg/kg, iv), or by (*B*) injection of phenylbiguanide coincident with inhibition of splanchnic SNA. Reproduced from Mobley et al. (2006)[76], with permission. Baro-activated CVLM neurons display prominent modulation of activity by the AP pulse (*C*) and their firing rate is tightly coupled to the level of mean AP (*D*). A biotinamide-labeled, baro-activated CVLM neuron (*E*) expresses GAD67 mRNA (*F*), suggesting it is GABAergic. Int, integrated. Reproduced from Schreihofer and Guyenet (2003)[98], with permission.

afferent nerves and is associated with a reduction in the activity of baro-activated GABAergic CVLM neurons coincident with increases in sympathetic nerve activity[97,98]. A firm tail pinch also activates sympathetic nerve activity and coincides with inhibition of baro-activated GABAergic CVLM neurons[98]. Likewise, activation of the peripheral chemoreflex inhibits some baro-activated GABAergic CVLM neurons; and blockade of GABA receptors in the CVLM by microinjection of gabazine greatly reduces the sympathoexcitatory response to hypoxia[67]. Thus, fluctuations in the activity of GABAergic CVLM neurons in either direction have profound effects upon the sympathetic nerve activity that regulates cardiovascular function.

### Activity of GABAergic CVLM Neurons: Baroreceptor-Dependent and Baroreceptor-Independent Regulation

GABAergic CVLM neurons are tonically activated by glutamate[37,99]. The NTS is a major source of this input[1,33,121], largely driven by arterial baroreceptor signals and acting upon *N*-methyl-D-aspartate (NMDA) and non-NMDA glutamate receptors in the CVLM[33,66,75,120]. Many baro-activated CVLM neurons are silenced by unloading baroreceptors, suggesting that they require this input for their tonic activity[46,98]. Other peripheral stimuli can be activated to excite CVLM neurons but have no apparent tonic influence on the activity of the neurons. For example, stimulation of $5HT_3$ receptors on cardiopulmonary vagal afferents to the NTS acutely activates CVLM neurons (Figure 5–4B), but this reflex is not tonically active.

Abundant evidence suggests that the critical GABAergic neurons of the CVLM are also tonically activated independent of arterial baroreceptor input. Consistent with baroreceptor-independent drive of CVLM neurons, inhibition of GABA receptors in the RVLM activates pre-sympathetic RVLM neurons even in the absence of baroreceptor input[26,107]. Likewise, inhibition of the CVLM continues to increase sympathetic nerve activity after lowering arterial pressure below baroreceptor threshold, acute denervation of baroreceptor afferent nerves, or inhibition of the NTS[22,26,66]. The baroreceptor-independent drive to the CVLM appears to be glutamatergic, because unloading baroreceptors by hypotension or blockade of glutamatergic inputs in the NTS produces a smaller rise in arterial pressure than blockade of glutamatergic inputs in the CVLM[24,37]. Furthermore, after inhibition or lesions of the NTS, arterial baroreceptor reflexes are abolished; but blockade of glutamate receptors in the CVLM by microinjection of kynurenate continues to increase sympathetic nerve activity and arterial pressure[66,99]. Collectively, these observations suggest that the critical GABAergic CVLM neurons are tonically activated by glutamate that is not derived from the NTS and does not depend on baroreceptor inputs.

One possible source of excitatory input to CVLM neurons is the paraventricular nucleus of the hypothalamus. Stimulation of this region can evoke depressor responses that coincide with the activation of baro-activated, pulse-modulated CVLM neurons[123]. Another source of excitatory input may be central respiratory–related neurons. Some individually recorded baro-activated GABAergic CVLM neurons show pre-inspiratory peaks in their activity reminiscent of adjacent excitatory respiratory-related neurons of the pre-Bötzinger complex[38],[65]. In addition, lesions of neurons in the pre-Bötzinger complex impair the ability of the CVLM to decrease arterial pressure[120]. (see Chapter 10 for further discussion of cardiorespiratory integration in the medulla oblongata.). Furthermore, under conditions of minimal baroreceptor inputs, increasing central respiratory drive by hypoventilation leads to larger sympathoexcitatory responses to the blockade of glutamatergic inputs to the CVLM. These data suggest that central respiratory–related neurons may provide a glutamatergic input to critical cardiovascular-related neurons in the CVLM[66].

Whether the baroreceptor-driven and baroreceptor-independent CVLM-mediated inhibition of the RVLM neurons arises from separate populations of CVLM neurons or the same population integrating both types of inputs is not known[67,119]. Many baro-activated GABAergic CVLM neurons are still tonically active after decreasing arterial pressure below baroreceptor threshold[65,97], suggesting that baroreceptor-independent inputs also drive their activity. Indeed, although these neurons no longer have pulse-modulated activity after unloading of baroreceptors, they do maintain respiratory-related activity[65], which is also observed in their putative target neurons in the RVLM and in sympathetic nerve activity[39].

## THE CAUDAL PRESSOR AREA

Stimulation or disinhibition of a discrete region in the medulla caudal to the depressor region of the CVLM has been shown consistently to increase arterial pressure and sympathetic nerve activity in anesthetized rats[16,34,81,108]. Conversely, inhibition of this region by local injection of $GABA_A$ agonists or, more prominently, glycine, markedly reduces arterial pressure[84], suggesting that this area plays an important role in the maintenance of sympathetic vasomotor tone. The large increase in arterial pressure produced by local injections of $GABA_A$ antagonists indicates that this area is normally under a high degree of tonic inhibition in anesthetized animals[84]. Nevertheless, how the caudal pressor area integrates into known circuits involved in the physiological control of the cardiovascular system remains a mystery. It is not known whether the caudal pressor area mediates any short-term cardiovascular reflexes. Anatomical data regarding the identity of the neurons in the caudal pressor area that are involved in cardiovascular regulation and their critical inputs are also lacking.

The RVLM is essential for pressor responses evoked from the caudal pressor area. Stimulation of this region excites pre-sympathetic neurons in the RVLM[15], and inhibition of the RVLM prevents the rise in arterial pressure evoked from the caudal pressor area[34,84], indicating that the pressor response initiated by the caudal pressor area requires activation of the RVLM. Inhibition of the caudal pressor area with glycinergic or GABAergic analogues significantly decreases the activity of pre-sympathetic RVLM neurons, sympathetic nerve activity, and arterial pressure[15,81,84], indicating that the caudal pressor area provides a necessary tonic excitatory input to pre-sympathetic RVLM neurons.

The mechanism underlying the caudal pressor area–evoked activation of the RVLM is not well understood. Direct projections from the region of the caudal pressor area to the RVLM are sparse[109], and stimulation of pre-sympathetic RVLM neurons by the caudal pressor area does not appear to require activation of glutamate receptors in the RVLM[16]. Instead, the pressor response from caudal pressor area stimulation appears to require a functional CVLM. Blockade of $GABA_A$ receptors within the CVLM reduces the increase in arterial pressure evoked from stimulation of the caudal pressor area[16], suggesting inhibition of the CVLM may contribute to the excitation of the RVLM. However, the pressor response does not appear to involve a reduction of GABAergic inputs to the RVLM[81]. The depressor response evoked by inhibition of the caudal pressor area is virtually abolished after blockade of glutamate receptors in the CVLM[16], suggesting CVLM activity is needed to reduce the drive to the RVLM. Although the region of the CVLM has been identified as important, the identities of the critical neurons within the CVLM are not known.

The caudal pressor area appears to have widespread connections to other autonomic regions of the brainstem and pons, and these may contribute to the complexity of the mechanisms underlying excitation of the RVLM mediated by the caudal pressor area. Projections from the caudal pressor area are most dense to the commissural NTS, A5 region, and lateral parabrachial nucleus, with sparse projections to the CVLM and the RVLM[109]. However, precise connections within these heterogeneous regions have not been established. It appears that neurons in the caudal pressor area are tonically inhibited by GABA[81], although the source of this input is not known. Given its impressive impact on the activity of pre-sympathetic RVLM neurons, one would expect that the caudal pressor area would affect reflex control of sympathetic nerve activity mediated by the RVLM. However, inhibition of the caudal pressor area does not alter the pressor response to carotid occlusion[84], suggesting that other inputs to the RVLM can function in the absence of an excitatory drive from the caudal pressor area. In contrast, stimulation of the nucleus raphé obscurus evokes a pressor response that requires the RVLM, and this response is virtually abolished after inhibition of glutamatergic inputs to the caudal pressor area[103]. The mechanisms underlying the pressor response of the caudal pressor area and its interactions with other regions of the ventrolateral medulla require further investigation.

## DIFFERENTIAL REGULATION OF SYMPATHETIC OUTFLOW TO PERIPHERAL VASCULAR BEDS

The ventrolateral medulla is clearly integral for the control of sympathetic vasomotor tone but the mechanisms underlying differential or selective regulation of distinct vascular beds is not well understood. Physiological conditions, such as muscle use, standing, fear, and food intake, result in unique patterns of sympathetic nerve activity to divert blood flow to where it is needed. If dedicated pathways to each tissue or for each situation exist, their points of origin within the CNS are not known. Furthermore, the distinction at the level of the ventrolateral medulla between control of sympathetic vasomotor outflow specifically versus control of other types of sympathetic nerve activity is not clear.

The rat RVLM is connected to virtually all sympathetically innervated targets, whether or not they are involved in cardiovascular regulation. For example, trans-synaptic retrograde transport of pseudorabies virus from the pineal gland[53] or interscapular brown adipose tissue[17] results in labeling of RVLM neurons with a time course consistent with direct innervation of sympathetic preganglionic neurons by the RVLM. At least in cat, the RVLM appears to be topographically organized, with distinct regions preferentially controlling muscle vasoconstrictors, visceral vasoconstrictors, or kidney[69]. In contrast, there is no clear topographical organization in the rat RVLM. Instead, RVLM sites that can elicit preferential responses in one sympathetic nerve or another after focal micro-stimulation are intermixed[8,40]. How these different clusters of RVLM neurons, whether topographically distinct as in the cat or intermixed as in the rat, are independently controlled is not known. Nevertheless, it is evident that certain populations are differentially regulated, and that stimuli yielding differential sympathetic responses are associated with heterogeneous responses in pre-sympathetic RVLM neurons. For example, systemic injection of cholecystokinin activates lumbar sympathetic nerve activity while inhibiting splanchnic sympathetic nerve activity; and individual pre-sympathetic RVLM neurons display either one or the other response[91]. Analogous heterogeneous responses in RVLM neurons have been observed with other stimuli that affect sympathetic nerve activity, such as stimulation of the nasopharyngeal reflex[70], and hypoxia[51].

The baro-activated GABAergic neurons in the CVLM also display heterogeneous patterns of activity under resting conditions and with sympathetic-altering stimuli, suggesting dedication to inhibition of particular RVLM neurons or sympathetic nerves. For instance, four patterns of respiratory-related activity have been observed in GABAergic baro-activated CVLM neurons that may be inversely related to the patterns previously reported in pre-sympathetic RVLM neurons and particular sympathetic nerves[65]. In addition, baro-activated GABAergic CVLM neurons are either inhibited, excited, or unaffected by systemic cholecystokinin[76], in agreement with the differential responses observed in their putative target neurons in the RVLM[92]. Thus, at the level of the ventrolateral medulla some individual neurons may be dedicated to particular sympathetic outflows or respond differentially to stimuli to produce complex patterning of individual sympathetic nerves. There are no known anatomical differences, such as phenotypic markers or morphology, that coincide with the differential physiological responses of these medullary neurons, suggesting perhaps that the specificity derives from the sources of the precise inputs to particular neurons of the CVLM and RVLM.

## THE VENTROLATERAL MEDULLA AND HYPERTENSION

Given the critical importance of the ventrolateral medulla in the regulation of arterial pressure, it is not surprising that this region of the brainstem has been considered in the pathophysiology of hypertension. Indeed, since the early studies on the role of the brain in animal models of hypertension, the CVLM and RVLM have been foci of attention, owing in large part to the presence of catecholamine neurons in these areas and the anti-hypertensive effects of drugs that alter catecholaminergic neural transmission in the central nervous system. Several types of data have supported the involvement of the ventrolateral medulla in hypertension. These include neurochemical differences between hypertensive animals and controls, impact of stimulation or inhibition of these regions on arterial pressure in hypertensive versus normotensive animals, differences in response to local injections of neurotransmitters or drugs, and differences in the firing rates or patterns of neurons in these areas.

Considering that the RVLM is a key site of pre-sympathetic vasomotor neurons, they may be expected to be more active in models of neurogenic hypertension, as a result of either more excitatory input or less inhibitory input. Although the few studies comparing the firing rates of these neurons between normotensive and hypertensive rats have provided inconsistent evidence, a shift in the balance between excitatory and inhibitory drive to the RVLM is apparent. There is a consistent decrease in arterial pressure in response to injection of glutamate antagonists into the RVLM in multiple models of hypertension in rats[113], which contrasts markedly with the lack of effect of such drugs in normotensive control rats. However, the fall in arterial pressure toward normotensive levels following injection of an ionotropic glutamate receptor antagonist, such as kynurenic acid, into the RVLM should not be interpreted as an increase in excitatory drive to this region. Similar results would be obtained if inhibitory inputs were decreased. Likewise, altered responses to CVLM manipulation in hypertension[103] point to a change without elucidating underlying mechanisms.

One difference observed in many hypertensive animal models is a decrease in arterial pressure toward normotensive levels following injection into the RVLM of angiotensin type 1 receptor antagonists[113]. This response, which contrasts with the lack of effect of these treatments in normotensive rats, suggests that angiotensin peptides in the RVLM may be involved in the pathophysiology of hypertension. Angiotensin in RVLM stimulates pre-sympathetic RVLM neurons[56], possibly the C1 neurons in particular[57]. Despite the robust nature of the response to blockade of angiotensin type 1 receptor in the RVLM of hypertensive rats, considerable work needs to be performed to establish a role for angiotensin in the RVLM in hypertension. The critical pieces of missing information include the source of angiotensin and whether it has the potential to chronically affect the RVLM pre-sympathetic neurons[3]. Interestingly, arterial pressure increases when angiotensin type 1 receptor signaling in the RVLM is increased through an adenoviral vector that causes over-expression of a constitutively active mutant of angiotensin type 1 receptors in astrocytes[3].

Two additional types of observations have focused attention on an important role of the RVLM in hypertension. First, the RVLM may be the brain site of action of clinically useful antihypertensive drugs, such as clonidine. While the debate about whether the key action of these drugs is at $\alpha_2$-adrenoceptors or imidazoline receptors continues[28,36], the more significant issue is whether the RVLM is indeed the critical site of action. Clonidine and related drugs decrease arterial pressure when injected directly into the RVLM, and the RVLM is necessary for the response to these drugs when given systemically[28]. However, intravenous clonidine has a more profound inhibitory effect on sympathetic nerve activity than on the activity of pre-sympathetic RVLM neurons[95], raising the possibility that regions other than the RVLM also contribute to the antihypertensive effects of clonidine and related drugs.

Second, clinical studies have suggested a relationship between pulsating arteries on the ventral surface of the brainstem in association with hypertension[54], and surgical removal of the pulsating artery has been reported to reverse hypertension[54]. Additionally, in an animal model of this association, pulse-synchronous pressure exerted on the rostral ventrolateral medullary surface in anesthetized rats increases arterial pressure; an effect reversed by local injection of a glutamate receptor antagonist[77].

Whereas most of the studies examining the role of the RVLM in hypertension have been carried out in acute anesthetized preparations, it is important to note that chronic changes in RVLM do result in lasting changes in arterial pressure in conscious rats. For example, Kishi et al.[50] report that chronic over-expression of the endothelial isoform of nitric oxide synthase, produced by injection into the RVLM of an adenoviral vector, leads to a chronic decrease in arterial pressure. Conversely, adenoviral vector-induced over-expression of inducible nitric oxide synthase produced a sustained increase in arterial pressure[49]. With current advances in viral vector technology, new information on the role of brainstem structures in the chronic control of arterial pressure and hypertension should be forthcoming. However, it is already clear that changes in the ventrolateral medulla can have profound consequences on the long-term control of arterial pressure related to hypertension.

## SUMMARY

Over the past 25 years, the ventrolateral medulla has been the focus of studies on the brain control of cardiovascular function and sympathetic vasomotor tone. Much has been learned about the functional organization of this complex region, and these findings have validated its importance. Although many aspects of its organization are now well understood and appreciated, such as the role of the RVLM in the maintenance of baseline arterial pressure and the function of the CVLM in relaying inhibitory baroreceptor signals to pre-sympathetic RVLM neurons, there is still much to learn. Tools to dissect complex heterogeneous brain structures and chronically manipulate subsets of neurons in ways that can be studied in the context of cardiovascular regulation in conscious animals will be critical for the development of new knowledge about these critical regions of the brainstem.

ACKNOWLEDGEMENTS Drs. Schreihofer and Sved are supported by grants from the National Institutes of Health (R01 HL075174 and R01 HL086759 to AMS, R01 HL055687 to AFS).

## References

1. Agarwal, S. K., and Calaresu, F. R. (1991). Monosynaptic connection from caudal to rostral ventrolateral medulla in the baroreceptor reflex pathway. *Brain Research* 555, 70–74.
2. Agarwal, S. K., Gelsema, A. J., and Calaresu, F. R. (1989). Neurons in rostral VLM are inhibited by chemical stimulation of caudal VLM in rats. *American Journal of Physiology* 257, R265–R270.
3. Allen, A. M., Dosanjh, J. K., Erac, M., Dassanayake, S., Hannan, R. D., and Thomas, W. G. (2006). Expression of constitutively active angiotensin receptors in the rostral ventrolateral medulla increases blood pressure. *Hypertension.* 47, 1054–1061.
4. Arango, V., Ruggiero, D. A., Callaway, J. L., Anwar, M., Mann, J. J., and Reis, D. J. (1988). Catecholaminergic neurons in the ventrolateral medulla and nucleus of the solitary tract in the human. *Journal of Comparative Neurology* 273, 224–240.
5. Bago, M., and Dean, C. (2001). Sympathoinhibition from ventrolateral periaqueductal gray mediated by 5-HT(1A) receptors in the RVLM. *American Journal of Physiology. Regulatory, Integrative and Comparative Physiology* 280, R976–R984.
6. Barman, S. M., and Gebber, G. L. (1985). Axonal projection patterns of ventrolateral medullospinal sympathoexcitatory neurons. *Journal of Neurophysiology* 53, 1551–1566.
7. Bazil, M. K., and Gordon, F. J. (1991). Spinal NMDA receptors mediate pressor responses evoked from the rostral ventrolateral medulla. *American Journal of Physiology* 260, H267–H275.

8. Beluli, D. J., and Weaver, L. C. (1991). Differential control of renal and splenic nerves without medullary topography. *American Journal of Physiology* 260, H1072–H1079.
9. Blessing, W. W. (1988). Depressor neurons in rabbit caudal medulla act via GABA receptors in rostral medulla. *American Journal of Physiology* 254, H686–H692.
10. Blessing, W. W. (1997). *The Lower Brain Stem and Bodily Homeostasis*. New York: Oxford University Press.
11. Blessing, W. W., and Reis, D. J. (1982). Inhibitory cardiovascular function of neurons in the caudal ventrolateral medulla of the rabbit: Relationship to the area containing A1 noradrenergic cells. *Brain Research* 253, 161–171.
12. Bourassa, E. A., Sved, A. F., and Speth, R. C. (2008). Angiotensin modulation of rostral ventrolateral medulla (RVLM) in cardiovascular regulation. *Molecular and Cellular Endocrinology* 302, 167–75.
13. Brooks, V. L., Freeman, K. L., and Clow, K. A. (2004). Excitatory amino acids in rostral ventrolateral medulla support blood pressure during water deprivation in rats. *American Journal of Physiology. Heart and Circulatory Physiology* 286, H1642– H1648.
14. Burman, K. J., Sartor, D. M., Verberne, A. J., and Llewellyn-Smith, I. J. (2004). Cocaine- and amphetamine-regulated transcript in catecholamine and noncatecholamine presympathetic vasomotor neurons of rat rostral ventrolateral medulla. *Journal of Comparative Neurology* 476, 19–31.
15. Campos, R. R., and McAllen, R. M. (1999). Tonic drive to sympathetic premotor neurons of rostral ventrolateral medulla from caudal pressor area neurons. *American Journal of Physiology* 276, R1209–R1213.
16. Campos, R. R., Possas, O. S., Cravo, S. L., Lopes, O. U., and Guertzenstein, P. G. (1994). Putative pathways involved in cardiovascular responses evoked from the caudal pressor area. *Brazilian Journal of Medical and Biological Research* 27, 2467–2479.
17. Cano, G., Passerin, A. M., Schiltz, J. C., Card, J. P., Morrison, S. F., and Sved, A. F. (2003). Anatomical substrates for the central control of sympathetic outflow to interscapular adipose tissue during cold exposure. *Journal of Comparative Neurology* 460, 303–326.
18. Card, J. P., Sved, J. C., Craig, B., Raizada, M., Vazquez, J., and Sved, A. F. (2006). Efferent projections of rat rostroventrolateral medulla C1 catecholamine neurons: Implications for the central control of cardiovascular regulation. *Journal of Comparative Neurology* 499, 840–859.
19. Chan, R. K. W., and Sawchenko, P. E. (1998). Organization and transmitter specificity of medullary neurons activated by sustained hypertension: Implications for understanding baroreceptor reflex circuitry. *Journal of Neuroscience* 18, 371–387.
20. Connor, H. E., and Drew, G. M. (1987). Do adrenaline-containing neurones from the rostral ventrolateral medulla excite preganglionic sympathetic cell bodies? *Journal of Autonomic Pharmacology* 7, 87–96.
21. Coote, J. H., and Lewis, D. I. (1995). Bulbospinal catecholamine neurones and sympathetic pattern generation. *Journal of Physiology and Pharmacology* 46, 259–271.
22. Cravo, S. L., and Morrison, S. F. (1993). The caudal ventrolateral medulla is a source of tonic sympathoinhibition. *Brain Research* 621, 133–136.
23. Dampney, R. A., Polson, J. W., Potts, P. D., Hirooka, Y., and Horiuchi, J. (2003). Functional organization of brain pathways subserving the baroreceptor reflex: Studies in conscious animals using immediate early gene expression. *Cellular and Molecular Neurobiology* 23, 597–616.
24. Dampney, R. A. L (1994). Functional organization of central pathways regulating the cardiovascular system. *Physiological Reviews* 74, 323–364.
25. Dampney, R. A. L (1994). The subretrofacial vasomotor nucleus: Anatomical, chemical and pharmacological properties and role in cardiovascular regulation. *Progress in Neurobiology* 42, 197–227.
26. Dampney, R. A. L, Blessing, W. W., and Tan, E (1988). Origin of tonic GABAergic inputs to vasopressor neurons in the subretrofacial nucleus of the rabbit. *Journal of the Autonomic Nervous System* 24, 227–239.
27. Dempesy, C. W., Richardson, D. E., and Fontana, C. J. (1993). Cardiovascular sympathoinhibitory neurons form an extended longitudinal column in cat lateral medulla. *Brain Research* 603, 328–332.
28. Ernsberger, P., and Haxhiu, M. A. (1997). The I1–imidazoline-binding site is a functional receptor mediating vasodepression via the ventral medulla. *American Journal of Physiology* 273, R1572– R1579.
29. Farnham, M. M., Li, Q., Goodchild, A. K., and Pilowsky, P. M. (2008). PACAP is expressed in sympathoexcitatory bulbospinal C1 neurons of the brain stem and increases sympathetic nerve activity in vivo. *American Journal of Physiology. Regulatory, Integrative and Comparative Physiology* 294, R1304–R1311.

30. Feldberg, W., and Guertzenstein, P. G. (1986). Blood pressure effects of leptazol applied to the ventral surface of the brain stem of cats. *Journal of Physiology* 372, 445–456.
31. Gieroba, Z. J., Li, Y. W., and Blessing, W. W. (1992). Characteristics of caudal ventrolateral medullary neurons antidromically activated from rostral ventrolateral medulla in the rabbit. *Brain Research* 582, 196–207.
32. Gilbey, M. P., Jordan, D., Richter, D. W., and Spyer, K. M. (1984). Synaptic mechanisms involved in the inspiratory modulation of vagal cardio-inhibitory neurones in the cat. *Journal of Physiology* 356, 65–78.
33. Gordon, F. J. (1987). Aortic baroreceptor reflexes are mediated by NMDA receptors in caudal ventrolateral medulla. *American Journal of Physiology* 252, R628–R633.
34. Gordon, F. J., and McCann, L. A. (1988). Pressor responses evoked by microinjections of L-glutamate into the caudal ventrolateral medulla of the rat. *Brain Research* 457, 251–258.
35. Guyenet, P. G. (1990). Role of the ventral medulla oblongata in blood pressure regulation. In A. D. Loewy and K. M. Spyer (Eds.), *Central Regulation of Autonomic Functions*, pp. 145–167. New York: Oxford University Press.
36. Guyenet, P. G. (1997). Is the hypotensive effect of clonidine and related drugs due to imidazoline binding sites? *American Journal of Physiology* 273, R1580–R1584.
37. Guyenet, P. G., Filtz, T. M., and Donaldson, S. R. (1987). Role of excitatory amino acids in rat vagal and sympathetic baroreflexes. *Brain Research* 407, 272–284.
38. Guyenet, P. G., Sevigny, C. P., Weston, M. C., and Stornetta, R. L. (2002). Neurokinin-1 receptor-expressing cells of the ventral respiratory group are functionally heterogeneous and predominantly glutamatergic. *Journal of Neuroscience* 22, 3806–3816.
39. Haselton, J. R., and Guyenet, P. G. (1989). Central respiratory modulation of medullary sympathoexcitatory neurons in rat. *American Journal of Physiology* 256, R739–R750.
40. Hayes, K., and Weaver, L. C. (1990). Selective control of sympathetic pathways to the kidney, spleen and intestine by the ventrolateral medulla in rats. *Journal of Physiology* 428, 371–385.
41. Horiuchi, J., Killinger, S., and Dampney, R. A. (2004). Contribution to sympathetic vasomotor tone of tonic glutamatergic inputs to neurons in the RVLM. *American Journal of Physiology. Regulatory, Integrative and Comparative Physiology* 287, R1335–R1343.
42. Ito, S., and Sved, A. F. (1997). Tonic glutamate-mediated control of rostral ventrolateral medulla and sympathetic vasomotor tone. *American Journal of Physiology* 273, R487–R494.
43. Ito, S., and Sved, A. F. (2000). Pharmacological profile of depressor response elicited by sarthran in rat ventrolateral medulla. *American Journal of Physiology. Heart and Circulatory Physiology* 279, H2961–H2966.
44. Jansen, A. S. P., and Loewy, A. D. (1997). Neurons lying in the white matter of the upper cervical spinal cord project to the intermediolateral cell column. *Neuroscience* 77, 889–898.
45. Jansen, A. S. P, Wessendorf, M. W., and Loewy, A. D. (1995). Transneuronal labeling of CNS neuropeptide and monoamine neurons after pseudorabies virus injections into the stellate ganglion. *Brain Research* 683, 1–24.
46. Jeske, I., Morrison, S. F., Cravo, S. L., and Reis, D. J. (1993). Identification of baroreceptor reflex interneurons in the caudal ventrolateral medulla. *American Journal of Physiology* 264, R169–R178.
47. Jordan, D., Khalid, M. E., Schneiderman, N., and Spyer, K. M. (1982). The location and properties of preganglionic vagal cardiomotor neurones in the rabbit. *Pflugers Archives* 395, 244–50.
48. Kiely, J. M., and Gordon, F. J. (1994). Role of rostral ventrolateral medulla in centrally mediated pressor responses. *American Journal of Physiology* 267, H1549–H1556.
49. Kimura, Y., Hirooka, Y., Sagara, Y., Ito, K., Kishi, T., Shimokawa, H., Takeshita, A., and Sunagawa, K. (2005). Overexpression of inducible nitric oxide synthase in rostral ventrolateral medulla causes hypertension and sympathoexcitation via an increase in oxidative stress. *Circulation Research* 96, 252–260.
50. Kishi, T., Hirooka, Y., Sakai, K., Shigematsu, H., Shimokawa, H., and Takeshita, A. (2001). Overexpression of eNOS in the RVLM causes hypotension and bradycardia via GABA release. *Hypertension* 38, 896–901.
51. Koganezawa, T., and Terui, N. (2006). Differential responsiveness of RVLM sympathetic premotor neurons to hypoxia in the rabbit. *American Journal of Physiology. Heart and Circulatory Physiology* 292, H408–H414.
52. Koshiya, N., Huangfu, D., and Guyenet, P. G. (1993). Ventrolateral medulla and sympathetic chemoreflex in the rat. *Brain Research* 609, 174–184.
53. Larsen, P. J., Enquist, L. W., and Card, J. P. (1998). Characterization of the multisynaptic neuronal control of the rat pineal gland using viral transneuronal

tracing. *European Journal of Neuroscience* 10, 128–145.

54. Levy, E. I., Scarrow, A. M., and Jannetta, P. J. (2001). Microvascular decompression in the treatment of hypertension: Review and update. *Surgical Neurology* 55, 2–10.
55. Li, Y.-W., Gieroba, Z. J., McAllen, R. M., and Blessing, W. W. (1991). Neurons in rabbit caudal ventrolateral medulla inhibit bulbospinal barosensitive neurons in rostral medulla. *American Journal of Physiology* 261, R44–R51.
56. Li, Y.-W., and Guyenet, P. G. (1995). Neuronal excitation by angiotensin II in the rostral ventrolateral medulla of the rat in vitro. *American Journal of Physiology* 268, R272–R277.
57. Li, Y.-W., and Guyenet, P. G. (1996). Angiotensin II decreases a resting $K^+$ conductance in rat bulbospinal neurons of the C1 area. *Circulation Research* 78, 274–282.
58. Lipski, J., Kanjhan, R., Kruszeska, B., and Rong, W. (1996). Properties of presympathetic neurones in the rostral ventrolateral medulla in the rat: An intracellular study "in vivo." *Journal of Physiology* 490, 729–744.
59. Lipski, J., Lin, J., Teo, M. Y., and van Wyk, M. (2002). The network vs. pacemaker theory of the activity of RVL presympathetic neurons—a comparison with another putative pacemaker system. *Autonomic Neuroscience: Basic and Clinical* 98, 85–89.
60. Llewellyn-Smith, I. J., Minson, J. B., Pilowsky, P. M., Arnolda, L. F., and Chalmers, J. P. (1995). The one hundred percent hypothesis: Glutamate or GABA in synapses on sympathetic preganglionic neurons. *Clinical and Experimental Hypertension* 17, 323–333.
61. Lovick, T. A. (1993). The periaqueductal grey-rostral medulla connection in the defence reaction: Efferent pathways and descending control mechanisms. *Behavioural Brain Research* 58, 19–25.
62. Madden, C. J., Stocker, S. D., and Sved, A. F. (2006). Attenuation of homeostatic responses to hypotension and glucoprivation after destruction of catecholaminergic rostral ventrolateral medulla neurons. *American Journal of Physiology. Regulatory, Integrative and Comparative Physiology* 291, R751–R759.
63. Madden, C. J., and Sved, A. F. (2003). Cardiovascular regulation after destruction of the C1 cell group of the rostral ventrolateral medulla in rats. *American Journal of Physiology. Heart and Circulatory Physiology* 285, H2734–H2748.
64. Malhotra, V., Kachroo, A., and Sapru, H. N. (1993). Role of alpha 1-adrenergic receptors in the intermediolateral column in mediating the pressor responses elicited by the stimulation of ventrolateral medullary pressor area. *Brain Research* 626, 278–286.
65. Mandel, D. A., and Schreihofer, A. M. (2006). Central respiratory modulation of barosensitive neurones in rat caudal ventrolateral medulla. *Journal of Physiology* 572, 881–896.
66. Mandel, D. A., and Schreihofer, A. M. (2008). Glutamatergic inputs to the CVLM independent of the NTS promote tonic inhibition of sympathetic vasomotor tone in rats. *American Journal of Physiology. Heart and Circulatory Physiology* 295, H1772–H1779.
67. Mandel, D. A., and Schreihofer, A. M. (2009). Modulation of the sympathetic response to acute hypoxia by the caudal ventrolateral medulla in rats. *Journal of Physiology* 587, 461–475.
68. Mayorov, D. N. (2007). Brain superoxide as a key regulator of the cardiovascular response to emotional stress in rabbits. *Experimental Physiology* 92, 471–479.
69. McAllen, R., May, C., and Campos, R. (1997). The supply of vasomotor drive to individual classes of sympathetic neuron. *Clinical and Experimental Hypertension* 19, 607–618.
70. McCulloch, P. F., Panneton, W. M., and Guyenet, P. G. (1999). The rostral ventrolateral medulla mediates the sympathoactivation produced by chemical stimulation of the rat nasal mucosa. *Journal of Physiology* 516 (Pt 2), 471–484.
71. Menezes, R. C., and Fontes, M. A. (2007). Cardiovascular effects produced by activation of GABA receptors in the rostral ventrolateral medulla of conscious rats. *Neuroscience* 144, 336–343.
72. Mills, E. H., Minson, J. B., and Chalmers, J. (1988). Effects of intrathecal administration of methysergide, phentolamine, and pindolol on pressor responses to electrical stimulation of the rostral ventrolateral medulla. *Journal of Cardiovascular Pharmacology* 11, 456–460.
73. Milner, T. A., Morrison, S. F., Abate, C., and Reis, D. J. (1988). Phenylethanolamine N-methyltransferase-containing terminals synapse directly on sympathetic preganglionic neurons in the rat. *Brain Research* 448, 205–222.
74. Miyawaki, T., Goodchild, A. K., and Pilowsky, P. M. (2002). Evidence for a tonic GABA-ergic inhibition of excitatory respiratory-related afferents to presympathetic neurons in the rostral ventrolateral medulla. *Brain Research* 924, 56–62.
75. Miyawaki, T., Suzuki, S., Minson, J., Arnolda, L., Chalmers, J., Llewellyn-Smith, I., and Pilowsky, P. (1997). Role of AMPA/kainate receptors in transmission of the sympathetic baroreflex in rat

CVLM. *American Journal of Physiology* 272, R800–R812.
76. Mobley, S. C., Mandel, D. A., and Schreihofer, A. M. (2006). Systemic cholecystokinin differentially affects baro-activated GABAergic neurons in rat caudal ventrolateral medulla. *Journal of Neurophysiology* 96, 2760–2768.
77. Morimoto, S., Sasaki, S., Miki, S., Kawa, T., Nakamura, K., Ichida, T., Itoh, H., Nakata, T., Takeda, K., Nakagawa, M., and Yamada, H. (1999). Pressor response to compression of the ventrolateral medulla mediated by glutamate receptors. *Hypertension* 33, 1207–1213.
78. Morrison, S. F. (2003). Glutamate transmission in the rostral ventrolateral medullary sympathetic premotor pathway. *Cellular and Molecular Neurobiology* 23, 761–772.
79. Morrison, S. F., Milner, T. A., and Reis, D. J. (1988). Reticulospinal vasomotor neurons in the rat rostral ventrolateral medulla: Relationship to sympathetic nerve activity and the C1 adrenergic cell group. *Journal of Neuroscience* 8, 1286–1301.
80. Natarajan, M., and Morrison, S. F. (1999). Adrenal epinephrine secretion is not regulated by sympathoinhibitory neurons in the caudal ventrolateral medulla. *Brain Research* 827, 169–175.
81. Natarajan, M., and Morrison, S. F. (2000). Sympathoexcitatory CVLM neurons mediate responses to caudal pressor area stimulation. *American Journal of Physiology. Regulatory, Integrative and Comparative Physiology* 279, R364–R374.
82. Paxinos, G., and Watson, C. (2007). *The Rat Brain in Stereotaxic Coordinates*, Amsterdam, Netherlands: Elsevier.
83. Peng, Y. J., Wang, N., Gong, Q. L., and Li, P. (2002). Caudal ventrolateral medulla mediates the depressor response elicited by the greater splanchnic nerve afferent stimulation in rats. *Neuroscience Letters* 325, 134–138.
84. Possas, O. S., Campos, R. R., Cravo, S. L., Lopes, O. U., and Guertzenstein, P. G. (1994). A fall in arterial blood pressure produced by inhibition of the caudalmost ventrolateral medulla: The caudal pressor area. *Journal of the Autonomic Nervous System* 49, 235–245.
85. Potts, P. D., Allen, A. M., Horiuchi, J., and Dampney, R. A. L. (2000). Does angiotensin II have a significant tonic action on cardiovascular neurons in the rostral and caudal VLM? *American Journal of Physiology. Regulatory, Integrative and Comparative Physiology* 279, R1392–R1402.
86. Rentero, N., Cividjian, A., Trevaks, D., Pequignot, J. M., Quintin, L., and McAllen, R. M. (2002). Activity patterns of cardiac vagal motoneurons in rat nucleus ambiguus. *American Journal of Physiology. Regulatory, Integrative and Comparative Physiology* 283, R1327–R1334.
87. Ritter, S., Dinh, T. T., and Li, A. J. (2006). Hindbrain catecholamine neurons control multiple glucoregulatory responses. *Physiology and Behavior* 89, 490–500.
88. Ross, C. A., Ruggiero, D. A., Park, D. H., Joh, T. H., Sved, A. F., Fernandez-Pardal, J., Saavedra, J. M., and Reis, D. J. (1984). Tonic vasomotor control by the rostral ventrolateral medulla: Effect of electrical or chemical stimulation of the area containing C1 adrenaline neurons on arterial pressure, heart rate and plasma catecholamines and vasopressin. *Journal of Neuroscience* 4, 474–494.
89. Ruggiero, D. A., Cravo, S. L., Golanov, E., Gomez, R., Anwar, M., and Reis, D. J. (1994). Adrenergic and non-adrenergic spinal projections of a cardiovascular-active pressor area of medulla oblongata: Quantitative topographic analysis. *Brain Research* 663, 107–120.
90. Saha, S., Drinkhill, M. J., Moore, J. P., and Batten, T. F. (2005). Central nucleus of amygdala projections to rostral ventrolateral medulla neurones activated by decreased blood pressure. *European Journal of Neuroscience* 21, 1921–1930.
91. Sartor, D. M., and Verberne, A. J. (2002). Cholecystokinin selectively affects presympathetic vasomotor neurons and sympathetic vasomotor outflow. *American Journal of Physiology. Regulatory, Integrative and Comparative Physiology* 282, R1174– R1184.
92. Sartor, D. M., and Verberne, A. J. (2003). Phenotypic identification of rat rostroventrolateral medullary presympathetic vasomotor neurons inhibited by exogenous cholecystokinin. *Journal of Comparative Neurology* 465, 467–479.
93. Sawchenko, P. E., Li, H. Y., and Ericsson, A. (2000). Circuits and mechanisms governing hypothalamic responses to stress: A tale of two paradigms. *Progress in Brain Research* 122, 61–78.
94. Schreihofer, A. M., and Guyenet, P. G. (1997). Identification of C1 presympathetic neurons in rat rostral ventrolateral medulla by juxtacellular labeling in vivo. *Journal of Comparative Neurology* 387, 524–536.
95. Schreihofer, A. M., and Guyenet, P. G. (2000). Role of presympathetic C1 neurons in the sympatholytic and hypotensive effects of clonidine in rats. *American Journal of Physiology. Regulatory, Integrative and Comparative Physiology* 279, R1753– R1762.
96. Schreihofer, A. M., and Guyenet, P. G. (2000). Sympathetic reflexes after depletion of

bulbospinal catecholaminergic neurons with anti-DβH-saporin. *American Journal of Physiology. Regulatory, Integrative and Comparative Physiology* 279, R729–R742.

97. Schreihofer, A. M., and Guyenet, P. G. (2002). The baroreflex and beyond: Control of sympathetic vasomotor tone by GABAergic neurons in the ventrolateral medulla. *Clinical and Experimental Pharmacology and Physiology* 29, 514–521.
98. Schreihofer, A. M., and Guyenet, P. G. (2003). Baro-activated neurons with pulse-modulated activity in the rat caudal ventrolateral medulla express GAD67 mRNA. *Journal of Neurophysiology* 89, 1265–1277.
99. Schreihofer, A. M., Ito, S., and Sved, A. F. (2005). Brain stem control of arterial pressure in chronic arterial baroreceptor-denervated rats. *American Journal of Physiology. Regulatory, Integrative and Comparative Physiology* 289, R1746–R1755.
100. Schreihofer, A. M., Stornetta, R. L., and Guyenet, P. G. (1999). Evidence for glycinergic respiratory neurons: Bötzinger neurons express mRNA for glycinergic transporter 2. *Journal of Comparative Neurology* 407, 583–597.
101. Schreihofer, A. M., Stornetta, R. L., and Guyenet, P. G. (2000). Regulation of sympathetic tone and arterial pressure by rostral ventrolateral medulla after depletion of C1 cells in rat. *Journal of Physiology* 529, 221–236.
102. Seyedabadi, M., Li, Q., Padley, J. R., Pilowsky, P. M., and Goodchild, A. K. (2006). A novel pressor area at the medullo-cervical junction that is not dependent on the RVLM: Efferent pathways and chemical mediators. *Journal of Neuroscience* 26, 5420–5427.
103. Silva, N. F., Pires, J. G., Dantas, M. A., and Futuro Neto, H. A. (2002). Excitatory amino acid receptor blockade within the caudal pressor area and rostral ventrolateral medulla alters cardiovascular responses to nucleus raphé obscurus stimulation in rats. *Brazilian Journal of Medical and Biological Research* 35, 1237–1245.
104. Smith, D. W., Sibbald, J. R., Khanna, S., and Day, T. A. (1995). Rat vasopressin cell responses to simulated hemorrhage: Stimulus-dependent role for A1 noradrenergic neurons. *American Journal of Physiology* 268, R1336–R1342.
105. Smith, J. K., and Barron, K. W. (1990). GABAergic responses in ventrolateral medulla in spontaneously hypertensive rats. *American Journal of Physiology* 258, R450–R456.
106. Stornetta, R. L., Sevigny, C. P., Schreihofer, A. M., Rosin, D. L., and Guyenet, P. G. (2002). Vesicular glutamate transporter DNPI/VGLUT2 is expressed by both C1 adrenergic and nonaminergic presympathetic vasomotor neurons of the rat medulla. *Journal of Comparative Neurology* 444, 207–220.
107. Sun, M.-K., and Guyenet, P. G. (1985). GABA-mediated baroreceptor inhibition of reticulospinal neurons. *American Journal of Physiology* 249, R672–R680.
108. Sun, W., and Panneton, W. M. (2002). The caudal pressor area of the rat: Its precise location and projections to the ventrolateral medulla. *American Journal of Physiology Regulatory, Integrative and Comparative Physiology* 283, R768–R778.
109. Sun, W., and Panneton, W. M. (2005). Defining projections from the caudal pressor area of the caudal ventrolateral medulla. *Journal of Comparative Neurology* 482, 273–293.
110. Sundaram, K., and Sapru, H. (1991). NMDA receptors in the intermediolateral column of the spinal cord mediate sympathoexcitatory cardiac responses elicited from the ventrolateral medullary pressor area. *Brain Research* 544, 33–41.
111. Sved, A. F. (1989). PNMT-containing catecholaminergic neurons are not necessarily adrenergic. *Brain Research* 481, 113–118.
112. Sved, A. F., Ito, S., and Madden, C. J. (2000). Baroreflex dependent and independent roles of the caudal ventrolateral medulla in cardiovascular regulation. *Brain Research Bulletin* 51, 129–133.
113. Sved, A. F., Ito, S., and Sved, J. C. (2003). Brainstem mechanisms of hypertension: Role of the rostral ventrolateral medulla. *Current Hypertension Reports* 5, 262–268.
114. Sved, A. F., Mancini, D. L., Graham, J. C., Schreihofer, A. M., and Hoffman, G. E. (1994). PNMT-containing neurons of the C1 cell group express c-Fos in response to changes in baroreceptor input. *American Journal of Physiology* 266, R361–R367.
115. Tagawa, T., and Dampney, R. A. L. (1999). AT1 receptors mediate excitatory inputs to rostral ventrolateral medulla pressor neurons from hypothalamus. *Hypertension* 34, 1301–1307.
116. Terui, N., Saeki, Y., and Kumada, M. (1986). Barosensory neurons in the ventrolateral medulla in rabbits and their responses to various afferent inputs from peripheral and central sources. *Japanese Journal of Physiology* 36, 1141–1164.
117. Verberne, A. J., Lam, W., Owens, N. C., and Sartor, D. (1997). Supramedullary modulation of sympathetic vasomotor function. *Clinical and Experimental Pharmacology and Physiology* 24, 748–754.

118. Verberne, A. J., Stornetta, R. L., and Guyenet, P. G. (1999). Properties of C1 and other ventrolateral medullary neurones with hypothalamic projections in the rat. *Journal of Physiology* 517, 477–494.
119. Verberne, A. J., and Guyenet, P. G. (1992). Medullary pathway of the Bezold-Jarisch reflex in the rat. *American Journal of Physiology* 263, R1195–R1202.
120. Wang, H., Weston, M. C., McQuiston, T. J., Stornetta, R. L., and Guyenet, P. G. (2003). Neurokinin-1 receptor-expressing cells regulate depressor region of rat ventrolateral medulla. *American Journal of Physiology. Heart and Circulatory Physiology* 285, H2757– H2769.
121. Weston, M., Wang, H., Stornetta, R. L., Sevigny, C. P., and Guyenet, P. G. (2003). Fos expression by glutamatergic neurons of the solitary tract nucleus after phenylephrine-induced hypertension in rats. *Journal of Comparative Neurology* 460, 525–541.
122. Willette, R. N., Punnen, S., Krieger, A. J., and Sapru, H. N. (1984). Interdependence of rostral and caudal ventrolateral medullary areas in the control of blood pressure. *Brain Research* 321, 169–174.
123. Yang, Z., and Coote, J. H. (1999). The influence of the paraventricular nucleus on baroreceptor dependent caudal ventrolateral medullary neurones of the rat. *Pflügers Archiv* 438, 47–52.
124. Zhou, W., Fu, L. W., Tjen-A-Looi, S. C., Guo, Z. L., and Longhurst, J. C. (2006). Role of glutamate in a visceral sympathoexcitatory reflex in rostral ventrolateral medulla of cats. *American Journal of Physiology. Heart and Circulatory Physiology* 291, H1309– H1318.

# 6

# Sympathetic Preganglionic Neurons

IDA J. LLEWELLYN-SMITH

Sympathetic preganglionic neurons are critical links in the central circuitry that regulates the activity of every organ in the body. The axons of sympathetic preganglionic neurons exit the central nervous system from thoracic and upper lumbar segments of the spinal cord to innervate post-ganglionic neurons in sympathetic ganglia and chromaffin cells in the medulla of the adrenal gland. Sympathetic preganglionic neurons are the source of all sympathetic outflow but are not just passive conduits that convey central drive to the periphery. They have different morphologies and heterogeneous physiological properties. They respond to neurotransmitters in different ways, and their innervation by axons that are capable of releasing different neurotransmitters is also variable. The ways in which they respond to normal and abnormal homeostatic challenges are also inconsistent. All of these differences probably reflect the fact that different populations of sympathetic preganglionic neurons are involved in controlling different autonomic functions.

This chapter will review information on sympathetic preganglionic neurons that has appeared since the publication of the first edition of this book in 1990. The first part of the chapter deals with the anatomy and electrophysiology of the sympathetic preganglionic neurons themselves. The second part covers the neuronal circuitry that influences the activity of these important neurons. Other chapters in this book provide insight into the involvement of sympathetic preganglionic neurons in the control of different autonomic functions, so that involvement will not examined in any detail here. Sympathetic preganglionic neurons in normal neonatal and adult animals are the focus of the chapter. Most of the information derives from studies on sympathetic preganglionic neurons in rats, and some of the data have been generated in cats, guinea pigs, and birds. To learn how sympathetic preganglionic neurons develop and age, readers are referred to the work of C. J. Forehand, P. E. Phelps, R. M. Santer, and Y. P. Yip.

## SYMPATHETIC PREGANGLIONIC NEURONS

### Distribution of Sympathetic Preganglionic Neurons

Unlike parasympathetic preganglionic neurons, which occur in both brainstem and spinal nuclei (see Chapter 7), the cell bodies of the sympathetic preganglionic neurons are restricted to the lateral horn of thoracic and upper lumbar segments of the spinal cord (caudal cervical spinal segment 8 through to lumbar segment 2 in rats) and are distributed between four "subnuclei" (Figure 6–1). The highest concentration of sympathetic preganglionic somata is found in the intermediolateral cell column. In this subnucleus, cell bodies are organized into closely spaced "nests" that are located at the boundary between the spinal gray and white matter. In the most rostral thoracic segments, these nests contain many somata, whereas only a few cell bodies occur in the nests at the caudal end of the preganglionic distribution. Many sympathetic preganglionic neurons also lie in the central autonomic area above the central canal (i.e., dorsal lamina X). Neurons with this subnuclear position are most numerous in caudal thoracic and rostral lumbar spinal segments[3,142]. The third subnucleus with preganglionic cell bodies is the intercalated nucleus, which is located between the intermediolateral cell column and the central autonomic area. The fourth subnucleus is the dorsolateral funiculus of the spinal white matter, which contains many neurons rostrally but few caudally (e.g., [55]).

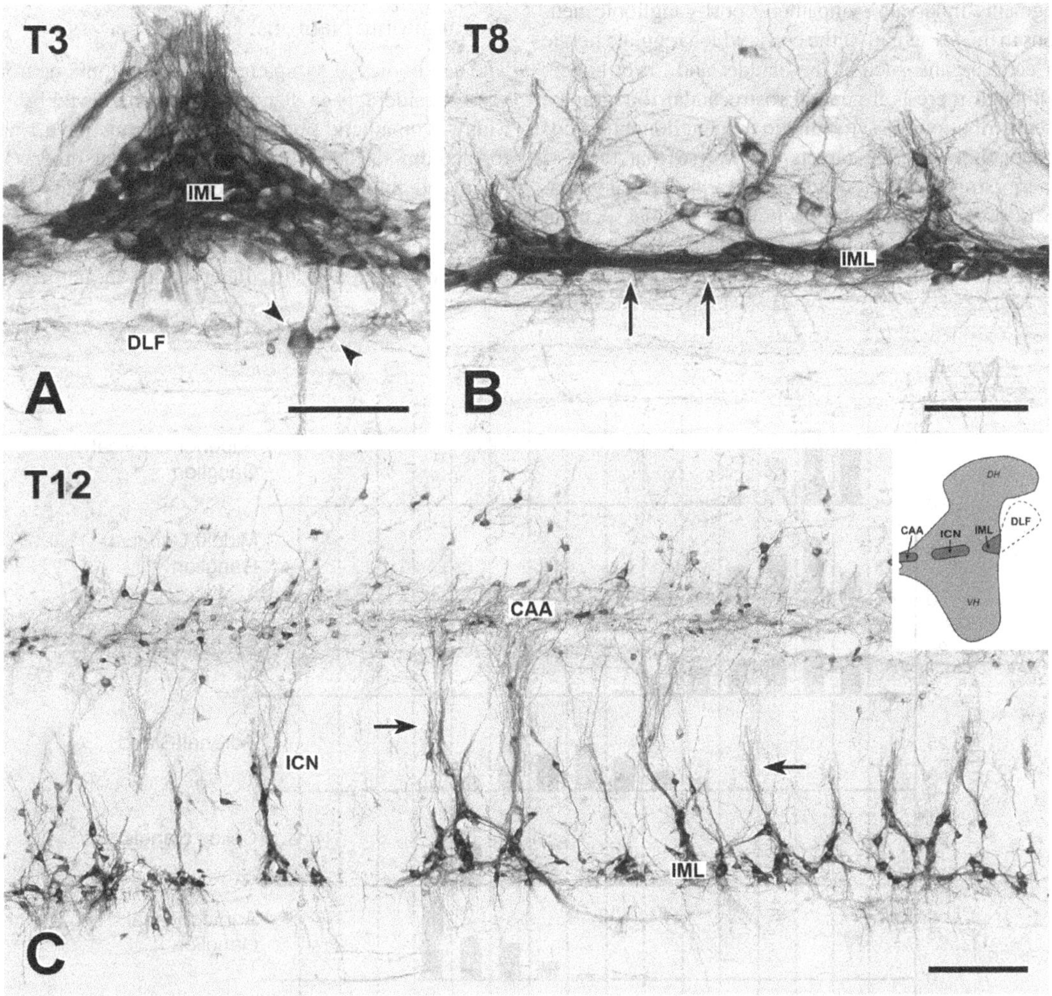


Figure 6–1 Organization of sympathetic preganglionic neurons. Sympathetic preganglionic neurons were visualized by immunoperoxidase staining for choline acetyltransferase in horizontal sections of rat thoracic spinal cord. The sympathetic preganglionic somata are distributed between four subnuclei in the lateral horn: the intermediolateral cell column (IML), the central autonomic area (CAA), the intercalated nucleus (ICN) and the dorsolateral funiculus (DLF). Inset in *C:* Diagram showing a transverse section through the gray matter of spinal segment T3 onto which these four autonomic subnuclei have been mapped. *A–C:* In the IML, sympathetic preganglionic neurons are clumped together in "nests" that are connected by their rostrocaudally running dendrites (*B, arrows*). The nests in rostral thoracic cord (*A*) contain more sympathetic preganglionic somata than the nests in the caudal thoracic cord (*C*). Bundles of labeled dendrites also travel medially (*C, arrows*) towards the central canal. The full trajectory of the dendrites in *B* is not apparent because they project ventrally as well as medially at this level of the cord. In *A:* two labeled cell bodies (*arrowheads*) occur in the white matter of the dorsolateral funiculus. Bars in *A* and *B:* 100 μm; bar in *C:* 250 μm.

An important feature of the organization of sympathetic preganglionic neurons is that they are topographically arranged within the lateral horn[142] (Figure 6–2). Neurons in rostral thoracic spinal segments send axons to sympathetic ganglia in the upper part of the body and are involved in regulating targets such as the pupils, salivary glands, and the heart. In contrast, neurons in caudal thoracic and upper lumbar segments innervate sympathetic post-ganglionic neurons in the lower part of the body, which regulate pelvic visceral organs, such as the bladder and lower bowel. Although there is a general rostrocaudal topography, the distributions of sympathetic preganglionic neurons innervating different targets overlap so that there is intermixing of different functional classes of sympathetic preganglionic neuron within each spinal segment (Figure 6–2). For example, in the rat, the intermediolateral cell column of thoracic segment 13 contains sympathetic preganglionic neurons that innervate the adrenal medulla and major pelvic ganglion as well as neurons supplying the coeliac ganglion[142]. These rostrocaudal and intrasegmental variations indicate that it is important to identify the innervation target of a sympathetic preganglionic neuron when studying it.

## Morphology of Sympathetic Preganglionic Neurons

The cell bodies of sympathetic preganglionic neurons vary considerably in size and shape (reviewed by [19]). Many sympathetic preganglionic neurons have small to medium-sized fusiform cell bodies but others are large and multipolar. Whether differences in somal morphology have any physiological significance[19] remains an unanswered question, but there may be some correlation with innervation target and/or

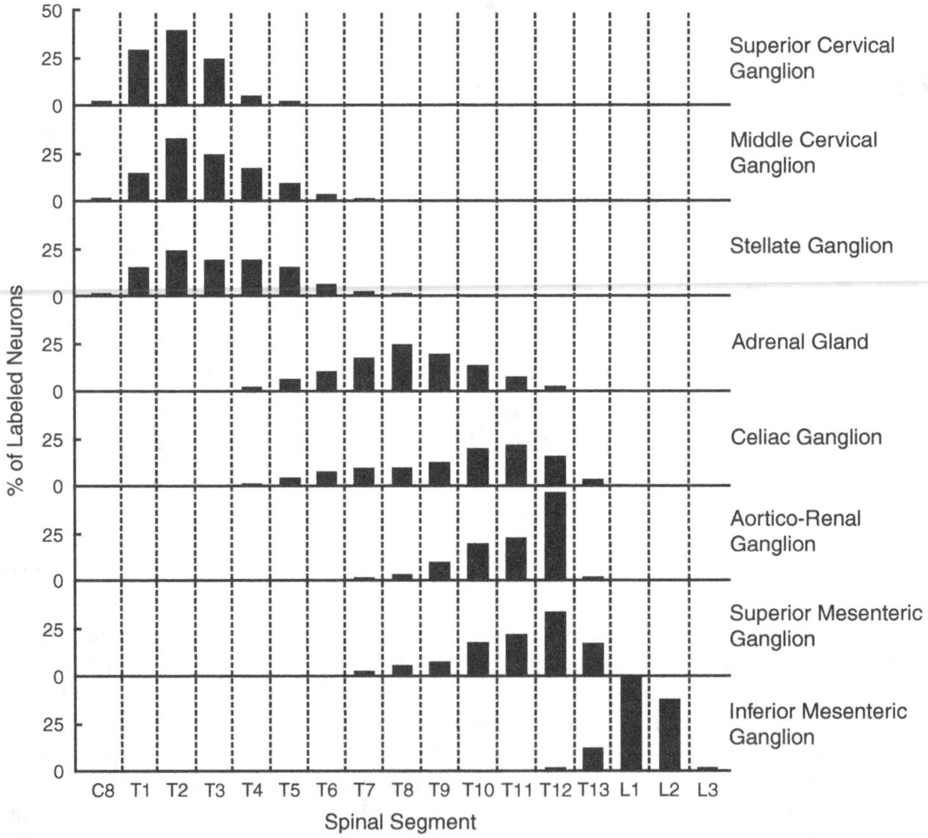


Figure 6–2 Segmental distribution of sympathetic preganglionic neurons. Histograms showing the distribution of rat sympathetic preganglionic neurons that were retrogradely labeled from injection of Fluorogold into the sympathetic ganglia indicated on the right and into the medulla of the adrenal gland. Reproduced from Strack et al. (1988)[142], with permission.

function. For example, sympathetic preganglionic neurons supplying the adrenal medulla are almost always fusiform, whereas large multipolar neurons are prominent caudally and some can be retrogradely labeled from the coeliac ganglion, suggesting that they may be involved in visceral regulation[55].

The axons of sympathetic preganglionic neurons can be either myelinated or unmyelinated. Preganglionic axons arise not only from cell bodies but also from primary dendrites and sometimes secondary dendrites[21,35,121] and can be the site of synaptic input[91]. Branching of preganglionic axons has been documented to occur within the spinal cord; but electrophysiological evidence suggests that sympathetic preganglionic neurons are unlikely to have collaterals that are part of recurrent inhibitory circuits, as found between motor neurons in the ventral horn (see [19]).

Intracellular dye-filling has shown that individual sympathetic preganglionic neurons in mammals and birds have very large dendritic arbors that extend rostrocaudally for hundreds of micrometers (Figure 6–3)[21,35,46,116]. In the intermediolateral cell column, dendrites from many sympathetic preganglionic neurons are tightly grouped together into thick bundles that run rostrocaudally and connect the nests containing the preganglionic cell bodies (e.g., [11]) (Figure 6–1). Mediolaterally oriented bundles of preganglionic dendrites that arise from neurons in the intermediolateral cell column and the intercalated nucleus also connect the intermediolateral column with the central autonomic area. Ultrastructural studies have shown that, within the dendritic bundles, individual dendrites are surrounded by astroglial processes, except at sites of synaptic contact[99]. Hence, the dendritic bundles

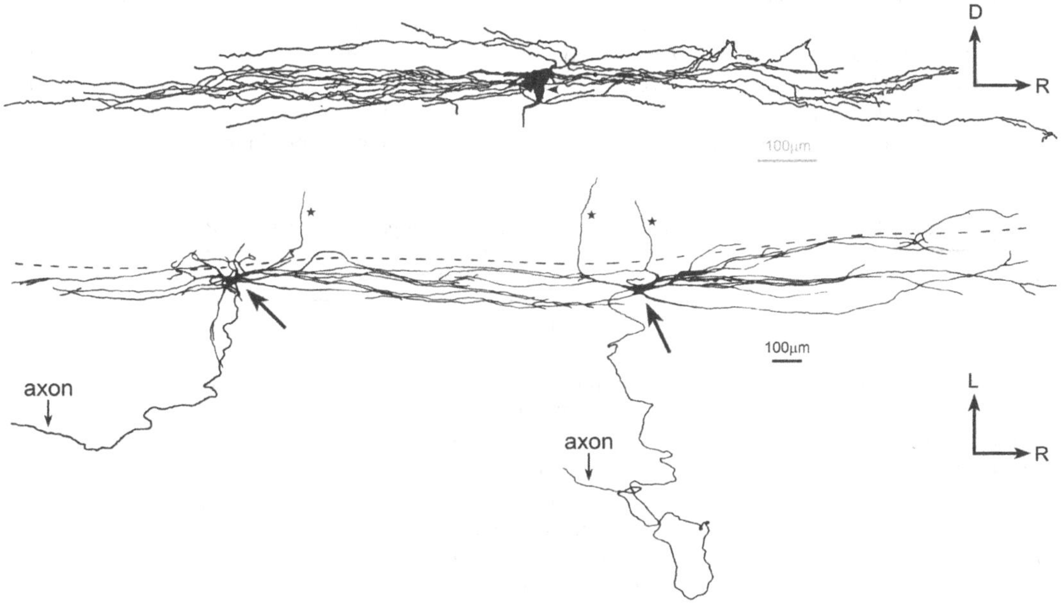


Figure 6–3 Morphology of sympathetic preganglionic neurons. *Top panel,* Camera lucida drawing of a sympathetic preganglionic neuron from cat lumbar spinal cord. The neuron was identified by antidromic activation from the lumbar sympathetic trunk, filled with biocytin, cut in the parasagittal plane and reconstructed. The conduction velocity of the axon was 7.0 m/sec. The *arrowhead* indicates the axon hillock. This neuron has many primary dendrites that are mostly confined to the intermediolateral cell column. *D:* dorsal; *R:* rostral. Modified from Pilowsky et al. (1994)[116], with permission. *Bottom panel,* Camera lucida drawings of two sympathetic preganglionic neurons (*arrows*) from cat upper thoracic spinal cord. The neurons were identified by antidromic activation from the T3 white ramus, filled with horseradish peroxidase, cut in the horizontal plane and reconstructed. The axons of both neurons arise from medially projecting primary dendrites. The rostrocaudal dendrites of the two adjacent neurons are bundled and each neuron has at least one dendrite (*stars*) that extends into the white matter. *Dashed line,* border between the gray and white matter at the level of the cell body. *L:* lateral; *R:* rostral. Modified from Dembowsky et al. (1985)[35], with permission.

may not be the site of electrotonic coupling that is thought to underlie the oscillating activity of some neonatal rat sympathetic preganglionic neurons[113], even though gap junction proteins occur on preganglionic dendrites[97]. The rostrocaudal and mediolateral preganglionic dendrites plus the preganglionic somata in the intermediolateral cell column form a ladder-like arrangement. This prominent organizational pattern is reflected in the immunohistochemical staining patterns of nerve fibers that innervate sympathetic preganglionic neurons. These extensive dendritic trees also mean that most of the synaptic input to sympathetic preganglionic neurons occurs on their dendrites.

## Neurochemical Phenotypes of Sympathetic Preganglionic Neurons

### *Chemical Neuroanatomy of Sympathetic Preganglionic Neurons*

Like cranial and sacral parasympathetic preganglionic neurons and somatic motor neurons in the ventral horn, all sympathetic preganglionic neurons are cholinergic. Activation of these neurons results in the release of acetylcholine from their terminals onto their innervation target, evoking effects mediated by both nicotinic and muscarinic receptors (reviewed by [76]). In anatomical studies, sympathetic preganglionic neurons are often identified by the presence of choline acetyltransferase, the enzyme that synthesizes acetylcholine (e.g., [11]).

The majority of sympathetic preganglionic neurons in the thoracic and upper lumbar cord are also capable of synthesizing nitric oxide (e.g., [1,54,55]), and these neurons may be the source of all of the nitric oxide–producing axons in sympathetic ganglia and the adrenal medulla (see [82]). Thus, most sympathetic preganglionic neurons may be able to influence sympathetic nerve activity through the release of not only acetylcholine but also nitric oxide. Nitric oxide released from one sympathetic preganglionic neuron could also influence the activity of surrounding sympathetic preganglionic neurons since this gaseous molecule has effects for up to 150 μm from its site of release. Because sympathetic preganglionic neurons robustly express nitric oxide synthase, the enzyme that produces nitric oxide, a number of studies have examined the spinal distribution of nitric oxide synthase-immunoreactive sympathetic preganglionic neurons or have used the ability to make nitric oxide as a way to identify large populations of these neurons in order to study their other features (see Table 6–1).

At least some sympathetic preganglionic neurons also have the ability to synthesize amino acid transmitters. Recent work has identified a population of preganglionic neurons in the rostral thoracic spinal

Table 6–1. Neurochemical Phenotypes of Different Functional Groups of Sympathetic Preganglionic Neurons

| Function | Phenotype of SPN | Identification of SPN Function | Species | Reference |
|---|---|---|---|---|
| Secretion of saliva | ACh+Calretinin | SPN terminals surround PGSN projecting to salivary gland | Rat | 52 |
| Secretion of saliva | ACh+NOS | SPN terminals surround PGSN projecting to salivary gland | Guinea pig | 30 |
| Sympathetic control of the heart | ACh+Calretinin+NOS | SPN terminals surround PGSN with the same neurochemistry as axons in the heart | Rat | 2,122 |
| Retraction of the upper eyelid | ACh+ENK+Calretinin | SPN terminals surround PGSN projecting to the tarsal muscle in the eyelid | Rat | 27 |
| | ACh+ENK+Calbindin | SPN terminals surround PGSN projecting to the tarsal muscle in the eyelid | | |
| | ACh+NOS, no ENK | SPN terminals surround PGSN projecting to the tarsal muscle in the eyelid | | |
| Sweating | ACh+CRF | SPN terminals surround PGSN projecting to paw pads AND SPN terminals surround PGSN with the same neurochemistry as sudomotor PGSN | Cat | 130 |
| Adrenaline release from chromaffin cells | ACh+Calretinin | SPN terminals surround adrenergic chromaffin cells AND IR in SPN projecting to adrenal medulla | Cat | 44 |

ACh, acetylcholine; CRF, corticotropin releasing factor; ENK, enkephalin and enkephalin-related peptides; IR, immunoreactivity; NOS, nitric oxide synthase; PGSN, postganglionic sympathetic neuron; SPN, sympathetic preganglionic neuron.

cord whose axons and cell bodies contain markers for synthesis of γ-aminobutyric acid (GABA)[63]. These neurons send axons to the superior cervical ganglion.

Surprisingly, peptide neurotransmitters that occur in sympathetic preganglionic neurons are not well characterized. In the 1980s, work on tissue from animals treated with colchicine, which stops axonal transport, demonstrated a variety of neuropeptides in sympathetic preganglionic somata (e.g., [33,72,154]); but these data could be compromised by the fact that colchicine can induce the expression of neuropeptide mRNA in neurons that do not usually contain neuropeptides[119]. A few peptides have subsequently been visualized in identified sympathetic preganglionic somata in animals that were not treated with colchicine (e.g., corticotropin-releasing factor in cat neurons[130] and cocaine- and amphetamine-regulated transcript in rat neurons[45]). Recently, a new approach has been successful at boosting cell-body levels of neuropeptides so that they can be detected with immunohistochemistry[125]. Immunoreactivity for enkephalin, somatostatin, calcitonin gene-related peptide, vasoactive intestinal peptide, and neurotensin were found in cat sympathetic preganglionic neurons after tying or cutting the sympathetic thoracic trunk. *In situ* hybridization is another alternative for determining the neuropeptide phenotypes of sympathetic preganglionic neurons and has been used to demonstrate that sympathetic preganglionic neurons projecting to the superior cervical ganglion are able to make pituitary adenylate cyclase–activating polypeptide[12]. Interestingly, this method has not yet been applied systematically to the question of which neuropeptides are synthesized by different groups of sympathetic preganglionic neurons.

Although electrophysiological studies have shown that sympathetic preganglionic neurons express receptors for a wide variety of amino acid, classical, and peptide transmitters (see below), only a limited number of receptor types have been demonstrated anatomically. Alpha-amino-3-hydroxy-5-methylisoxazole-4-propionate (AMPA)–type glutamate receptor subunits have been examined in sympathetic preganglionic neurons in thoracic segment 8. Virtually all of these neurons are immunoreactive for GLUR1; two-thirds or more contain GLUR2 and GLUR3; but GLUR4 is absent[100]. Neurokinin-1 receptors, which bind substance P, are widely distributed amongst sympathetic preganglionic neurons, including some of those that respond to hypotension with activation of the immediate early gene, *c-fos*[18,53,88].

Other neurochemicals that are not directly related to neurotransmission have also been identified in sympathetic preganglionic neurons, including the gap junction protein, connexin 36; and the calcium-binding proteins, calbindin and calretinin[52,54,97].

### *Relationship of Neurochemical Phenotype to Innervation Target and/or Function*

Several studies involving retrograde tracing from sympathetic ganglia and the adrenal medulla have demonstrated that the neurochemical phenotypes of sympathetic preganglionic neurons vary depending on their innervation target. In guinea pigs, sympathoadrenal neurons contain leu-enkephalin[32]. In rats, the ability to synthesize GABA occurs in sympathetic preganglionic neurons that project to the superior cervical ganglion[63], and some of these neurons also contain pituitary adenylate cyclase–activating polypeptide[12]. The proportions of neurons containing immunoreactivity for calbindin D28K or cocaine- and amphetamine-regulated transcript correlate with where the neurons send their axons[45,54]. Between 70% and 90% of sympathoadrenal neurons express the neurokinin-1 receptor, but this receptor is found in only about 15% of sympathetic preganglionic neurons supplying the lumbar 5 sympathetic chain ganglion[53,88]. Nitric oxide synthase occurs in all sympathoadrenal preganglionic neurons but in only about 55% of coeliac-projecting neurons and about 45% of neurons that send axons to the superior mesenteric ganglion[54,55]. Interestingly, among sympathetic preganglionic neurons that innervate the superior cervical ganglion, the proportion of cell bodies with immunoreactivity for nitric oxide synthase even varies between different lateral horn subnuclei[55].

There is also a link between the neurochemical phenotypes of sympathetic preganglionic neurons and their functions. Demonstrating this link relies upon correlating the neurochemistry of a preganglionic axon with the neurochemistry and innervation target of the post-ganglionic neuron that the axon innervates. During the 1980s, it became clear that populations of peripheral autonomic neurons with different functions, including sympathetic post-ganglionic neurons[48], contained distinctive combinations of neuropeptides and other neurochemicals. Furthermore, these combinations of neurochemical markers correlated well with the innervation targets and therefore functions of the peripheral autonomic neurons. These observations led to the concept that the chemical coding of sympathetic post-ganglionic neurons could be used to identify their function[49,65]. Anderson, Grkovic, and others have used information about the neurochemistry and projection patterns of post-ganglionic neurons to pinpoint the neurochemical phenotypes of different functional groups of preganglionic neurons. As Table 6–1 shows, only a small fraction of the functional circuits involving sympathetic preganglionic neurons have been investigated, and there is much more work to be done on defining the chemical coding of sympathetic preganglionic neurons.

## Electrophysiological Properties of Sympathetic Preganglionic Neurons

When the first edition of this book appeared in 1990, the electrophysiological properties of sympathetic preganglionic neurons were relatively well characterized as a result of intracellular and extracellular recordings in adult animals *in vivo* and in neonatal spinal cord slices *in vitro* (reviewed by [19,118]). There had been work showing that more than half of these neurons in rats and cats have unmyelinated axons, that their conduction velocities vary widely among vertebrate species, and that there was considerable convergence and divergence of preganglionic axons. The resting membrane potential of sympathetic preganglionic neurons was known to be about -60 mV both *in vivo* and *in vitro*, and steady-state current-voltage relations had been defined. Sympathetic preganglionic action potentials and their underlying ionic conductances (Figure 6–4) had also been characterized. The long durations and prominent after-hyperpolarizations of their action potentials are features that allow electrophysiologists to distinguish sympathetic preganglionic neurons from nearby interneurons (e.g., [36]). More recent investigations *in vitro* have revealed that sympathetic preganglionic neurons are electrically coupled[113]. These electrical synapses may be important for the generation of sympathetic rhythms and for the summation of inputs to postganglionic neurons. Rhythmic activity has also been demonstrated in individual sympathetic preganglionic neurons; this activity occurs spontaneously but can also be evoked by synaptic input or the application of serotonin (5-hydroxytryptamine, 5-HT) or noradrenaline (e.g., [131]). A subset of lower lumbar and upper thoracic neurons, which have activity that is correlated with the respiratory cycle, has also been identified[156]. These neurons and those in the upper thoracic cord with respiratory-related activity may be involved in vasomotor control. Since 1990, new preparations have also been important for elucidating the electrophysiological properties of sympathetic preganglionic neurons and their inputs. Work on horizontal slices, in which rostrocaudal dendrites and most of their descending inputs are intact, has allowed a better correlation to be made between structure and function[58], has revealed new membrane conductances, and has suggested the presence of a slow transmitter in descending inputs that was not noradrenaline[124]. Studies in the neonatal rat brainstem-spinal cord preparation have shed light on the origins and effects of supraspinal inputs that influence preganglionic neuronal activity[38,39,40] (see below). Patch clamping has also superseded sharp electrodes and yielded a number of new findings, in particular about the effects of neurotransmitters on the activity of sympathetic preganglionic neurons (see below).

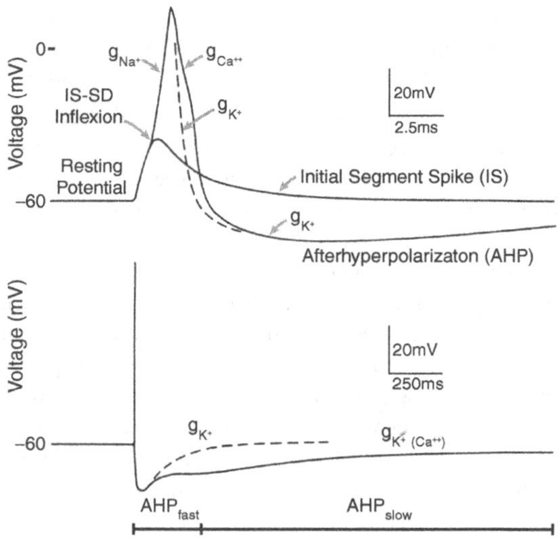


Figure 6–4 Action potentials in sympathetic preganglionic neurons. The action potentials in sympathetic preganglionic neuron are of long duration. Often there is an inflexion on the rising phase, which reflects depolarization of the axon initial segment (IS). The remainder of the upstroke reflects somato-dendritic (SD) depolarization. The depolarization is due to an increase in membrane permeability for sodium (i.e., increase in membrane conductance $g_{Na+}$). The falling phase of the action potential involves increases in membrane permeability for potassium ions and calcium ions (i.e., increases in membrane conductances $g_{K+}$ and $g_{Ca++}$) and a decrease in permeability for sodium ions (i.e., decrease in membrane conductance $g_{Na+}$). The hump on the falling phase of the action potential reflects slowing in the rate of depolarization due to the movement of calcium ions from the extracellular space into the neuron. The resultant splaying of the action potential is the cause of its prolonged duration. The afterhyperpolarization (AHP) of the action potential has two phases. The fast phase is due to voltage-dependent delayed rectifier potassium channels. The subsequent slow phase relies upon the opening of calcium-activated potassium channels. For more details, see Cabot (1990)[19], from which the diagram was reproduced with permission.

Electrophysiological properties have mainly been studied in sympathetic preganglionic neurons whose function and/or innervation target had not been defined. However, by 1990, Janig and colleagues had done an extensive series of experiments to assess the properties of vasoconstrictor sympathetic pre- and post-ganglionic neurons *in vivo* (reviewed by [64]).

These studies revealed that vasoconstrictor neurons showed cardiac- and respiratory-related activity but that conduction velocity was not a reliable indicator of function. Although vasoconstrictor neurons showed ongoing activity, many other neurons were silent, probably reflecting the fact that many sympathetic circuits control targets that are only intermittently active. There is also now some information about the properties of sympathetic preganglionic neurons that control catecholamine release from chromaffin cells[149]. Patch clamping of neurons retrogradely labeled from the adrenal medulla showed that the active membrane properties of all of the recorded neurons were similar. Nevertheless, the range of active membrane conductances was sufficient to ensure that sympathoadrenal neurons were capable of providing the differentiated output that has been observed with extracellular recording *in vivo* (e.g., [25]).

## CIRCUITS CONTROLLING THE ACTIVITY OF SYMPATHETIC PREGANGLIONIC NEURONS

### Origin of Synaptic Inputs to Sympathetic Preganglionic Neurons

Sympathetic preganglionic neurons receive synapses from neurons in the brain and from neurons in the spinal cord (reviewed by [82]). The neurons that provide this synaptic input are often referred to as *presympathetic* neurons because they are likely to be directly involved in regulating the activity of sympathetic preganglionic neurons.

Attenuated strains of neurotropic viruses, which cross synapses and label chains of synaptically connected neurons, have been used extensively to determine the locations of brain presympathetic neurons. Injections of these viral tracers into sympathetic ganglia, tissues, or organs have revealed that five main brain regions provide monosynaptic input to sympathetic preganglionic neurons. These brain regions are the rostral ventrolateral medulla (RVLM); the rostral ventromedial medulla; the caudal raphé nuclei (i.e., raphé pallidus, raphé magnus, and raphé obscurus); the A5 region; and the paraventricular nucleus (PVN) of the hypothalamus. Some synapses on sympathetic preganglionic neurons also originate from orexin-immunoreactive neurons in the lateral hypothalamus[47]. Ultrastructural studies have confirmed that terminals anterogradely labeled from the RVLM, caudal raphé nuclei, and PVN[10,110,155] and orexin-immunoreactive terminals[87] synapse on sympathetic preganglionic neurons. However, the only pathway that has been confirmed electrophysiologically is the one from the RVLM to sympathetic preganglionic neurons (e.g., [38,40]). Neurons in the locus coeruleus, arcuate nucleus, and cortex also supply axons to the lateral horn of the spinal cord; but it remains to be determined whether these supraspinal neurons synapse on sympathetic preganglionic neurons or on other types of neurons in spinal autonomic regions.

Sympathetic preganglionic neurons are also innervated by spinal neurons, which have been identified through both trans-synaptic viral tracing and electrophysiological studies. The intraspinal presympathetic neurons occur within the intermediolateral cell column, around this subnucleus in spinal cord laminae V and VII, and also in lamina X above the central canal (see Chapter 8 for more details).

Information about the sources of synaptic input to sympathetic preganglionic neurons has also been derived from comparisons of intact spinal cords and cords at two weeks after a complete spinal cord transection. At this time after transection, preganglionic neuronal morphology has returned to normal and all severed axons have been cleared from the lateral horn. These comparisons can distinguish intraspinal from supraspinal synapses because at two weeks post-transection, supraspinal synapses are absent, and only intraspinal synapses persist. Sensory neurons cannot be the source of the surviving synapses because the first spinal neurons that become virus-labeled after sympathetic preganglionic neurons are interneurons, not dorsal horn neurons.

### Neurotransmitters that Affect the Activity of Sympathetic Preganglionic Neurons

Circuits that control the activity of sympathetic preganglionic neurons use a diverse array of neurotransmitters and neuromodulators, including amino acids, monoamines, and neuropeptides (reviewed by [82]; also see Table 6–2). Electrophysiological studies have shown that many of these neurochemicals directly affect the activity of sympathetic preganglionic neurons, and light and electron microscopic immunocytochemistry have demonstrated that the same chemicals occur in terminals that synapse on sympathetic preganglionic neurons and/or in axons in the lateral horn. Sympathetic preganglionic neurons receive inputs that contain amino acids and neuropeptides from both supraspinal and intraspinal sources. In contrast, the monoaminergic innervation of preganglionic neurons arises only from neurons in the brainstem. Many of the transmitters discussed in this section affect autonomic function when injected into the subarachnoid space surrounding the thoracic spinal cord. More information about these effects can be found in other chapters of this book, which deal with the control of individual autonomic functions (e.g., Chapter 5).

### *Amino Acids*

The most important neurotransmitters involved in controlling the activity of sympathetic preganglionic neurons are the amino acids, glutamate, GABA, and glycine (Table 6–2; Figure 6–5).

Glutamate produces fast excitatory responses in sympathetic preganglionic neurons through actions on ionotropic receptors, which are directly linked to ion channels. Ionotropic *N*-methyl-D-aspartate (NMDA) receptors and non-NMDA receptors are involved in glutamatergic transmission to preganglionic neurons and also in the excitatory pathway from the RVLM to sympathetic preganglionic neurons that project through the splanchnic and adrenal nerves[74,108,135]. Activation of metabotropic receptors, which link to ion channels via other signaling mechanisms, usually G-proteins, also influences the activity of sympathetic preganglionic neurons. Group I metabotropic glutamate receptors produce depolarization, whereas group II receptors, which occur on only a few preganglionic neurons, cause hyperpolarization[112,134,151].

In contrast to glutamate, GABA and glycine elicit fast inhibitory responses. The ionotropic $GABA_A$ receptors and metabotropic $GABA_B$ receptors are responsible for the effects of GABA on sympathetic preganglionic neurons[150]. GABAergic inputs provide strong tonic inhibition to sympathetic preganglionic neurons[148], indicating that GABA is likely to be very important for setting the overall level of excitability of these neurons. There is only one type of glycine receptor, and it mediates the effects of this amino acid. It is possible that a small subset of sympathetic preganglionic neurons may not respond to glycine, because in cats some of these neurons appear to lack glycine receptors[61].

Axons that are immunoreactive for glutamate (Figure 6–5A), GABA (Figure 6–5B), and glycine[9,14,20] form synapses on sympathetic preganglionic neurons; and either glutamate or GABA is present in around 95% of the terminals that provide synaptic input to these neurons[83,89,90]. The proportion of sympathetic preganglionic synapses that contain glycine is not

Table 6–2 Neurotransmitters that Affect the Activity of Sympathetic Preganglionic Neurons

| Neurotransmitter | Exogenous Application Affects SPN | Axons in Lateral Horn | Synapses on Identified SPN |
|---|---|---|---|
| Glutamate | Excitation [a] [62,74,108,132,134,135 reviewed by 76] | Yes [109] | Yes [83,84,90] |
| GABA | Inhibition [61,148,150 reviewed by 76] | Yes [14] | Yes [9,14,22,83,84] |
| Glycine | Inhibition [61,73,133,153 reviewed by 76] | Yes [136] | Yes [20] |
| Noradrenaline | Excitation OR Inhibition [59,77 reviewed by 76] | Yes [a e.g., 103] | Yes [a 29] |
| Adrenaline | Excitation OR Inhibition [77,106 reviewed by 76] | Yes [b, e.g., 103] | Yes [b 13,101] |
| Serotonin | Excitation, Inhibition, No effect [51,78,80,115 reviewed by 76] | Yes [e.g., 67] | Yes [9,28,67,147] |
| Angiotensin II | Excitation [79] | Yes [e.g., 81] | ? |
| CART | ? | Yes [reviewed by 43] | Yes [reviewed by 43] |
| Enkephalin | ? | Yes [e.g., 103] | Yes [85,147] |
| NPY | ? | Yes [e.g., 103] | Yes [28] |
| Orexin | Excitation [4,146] | Yes [e.g., 145] | Yes [87] |
| Oxytocin | Excitation [7,128] | Yes [reviewed by 120] | Yes [57] |
| PACAP | Excitation [75,152] | | Yes [31] |
| Somatostatin | ? | Yes [inferred from 31] | Yes [28] |
| Substance P | Excitation [23,60] | Yes [e.g., 103] | Yes [9,117,147] |
| TRH | Excitation [8,70] | Yes [e.g., 6] | ? |
| Vasopressin | Excitation [68,69,128] | Yes [reviewed by 120] | ? |

Excitation = Depolarization, excitatory post-synaptic potentials, excitatory post-synaptic currents and/or increased activity
Inhibition = Hyperpolarization, inhibitory post-synaptic potentials, inhibitory post-synaptic currents and/or decreased activity
[a] Metabotropic receptors on some sympathetic preganglionic neurons cause hyperpolarization; see text for details
[b] Detected by immunoreactivity for tyrosine hydroxylase
[c] Detected by immunoreactivity for phenylethanolamine *N*-methyltransferase
CART, cocaine and amphetamine regulated transcript; NPY, neuropeptide Y; PACAP, pituitary adenylate cyclase-activating polypeptide; SPN, sympathetic preganglionic neuron; TRH, thyrotropin releasing hormone; VIP, vasoactive intestinal peptide.
The review by Laskey et al. (1988)[76] contains references to work published before 1987.

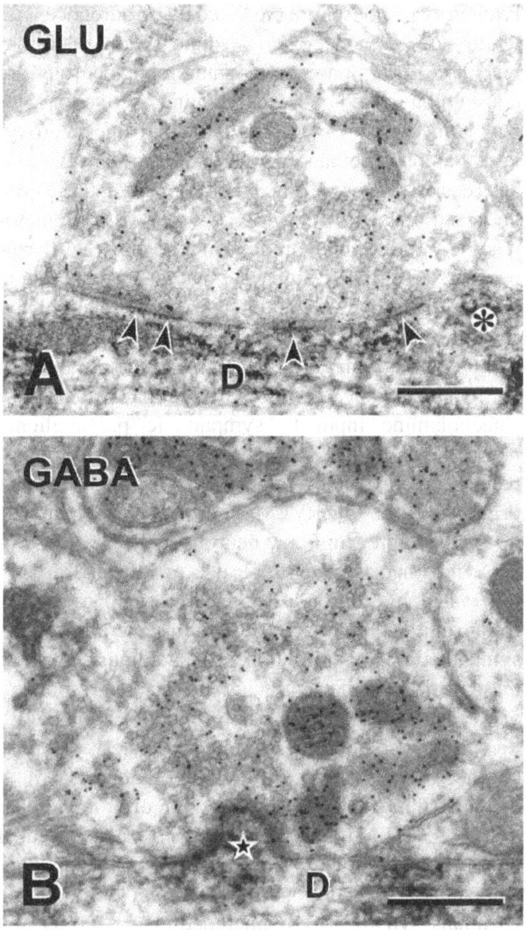


Figure 6–5 Amino acid immunoreactivity in axon terminals that synapse on sympathetic preganglionic neurons. Glutamate- and GABA-immunoreactive terminals synapse on choline acetyltransferase-immunoreactive rat sympathetic preganglionic neurons in the intermediolateral cell column of spinal cord segment T8. *A:* An axon terminal showing glutamate (GLU)-immunoreactivity forms a synapse with multiple small asymmetrical active zones (*arrowheads*) on the dendrite (D) of a sympathetic preganglionic neuron. The dendrite contains immunoreactivity for choline acetyltransferase (*asterisk*). Immunogold staining for GABA in a serial section showed that this terminal was negative for GABA. *B:* An axon terminal showing GABA-immunoreactivity directly contacts a spine (*star*) that arises from the dendrite (D) of a sympathetic preganglionic neuron. This GABA-positive terminal formed a synapse on the spine in another ultrathin section. Immunogold staining for glutamate in a serial section showed that this terminal was negative for glutamate. Bars, 500 nm. Reproduced from Llewellyn-Smith and Weaver (2001)[92], with permission.

known, so glycine could occur in inputs that do not contain glutamate or GABA. However, glycine could also coexist with GABA because the same transporter packages these two amino acids into synaptic vesicles[41]. The data showing that virtually all axons that synapse on sympathetic preganglionic neurons contain either GABA or glutamate has important implications for understanding the regulation of the activity of sympathetic preganglionic neurons. If an amino acid is present in every terminal that synapses on a sympathetic preganglionic neuron, then any other transmitters in the terminal must coexist with, and will probably be co-released with, an amino acid. If the required post-synaptic receptors are present, then the amino acid transmitter will drive the sympathetic preganglionic neuron, and the co-localized transmitter(s) will modulate the effects of the amino acid.

Normally, only one amino acid occurs in terminals that form synapses on preganglionic neurons; i.e., either glutamate or GABA. However, immunoreactivity for both of these amino acids can be found in synaptic terminals two weeks after a complete spinal cord transection[92]. It is possible that these terminals could actually release both glutamate and GABA because synaptic vesicles can co-store and co-release these two amino acids. However, the terminals that contain both GABA and glutamate could also be GABAergic, since glutamate is a precursor for GABA synthesis.

Transporters package neurotransmitters into vesicles; and, consistent with the extensive glutamatergic input to sympathetic preganglionic neurons, axons containing all three vesicular glutamate transporters occur in spinal autonomic regions. Innervation by axons containing immunoreactivity for vesicular glutamate transporter 1 is sparse in the lateral horn; but there are abundant axons with immunoreactivity for vesicular glutamate transporter 2[86]. These axons closely appose sympathetic preganglionic neurons retrogradely labeled from a variety of peripheral targets and form synapses on sympathetic preganglionic neurons retrogradely labeled from intraperitoneal injections of Fluorogold[86]. Axons and synaptic terminals in the lateral horn also show immunoreactivity for vesicular glutamate transporter 3[111,140]. These axons and terminals may not, in fact, contain glutamate, since GABA occurs in terminals with vesicular glutamate transporter 3-immunoreactivity in the intermediolateral cell column[140].

As expected, supraspinal neurons that provide synaptic input to sympathetic preganglionic neurons also contain neurochemical markers of amino acid neurotransmission. Bulbospinal neurons in the RVLM and caudal raphé nuclei express mRNA for vesicular glutamate transporter 2 and immunoreactivity for phosphate-activated glutaminase, which synthesizes glutamate[102,141]. Vesicular glutamate transporter 2 mRNA also occurs in autonomic neurons in the PVN[137]. Expression of mRNA for glutamic acid decarboxylase, which synthesizes GABA, occurs in spinally projecting medullary raphé neurons, including those with immunoreactivity for vesicular glutamate transporter 3[139,140]. Furthermore, anterogradely labeled terminals in the intermediolateral cell column that come from the ventral medulla contain immunoreactivity for GABA or glutamate[89].

As well as supraspinal amino acid input, sympathetic preganglionic neurons receive synapses from intraspinal neurons that use amino acid transmitters. In slice preparations *in vitro*, which lack input from the brain, sympathetic preganglionic neurons have ongoing inhibitory and excitatory synaptic activity that is blocked by amino acid antagonists (e.g., [74,133,135]). In addition, synaptic terminals with glutamate- or GABA-immunoreactivity are still found on these neurons two weeks after a complete spinal cord transection, when the only input comes for intraspinal neurons[84,92]. GABAergic spinal interneurons are clearly part of the spinal circuitry regulating the activity of sympathetic preganglionic neurons. Not only does viral tracing from the adrenal medulla label spinal interneurons that express glutamic acid decarboxylase mRNA; but bicuculline-sensitive, inhibitory post-synaptic potentials can also be evoked by stimulating the spinal regions where the virus-labeled inhibitory interneurons lie[37]. The location of the excitatory spinal interneurons that release glutamate onto sympathetic preganglionic neurons has not been identified. Spinal neurons that express mRNA for vesicular glutamate transporter 2 occur in regions where sympathetic interneurons are located[86]; but it is not known whether any synapses on sympathetic preganglionic neurons arise from these glutamatergic spinal neurons.

Another potential source of glutamatergic input to sympathetic preganglionic neurons is primary afferents, but there is no evidence for such a connection. There are no degenerating terminals in the intermediolateral cell column after dorsal roots are cut[114], and viral tracing studies indicate that spinal interneurons are immediately antecedent to sympathetic preganglionic neurons[24,143]. These data suggest that the central processes of sensory neurons do not provide any of the amino acid–containing input to sympathetic preganglionic neurons, and that these neurons must receive sensory information via spinal interneurons.

### Monoamines

Sympathetic preganglionic neurons show both excitatory and inhibitory responses when noradrenaline or adrenaline are applied exogenously (Table 6–2). Excitatory responses are mediated by $\alpha_1$-adrenoceptors while $\alpha_2$-adrenoceptors mediate the inhibitory responses[59]. Sympathetic preganglionic neurons are densely innervated by axons immunoreactive for catecholamine synthesizing enzymes—tyrosine hydroxylase and phenylethanolamine *N*-methyltransferase—and receive synapses from axons containing these imm unoreactivities[13,29,94,101,103]. Since axons with immunoreactivity for catecholamine synthetic enzymes disappear caudal to a transection[94], sympathetic preganglionic neurons must receive all of their catecholaminergic input from the brain. Viral tracing indicates that the C1 adrenergic neurons of the RVLM and the noradrenergic neurons of the A5 group are the major sources of catecholamine input to sympathetic preganglionic neurons[66]. Consistent with these data, axons immunoreactive for vesicular monoamine transporter 2, which originate from C1 RVLM neurons, closely appose sympathetic preganglionic neurons[129].

Sympathetic preganglionic neurons are also directly innervated by neurons that use serotonin as a neurotransmitter (Table 6-2). Serotonin generally excites sympathetic preganglionic neurons, although some of these neurons in the central autonomic area respond to 5-HT by hyperpolarizing before they depolarize[115]. Serotonin also increases sympathetic nerve activity and has been implicated in the generation of sympathetic rhythmic activity[96,98]. Detection of immunoreactivity for 5-HT or the serotonin transporter has revealed dense plexuses of serotonergic axons surrounding sympathetic preganglionic neurons, and serotonergic terminals synapse on sympathoadrenal neurons and neurons that project to the superior cervical ganglion[9,67,94,147]. The medullary raphé nuclei are the main source of the serotonergic input to sympathetic preganglionic neurons[16,66,95].

### Neuropeptides

A variety of peptide neurotransmitters are likely to be involved in controlling the activity of sympathetic preganglionic neurons (Table 6-2). Some of these neuropeptides are known to affect preganglionic neuronal activity when applied exogenously, and terminals that contain immunoreactivity for the peptides have been verified to synapse on sympathetic preganglionic neurons by electron microscopic immunocytochemistry. Neuropeptides that fall into this group are orexin, oxytocin, pituitary adenylate cyclase–activating polypeptide, and substance P (Table 6-2). For other neuropeptides, including angiotensin II, thyrotropin releasing hormone, and vasopressin, electrophysiological studies have demonstrated effects on sympathetic preganglionic neurons, and there are immunoreactive axons in the lateral horn but evidence for synapses is lacking (Table 6-2). In general, when applied to slice preparations of mammalian spinal cord, all of the neuropeptides that have been tested electrophysiologically excite sympathetic preganglionic neurons, either depolarizing them, causing them to fire, or increasing their firing rate. The involvement of a third group of neuropeptides in spinal preganglionic regulation is suggested by their presence in axons that synapse on sympathetic preganglionic neurons, but the effects of these peptides have not yet been tested on sympathetic preganglionic neurons. This group includes cocaine- and amphetamine-regulated transcript, enkephalin, neuropeptide Y, and somatostatin (Table 6-2). Finally, there are neuropeptides that occur in axons in the lateral horn or in axons that closely appose sympathetic preganglionic neurons and that may or may not have direct effects on sympathetic preganglionic neurons and may or may not be in synaptic contact with them. This group of peptides includes avian pancreatic peptide, calcitonin gene-related peptide, cholecystokinin, corticotropin-releasing factor, galanin, nociceptin, and vasoactive intestinal peptide[19,42,103].

Some of the neuropeptide-containing inputs to spinal sympathetic regions come exclusively from neurons in the brain, including the oxytocin-, vasopressin-, and orexin-immunoreactive axons. Intraspinal as well as supraspinal neurons provide axons to the lateral horn that contain other neuropeptides, including substance P, enkephalin, and neuropeptide Y. Brainstem serotonin neurons that contain substance P innervate the spinal cord[126]; some spinally projecting RVLM neurons contain preproenkephalin mRNA[138], and medullospinal neurons show markers for neuropeptide Y synthesis[105,138]. Nevertheless, the survival of axons and the persistence of synapses immunoreactive for these three neuropeptides caudal to a complete transection indicate that spinal neurons must also provide some of the substance P-, enkephalin-, and neuropeptide Y-containing inputs to sympathetic preganglionic neurons[26,34,93,123]. Neurons in spinal cord laminae V and VII that express neuropeptide Y mRNA could be the source of the neuropeptide Y-containing axons that remain after transection[104], and the enkephalin immunoreactive innervation that is not affected by transection could come from neurons in lamina X above the central canal[85], where interneurons immediately antecedent to sympathetic preganglionic neurons are located[144]. The location of the neurons that supply the intraspinal substance P-immunoreactive input to sympathetic preganglionic neuron has yet to be identified.

### *Other Neurotransmitters*

Acetylcholine either depolarizes or hyperpolarizes sympathetic preganglionic neurons, depending on whether nicotinic or muscarinic receptors are activated[15,50]. Whether or not these neurons receive synapses or close appositions from nerve terminals capable of releasing acetylcholine needs to be clarified. Apparently, there are no terminals immunoreactive for the vesicular acetylcholine transporter around sympathetic preganglionic somata[127], but there could be input to dendrites.

Purines affect the activity of sympathetic preganglionic neurons. In the intermediolateral cell column, these neurons are surrounded by a dense network of axons that are immunoreactive for the adenosine 2A receptor. Some of these axons make synapses[17], but the post-synaptic targets of these synapses remain unclear. Nevertheless, at least some synapses are likely to occur on sympathetic preganglionic neurons, since activation of pre-synaptic adenosine 2A receptors increased the amplitude of inhibitory post-synaptic potentials at preganglionic neurons, an effect that was blocked by a specific antagonist against these receptors[17].

## Variations in the Innervation of Sympathetic Preganglionic Neurons

Many of the chapters in this book make it clear that the central control of different sympathetic outflows is not uniform. Hence, the same physiological challenge evokes different responses in different functional groups of sympathetic preganglionic neurons (reviewed by [107]). Differences in the innervation of different functional classes of sympathetic preganglionic neuron by the various groups of neurochemically identified axons discussed above are likely to underpin these differentiated physiological responses.

As discussed above, different functional groups of sympathetic preganglionic neurons are organized topographically within the lateral horn. This organizational pattern is probably the reason that the distribution of various types of immunoreactive axons varies rostrocaudally along the length of the intermediolateral cell column (Figure 6–6A). Axons containing immunoreactivity for 5-HT, substance P, somatostatin, oxytocin, neurotensin, or neurophysin are distributed non-uniformly through the lateral horn of thoracic and upper lumbar segments of the cat spinal cord, as are serotonergic axons in the rabbit[67,71]. The innervation of sympathetic preganglionic neurons that respond to a hypotensive stimulus with *c-fos* activation is also heterogeneous; and there are rostrocaudal variations in the innervation of these neurons by axons immunoreactive for neuropeptide Y, phenylethanolamine *N*-methyltransferase, or galanin[103] (Figure 6–6D). Somatostatin-immunoreactive axons preferentially innervate sympathetic preganglionic neurons that supply the adrenal medulla[56], whereas galanin-immunoreactive axons seem to avoid sympathetic

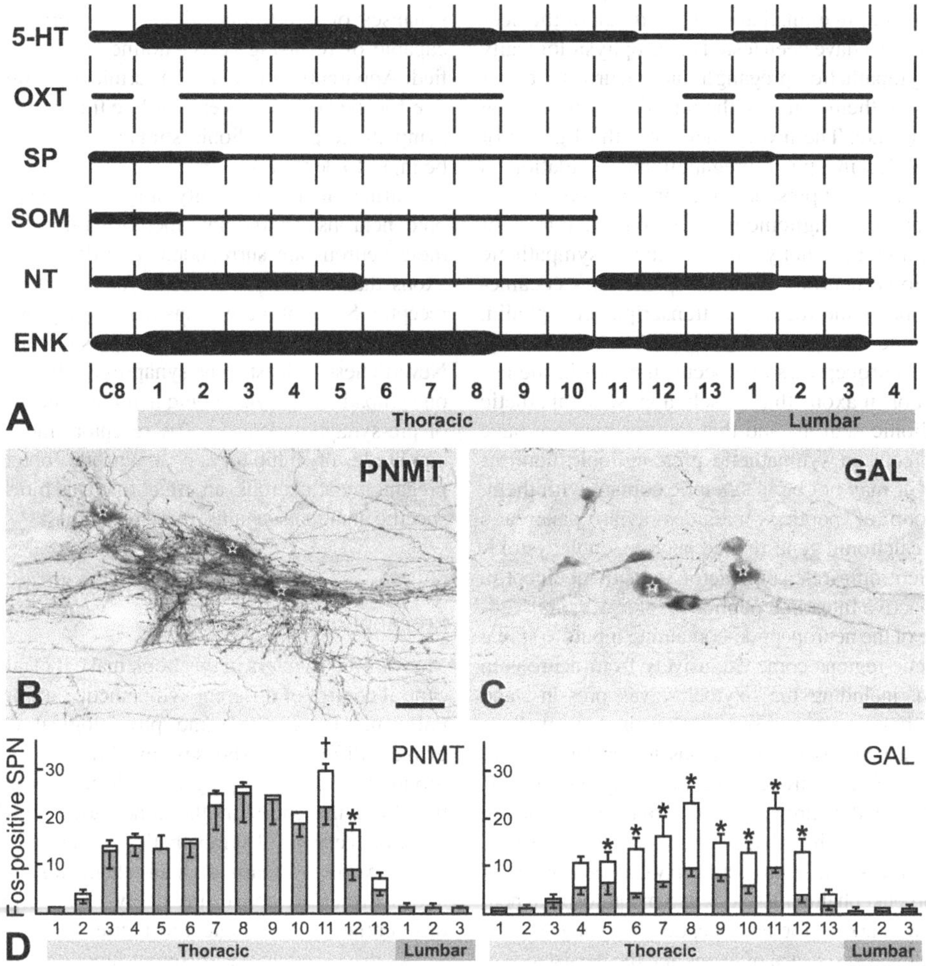


Figure 6–6 Variations in the innervation of sympathetic preganglionic neurons. *A*: Diagram showing rostrocaudal variations in the innervation of the cat intermediolateral cell column by nerve fibers immunoreactive for serotonin (5-hydroxytryptamine, 5-HT), oxytocin (OXT), substance P (SP), somatostatin (SOM), neurotensin (NT) and enkephalin (ENK). Bar width represents axon density at each spinal segmental level (i.e., very dense, dense, moderate and sparse), with the thickest bar width indicating where axons are densest. C8, cervical segment 8. Modified from Krukoff et al. (1985)[71], with permission. *B* and *C:* Micrographs showing sympathetic preganglionic neurons (*stars*) retrogradely labeled with cholera toxin B subunit from the coeliac ganglion. *B:* The retrogradely labeled neurons lie in a dense network of axons immunoreactive for phenylethanolamine *N*-methyltransferase (PNMT). *C:* Axons immunoreactive for galanin (GAL) avoid these neurons. Scale bars, 50 μm. *D:* Segmental frequency distribution histograms of barosensitive Fos-positive sympathetic preganglionic neurons in the intermediolateral cell column with and without close appositions from immunoreactive axons on somata or proximal dendrites. *Shaded bars,* numbers of Fos-positive neurons with close appositions from varicose immunoreactive axons. *Open bars,* Fos-positive neurons lacking close appositions from varicose immunoreactive axons.*Significant differences at the same segmental level in the proportion of Fos-positive sympathetic preganglionic neuron contacted by appositions of this immunoreactivity compared with the proportion of Fos-positive sympathetic preganglionic neuron receiving other immunoreactive appositions ($P < 0.05$). †Significant difference at the same segmental level in the proportion of Fos-positive sympathetic preganglionic neurons contacted by appositions from axons immunoreactive for PNMT compared with the proportion of Fos-positive sympathetic preganglionic neurons receiving GAL-immunoreactive appositions ($P < 0.05$). Modified from Minson et al. (2002)[103], with permission.

preganglionic neurons that project to the coeliac ganglion (Figure 6–6B and C).

Immunocytochemically defined synaptic inputs to sympathetic preganglionic neurons have been quantified in only a few electron microscopic immunocytochemical studies. Like the light microscopic studies, these ultrastructural analyses show that different groups of sympathetic preganglionic neurons vary with respect to the proportion of synaptic input that they receive from different types of neurotransmitter-identified axons. Sympathoadrenal neurons receive about 70% of their synaptic input from glutamate-containing terminals, whereas glutamate occurs in only half of the input to sympathetic preganglionic neurons that innervate the superior cervical ganglion[83,90]. As expected, if an amino acid is present in all terminals that synapse on sympathetic preganglionic neurons (see above), about 30% and about 50% of the synaptic input to these two groups of neurons, respectively, is GABA-immunoreactive[9,83]. More than half of the synaptic input to sympathetic preganglionic neurons that project to the major pelvic ganglion, which are involved in regulating the pelvic viscera, is immunoreactive for enkephalin[85]. The intermediolateral cell column is heavily innervated by enkephalin-immunoreactive axons, but whether enkephalin axons provide an equivalently large proportion of synaptic input to other groups of sympathetic preganglionic neurons remains an open question.

As well as these rostrocaudal differences in neurotransmitter-identified innervation, sympathetic preganglionic neurons at different rostrocaudal levels of the lateral horn probably also receive different proportions of their input from supraspinal versus intraspinal sources. In rats, significantly more than half of the synaptic input to choline acetyltransferase-immunoreactive sympathetic preganglionic neurons in thoracic spinal segment 8 is lost following a complete spinal cord transection[92]. This finding indicates that neurons above the lesion, likely supraspinal neurons, supply most of the synaptic input to sympathetic preganglionic neurons at this level of the spinal cord. In contrast, in thoracic spinal segment 12 to lumbar segment 2, the innervation of sympathetic preganglionic neurons that project to the major pelvic ganglion seems to be almost identical in rats with intact and rats with completely transected cords[85]. These observations suggest that most of the synaptic input to sympathetic preganglionic neurons that control the activity of the pelvic viscera comes from spinal rather than supraspinal sources.

## Looking to the Future

There have been dramatic advances in our understanding of the structure and function of sympathetic preganglionic neurons since the first edition of this book was published in 1990. A flurry of research activity in the 1980s and 1990s defined the direct effects of a variety of neurotransmitters and neuromodulators on sympathetic preganglionic neurons. Antibody-labeling and tract-tracing studies at light and electron microscopic levels have also clarified some of the central circuits in which sympathetic preganglionic neurons participate. It is now obvious that the functions and innervation patterns of sympathetic preganglionic neurons are much more finely differentiated than might have been suspected in 1990. Nevertheless, as Tables 6-1 and 6-2 highlight, there is still a host of questions to be answered about these important neurons. Many neuroactive substances that are known to be involved in central autonomic control at the spinal cord level, and neurochemicals that may be discovered in the future, need to be tested electrophysiologically to determine their direct effects on sympathetic preganglionic neurons. The neurochemical phenotypes of all of the different functional types of sympathetic preganglionic neurons are still very poorly understood. This wide gap in our knowledge would benefit from systematic studies to detect neuropeptides and other neurochemicals in sympathetic preganglionic neurons combined with chemical coding of the post-ganglionic neurons that they innervate. A very large amount of research with anatomical and physiological techniques is also required to understand how synaptic inputs vary between different functional groups of sympathetic preganglionic neurons. The other chapters in this book underline that neurons in many regions of the central nervous system project to the lateral horn of the spinal cord, where they influence sympathetic outflow. However, for most of these circuits, it is unclear whether the inputs occur on sympathetic preganglionic neurons or spinal sympathetic interneurons, or both. Quantitative electron microscopic immunocytochemical studies would also clarify the differential innervation patterns of sympathetic preganglionic neurons that project to different targets and have different functions. Finally, since many synaptic inputs to sympathetic preganglionic neurons are likely to contain an amino acid plus at least one other neurotransmitter, it would be worthwhile for physiological and electrophysiological studies to assess how cocktails of antagonists affect the activity of sympathetic preganglionic neurons *in vitro* and sympathetic outflow *in vivo*.

ACKNOWLEDGEMENTS A Project Grant (#480414) and a Research Fellowship (#229921) from the National Health and Medical Research Council of Australia supported this work. Lee Travis provided valuable assistance.

## References


1. Anderson, C. R. (1992). NADPH diaphorase-positive neurons in the rat spinal cord include a subpopulation of autonomic preganglionic neurons. *Neuroscience Letters* 139, 280–284.
2. Anderson, C. R. (1998). Identification of cardiovascular pathways in the sympathetic nervous system. *Clinical and Experimental Pharmacology and Physiology* 25, 449–452.
3. Anderson, C. R., McLachlan, E. M., and Srb-Christie, O. (1989). Distribution of sympathetic preganglionic neurons and monoaminergic nerve terminals in the spinal cord of the rat. *Journal of Comparative Neurology* 283, 269–284.
4. Antunes, V. R., Brailoiu, G. C., Kwok, E. H., Scruggs, P., and Dun, N. J. (2001). Orexins/hypocretins excite rat sympathetic preganglionic neurons in vivo and in vitro. *American Journal of Physiology. Regulatory, Comparative and Integrative Physiology* 281, R1801–R1807.
5. Appel, N. M., and Elde, R. P. (1988). The intermediolateral cell column of the thoracic spinal cord is comprised of target-specific subnuclei: Evidence from retrograde transport studies and immunohistochemistry. *Journal of Neuroscience* 8, 1767–1775.
6. Appel, N. M., Wessendorf, M. W., and Elde, R. P. (1987). Thyrotropin-releasing hormone in spinal cord: Coexistence with serotonin and with substance P in fibers and terminals apposing identified preganglionic sympathetic neurons. *Brain Research* 415, 137–143.
7. Backman, S. B., and Henry, J. L. (1984). Effects of oxytocin and vasopressin on thoracic sympathetic preganglionic neurones in the cat. *Brain Research Bulletin* 13, 679–684.
8. Backman, S. B., and Henry, J. L. (1984). Effects of substance P and thyrotropin-releasing hormone on sympathetic preganglionic neurones in the upper thoracic intermediolateral nucleus of the cat. *Canadian Journal of Physiology and Pharmacology* 62, 248–251.
9. Bacon, S. J., and Smith, A. D. (1988). Preganglionic sympathetic neurones innervating the rat adrenal medulla: Immunocytochemical evidence of synaptic input from nerve terminals containing substance P, GABA or 5-hydroxytryptamine. *Journal of the Autonomic Nervous System* 24, 97–122.
10. Bacon, S. J., Zagon, A., and Smith, A. D. (1990). Electron microscopic evidence of a monosynaptic pathway between cells in the caudal raphé nuclei and sympathetic preganglionic neurons in the rat spinal cord. *Experimental Brain Research* 79, 589–602.
11. Barber, R. P., Phelps, P. E., Houser, C. R., Crawford, G. D., Salvaterra, P. M., and Vaughn, J. E. (1984). The morphology and distribution of neurons containing choline acetyltransferase in the adult rat spinal cord: An immunocytochemical study. *Journal of Comparative Neurology* 229, 329–346.
12. Beaudet, M. M., Braas, K. M., and May, V. (1998). Pituitary adenylate cyclase activating polypeptide (PACAP) expression in sympathetic preganglionic projection neurons to the superior cervical ganglion. *Journal of Neurobiology* 36, 325–336.
13. Bernstein-Goral, H., and Bohn, M. C. (1989). Phenylethanolamine *N*-methyltransferase-immunoreactive terminals synapse on adrenal preganglionic neurons in the rat spinal cord. *Neuroscience* 32, 521–537.
14. Bogan, N., Mennone, A., and Cabot, J. B. (1989). Light microscopic and ultrastructural localization of GABA-like immunoreactive input to retrogradely labeled sympathetic preganglionic neurons. *Brain Research* 505, 257–270.
15. Bordey, A., Feltz, P., and Trouslard, J. (1996). Nicotinic actions on neurones of the central autonomic area in rat spinal cord slices. *Journal of Physiology* 497, 175–187.
16. Bowker, R. M., Westlund, K. N., Sullivan, M. C., and Coulter, J. D. (1982). Organization of descending serotonergic projections to the spinal cord. *Progress in Brain Research* 57, 239–265.
17. Brooke, R. E., Deuchars, J., and Deuchars, S. A. (2004). Input-specific modulation of neurotransmitter release in the lateral horn of the spinal cord via adenosine receptors. *Journal of Neuroscience* 24, 127–137.
18. Burman, K. J., McKitrick, D. J., Minson, J. B., West, A., Arnolda, L. F., and Llewellyn-Smith, I. J. (2001). Neurokinin-1 receptor immunoreactivity in hypotension sensitive sympathetic preganglionic neurons. *Brain Research* 915, 238–243.
19. Cabot, J. B. (1990). Sympathetic preganglionic neurons: Cytoarchitecture, ultrastructure and biophysical properties. In A. D. Loewy and K. M. Spyer (Eds), *Central Regulation of Autonomic Functions,* pp. 44–67. Oxford, UK: Oxford University Press.
20. Cabot, J. B., Alessi, V., and Bushnell, A. (1992). Glycine-like immunoreactive input to sympathetic preganglionic neurons. *Brain Research* 571, 1–18.
21. Cabot, J. B., and Bogan, N. (1987). Light microscopic observations on the morphology of sympathetic preganglionic neurons in the pigeon, *Columba livia*. *Neuroscience* 20, 467–486.

22. Cabot, J. B., Bushnell, A., Alessi, V., and Mendell, N. R. (1995). Postsynaptic gephyrin immunoreactivity exhibits a nearly one-to-one correspondence with gamma-aminobutyric acid-like immunogold-labeled synaptic inputs to sympathetic preganglionic neurons. *Journal of Comparative Neurology* 356, 418–432.
23. Cammack, C., and Logan, S. D. (1996). Excitation of rat sympathetic preganglionic neurones by selective activation of the NK1 receptor. *Journal of the Autonomic Nervous System* 57, 87–92.
24. Cano, G., Sved, A. F., Rinaman, L., Rabin, B. S., and Card, J. P. (2001). Characterization of the central nervous system innervation of the rat spleen using viral transneuronal tracing. *Journal of Comparative Neurology* 439, 1–18.
25. Cao, W. H., and Morrison, S. F. (2001). Differential chemoreceptor reflex responses of adrenal preganglionic neurons. *American Journal of Physiology. Regulatory, Integrative and Comparative Physiology* 281, R1825–R1832.
26. Cassam, A. K., Llewellyn-Smith, I. J., and Weaver, L. C. (1997). Catecholamine enzymes and neuropeptides are expressed in fibres and somata in the intermediate gray matter in chronic spinal rats. *Neuroscience* 78, 829–841.
27. Chanthaphavong, R. S., Murphy, S. M., and Anderson, C. R. (2003). Chemical coding of sympathetic neurons controlling the tarsal muscle of the rat. *Autonomic Neuroscience* 105, 77–89.
28. Chiba, T. (1989). Direct synaptic contacts of 5-hydroxytryptamine-, neuropeptide Y-, and somatostatin-immunoreactive nerve terminals on the preganglionic sympathetic neurons of the guinea pig. *Neuroscience Letters* 105, 281–286.
29. Chiba, T., and Masuko, S. (1986). Direct synaptic contacts of catecholamine axons on the preganglionic sympathetic neurons in the rat thoracic spinal cord. *Brain Research* 380, 405–408.
30. Chiba, T., and Tanaka, K. (1998). A target specific pathway from nitric oxide synthase immunoreactive preganglionic sympathetic to superior cervical ganglion neurons innervating the submandibular salivary gland. *Journal of the Autonomic Nervous System* 71, 139–147.
31. Chiba, T., Tanaka, K., Tatsuoka, H., Dun, S. L., and Dun, N. J. (1996). The synaptic structure of PACAP immunoreactive axons in the intermediolateral nucleus of the rat. *Neuroscience Letters* 214, 65–68.
32. Colombo-Benkmann, M., Heym, C., and Schemann, M. (1995). Preganglionic sympathetic neurones, innervating the guinea pig adrenal medulla, immunohistochemically contain choline acetyltransferase and also leu-enkephlain. *Neuroscience Letters* 190, 155–158.
33. Dalsgaard, C.-J., Hokfelt, T., Elfvin, L.-G., and Terenius, L. (1982). Enkephalin-containing sympathetic preganglionic neurons projecting to the inferior mesenteric ganglion: Evidence from combined retrograde tracing and immunohistochemistry. *Neuroscience* 7, 2039–2050.
34. Davis, B. M., and Cabot, J. B. (1984). Substance P-containing pathways to avian sympathetic preganglionic neurons: Evidence for major spinal-spinal circuitry. *Journal of Neuroscience* 4, 2145–2159.
35. Dembowsky, K., Czachurski, J., and Seller, H. (1985). Morphology of sympathetic preganglionic neurons in the thoracic spinal cord of the cat: An intracellular horseradish peroxidase study. *Journal of Comparative Neurology* 238, 453–465.
36. Deuchars, S. A., Brooke, R. E., Frater, B., and Deuchars, J. (2001). Properties of interneurones in the intermediolateral cell column of the rat spinal cord: Role of the potassium channel subunit Kv3.1. *Neuroscience* 106, 433–446.
37. Deuchars, S. A., Milligan, C. J., Stornetta, R. L., and Deuchars, J. (2005). GABAergic neurons in the central region of the spinal cord: A novel substrate for sympathetic inhibition. *Journal of Neuroscience* 25, 1063–1070.
38. Deuchars, S. A., Morrison, S. F., and Gilbey, M. P. (1995). Medullary-evoked EPSPs in neonatal rat sympathetic preganglionic neurones in vitro. *Journal of Physiology* 487, 453–463.
39. Deuchars, S. A., Spyer, K. M., Brooks, P. A., and Gilbey, M. P. (1995). A study of sympathetic preganglionic neuronal activity in a neonatal rat brainstem-spinal cord preparation. *Journal of the Autonomic Nervous System* 52, 51–63.
40. Deuchars, S. A., Spyer, K. M., and Gilbey, M. P. (1997). Stimulation within the rostral ventrolateral medulla can evoke monosynaptic GABAergic IPSPs in sympathetic preganglionic neurons in vitro. *Journal of Neurophysiology* 77, 229–235.
41. Dumoulin, A., Rostaing, P., Bedet, C., Levi, S., Isambert, M. F., Henry, J. P., Triller, A., and Gasnier, B. (1999). Presence of the vesicular inhibitory amino acid transporter in GABAergic and glycinergic synaptic terminal boutons. *Journal of Cell Science* 112, 811–823.
42. Dun, N. J., Dun, S. L., and Hwang, L. L. (1997). Nociceptin-like immunoreactivity in autonomic nuclei of the rat spinal cord. *Neuroscience Letters* 234, 95–98.
43. Dun, S. L., Brailoiu, G. C., Yang, J., Chang, J. K., and Dun, N. J. (2006). Cocaine- and amphetamine-

regulated transcript peptide and sympatho-adrenal axis. *Peptides* 27, 1949–1955.

44. Edwards, S. L., Anderson, C. R., Southwell, B. R., and McAllen, R. M. (1996). Distinct preganglionic neurons innervate noradrenaline and adrenaline cells in the cat adrenal medulla. *Neuroscience* 70, 825–832.
45. Fenwick, N. M., Martin, C. L., and Llewellyn-Smith, I. J. (2006). Immunoreactivity for cocaine- and amphetamine-regulated transcript in rat sympathetic preganglionic neurons projecting to sympathetic ganglia and the adrenal medulla. *Journal of Comparative Neurology* 495, 422–433.
46. Forehand, C. J. (1990). Morphology of sympathetic preganglionic neurons in the neonatal rat spinal cord: An intracellular horseradish peroxidase study. *Journal of Comparative Neurology* 298, 334–342.
47. Geerling,J.C.,Mettenleiter,T.C.,andLoewy,A.D. (2003). Orexin neurons project to diverse sympathetic outflow systems. *Neuroscience* 122, 541–550.
48. Gibbins, I. (1995). Chemical neuroanatomy of sympathetic ganglia. In E. M. McLachlan (Ed.), *Autonomic Ganglia*, pp. 73–121. Luxembourg: Harwood Academic Publishers.
49. Gibbins, I. L. (1992). Vasoconstrictor, vasodilator and pilomotor pathways in sympathetic ganglia of guinea pigs. *Neuroscience* 47, 657–672.
50. Gibson, I. C., and Logan, S. D. (1995). Effects of muscarinic receptor stimulation of sympathetic preganglionic neurones of neonatal rat spinal cord *in vitro*. *Neuropharmacology* 34, 309–318.
51. Gilbey, M. P., and Stein, R. D. (1991). Characteristics of sympathetic preganglionic neurones in the lumbar spinal cord of the cat. *Journal of Physiology* 432, 427–443.
52. Grkovic, I., and Anderson, C. R. (1995). Calretinin-containing preganglionic nerve terminals in the rat superior cervical ganglion surround neurons projecting to the submandibular salivary gland. *Brain Research* 684, 127–135.
53. Grkovic, I., and Anderson, C. R. (1996). Distribution of immunoreactivity for the NK1 receptor on different subpopulations of sympathetic preganglionic neurons in the rat. *Journal of Comparative Neurology* 374, 376–386.
54. Grkovic, I., and Anderson, C. R. (1997). Calbindin D28K-immunoreactivity identifies distinct subpopulations of sympathetic pre- and post-ganglionic neurons in the rat. *Journal of Comparative Neurology* 386, 245–259.
55. Hinrichs, J. M., and Llewellyn-Smith, I. J. (2009). Variability in the occurrence of nitric oxide synthase immunoreactivity in different populations of rat sympathetic preganglionic neurons. *Journal of Comparative Neurology* 514, 492–506.
56. Holets, V., and Elde, R. (1982). The differential distribution and relationship of serotonergic and peptidergic fibers to sympathoadrenal neurons in the intermediolateral cell column of the rat: A combined retrograde axonal transport and immunofluorescence study. *Neuroscience* 7, 1155–1174.
57. Hosoya, Y., Matsukawa, Okado, N., Sugiura, Y., and Kohno, K. (1995). Oxytocinergic innervation to the upper thoracic sympathetic preganglionic neurons in the rat. A light and electron microscopical study using a combined retrograde transport and immunocytochemical technique. *Experimental Brain Research* 107, 9–16.
58. Inokuchi,H.,Masuko,S.,Chiba,T.,Yoshimura,M., Polosa, C., and Nishi, S. (1993). Membrane properties and dendritic arborization of the intermediolateral nucleus neurons in the guinea pig thoracic spinal cord in vitro. *Journal of the Autonomic Nervous System* 43, 97–106.
59. Inokuchi, H., and Yoshimura, M. (1992). Adrenergic receptors ($\alpha_1$ and $\alpha_2$) modulate different potassium conductances in sympathetic preganglionic neurones. *Canadian Journal of Physiology and Pharmacology* 70, S92–S97.
60. Inokuchi, H., Yoshimura, M., Polosa, C., and Nishi, S. (1993). Tachykinins depress a calcium-dependent potassium conductance in sympathetic preganglionic neurons. *Regulatory Peptides* 46, 367–369.
61. Inokuchi, H., Yoshimura, M., Trzebski, A., Polosa, C., and Nishi, S. (1992). Fast inhibitory postsynaptic potentials and responses to inhibitory amino acids of sympathetic preganglionic neurons in the adult cat. *Journal of the Autonomic Nervous System* 41, 53–60.
62. Inokuchi,H.,Yoshimura,M.,Yamada,S.,Polosa,C., and Nishi, S. (1992). Fast excitatory postsynaptic potentials and the responses to excitant amino acids of sympathetic preganglionic neurons in the slice of the cat spinal cord. *Neuroscience* 46, 657–667.
63. Ito, T., Hioki, H., Nakamura, K., Tanaka, Y., Nakade, H., Kaneko, T., Iino, S., and Nojyo, Y. (2007). Gamma-aminobutyric acid-containing sympathetic preganglionic neurons in rat thoracic spinal cord send their axons to the superior cervical ganglion. *Journal of Comparative Neurology* 502, 113–125.
64. Janig, W. (1988). Pre- and postganglionic vasoconstrictor neurons: Differentiation, types, and discharge properties. *Annual Review of Physiology* 50, 525–539.

65. Janig, W., and McLachlan, E. M. (1992). Characteristics of function-specific pathways in the sympathetic nervous system. *Trends in Neuroscience* 15, 475–481.
66. Jansen, A. S., Wessendorf, M. W., and Loewy, A. D. (1995). Transneuronal labeling of CNS neuropeptide and monoamine neurons after pseudorabies virus injections into the stellate ganglion. *Brain Research* 683, 1–24.
67. Jensen, I., Llewellyn-Smith, I. J., Minson, J. B., Pilowsky, P. M., and Chalmers, J. P. (1995). Serotonin inputs to rabbit sympathetic preganglionic neurons projecting to the superior cervical ganglion or adrenal medulla. *Journal of Comparative Neurology* 353, 427–438.
68. Kolaj, M., and Renaud, L. P. (1998). Vasopressin acting at V1–type receptors produces membrane depolarization in neonatal rat spinal lateral column neurons. *Progress in Brain Research* 119, 275–284.
69. Kolaj, M., and Renaud, L. P. (1998). Vasopressin-induced currents in rat neonatal spinal lateral horn neurons are G-protein mediated and involve two conductances. *Journal of Neurophysiology* 80, 1900–1910.
70. Kolaj, M., Shefchyk, S. J., and Renaud, L. P. (1997). Two conductances mediate thyrotropin-releasing-hormone-induced depolarization of neonatal rat spinal preganglionic and lateral horn neurons. *Journal of Neurophysiology* 78, 1726–1729.
71. Krukoff, T. L., Ciriello, J., and Calaresu, F. R. (1985). Segmental distribution of peptide- and 5HT-like immunoreactivity in nerve terminals and fibres of the thoracolumbar sympathetic nuclei of the cat. *Journal of Comparative Neurology* 240, 103–116.
72. Krukoff, T. L., Ciriello, J., and Calaresu, F. R. (1985). Segmental distribution of peptide-like immunoreactivity in cell bodies of the thoracolumbar sympathetic nuclei of the cat. *Journal of Comparative Neurology* 240, 90–102.
73. Krupp, J., Bordey, A., and Feltz, P. (1997). Electrophysiological evidence for multiple glycinergic inputs to neonatal rat sympathetic preganglionic neurons in vitro. *European Journal of Neuroscience* 9, 1711–1719.
74. Krupp, J., and Feltz, P. (1995). Excitatory postsynaptic currents and glutamate receptors in neonatal rat sympathetic preganglionic neurons in vitro. *Journal of Neurophysiology* 72(4), 1503–1512.
75. Lai, C. C., Wu, S. Y., Lin, H. H., and Dun, N. J. (1997). Excitatory action of pituitary adenylate cyclase activating polypeptide on rat sympathetic preganglionic neurons in vivo and in vitro. *Brain Research* 748, 189–194.
76. Laskey, W., and Polosa, C. (1988). Characteristics of the sympathetic preganglionic neuron and its synaptic input. *Progress in Neurobiology* 31, 47–84.
77. Lewis, D. I., and Coote, J. H. (1990). Excitation and inhibition of rat sympathetic preganglionic neurons by catecholamines. *Brain Research* 530, 229–234.
78. Lewis, D. I., and Coote, J. H. (1990). The influence of 5-hydroxytryptamine agonists and antagonists on identified sympathetic preganglionic neurons in the rat, in vivo. *British Journal of Pharmacology* 99, 667–672.
79. Lewis, D. I., and Coote, J. H. (1993). Angiotensin II in the spinal cord of the rat and its sympatho-excitatory effects. *Brain Research* 614, 1–9.
80. Lewis, D. I., Sermasi, E., and Coote, J. H. (1993). Excitatory and indirect actions of 5-hydroxytryptamine on sympathetic preganglionic neurones in the neonate rat spinal cord in vitro. *Brain Research* 610, 267–275.
81. Lind, R. W., Swanson, L. W., and Ganten, D. (1985). Organization of angiotensin II immunoreactive cells and fibers in the rat central nervous system. An immunohistochemical study. *Neuroendocrinology* 40, 2–24.
82. Llewellyn-Smith, I. J. (2009). Anatomy of synaptic circuits controlling the activity of sympathetic preganglionic neurons. *Journal of Chemical Neuroanatomy* 38, 231–239.
83. Llewellyn-Smith, I. J., Arnolda, L. F., Pilowsky, P. M., Chalmers, J. P., and Minson, J. B. (1998). GABA- and glutamate-immunoreactive synapses on sympathetic preganglionic neurons projecting to the superior cervical ganglion. *Journal of the Autonomic Nervous System* 71, 96–110.
84. Llewellyn-Smith, I. J., Cassam, A. K., Krenz, N. R., Krassioukov, A. V., and Weaver, L. C. (1997). Glutamate- and GABA-immunoreactive synapses on sympathetic preganglionic neurons caudal to a spinal cord transection in rats. *Neuroscience* 80, 1225–1235.
85. Llewellyn-Smith, I. J., DiCarlo, S. E., Collins, H. L., and Keast, J. R. (2005). Enkephalin-immunoreactive interneurons extensively innervate sympathetic preganglionic neurons regulating the pelvic viscera. *Journal of Comparative Neurology* 488, 278–289.
86. Llewellyn-Smith, I. J., Martin, C. L., Fenwick, N. M., DiCarlo, S. E., Lujan, H. L., and Schreihofer, A. M. (2007). VGLUT1 and VGLUT2 innervation in autonomic regions of intact and transected rat spinal cord. *Journal of Comparative Neurology* 503, 741–767.

87. Llewellyn-Smith, I. J., Martin, C. L., Marcus, J. N., Yanagisawa, M., Minson, J. B., and Scammell, T. E. (2003). Orexin-immunoreactive inputs to rat sympathetic preganglionic neurons. *Neuroscience Letters* 351, 115–119.
88. Llewellyn-Smith, I. J., Martin, C. L., Minson, J. B., Pilowsky, P. M., Arnolda, L. F., Basbaum, A. I., and Chalmers, J. P. (1997). Neurokinin-1 receptor-immunoreactive sympathetic preganglionic neurons: Target specificity and ultrastructure. *Neuroscience* 77, 1137–1149.
89. Llewellyn-Smith, I. J., Minson, J. B., Pilowsky, P. M., Arnolda, L. F., and Chalmers, J. P. (1995). The one hundred percent hypothesis: Glutamate or GABA in synapses on sympathetic preganglionic neurons. *Clinical and Experimental Hypertension* 17, 323–334.
90. Llewellyn-Smith, I. J., Phend, K. D., Minson, J. B., Pilowsky, P. M., and Chalmers, J. P. (1992). Glutamate-immunoreactive synapses on retrogradely labeled sympathetic preganglionic neurons in rat thoracic spinal cord. *Brain Research* 581, 67–80.
91. Llewellyn-Smith, I. J., Pilowsky, P., Minson, J. B., and Chalmers, J. (1995). Synapses on axons of sympathetic preganglionic neurons in rat and rabbit spinal cord. *Journal of Comparative Neurology* 354, 193–208.
92. Llewellyn-Smith, I. J., and Weaver, L. C. (2001). Changes in synaptic inputs to sympathetic preganglionic neurons after spinal cord injury. *Journal of Comparative Neurology* 435, 226–240.
93. Llewellyn-Smith, I. J., and Weaver, L. C. (2004). Interneuronal inputs to sympathetic preganglionic neurons: Evidence from transected spinal cord. In N. J. Dun, B. H. Machado, and P. M. Pilowsky (Eds.), *Neural Mechanisms of Cardiovascular Regulation*, pp. 265–283. Boston: Kluwer.
94. Llewellyn-Smith, I. J., Weaver, L. C., and Keast, J. R. (2006). Effects of spinal cord injury on synaptic inputs to sympathetic preganglionic neurons. *Progress in Brain Research* 152, 11–26.
95. Loewy, A. D., and McKeller, S. (1981). Serotonergic projections from the ventral medulla to the intermediolateral cell column in the rat. *Brain Research* 211, 146–152.
96. Madden, C. J., and Morrison, S. F. (2006). Serotonin potentiates sympathetic responses evoked by spinal NMDA. *Journal of Physiology* 577, 525–537.
97. Marina, N., Becker, D. L., and Gilbey, M. P. (2008). Immunohistochemical detection of connexin36 in sympathetic preganglionic and somatic motoneurons in the adult rat. *Autonomic Neuroscience* 139, 15–23.
98. Marina, N., Taheri, M., and Gilbey, M. P. (2006). Generation of a physiological sympathetic motor rhythm in the rat following spinal application of 5-HT. *Journal of Physiology* 571, 441–450.
99. Markham, J. A., and Vaughn, J. E. (1990). Ultrastructural analysis of choline acetyltransferase-immunoreactivite sympathetic preganglionic neurons and their dendritic bundles in rat thoracic spinal cord. *Synapse* 5, 299–312.
100. McNair, C. J., Baxter, G. J., Kerr, R., and Maxwell, D. J. (1998). Glutamate receptor subunits associated with rat sympathetic preganglionic neurons. *Neuroscience Letters* 256, 29–32.
101. Milner, T. A., Morrison, S. F., Abate, C., and Reis, D. J. (1988). Phenylethanolamine *N*-methyltransferase-containing terminals synapse directly on sympathetic preganglionic neurons in the rat. *Brain Research* 448, 205–222.
102. Minson, J., Pilowsky, P., Llewellyn-Smith, I., Kaneko, T., Kapoor, V., and Chalmers, J. (1991). Glutamate in spinally projecting neurons of the rostral ventral medulla. *Brain Research* 555, 326–331.
103. Minson, J. B., Arnolda, L. F., and Llewellyn-Smith, I. J. (2002). Neurochemistry of nerve fibers apposing sympathetic preganglionic neurons activated by sustained hypotension. *Journal of Comparative Neurology* 449, 307–318.
104. Minson, J. B., Llewellyn-Smith, I. J., and Arnolda, L. F. (2001). Neuropeptide Y mRNA expression in interneurons in rat spinal cord. *Autonomic Neuroscience* 93, 14–20.
105. Minson, J. B., Llewellyn-Smith, I. J., Pilowsky, P. M., and Chalmers, J. P. (1994). Bulbospinal neuropeptide Y-immunoreactive neurons in the rat comparison with adrenaline-synthesizing neurons. *Journal of the Autonomic Nervous System* 47, 233–243.
106. Miyazaki, T., Coote, J. H., and Dun, N. J. (1989). Excitatory and inhibitory effects of epinephrine on neonatal rat sympathetic preganglionic neurons in vitro. *Brain Research* 497, 108–116.
107. Morrison, S. F. (2001). Differential control of sympathetic outflow. *American Journal of Physiology. Regulatory, Integrative and Comparative Physiology* 281, R683–R698.
108. Morrison, S. F. (2003). Glutamate transmission in the rostral ventrolateral medullary sympathetic premotor pathway. *Cellular and Molecular Neurobiology* 23, 761–772.
109. Morrison, S. F., Callaway, J., Milner, T. A., and Reis, D. J. (1991). Rostral ventrolateral medulla: A source of the glutamatergic innervation of the sympathetic intermediolateral nucleus. *Brain Research* 562, 126–135.

110. Motawei, K., Pyner, S., Ranson, R. N., Kamel, M., and Coote, J. H. (1999). Terminals of paraventricular spinal neurones are closely associated with adrenal medullary sympathetic preganglionic neurones: Immunocytochemical evidence for vasopressin as a possible neurotransmitter in this pathway. *Experimental Brain Research* 126, 68–76.
111. Nakamura, K., Wu, S. X., Fujiyama, F., Okamoto, K., Hioki, H., and Kaneko, T. (2004). Independent inputs by VGLUT2- and VGLUT3-positive glutamatergic terminals onto rat sympathetic preganglionic neurons. *NeuroReport* 15, 431–436.
112. Nolan, M. F., and Logan, S. D. (1998). Metabotropic glutamate receptor-mediated excitation and inhibition of sympathetic preganglionic neurones. *Neuropharmacology* 37, 13–24.
113. Nolan, M. F., Logan, S. D., and Spanswick, D. (1999). Electrophysiological properties of electrical synapses between rat sympathetic preganglionic neurones in vitro. *Journal of Physiology* 519 Pt 3, 753–764.
114. Petras, J. M., and Cummings, J. F. (1972). Autonomic neurones in the spinal cord of the rhesus monkey. A correlation of the cytoarchitectonics and sympathectomy with fibre degeneration following dorsal rhizotomy. *Journal of Comparative Neurology* 146, 189–218.
115. Pickering, A. E., Spanswick, D., and Logan, S. D. (1994). 5-Hydroxytryptamine evokes depolarizations and membrane potential oscillations in rat sympathetic preganglionic neurones. *Journal of Physiology* 480, 109–121.
116. Pilowsky, P., Llewellyn-Smith, I. J., Arnolda, L., Minson, J., and Chalmers, J. (1994). Intracellular recording from sympathetic preganglionic neurons in cat lumbar spinal cord. *Brain Research* 656, 319–328.
117. Pilowsky, P., Llewellyn-Smith, I. J., Lipski, J., and Chalmers, J. (1992). Substance P immunoreactive boutons form synapses with feline sympathetic preganglionic neurons. *Journal of Comparative Neurology* 320, 121–135.
118. Polosa, C., Yoshimura, M., and Nishi, S. (1988). Electrophysiological properties of sympathetic preganglionic neurons. *Annual Review of Physiology* 50, 541–551.
119. Pu, S., Dube, M. G., Edwards, T. G., Kalra, S. P., and Kalra, P. S. (1999). Disruption of neural signaling within the hypothalamic ventromedial nucleus upregulates galanin gene expression in association with hyperphagia: An *in situ* hybridization analysis. *Molecular Brain Research* 64, 85–91.
120. Pyner, S. (2009). Neurochemistry of the paraventricular nucleus of the hypothalamus: Implications for cardiovascular regulation. *Journal of Chemical Neuroanatomy* 38, 197–208.
121. Rethelyi, M. (1972). Cell and neuropil architecture of the intermediolateral (sympathetic) nucleus of cat spinal cord. *Brain Research* 46, 203–213.
122. Richardson, R. J., Grkovic, I., Allen, A. M., and Anderson, C. R. (2006). Separate neurochemical classes of sympathetic postganglionic neurons project to the left ventricle of the rat heart. *Cell and Tissue Research* 324, 9–16.
123. Romagnano, M. A., Braiman, J., Loomis, M., and Hamill, R. W. (1987). Enkephalin fibers in autonomic nuclear regions: Intraspinal vs. *supraspinal* origin. *Journal of Comparative Neurology* 266, 319–331.
124. Sah, P., and McLachlan, E. M. (1995). Membrane properties and synaptic potentials of sympathetic preganglionic neurons studied in horizontal spinal cord slices *in vitro*. *Journal of the Autonomic Nervous System* 53, 1–14.
125. Samano, C., Zetina, M. E., Cifuentes, F., and Morales, M. A. (2009). Segregation of met-enkephalin from vesicular acetylcholine transporter and choline acetyltransferase in sympathetic preganglionic varicosities mostly lacking synaptophysin and synaptotagmin. *Neuroscience* 163, 180–189.
126. Sasek, C. A., Wessendorf, M. W., and Helke, C. J. (1990). Evidence for coexistence of thyrotropin-releasing hormone, substance P and serotonin in ventral medullary neurons that project to the intermediolateral cell column in the rat. *Neuroscience* 35, 105–119.
127. Schafer, M. K., Eiden, L. E., and Weihe, E. (1998). Cholinergic neurons and terminal fields revealed by immunohistochemistry for the vesicular acetylcholine transporter. I. Central nervous system. *Neuroscience* 84, 331–359.
128. Sermasi, E., and Coote, J. H. (1994). Oxytocin acts at V1 receptors to excite sympathetic preganglionic neurones in neonate rat spinal cord in vitro. *Brain Research* 647, 323–332.
129. Sevigny, C. P., Bassi, J., Teschemacher, A. G., Kim, K. S., Williams, D. A., Anderson, C. R., and Allen, A. M. (2008). C1 neurons in the rat rostral ventrolateral medulla differentially express vesicular monoamine transporter 2 in soma and axonal compartments. *European Journal of Neuroscience* 28, 1536–1544.
130. Shafton, A. D., Oldfield, B. J., and McAllen, R. M. (1992). CRF-like immunoreactivity selectively labels preganglionic sudomotor neurons in cat. *Brain Research* 599, 253–260.

131. Shen, E., Wu, S. Y., and Dun, N. J. (1994). Spontaneous and transmitter-induced rhythmic activity in neonatal rat sympathetic preganglionic neurons in vitro. *Journal of Neurophysiology* 71(3), 1197–1205.
132. Spanswick, D., and Logan, S. D. (1990). Sympathetic preganglionic neurones in neonatal rat spinal cord in vitro: Electrophysiological characteristics and the effects of selective excitatory amino acid receptor agonists. *Brain Research* 525, 181–188.
133. Spanswick, D., Pickering, A. E., Gibson, I. C., and Logan, S. D. (1994). Inhibition of sympathetic preganglionic neurons by spinal glycinergic interneurons. *Neuroscience* 62, 205–216.
134. Spanswick, D., Pickering, A. E., Gibson, I. C., and Logan, S. D. (1995). Excitation of sympathetic preganglionic neurons via metabotropic excitatory amino acid receptors. *Neuroscience* 68, 1247–1261.
135. Spanswick, D., Renaud, L. P., and Logan, S. D. (1998). Bilaterally evoked monosynaptic EPSPs, NMDA receptors and potentiation in rat sympathetic preganglionic neurones in vitro. *Journal of Physiology* 509, 195–209.
136. Spike, R. C., Todd, A. J., and Johnston, H. M. (1993). Coexistence of NADPH diaphorase with GABA, glycine, and acetylcholine in rat spinal cord. *Journal of Comparative Neurology* 335, 320–333.
137. Stocker, S. D., Simmons, J. R., Stornetta, R. L., Toney, G. M., and Guyenet, P. G. (2006). Water deprivation activates a glutamatergic projection from the hypothalamic paraventricular nucleus to the rostral ventrolateral medulla. *Journal of Comparative Neurology* 494, 673–685.
138. Stornetta, R. L., Akey, P. J., and Guyenet, P. G. (1999). Location and electrophysiological characterization of rostral medullary adrenergic neurons that contain neuropeptide Y mRNA in rat medulla. *Journal of Comparative Neurology* 415, 482–500.
139. Stornetta, R. L., McQuiston, T. J., and Guyenet, P. G. (2004). GABAergic and glycinergic presympathetic neurons of rat medulla oblongata identified by retrograde transport of pseudorabies virus and *in situ* hybridization. *Journal of Comparative Neurology* 479, 257–270.
140. Stornetta, R. L., Rosin, D. L., Simmons, J. R., McQuiston, T. J., Vujovic, N., Weston, M. C., and Guyenet, P. G. (2005). Coexpression of vesicular glutamate transporter-3 and gamma-aminobutyric acidergic markers in rat rostral medullary raphé and intermediolateral cell column. *Journal of Comparative Neurology* 492, 477–494.
141. Stornetta, R. L., Sevigny, C. P., Schreihofer, A. M., Rosin, D. L., and Guyenet, P. G. (2002). Vesicular glutamate transporter DNPI/VGLUT2 is expressed by both C1 adrenergic and nonaminergic presympathetic vasomotor neurons of the rat medulla. *Journal of Comparative Neurology* 444, 207–220.
142. Strack, A. M., Sawyer, W. B., Marubio, L. M., and Loewy, A. D. (1988). Spinal origin of sympathetic preganglionic neurons in the rat. *Brain Research* 455, 187–191.
143. Tang, X., Neckel, N. D., and Schramm, L. P. (2003). Locations and morphologies of sympathetically correlated neurons in the T(10) spinal segment of the rat. *Brain Research* 976, 185–193.
144. Tang, X., Neckel, N. D., and Schramm, L. P. (2004). Spinal interneurons infected by renal injection of pseudorabies virus in the rat. *Brain Research* 1004, 1–7.
145. van Den Pol, A. N. (1999). Hypothalamic hypocretin (orexin): Robust innervation of the spinal cord. *Journal of Neuroscience* 19, 3171–3182.
146. van den Top, M., Nolan, M. F., Lee, K., Richardson, P. J., Buijs, R. M., Davies, C. H., and Spanswick, D. (2003). Orexins induce increased excitability and synchronisation of rat sympathetic preganglionic neurones. *Journal of Physiology* 549, 809–821.
147. Vera, P. L., Holets, V. R., and Miller, K. E. (1990). Ultrastructural evidence of synaptic contacts between substance P-, enkephalin-, and serotonin-immunoreactive terminals and retrogradely labeled sympathetic preganglionic neurons in the rat: A study using a double-peroxidase procedure. *Synapse* 6, 221–229.
148. Wang, L., Spary, E., Deuchars, J., and Deuchars, S. A. (2008). Tonic GABAergic inhibition of sympathetic preganglionic neurons: A novel substrate for sympathetic control. *Journal of Neuroscience* 28, 12445–12452.
149. Wilson, J. M., Coderre, E., Renaud, L. P., and Spanswick, D. (2002). Active and passive membrane properties of rat sympathetic preganglionic neurones innervating the adrenal medulla. *Journal of Physiology* 545, 945–960.
150. Wu, S. Y., and Dun, N. J. (1992). Presynaptic $GABA_B$ receptor activation attenuates synaptic transmission to rat sympathetic preganglionic neurons in vitro. *Brain Research* 572, 94–102.
151. Wu, S. Y., and Dun, N. J. (1993). Excitatory amino acids depress synaptic currents in neonate rat sympathetic preganglionic neurons. *Journal of Neurophysiology* 69, 2030–2038.
152. Wu, S. Y., and Dun, N. J. (1997). Potentiation of NMDA currents by pituitary adenylate cyclase

activating polypeptide in neonatal rat sympathetic preganglionic neurons. *Journal of Neurophysiology* 78, 1175–1179.

153. Wu, S. Y., Miyazaki, T., and Dun, N. J. (1995). Glycine induces two distinct membrane currents in neonatal rat sympathetic preganglionic neurones in vitro. *Journal of Physiology* 483, 385–396.
154. Yamamoto, K., Senba, E., Matsunaga, T., and Tohyama, M. (1989). Calcitonin gene-related peptide containing sympathetic preganglionic and sensory neurons projecting to the superior cervical ganglion of the rat. *Brain Research* 487, 158–164.
155. Zagon, A., and Smith, A. D. (1993). Monosynaptic projections from the rostral ventrolateral medulla oblongata to identified sympathetic preganglionic neurons. *Neuroscience* 54, 729–743.
156. Zhou, S.-Y., and Gilbey, M. P. (1992). Respiratory-regulated activity of lower thoracic and upper sympathetic preganglionic neurones in the rat. *Journal of Physiology* 451, 631–642.

# 7

# Parasympathetic Preganglionic Neurons

DAVID JORDAN

Parasympathetic preganglionic neurons innervate most of the tissues of the body (excluding skeletal muscle and adipose tissue) and are therefore essential for maintaining homoeostasis. These neurons are involved in controlling functions as diverse as cardiac rate, changes in gut motility, and micturition. In concert with sympathetic outflows, they respond to environmental as well as internal physiological changes. Most of the literature considers each parasympathetic outflow in isolation, and the sympathetic and parasympathetic outflows individually. However, there is accumulating evidence that these outflows are regulated in highly complex and organized manners by regions of the central nervous system (CNS) so that the overall autonomic output is appropriate for the response required at any particular time. There is also evidence of parallel systems mediating autonomic behavioral and endocrine responses. As the source of all parasympathetic outflow, parasympathetic preganglionic neurons are important sites of integration and modulation. Each preganglionic neuron synapses with its post-ganglionic neuronal counterpart in the relevant peripheral ganglion. There is evidence for some integration within ganglia, but most of the integration and organization of parasympathetic outflow occurs within the CNS, at the level of the parasympathetic preganglionic neurons themselves, or at antecedent CNS sites. This chapter will describe the properties of preganglionic neurons of the different parasympathetic outflows, including their location, anatomical organization, synaptic inputs, and properties. Since much more detailed information is available about vagal preganglionic neurons than about those of the other parasympathetic outflows, this chapter will focus on these neurons and highlight the aspects of their organization that are likely to be common to other parasympathetic outflows. A chapter in the first edition of this book was devoted to vagal preganglionic neurons[74]. Consequently, only the areas that have shown major developments since 1990 will be dealt with in detail here.

## VAGAL PREGANGLIONIC NEURONS

Vagal preganglionic neurons provide the most extensive parasympathetic outflow. They innervate many structures, including the upper and lower airways, heart, liver, pancreas, gall bladder, and the entire gastrointestinal tract from the esophagus to the transverse colon. In higher mammals, vagal preganglionic neurons are located in the medulla oblongata in two distinct nuclei, the dorsal motor nucleus of the vagus (dorsal vagal nucleus [DVN]) and the nucleus ambiguus. There are also preganglionic neurons scattered in the reticular formation between these two nuclei. Vagal preganglionic neurons in the nucleus ambiguus have small myelinated (B fiber) axons, whilst those in the DVN have mainly unmyelinated (C fiber) axons. The location of vagal preganglionic neurons innervating the different viscera has been documented by transport of retrograde tracers from injections into branches of the vagus nerve or into discrete sites in vagally innervated tissues. It is now clear that in both nuclei there is a somatotopic organization of neurons that is target organ–dependent.

The nucleus ambiguus is a diffuse structure extending rostrally in a column from the caudal medulla to the facial nucleus. The organization of the nucleus ambiguus is still not well defined. The current nomenclature is based on both morphological differences between the subnuclear groups and target-based somatotopy[15]. The dorsal division, comprising the compact, semi-compact, and loose formations, contains neurons innervating the pharynx, larynx, upper airway accessory muscles, and striated muscles of the esophagus and upper esophageal sphincter. The more ventral and diffuse external formation is the location of vagal preganglionic neurons innervating the heart and airways. Neurons innervating the heart form a column at obex level, whilst those innervating lungs and airways occur in two separate clusters rostral and caudal to the cardiac projecting neurons[126].

Most neurons in the DVN are cholinergic preganglionic neurons, but the DVN also contains interneurons (possibly GABAergic inhibitory interneurons) and neurons that project to other central sites. The nucleus ambiguus contains few, if any, vagal preganglionic neurons projecting to subdiaphragmatic structures. Thus, the DVN is the sole location of these neuronal cell bodies, which innervate the gastrointestinal tract from the stomach as far caudal as the transverse colon, the liver, and the pancreas. Thoracic viscera (heart, airways, lungs, and esophagus) also receive innervation from DVN neurons. However, in most species the nucleus ambiguus provides the bulk of the parasympathetic innervation to these organs. Compared to the nucleus ambiguus, anatomical differences between regions of the DVN are less clear-cut. Nevertheless, the DVN has an obvious viscerotopic organization[41,42]. Neurons projecting to the thorax are found laterally in caudal DVN. Those innervating subdiaphragmatic structures are found in parallel longitudinal columns with gastric-innervating neurons more medially and intestinal-projecting neurons more laterally, especially in the rostral DVN[74]. Even for neurons innervating different regions within an organ, such as the stomach, there is topography in the DVN. This organization may relate to function (e.g., gastric acid secretion versus motility) or may simply reflect the embryological development of the gut[41]. Indeed, the presence of two separate vagal preganglionic nuclei has been ascribed to embryology/phylogeny. In lower vertebrates, the DVN is the primary site of vagal preganglionic neurons, and a ventrolateral nucleus only becomes prominent with the development of air breathing[126]. This probably reflects the changing function of the branchial innervation from moving water through the gills to controlling air movements in and out of the lungs.

## Gastro-Intestinal Innervation (See also Chapters 14 And 15)

The abdominal vagus splits into five major branches in the rat. These are the anterior and posterior gastric and coeliac branches, and a hepatic branch. Each originates from a separate longitudinal column in the DVN. Gastric branches originate in longitudinal columns that span the length of the DVN and fill the medial two-thirds of the nucleus. The lateral third comprises a column supplying the coeliac branches. The hepatic branch arises from neurons interspersed with the gastric neurons in the left DVN[41]. Injection of retrograde tracers into individual viscera has essentially confirmed this arrangement (e.g., [5,108]) (Figure 7–1). The gastric branches regulate gastric and duodenal motility and gastric acid secretion. The coeliac branches regulate motility in the small intestine and colon. Axons in the gastric and hepatic branches innervate the pancreas. Both insulin and glucagon are released by stimulation of either of these branches, but not the coeliac branches[13]; and the rise in insulin following ingestion of food occurs only with intact hepatic or gastric branches[14]. Consistent with these data, vagal preganglionic neurons innervating the pancreas occur in both rostral and caudal DVN, predominantly medially[22,108,121]. At least some vagal preganglionic neurons project to both stomach and pancreas[116].

A separate rostrocaudal functional topography is superimposed upon the organ-based mediolateral topography in the DVN. The DVN gives rise to parallel excitatory and inhibitory pathways to gastrointestinal muscles and the lower esophageal sphincter. Excitatory pathways originate in rostral areas; and inhibitory pathways, caudal to obex. These two pathways innervate neurochemically distinct excitatory and inhibitory post-ganglionic neurons[23] (Figure 7–2). These two functionally opposed outflows allow for discrete and independent reflex control of sphincter and motility. This occurs during swallowing, where activating vagal preganglionic neurons evokes the primary peristaltic response, and non-adrenergic, non-cholinergic nerves mediate the intrinsic peristaltic response. The inhibitory innervation of the stomach is important for fundic relaxation to accommodate food. Excitation in the corpus/antrum and pyloric sphincter is important for increased motility, which leads to more effective food breakdown. Pyloric sphincter relaxation is required for gastric emptying. The gall bladder and sphincter of Oddi also have a dual innervation, but gastric secretion appears to be under only excitatory control.

### *Inputs to the Dorsal Vagal Nucleus*

The somatotopic organization in the vagal motor nuclei is even expressed in the distribution of sensory afferents in the nucleus of the solitary tract (NTS; see

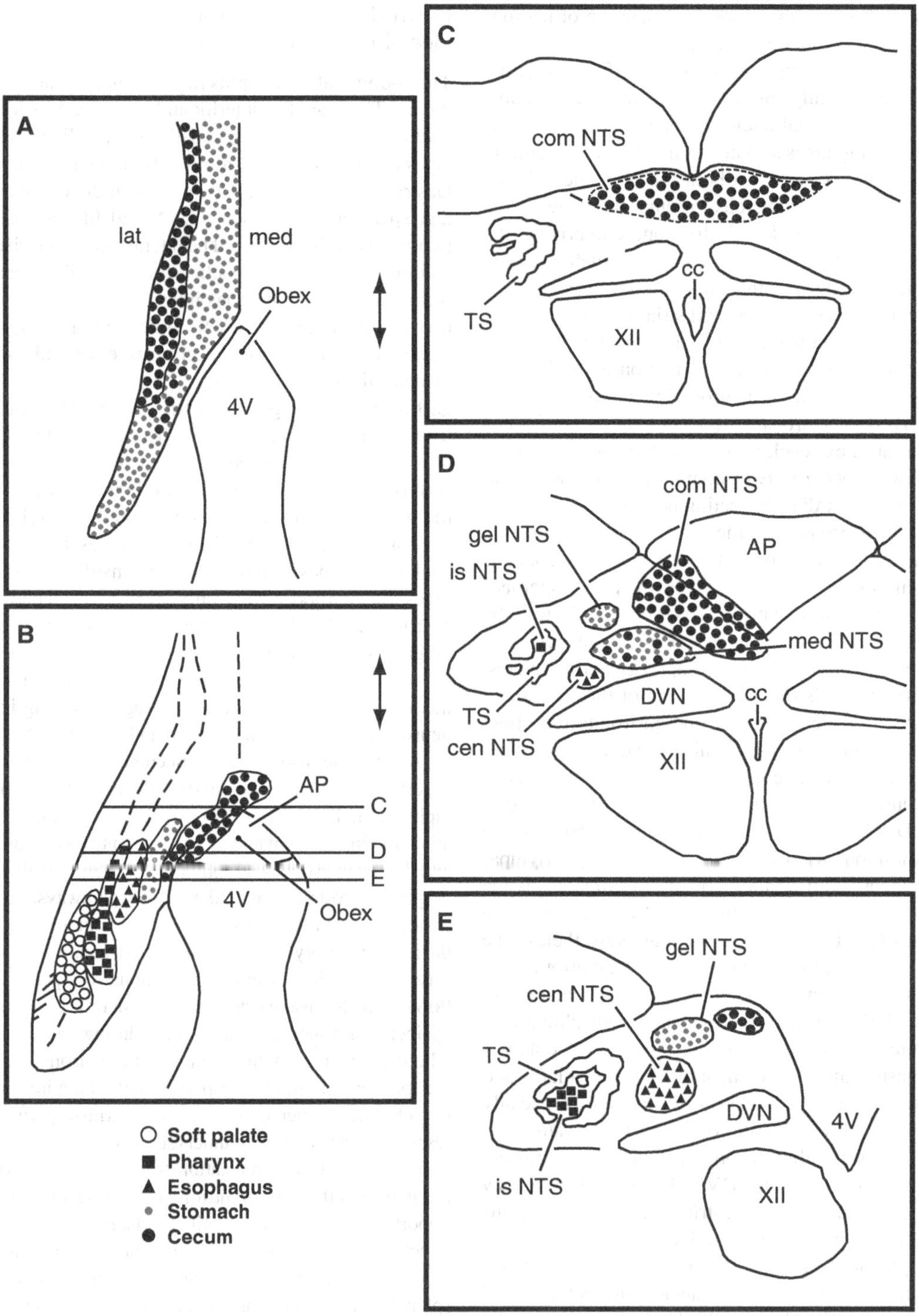


Figure 7–1 Viscerotopic organization in the dorsal vagal nucleus and nucleus of the solitary tract. Schematic representations in the horizontal plane of the DVN (*A*) and NTS (*B*). In *A:* cecal and gastric preganglionic neurons occupy lateral and medial longitudinal columns, respectively, within the DVN. Duodenal preganglionic neurons occupy the same column as gastric preganglionic neurons; those innervating the jejunum, ileum and ascending colon are found in the lateral columns with the cecal preganglionic neurons. *B–E* show that afferent terminals from different abdominal viscera project to different subnuclei within the NTS. Reproduced from Altschuler et al. (1991)[5], with permission.

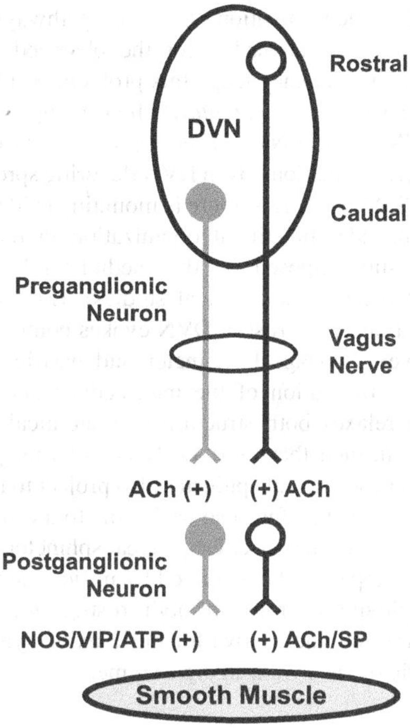


Figure 7–2 Parallel functional organization within the dorsal vagal nucleus. Vagal preganglionic neurons innervating the gut form two parallel rostrocaudal pathways in the DVN. This organization is superimposed on the viscerotopic organization shown in Figure 7–1. The excitatory and inhibitory pathways originate in the rostral and caudal DVN, respectively. Both sets of preganglionic neurons and the excitatory post-ganglionic neurons are cholinergic whilst the inhibitory post-ganglionic neurons may contain a variety of inhibitory neurotransmitters. Reproduced from Chang et al. (2003)[23], with permission.

Chapter 2). This longitudinal bilateral nucleus spans the length of the dorsal medulla and is the major termination site for visceral afferents running in the vagus and glossopharyngeal nerves. It also receives ascending inputs from spinal afferents and descending control from sites in the midbrain, hypothalamus, and forebrain, including the prefrontal cortex (see Chapter 11). Thus, the NTS is ideally positioned for integration of sensory input. Afferent terminals overlap to some extent, providing the basis for integration, but there is a general topography. Gastric afferents project to the medial subnucleus, esophageal afferents to the central subnucleus, and intestinal afferents to the commissural region[4,5] (Figure 7–1). Cardiovascular and respiratory afferents in the NTS have a similar organization[126]. This topography persists in NTS projection sites. For example, neurons in the central subnucleus project widely through the DVN and to the compact region of nucleus ambiguus, where esophageal and pharyngeal motor neurons are found. This pathway is thought to be involved in the complex motor act of swallowing.

Throughout the DVN, neurons have predominantly horizontal dendrites that stay within their own longitudinal columns, suggesting preservation of function within the columnar organization[42]. However, some dendrites do project into neighboring columns and even into the adjacent NTS[42]. For example, stomach- or pancreas-projecting DVN neurons have some dendrites that spread dorsally into the medial and gelatinosus NTS subnuclei[107,108]. This arrangement suggests that vagal afferents could synapse on preganglionic neurons in the DVN, providing the substrate for a monosynaptic vago-vagal reflex[102]. Although a few sensory afferents from the stomach synapse on gastric preganglionic dendrites in the DVN[107], a much larger monosynaptic input occurs on dendrites of gastric preganglionic neurons in the gelatinosus NTS subnucleus (Figure 7–3). Whether specific functional groups of afferent and/or efferent neurons are involved in this reflex arc is unclear; but retrograde tracing from the entire cervical vagus did not extend the areas of interaction, suggesting that this monosynaptic vago-vagal pathway was specific to the gastric reflex. Neurons responding to duodenal distension also have dendrites spreading into the NTS, including the medial and subpostremal regions and the gelatinosus subnucleus. Dendrites that extend into the contralateral DVN are a feature of both neurons that respond to duodenal distension and pancreas-projecting neurons[108].

Although reflex pathways are present in the brainstem, integrated patterns of response are organized at higher levels in the midbrain and forebrain. Activation of neurons in the lateral hypothalamus, which project to both the NTS and DVN to regulate food intake, modifies the activity of DVN neurons responsive to gastrointestinal distension[55]. Viral tracing has revealed brain regions involved in controlling specific groups of vagal preganglionic neurons. Pancreatic preganglionic neurons receive inputs from a range of hypothalamic nuclei, including nuclei in the dorsomedial and lateral hypothalamus, the paraventricular nucleus (PVN), and the suprachiasmatic nucleus. These hypothalamic neurons contain either oxytocin, orexin, or melanin-concentrating hormone[22]. Pancreatic preganglionic neurons receive monoamine inputs from a variety of cell groups. There is noradrenergic input from A5 and some from A1 and A2, and adrenergic input from C1, C2, and C3. Adrenergic axons surround both gastric and pancreatic preganglionic neurons and make synaptic contact[116]. Surprisingly, most 5-HT inputs came from the gigantocellular reticular nucleus with fewer from brainstem raphé nuclei[73].

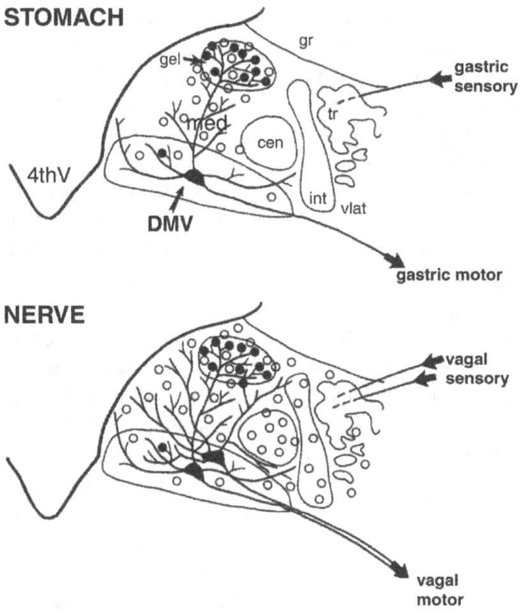


Figure 7–3 Organization of gastric vago-vagal reflexes within the dorsal vagal complex. *Top*, The distribution of vagal sensory and motor labeling in the DVN and NTS after injections of cholera toxin-horseradish peroxidase into the stomach. Gastric preganglionic neurons have dendrites that spread outside the DVN into the medial and gelatinosus subnuclei of the NTS. Gastric afferents terminate in the medial and gelatinosus subnuclei. Within the gelatinosus subnucleus, some gastric afferents make synapses with dendrites of gastric preganglionic neurons (*black circles*). *Open circles* show gastric afferent terminals that are not in contact with but may be adjacent to preganglionic dendrites. *Bottom,* After injections into the vagus that label a larger afferent field and more preganglionic neurons, the distribution of vago-vagal contacts does not differ from that seen after stomach injections. cen, subnucleus centralis; gel, subnucleus gelatinosus; int, intermediate subnucleus; med, medial subnucleus; tr, solitary tract; 4$^{th}$ V: fourth ventricle. Reproduced from Rinaman et al. (1989)[107,108], with permission.

For more information about autonomic processing in the NTS, see Chapter 2.

### *Functional Studies*

Functional studies of the role of the DVN have been complicated by its proximity to the NTS. Results from electrical and chemical stimulation must be interpreted carefully, since activation of sensory pathways in the NTS may be responsible for the observed effects. Many authors acknowledge this problem by referring to the *dorsal vagal complex*, which comprises both the DVN and the NTS. This is probably wise when considering function, given DVN dendritic spread into the NTS. Nevertheless, there is mounting evidence for a rostrocaudal functional organization in the DVN that is superimposed on the mediolateral viscerotopy revealed by anatomical studies[23] (Figure 7–2). Stimulation of the rostral DVN evokes contraction of the lower esophageal sphincter and gastric fundus, whereas stimulation of the intermediate and caudal regions relaxes both structures[1]. Anatomical studies have confirmed that most DVN neurons innervating the lower esophageal sphincter also project to the gastric fundus, with a few also projecting to the antrum[53]. Relaxations of the lower esophageal sphincter and the stomach appear to be mediated by nitric oxide. Vagal preganglionic neurons in both rostral and caudal DVN are immunoreactive for nitric oxide synthase[69], the nitric oxide–synthesizing enzyme.

## Intrathoracic Innervation

Preganglionic neurons projecting to intrathoracic structures are found in both the DVN and nucleus ambiguus. Vagal efferents innervating the heart slow the heart rate and cardiac electrical conduction and probably reduce the strength of contraction and cause vasodilatation. Those innervating the airways cause contraction of airway smooth muscles and mucus secretion. Recent reviews have discussed the organization of afferent and efferent neurons mediating ongoing and reflex control of the airways[59] (see also Chapter 13) and heart[61,126].

Early electrical stimulation studies produced contradictory evidence about the location of cardiac vagal preganglionic neurons, but it is now clear that they occur in the DVN, the nucleus ambiguus, and the reticular formation between them. Cardiac vagal preganglionic neurons in these locations have different biophysical, synaptic, and functional properties. Considerable information is available about DVN neurons, but much less is known about cardiomotor neurons in the nucleus ambiguus. DVN neurons projecting to the heart or cardiac vagal branches are in a lateral column spanning the obex level. In the nucleus ambiguus, they are mainly located ventrolaterally in the external formation[28,120] (Figure 7–4). In mammals, the nucleus ambiguus contains the majority of cardiomotor neurons, but the relative importance of the two nuclei varies between vertebrate groups[126]. Cardiac vagal preganglionic neurons in the lateral DVN have many mediolaterally oriented dendrites that do not extend into the NTS[28]. The dendritic arbors of these cardiac vagal preganglionic neurons are often intertwined. This organization may be responsible for dye-coupling between nucleus ambiguus neurons[71] and would be a mechanism for synchronizing control of the heartbeat. The total number of cardiac vagal preganglionic neurons is relatively small, and it has been argued that chemically activating a single cardiac vagal preganglionic neuron can slow the heart[87]. However, an alternate explanation would be that, after activation of one neuron, activity could spread through connections between dendrites. Additionally, cardiac vagal preganglionic axons diverge extensively in cardiac ganglia. Tracer injections into the nucleus ambiguus or DVN anterogradely label terminals around post-ganglionic neurons in all cardiac ganglia[25]. Single preganglionic axons appose on average about 30 post-ganglionic neurons, about three times more neurons than DVN axons. Interestingly, axons originating from the nucleus ambiguus and DVN target different populations of post-ganglionic neurons in the same ganglion[26], consistent with different cardiac functions for preganglionic neurons.

Little is known about synaptic inputs specifically to cardiomotor neurons. Viral tracing from the heart muscle or cardiac ganglia labels interneurons in the

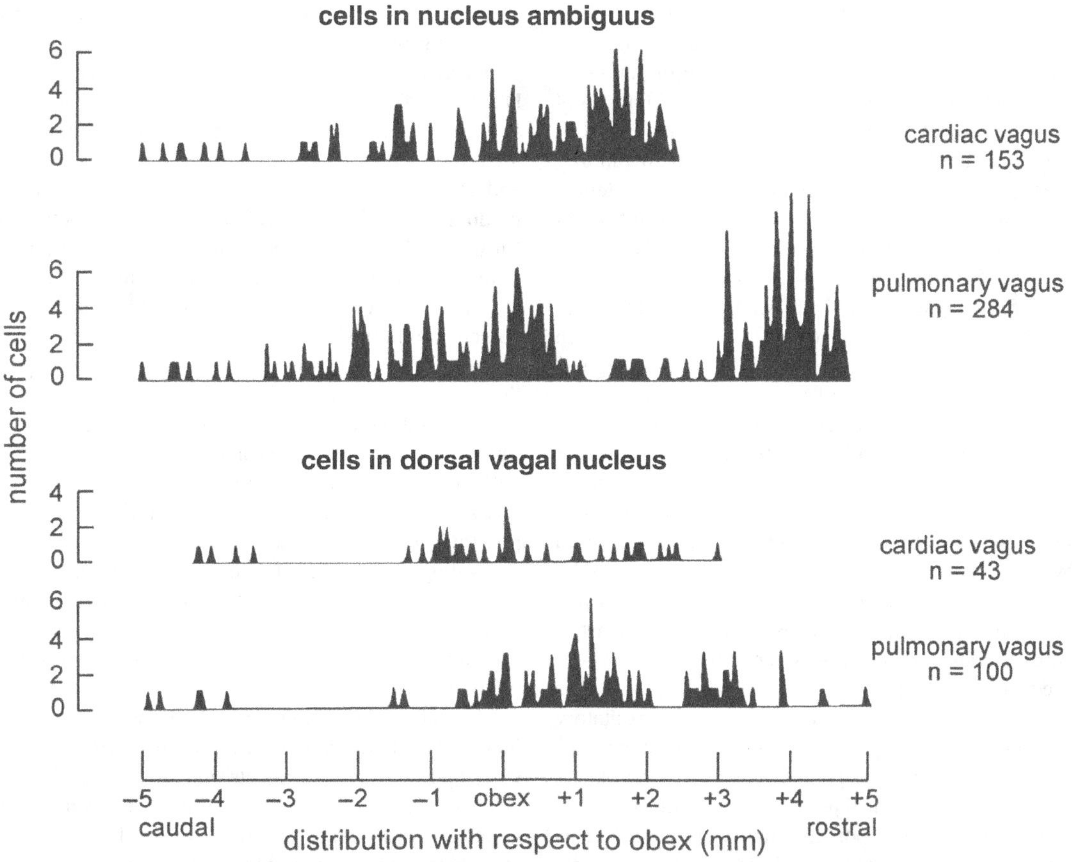


Figure 7–4 Rostrocaudal distribution of cardiac and pulmonary vagal preganglionic neurons in cat. Histograms of the number of labeled preganglionic neurons at each rostrocaudal level in the dorsal vagal nucleus and nucleus ambiguus after application of horseradish peroxidase to the cardiac or pulmonary branches of the vagus nerve. In the DVN, cardiac and pulmonary preganglionic neurons are found over a similar rostrocaudal extent around obex level. In the nucleus ambiguus, cardiac preganglionic neurons form a column spanning obex level. Pulmonary preganglionic neurons form two groups rostral and caudal to the cardiac preganglionic neurons. Reproduced from Taylor et al. (1999)[126], with permission.

nucleus ambiguus and neurons in medial and lateral NTS, raphé pallidus and obscurus, the parapyramidal nucleus, A5, locus coeruleus, and PVN[120]. In the nucleus ambiguus and DVN, GABA-immunoreactive synapses occur on somata and dendrites of cardiac vagal preganglionic neurons[75]. In the nucleus ambiguus, 5-HT immunoreactive terminals make close contact with dendrites of cardiac vagal preganglionic neurons[54]. In the DVN, a dense network of 5-HT axons envelops vagal preganglionic neurons, but whether these axons make synapses is unknown. Application of 5-HT or its selective receptor ligands can markedly modulate reflex-evoked changes in heart rate[61], and depletion of 5-HT attenuates baroreceptor reflexes[65]. Substance P-immunoreactive terminals make synaptic contact with chronotropic[85] but not dromotropic[84] cardiac vagal preganglionic neurons in the nucleus ambiguus. Oxytocin-immunoreactive axons are present in the DVN[49], and they closely appose the dendrites of vagal preganglionic neurons[104]. These inputs probably derive from parvocellular PVN neurons, since oxytocin-containing PVN neurons project to the DVN and/or spinal cord[113]. Vagal preganglionic neurons with oxytocin binding sites lie mainly in the anterior and mid-DVN[39]. Hence, these inputs may be more important in gastrointestinal than cardiac function, although there is functional evidence for a role in both (see below).

Cardiac vagal preganglionic neurons in the DVN and nucleus ambiguus are clearly different in function. In anesthetized animals, neurons in the nucleus ambiguus, which form the bulk of cardiac vagal preganglionic neurons, have small myelinated axons and little, if any, ongoing activity. This lack of activity is one reason for the paucity of studies on these neurons *in vivo*. When induced to fire, cardiac vagal preganglionic neurons show activity with a pulse-related component imposed by excitatory input from arterial baroreceptors[86]. Activity is also modulated in phase with ventilation, and this modulation is greatest during expiration[45,87]. This respiratory modulation is imposed partly by inspiratory-related inhibition, probably via muscarinic receptors (Figure 7–5). The neurons may also receive excitatory input during post-inspiration[45]. Some laryngeal neurons in the nucleus ambiguus fire during post-inspiration and synapse on cardiac vagal preganglionic neurons, so they may be one source of post-inspiratory excitation[91]. This circuit could explain the central component of respiratory sinus arrhythmia, where heart rate increases during each inspiration. Moreover, many reflex stimuli that influence the heart are more effective during the expiratory phase or when inspiration is suppressed.

The other group of vagal preganglionic neurons in the nucleus ambiguus innervates the airways and is responsible for bronchoconstriction and mucous secretion in a variety of airway reflexes. These neurons also have small myelinated axons and activity and firing patterns distinct from cardiac vagal preganglionic neurons. In anesthetized animals, airway preganglionic neurons have higher ongoing activity that is unaffected by arterial baroreceptors. They also have respiratory-related activity that is greatest during inspiration; i.e., out of phase with the cardiac vagal preganglionic neurons. Cardiac preganglionic neurons are located in the external nucleus ambiguus around obex level, and airway neurons lie rostral and caudal to the cardiac neurons[126] (Figure 7–4). This distribution mirrors that of neurons in the ventral respiratory group. A group of inspiratory-firing neurons occur around obex, like cardiac vagal preganglionic neurons. Expiratory neurons lie caudal and rostral to the inspiratory neurons, like airway preganglionic neurons. This organization may reflect a linkage between autonomic and respiratory regulatory mechanisms and control by common groups of neurons[106].

Heart-projecting preganglionic neurons in the DVN have features distinct from those in the nucleus ambiguus. They have unmyelinated axons, they do not receive baroreceptor or chemoreceptor inputs, and their ongoing firing shows no respiratory modulation[40,58]. The only reflex stimulus that activates cardiac DVN neurons powerfully is stimulation of unmyelinated pulmonary sensory afferents[58], which also activates cardiac preganglionic neurons in the nucleus ambiguus[135]. Myelinated vagal efferent fibers powerfully slow heart rate, consistent with the properties of cardiac vagal preganglionic neurons in the nucleus ambiguus. However, selective stimulation of ***un***myelinated vagal fibers also slows the heart, but with a slower onset and different pharmacology to that seen following stimulation of myelinated fibers[57], possibly due to different ganglionic connections[26]. Activating unmyelinated fibers also slows electrical conduction between the atria and ventricles and reduces cardiac contractility[43]. The fibers responsible for vagally mediated changes in coronary flow are unknown.

Arterial baroreceptors provide a major excitatory input to vagal preganglionic neurons involved in cardiac slowing. Baroreceptor afferents synapse on second-order neurons in the dorsomedial NTS. Other sensory afferents affecting heart rate, including those from arterial chemoreceptors and upper and lower airway receptors, also terminate in the NTS. Their terminals show a degree of functional topography but also some overlap[59]. The ongoing level of vagal tone derives from activity in these afferents as well as inputs from other CNS regions (Figure 7–5). At least some descending input is inhibitory since decerebration or lesions of the hypothalamus cause vagally mediated falls in heart rate. These inhibitory

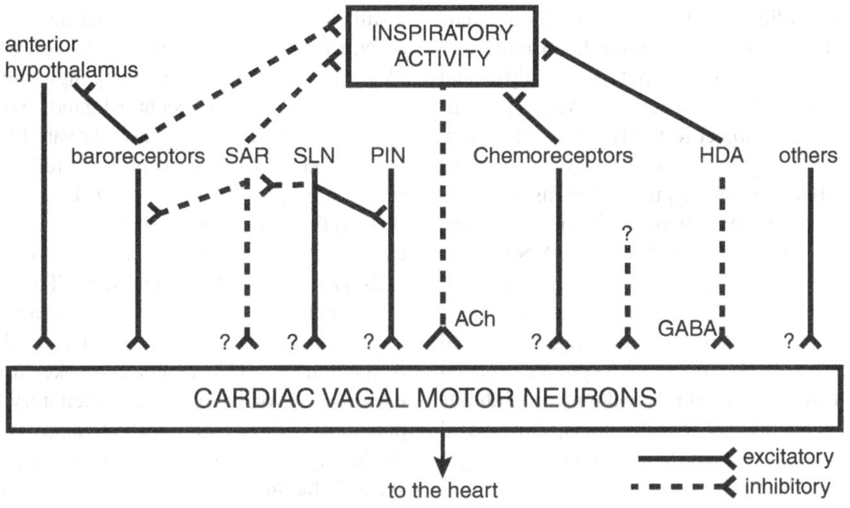


Figure 7–5 Possible mechanisms that interact at the level of cardiac preganglionic neurons. Cardiac preganglionic neurons are the final integrative site within the CNS for inputs regulating heart rate. Excitatory mechanisms are shown as solid lines, inhibitory mechanisms as dotted lines. Each line indicates a pathway of unknown synaptic complexity, not an individual neuron. GABA, γ-amino-butyric acid; HDA, hypothalamic defense area; PIN, subpopulation of post-inspiratory neurons; SAR, slowly adapting lung stretch receptor afferents; SLN, superior laryngeal nerve afferents;?, postulated pathways. Reproduced from Taylor et al. (1999)[126], with permission.

pathways are GABAergic. GABA receptor antagonists cause cardiac slowing in intact but not decerebrate animals and attenuate the tachycardia evoked by hypothalamic stimulation.

Because the dendrites of cardiac preganglionic neurons do not ramify in the NTS, one or more interneurons must be interposed between second-order NTS neurons receiving baroreceptor and other afferent inputs and cardiac preganglionic neurons. Viral tracing studies confirm this organization[120]. Measurements of central reflex delay indicate that baroreceptor inputs excite some cardiac vagal preganglionic neurons with a relatively short latency and others with a much longer delay[86], suggesting at least two separate pathways, with some neurons receiving input from both. Neurons in the medial NTS are retrogradely labeled from cardioinhibitory regions of the nucleus ambiguus[122], and axons anterogradely labeled from the NTS make synaptic contact with nucleus ambiguus preganglionic neurons[37]. Thus, a monosynaptic pathway carries information from the NTS to the nucleus ambiguus.

## Pharmacology of Vagal Preganglionic Neurons

Glutamate is a major excitatory neurotransmitter in the CNS. Most vagal preganglionic neurons in the nucleus ambiguus and DVN, including those projecting to the heart, express the α-amino-3-hydroxy-5-methylisoxazole-4-propionic acid (AMPA) receptor subunits GLUR2, GLUR3, and GLUR4 and the *N*-methyl-D-aspartate (NMDA) receptor subunits NR1 and NR2A[29]. Both dorsal vagal preganglionic neurons[129] and cardiac vagal preganglionic neurons in the nucleus ambiguus[87] show spontaneous and vagally evoked NMDA and non-NMDA excitatory responses. These pathways may mediate baroreceptor responses in cardiac vagal preganglionic neurons since NTS-evoked excitation of these neurons is attenuated by NMDA and non-NMDA receptor antagonists[101]. Microinjection of acetylcholine into the nucleus ambiguus produces bradycardia[2]. *In vitro* application of acetylcholine and nicotine excites cardiac vagal preganglionic neurons directly and by presynaptic facilitation of excitatory glutamatergic input[100]. However, iontophoresis of acetylcholine *in vivo* has a predominantly inhibitory effect through muscarinic receptors, which could be direct or via activation of local inhibitory interneurons. Muscarinic receptor antagonists also attenuate inspiratory-related inhibition in these neurons[45]. Nicotine applied to the ventral medullary surface induces bronchoconstriction and mucosal gland secretion[47,48], and airway projecting vagal preganglionic neurons in the nucleus ambiguus express nicotinic receptor subunits[36].

The major inhibitory neurotransmitter in the CNS is GABA. Microinjections of the $GABA_A$ receptor antagonist bicuculline into the region of the nucleus ambiguus and DVN produces falls in heart rate[38] and increases in gastric pressure, pyloric motility, and pancreatic secretion[95,119], respectively. Vagal preganglionic neurons are subject to GABAergic inhibition. Spontaneous and vagally evoked $GABA_A$ receptor-mediated inhibitory postsynaptic potentials occur in dorsal vagal preganglionic neurons[129] and in cardiac vagal preganglionic neurons in both the DVN and the nucleus ambiguus[133]. *In vivo*, $GABA_A$ receptor antagonists raised the ongoing firing rate of cardiac vagal preganglionic neurons and attenuated vagally evoked inhibition[63] but had no effect on inspiratory-related inhibition[62]. $GABA_B$ receptor activation also inhibits about 50% of gastric- and intestinal-projecting vagal preganglionic neurons[19], but $GABA_B$ receptor antagonists do not affect vagally evoked inhibition[134].

Monoamine neurotransmitters also affect vagal preganglionic neurons. Dopamine injected into the nucleus ambiguus acts at D2 receptors to reduce heart rate[27]. Noradrenaline (NA) applied to the dorsal vagal complex inhibits secretion of both gastric acid and insulin[116]. In the DVN, NA, acting on $\alpha_1$- and $\alpha_2$-adrenoceptors, respectively, excites (50%) and inhibits 25% of gastric vagal preganglionic neurons[83]. Application of 5-HT receptor ligands has a variety of effects on baseline cardiovascular variables and differential effects on cardiorespiratory reflexes[61] and gastric secretion and motility[124]. 5-HT excites some vagal preganglionic neurons and inhibits others. Excitation can be evoked by selective activation of several types of 5-HT receptors. In the DVN, $5\text{-HT}_2$-receptor activation depolarizes vagal preganglionic neurons, including those projecting to the stomach and intestine[3,18]. Activation of $5\text{-HT}_3$ receptors evokes a depolarizing response and/or an increase in excitatory postsynaptic potentials (ESPSs)[3], due partly to a postsynaptic action on the vagal preganglionic neurons and partly to a presynaptic facilitation of glutamatergic NMDA and non-NMDA inputs[138] (Figure 7–6). Activation of $5\text{-HT}_{1A}$ receptors excites DVN preganglionic neurons and cardiac and pulmonary preganglionic neurons in the nucleus ambiguus[136,137]. However, gastric and intestinal preganglionic neurons show no postsynaptic response

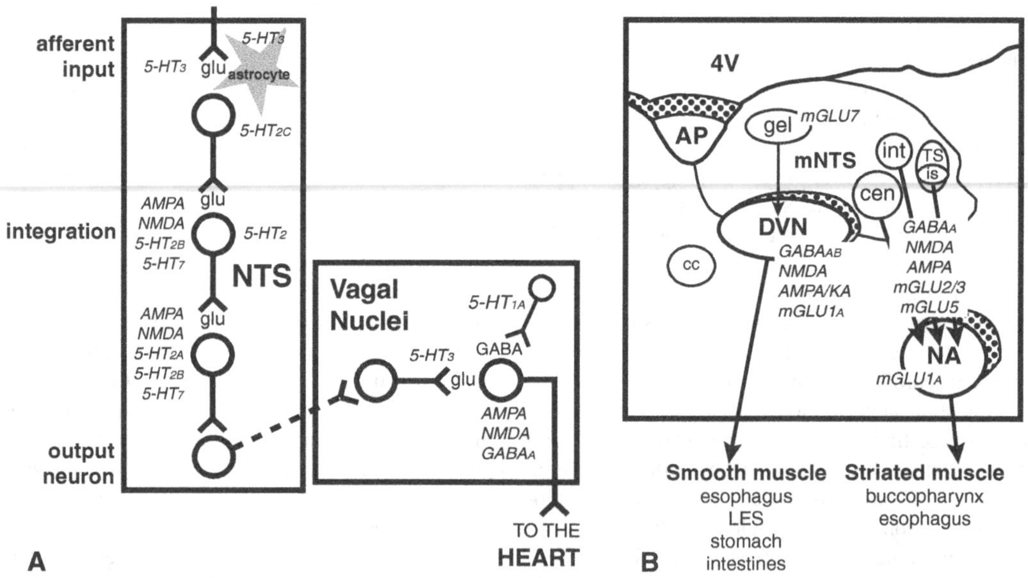


Figure 7–6 Possible sites and receptors in the NTS and DVN that could modify cardiac and gastrointestinal reflexes. *A:* Cardiac reflex function. In the NTS and vagal nuclei, a variety of 5-HT and glutamate receptors have differing actions on neuronal excitability. NTS neurons are classed as monosynaptic (receiving afferent inputs), polysynaptic (close to and including the output neurons) and intermediate (those in between). *B:* Gastrointestinal vagal reflexes. NTS subnuclei that are important in mediating gastrointestinal reflexes, and some of the amino acid transmitters that may function at these sites. cen, central subnucleus; gel, gelatinosus subnucleus; int, intermediate subnucleus; is, interstitial subnucleus, mNTS, medial NTS; NA, nucleus ambiguus; AMPA, amino-3-hydroxy-5-methyl-4-isoxazole; NMDA, *N*-methyl-D-aspartate. Reproduced from Jordan (2005b)[60] and Hornby (2001)[52], with permission.

to $5\text{-HT}_{1A}$ receptor agonists, though they do reduce NTS-evoked synaptic currents[18]. The effects of the other 5-HT receptors have not been studied at the cellular level, but antagonism of $5\text{-HT}_7$ receptors robustly attenuates bradycardia evoked by stimulation of arterial baroreceptors, chemoreceptors, and unmyelinated pulmonary receptors[64].

Numerous neuropeptides and their receptors are associated with vagal preganglionic neurons and affect gastrointestinal function[123]. One example is thyrotropin-releasing hormone, which is co-localized with 5-HT and/or substance P in inputs originating in the raphé nuclei[56]. When injected *in vivo,* thyrotropin-releasing hormone and 5-HT both evoke gastric acid secretion and motility and facilitate each other's action when given together. However, no such augmentation occurs at the level of the vagal preganglionic neurons[128], suggesting interactions at a presynaptic site. More recently, activation of presynaptic thyroid-releasing hormone receptors has been shown to uncover $5\text{-HT}_{1A}$ receptors on terminals presynaptic to gastric vagal preganglionic neurons[20]. Substance P-immunoreactive axons surround gastric vagal preganglionic neurons in the DVN[70] and chronotropic, but not dromotropic, cardiac vagal preganglionic neurons in the nucleus ambiguus[84,85]. Substance P, acting on neurokinin 1 receptors, induces decreases in gastric pressure and motility[68] and bradycardia but no change in atrio-ventricular conduction[84]. All gastrointestinal vagal preganglionic neurons except cecal neurons are activated by substance P acting at both neurokinin 1 and neurokinin 2 receptors[72]. Neuropeptide Y, another peptide in vagal afferents, inhibits gastric motility, acid secretion, and pancreatic secretion. Neuropeptide Y acts by presynaptically reducing the NTS-evoked excitatory input to gastrointestinal preganglionic neurons[21]. Oxytocin in the dorsal vagal complex has been implicated in regulating cardiovascular, gastric, and pancreatic functions and food intake. Microinjecting oxytocin in the DVN augmented baroreflexes[49] and stimulated gastric acid secretion[109] but decreased gastric motility[110] and pancreatic insulin secretion[117]. Oxytocin directly excites vagal preganglionic neurons[39], including those responding to gastric distension[88]. Hypothalamic orexin neurons are thought to be involved in energy homeostasis and regulation of feeding. Gastric vagal preganglionic neurons express orexin 1 receptors, and microinjecting orexin A and B into the DVN increases gastric pressure and antral motility[67], acid secretion, and changes pancreatic activity (see also Chapter 15). Orexins A and B excite DVN neurons projecting to the gastric corpus and fundus but not those projecting to duodenum or cecum[46]. Somatostatin, ghrelin, insulin, pancreatic polypeptide, and peptide YY are all thought to modify various aspects of pancreatic function by an action at the dorsal vagal complex (see Chapter 15).

DVN neurons contain nitric oxide synthase and are therefore capable of releasing nitric oxide. Microinjection of l-arginine into the DVN has been reported to increase[103] or decrease gastric motility[69]. The discrepancy is most likely due to injection spread to NTS sites, since nitric oxide synthase in vagal preganglionic neurons mediates at least part of their NMDA-evoked excitation[103].

## SACRAL PREGANGLIONIC NEURONS

Parasympathetic neurons in the sacral spinal cord regulate a variety of lower gastrointestinal and urogenital functions, including micturition, penile erection and ejaculation, and female sexual function. A common feature of the systems controlled by sacral outflows is that they perform two functions: storage, and then evacuation. In each system, the activity of autonomic (both parasympathetic and sympathetic) and somatic outflows are also coordinated. The neural organization in the CNS that allows this coordination is the focus of this section. For a wider perspective on autonomic control of the bladder and reproductive organs, see Chapters 19 and 20 and recent reviews[50,89].

### Urinary System

Parasympathetic preganglionic axons traveling in the pelvic nerves provide the major excitatory input to the bladder. These neurons are quiescent until the onset of micturition, when they are activated by spinal reflexes and descending voluntary control. Somatic motor neurons that have cell bodies in Onuf's nucleus in the ventral horn and innervate the external urethral sphincter are inhibited. Low (A-δ) and high (C-fiber) threshold sensory afferent fibers that respond to bladder distension and inflammation or noxious stimuli (C-fiber) travel mainly in the pelvic nerve (see Chapter 19). Stimulation of these sensory afferents activates pelvic preganglionic neurons through both spinal and supraspinal reflexes. At least one group of interneurons receives inputs from multiple visceral sites and may mediate, at the spinal level, antagonistic effects of these inputs on bladder reflexes.

The parasympathetic preganglionic neurons lie in laminae V-VII of the sacral (and in some species such as rat, also lowest lumbar) segments of the spinal cord. In the sacral parasympathetic nucleus, there is an organotopic organization. Bladder neurons are located laterally[93,94,96], and colonic neurons form a dorsal band[33] (Figure 7–7). Lateral neurons are organized in a dorsoventral fashion, whilst dorsal neurons have a mediolateral organization. Dendrites of the lateral neurons project to the region of the dorsal group. The dendrites of both dorsal and lateral neurons extend along the lateral edge of the dorsal horn. Dorsal preganglionic neurons also have dorsally projecting dendrites and dendrites that extend horizontally towards the midline[96]. Moreover, sacral preganglionic neurons have axon collaterals that could be the basis for recurrent inhibition[34]

Interneurons involved in regulating micturition have been trans-synaptically labeled from the bladder or urethra. Their cell bodies intermingle with preganglionic somata and occur in the same locations as the dendrites of preganglionic neurons, including on the lateral edge of the dorsal horn[99,132]. Both glycine- and GABA-containing interneurons are found in the dorsal commissure, and about 50% show co-localization of the two transmitters[118]. Interneurons located either dorsal or medial to the preganglionic neurons make monosynaptic connections using NMDA and non-NMDA receptors[7,8]. Some medial interneurons make inhibitory connections mediated by $GABA_A$ or glycine

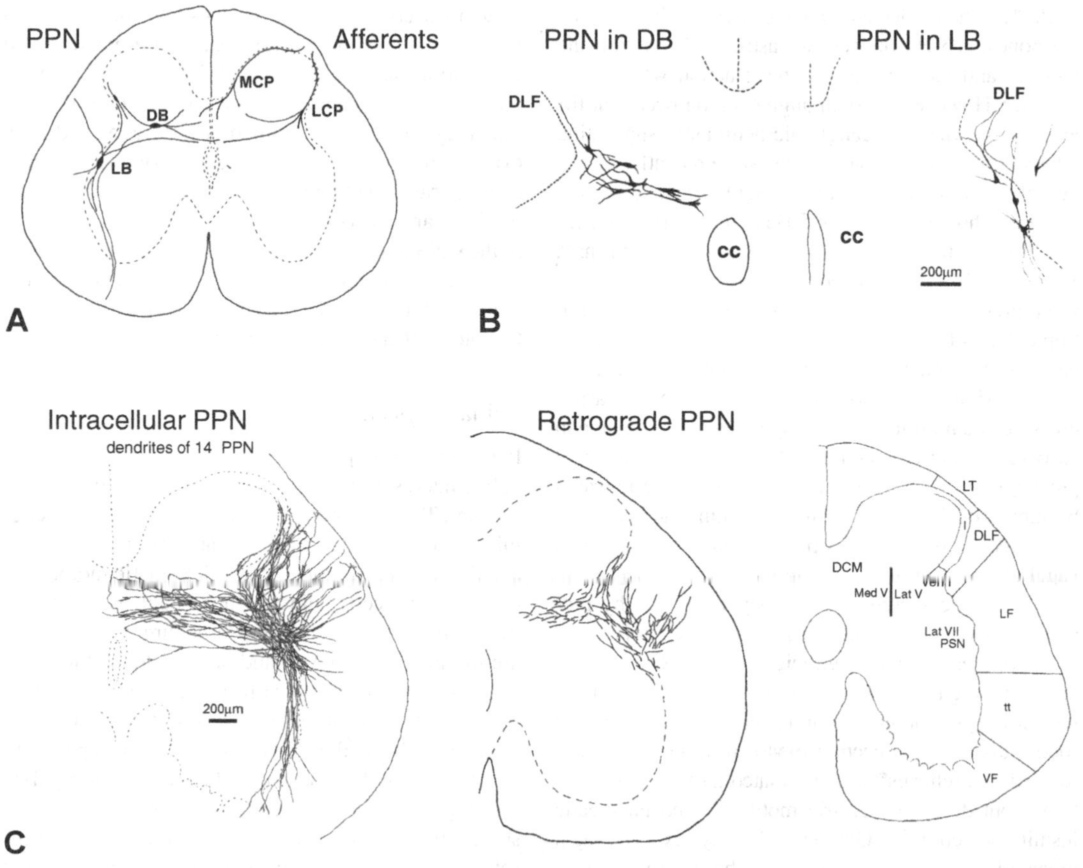


Figure 7–7 Distribution of pelvic nerve sensory afferents, pelvic preganglionic neurons and their dendritic fields in the sacral spinal cord. Transverse sections of sacral spinal cord showing the location and dendritic fields of preganglionic neurons and primary sensory afferent axons retrogradely labeled from the pelvic nerve. *A Left,* Sacral pelvic preganglionic neurons (PPN) occur in a lateral band (LB) and a dorsal band (DB). Dendrites of DB neurons extend horizontally in both medial and lateral directions. Dendrites of LB neurons project dorsolaterally into lamina I of the dorsal horn and dorsomedially into the dorsal gray commissure. *A Right,* Pelvic nerve afferents project in a medial collateral pathway (MCP) and a lateral collateral pathway (LCP). These terminal fields overlap the dendrites of DB & LB neurons. *B:* Detailed structure of DB and LB pelvic preganglionic dendrites. *C:* Dendritic fields of pelvic preganglionic neurons labeled by intracellular injection of neurobiotin (*left*) or retrograde transport of horseradish peroxidase (*middle*). Intracellular labeling shows a much greater dendritic spread than retrograde labeling and reveals an additional group of ventrally projecting dendrites. The diagram at the right shows anatomical features of the sacral cord at the level shown in the other two panels in *C*. Reproduced from Morgan et al. (1981, 1993)[93,94] and Nadelhaft et al. (1980)[96], with permission.

receptors[6]. Because some of the dorsal interneurons receive synapses from primary afferents[8], there is the basis for a disynaptic spinal reflex pathway.

Suprabulbar neurons are important in controlling sacral outflows. The pontine micturition center (Barrington's nucleus) is thought to be the integrating site and switch between storage and evacuation through a long spino-pontine-spinal reflex (see Chapter 19). Neurons in the pontine micturition center project to the spinal cord, with those in the medial region innervating the area containing sacral preganglionic neurons[51]. At least some of the axons from the pontine micturition center synapse on bladder preganglionic neurons[17] and also on dendrites of the GABA- and glycine-containing interneurons in the dorsal commissure[16,118].

Viral tracing from the bladder[99], urethra[132], colon[130], or prostate[97] labels neurons in the pontine micturition center, periaqueductal gray, midline raphé nuclei, locus coeruleus, and A5. In the pontine micturition center, there are neurons that selectively project to bladder and colon preganglionic neurons, but most are labeled from both sites[111]. Dorsal commissure interneurons are also double-labeled. Injection of different viruses into the bladder and external urethral sphincter labels the dorsal commissure, medullary raphé, and parapyramidal region, but not the pontine micturition center[98]. Interestingly, the pontine micturition center contained few prostate-projecting neurons, but neurons labeled from both bladder and prostate occurred in raphé, A5, locus coeruleus, and PVN[97].

### Pharmacology

There is little unequivocal evidence regarding the pharmacology of inputs to sacral preganglionic neurons, because most studies have applied ligands systemically, intracerebroventricularly, intrathecally, or by surperfusion, so that determining the actual site of action is impossible.

Glutamate is the major excitatory neurotransmitter affecting sacral preganglionic neurons[35,112]. Preganglionic neurons express high levels of various AMPA and NMDA receptor subunits[115], and local interneurons mediate EPSPs through NMDA and non-NMDA receptors[7,8]. Acetylcholine, NA, or 5-HT[35] do not have direct excitatory effects. Iontophoresis of GABA or glycine depresses spontaneous and evoked activity in sacral preganglionic neurons[30], and local spinal interneurons provide both GABAergic and glycinergic inhibitory inputs[6] with extensive co-localization of the two transmitters[118]. Some of these interneurons may mediate recurrent inhibition in sacral preganglionic neurons, since this was attenuated but not abolished by strychnine[34].

The sacral parasympathetic nucleus receives a dense 5-HT innervation, probably from raphé neurons[98]. The sacral cord, and particularly the dorsal commissure and sacral parasympathetic nucleus, contains binding sites for a range of 5-HT receptor ligands, including those selective for 5-$HT_{1A}$, 5-$HT_2$, and 5-$HT_3$ receptors[127]. Although there is no specific evidence for receptor localization on bladder preganglionic neurons, pelvic preganglionic neurons and dorsal commissural neurons are almost always apposed by varicosities containing 5-HT and thyrotropin-releasing hormone or substance P[125,140]. When applied directly, 5-HT is never excitatory but weakly inhibits dl-homocystate-evoked activity in a few bladder preganglionic neurons[35,90]. There is a wealth of information on the spinal and supraspinal effects of a range of 5-HT receptor ligands on sacral parasympathetic reflexes and activity[31,105], but it is unclear on which specific neurons the ligands act.

Many neuropeptides have been localized in the sacral cord and can modulate sacral reflexes. Leu-enkephalin occurs in nerve terminals and in the lateral preganglionic cell bodies in the parasympathetic nucleus[32]. Substance P-immunoreactive varicosities also appose preganglionic neurons[140]. Oxytocin-immunoreactive axons occur in both the dorsal commissure and parasympathetic nucleus, where they synapse on the somata and dendrites of pelvic-projecting neurons[125]. Other neuropeptides, such as vasoactive intestinal peptide and cholecystokinin, are probably restricted to the afferent side of the reflex. Finally, there is evidence that prostaglandin E2 may be an excitatory modulator of pelvic reflexes since *in vitro* it has been shown to directly excite preganglionic neurons[92].

## Sexual Organs

Unlike the control of many systems, where parasympathetic and sympathetic outflows are antagonistic, these outflows act in a synergistic and highly coordinated fashion in controlling the sex organs. For example, parasympathetic activity stimulates seminal fluid secretion; and sympathetic activity, its expulsion. Since Chapter 20 and a number of recent reviews have dealt with the reflex pathways responsible for various aspects of sexual responses in both males and females, these aspects will not be dealt with here.

The cell bodies of preganglionic neurons innervating the sexual organs lie in the sacral parasympathetic nucleus, and their axons travel in the pelvic nerve[96]. Penile injections of viral tracers in rats labeled preganglionic neurons in the parasympathetic nucleus from L5-S3, with most in L5-S1. Interneurons occurred mainly in the region surrounding the central canal and particularly dorsal to it, and more laterally in the region dorsal and medial to the preganglionic neurons[82]. Urethral injections first labeled neurons in the sacral parasympathetic nucleus and then in the dorsal commissure, dorsal horn, around the central canal, and in a band extending from there towards the preganglionic neurons[132]. Labeling occurred with similar patterns and timing after viral injections into the vagina and clitoris[81] or cauda epididymis[44].

Although readily recorded in spinal animals, urethrogenital spinal reflexes are difficult to evoke in intact animals, suggesting that a powerful descending inhibition normally suppresses them. Several brainstem and midbrain sites are labeled following viral injections into the penis, including the nucleus paragigantocellularis, parapyramidal nucleus, raphé pallidus and magnus, A5, and the pontine micturition center. In nucleus paragigantocellularis, parapyramidal nucleus, and raphé pallidus and magnus, many virus-labeled cells contained 5-HT, whilst the A5 neurons were immunoreactive for dopamine β-hydroxylase. Neurons in the parvocellular PVN and medial preoptic area were also labeled[82]. Vaginal injections labeled similar regions, but the medial preoptic area was unlabeled, suggesting that neurons in this region affect vaginal preganglionic neurons indirectly via neurons in the PVN, periaqueductal gray, and/or nucleus paragigantocellularis (e.g., [81]). The 5-HT-containing neurons in nucleus paragigantocellularis are one likely source of descending inhibition, since intrathecal administration of 5-HT in rats abolishes the coital reflex evoked by urethral stimulation[78]. 5-HT-immunoreactive terminals, many containing thyrotropin-releasing hormone, almost always appose pelvic preganglionic neurons and dorsal commissural neurons[140]. 5-HT$_2$ binding sites occur in the parasympathetic nucleus; and 5-HT$_{1A}$ binding sites occur in the dorsal commissure[127]. Immunoreactivity for the 5-HT$_{2C}$ receptor is present in all preganglionic neurons and in the dorsal interneurons retrogradely labeled from the penis[12]. Killing 5-HT neurons with 5,7-dihydroxytryptamine or bilateral lesions of the rostral nucleus paragigantocellularis facilitated urethrogenital reflexes[77,79]. Finally, axons labeled by anterograde tracer injections into the nucleus paragigantocellularis surround preganglionic neurons and interneurons activated by the urethrogenital reflex[76].

Catecholamine-containing axons also innervate the dorsal commissure and the sacral parasympathetic nucleus[114]. Dopamine β hydroxylase-immunoreactive terminals have been localized to the sacral parasympathetic nucleus[139] and make synapses on proximal dendrites and somata of most sacral preganglionic neurons, including those projecting to the penis. Adrenergic axons appose about half of sacral preganglionic neurons[141] and sacral parasympathetic preganglionic neurons receive synapses from adrenergic terminals[66].

Lesion studies suggest that descending excitatory inputs originate rostral to the inferior colliculus. Stimulation in the medial preoptic area facilitates urethrogenital reflexes[80], whilst direct stimulation of the PVN increased intracavernosus pressure and evoked erection and ejaculation[24], possibly through an oxytocin-containing PVN-spinal pathway. Oxytocin-binding sites and oxytocin-immunoreactive axons are present in the dorsal horn, around the central canal, and in the sacral parasympathetic nucleus[131], and these axons synapse on pelvic-projecting neurons[125] and on neurons virus-labeled from the penis[131]. Oxytocin induces penile erection in rats[10], whilst an oxytocin receptor antagonist decreases copulatory behavior and ejaculation[9]. These effects are most likely mediated by the PVN, since they were abolished following PVN lesions[11].

## CONCLUDING REMARKS

Major advances in our understanding of parasympathetic preganglionic neurons have occurred since the publication of the first edition of *Central Regulation of Autonomic Functions* in 1990. The research reviewed in this chapter and others in the current edition shows that these neurons are organized somatotopically in a target organ–dependent fashion and participate in the control of a variety of autonomic functions, including gastrointestinal motility and secretion, digestion, respiration, cardiac function, visceral blood flow, and control of the bladder, lower bowel, and sexual organs. However, parasympathetic preganglionic neurons are much more than simple sources of motor outflow to the thoracic and abdominal viscera. These neurons are important sites of integration and modulation of centrally generated signals that regulate autonomic outflow. Many recent *in vitro* studies have examined the morphological properties, synaptic inputs, and pharmacological responsiveness of target-identified, parasympathetic preganglionic neurons. However, modulation of parasympathetic outflow by supramedullary inputs is an area of research that has been barely touched. Furthermore, very little work has examined the structure and function of parasympathetic preganglionic neurons *in vivo*. To further our understanding of these important neurons, *in vivo* studies that identify them using a combination of antidromic activation from isolated vagal branches, responsiveness to specific stimuli, and, ideally, juxtacellular neuronal labeling, are essential. Although these methods are limited by the requirement for general anesthesia, only *in vivo* studies can provide information about how physiologically relevant stimuli affect parasympathetic preganglionic neurons and the autonomic outflow that they provide to their innervation targets in the periphery.

## References


1. Abrahams, T. P., Partosoedarso, E. R., and Hornby, P. J. (2002). Lower oesophageal sphincter relaxation evoked by stimulation of the dorsal motor nucleus of the vagus in ferrets. *Neurogastroenterology and Motility* 14, 295–304.
2. Agarwal, S. K., and Calaresu, F. R. (1991). Enkephalins, substance P and acetylcholine microinjected into the nucleus ambiguus elicit vagal bradycardia in rats. *Brain Research* 563, 203–208.
3. Albert, A. P., Spyer, K. M., and Brooks, P. A. (1996). The effect of 5-HT and selective 5-HT receptor agonists and antagonists on rat dorsal vagal preganglionic neurones in vitro. *British Journal of Pharmacology* 119, 519–526.
4. Altschuler, S. M., Bao, X. M., Bieger, D., Hopkins, D. A., and Miselis, R. R. (1989). Viscerotopic representation of the upper alimentary tract in the rat: Sensory ganglia and nuclei of the solitary and spinal trigeminal tracts. *Journal of Comparative Neurology* 283, 248–268.
5. Altschuler, S. M., Ferenci, D. A., Lynn, R. B., and Miselis, R. R. (1991). Representation of the cecum in the lateral dorsal motor nucleus of the vagus nerve and commissural subnucleus of the nucleus tractus solitarii in rat. *Journal of Comparative Neurology* 304, 261–274.
6. Araki, I. (1994). Inhibitory postsynaptic currents and the effects of GABA on visually identified sacral parasympathetic preganglionic neurons in neonatal rats. *Journal of Neurophysiology* 72, 2903–2910.
7. Araki, I., and De Groat, W. C. (1996). Unitary excitatory synaptic currents in preganglionic neurons mediated by two distinct groups of interneurons in neonatal rat sacral parasympathetic nucleus. *Journal of Neurophysiology* 76, 215–226.
8. Araki, I., and De Groat, W. C. (1997). Developmental synaptic depression underlying reorganization of visceral reflex pathways in the spinal cord. *Journal of Neuroscience* 17, 8402–8407.
9. Argiolas, A., Collu, M., Gessa, G. L., Melis, M. R., and Serra, G. (1988). The oxytocin antagonist d(CH2)5Tyr(Me)-Orn8-vasotocin inhibits male copulatory behaviour in rats. *European Journal of Pharmacology* 149, 389–392.
10. Argiolas, A., Melis, M. R., and Gessa, G. L. (1986). Oxytocin: An extremely potent inducer of penile erection and yawning in male rats. *European Journal of Pharmacology* 130, 265–272.
11. Argiolas, A., Melis, M. R., Mauri, A., and Gessa, G. L. (1987). Paraventricular nucleus lesion prevents yawning and penile erection induced by apomorphine and oxytocin but not by ACTH in rats. *Brain Research* 421, 349–352.
12. Bancila, M., Verge, D., Rampin, O., Backstrom, J. R., Sanders-Bush, E., McKenna, K. E., Marson, L., Calas, A., and Giuliano, F. (1999). 5-Hydroxytryptamine2C receptors on spinal neurons controlling penile erection in the rat. *Neuroscience* 92, 1523–1537.
13. Berthoud, H. R., Fox, E. A., and Powley, T. L. (1990). Localization of vagal preganglionics that stimulate insulin and glucagon secretion. *American Journal of Physiology* 258, R160–R168.
14. Berthoud, H. R., and Powley, T. L. (1990). Identification of vagal preganglionics that mediate cephalic phase insulin response. *American Journal of Physiology* 258, R523–R530.
15. Bieger, D., and Hopkins, D. A. (1987). Viscerotopic representation of the upper alimentary tract in the medulla oblongata in the rat: The nucleus ambiguus. *Journal of Comparative Neurology* 262, 546–562.
16. Blok, B. F., de Weerd, H., and Holstege, G. (1997). The pontine micturition center projects to sacral cord GABA immunoreactive neurons in the cat. *Neuroscience Letters* 233, 109–112.
17. Blok, B. F., and Holstege, G. (1997). Ultrastructural evidence for a direct pathway from the pontine micturition center to the parasympathetic preganglionic motoneurons of the bladder of the cat. *Neuroscience Letters* 222, 195–198.
18. Browning, K. N., and Travagli, R. A. (1999). Characterization of the in vitro effects of 5-hydroxytryptamine (5-HT) on identified neurones of the rat dorsal motor nucleus of the vagus (DMV). *British Journal of Pharmacology* 128, 1307–1315.
19. Browning, K. N., and Travagli, R. A. (2001). Mechanism of action of baclofen in rat dorsal motor nucleus of the vagus. *American Journal of Physiology. Gastrointestinal and Liver Physiology* 280, G1106–G1113.
20. Browning, K. N., and Travagli, R. A. (2001). The peptide TRH uncovers the presence of presynaptic 5-HT1A receptors via activation of a second messenger pathway in the rat dorsal vagal complex. *Journal of Physiology* 531, 425–435.
21. Browning, K. N., and Travagli, R. A. (2003). Neuropeptide Y and peptide YY inhibit excitatory synaptic transmission in the rat dorsal motor nucleus of the vagus. *Journal of Physiology* 549, 775–785.
22. Buijs, R. M., Chun, S. J., Niijima, A., Romijn, H. J., and Nagai, K. (2001). Parasympathetic and

sympathetic control of the pancreas: A role for the suprachiasmatic nucleus and other hypothalamic centers that are involved in the regulation of food intake. *Journal of Comparative Neurology* 431, 405–423.

23. Chang, H. Y., Mashimo, H., and Goyal, R. K. (2003). Musings on the wanderer: What's new in our understanding of vago-vagal reflex? IV. Current concepts of vagal efferent projections to the gut. *American Journal of Physiology. Gastrointestinal and Liver Physiology* 284, G357–G366.
24. Chen, K. K., Chan, S. H., Chang, L. S., and Chan, J. Y. (1997). Participation of paraventricular nucleus of hypothalamus in central regulation of penile erection in the rat. *Journal of Urology* 158, 238–244.
25. Cheng, Z., and Powley, T. L. (2000). Nucleus ambiguus projections to cardiac ganglia of rat atria: An anterograde tracing study. *Journal of Comparative Neurology* 424, 588–606.
26. Cheng, Z., Zhang, H., Guo, S. Z., Wurster, R., and Gozal, D. (2004). Differential control over postganglionic neurons in rat cardiac ganglia by NA and DmnX neurons: Anatomical evidence. *American Journal of Physiology. Regulatory, Integrative and Comparative Physiology* 286, R625–R633.
27. Chitravanshi, V. C., and Calaresu, F. R. (1992). Dopamine microinjected into the nucleus ambiguus elicits vagal bradycardia in spinal rats. *Brain Research* 583, 308–311.
28. Corbett, E. K., Batten, T. F., Kaye, J. C., Deuchars, J., and McWilliam, P. N. (1999). Labelling of rat vagal preganglionic neurones by carbocyanine dye DiI applied to the heart. *Neuroreport* 10, 1177–1181.
29. Corbett, E. K., Saha, S., Deuchars, J., McWilliam, P. N., and Batten, T. F. (2003). Ionotropic glutamate receptor subunit immunoreactivity of vagal preganglionic neurones projecting to the rat heart. *Autonomic Neuroscience* 105, 105–117.
30. De Groat, W. C. (1970). The effects of glycine, GABA and strychnine on sacral parasympathetic preganglionic neurones. *Brain Research* 18, 542–544.
31. De Groat, W. C. (2002). Influence of central serotonergic mechanisms on lower urinary tract function. *Urology* 59, 30–36.
32. De Groat, W. C., Kawatani, M., Hisamitsu, T., Lowe, I., Morgan, C., Roppolo, J., Booth, A. M., Nadelhaft, I., Kuo, D., and Thor, K. (1983). The role of neuropeptides in the sacral autonomic reflex pathways of the cat. *Journal of the Autonomic Nervous System* 7, 339–350.
33. De Groat, W. C., Nadelhaft, I., Milne, R. J., Booth, A. M., Morgan, C., and Thor, K. (1981). Organization of the sacral parasympathetic reflex pathways to the urinary bladder and large intestine. *Journal of the Autonomic Nervous System* 3, 135–160.
34. De Groat, W. C., and Ryall, R. W. (1968). Recurrent inhibition in sacral parasympathetic pathways to the bladder. *Journal of Physiology* 196, 579–591.
35. De Groat, W. C., and Ryall, R. W. (1968). The identification and characteristics of sacral parasympathetic preganglionic neurones. *Journal of Physiology* 196, 563–577.
36. Dehkordi, O., Kc, P., Balan, K. V., and Haxhiu, M. A. (2006). Airway-related vagal preganglionic neurons express multiple nicotinic acetylcholine receptor subunits. *Autonomic Neuroscience* 128, 53–63.
37. Deuchars, J., and Izzo, P. N. (1987). Demonstration of a monosynaptic pathway from the nucleus tractus solitarius to regions of the ventrolateral medulla with specific reference to vagal motoneurones in the nucleus ambiguus and brainstem localization. *Journal of Physiology* 438 80P–81P.
38. DiMicco, J. A., Gale, K., Hamilton, B., and Gillis, R. A. (1979). GABA receptor control of parasympathetic outflow to heart: Characterization and brainstem localization. *Science* 204, 1106–1109.
39. Dubois-Dauphin, M., Raggenbass, M., Widmer, H., Tribollet, E., and Dreifuss, J. J. (1992). Morphological and electrophysiological evidence for postsynaptic localization of functional oxytocin receptors in the rat dorsal motor nucleus of the vagus nerve. *Brain Research* 575, 124–131.
40. Ford, T. W., Bennett, J. A., Kidd, C., and McWilliam, P. N. (1990). Neurones in the dorsal motor vagal nucleus of the cat with non-myelinated axons projecting to the heart and lungs. *Experimental Physiology* 75, 459–473.
41. Fox, E. A., and Powley, T. L. (1985). Longitudinal columnar organization within the dorsal motor nucleus represents separate branches of the abdominal vagus. *Brain Research* 341, 269–282.
42. Fox, E. A., and Powley, T. L. (1992). Morphology of identified preganglionic neurons in the dorsal motor nucleus of the vagus. *Journal of Comparative Neurology* 322, 79–98.
43. Garcia, P. M., and Jordan, D. (2001). Effect of stimulating non-myelinated vagal axons on atrio-ventricular conduction and left ventricular function in anaesthetized rabbits. *Autonomic Neuroscience* 86, 183–191.
44. Gerendai, I., Toth, I. E., Kocsis, K., Boldogkoi, Z., Rusvai, M., and Halasz, B. (2001). Identification of CNS neurons involved in the innervation of the

epididymis: A viral transneuronal tracing study. *Autonomic Neuroscience* 92, 1–10.

45. Gilbey, M. P., Jordan, D., Richter, D. W., and Spyer, K. M. (1984). Synaptic mechanisms involved in the inspiratory modulation of vagal cardio-inhibitory neurones in the cat. *Journal of Physiology* 356, 65–78.
46. Grabauskas, G., and Moises, H. C. (2003). Gastrointestinal-projecting neurones in the dorsal motor nucleus of the vagus exhibit direct and viscerotopically organized sensitivity to orexin. *Journal of Physiology* 549, 37–56.
47. Haxhiu, M. A., Deal, E. C., Jr., Norcia, M. P., Van Lunteren, E., Mitra, J., and Cherniack, N. S. (1986). Medullary effects of nicotine and GABA on tracheal smooth muscle tone. *Respiratory Physiology* 64, 351–363.
48. Haxhiu, M. A., Van Lunteren, E., and Cherniack, N. S. (1991). Influence of ventrolateral surface of medulla on tracheal gland secretion. *Journal of Applied Physiology* 71, 1663–1668.
49. Higa, K. T., Mori, E., Viana, F. F., Morris, M., and Michelini, L. C. (2002). Baroreflex control of heart rate by oxytocin in the solitary-vagal complex. *American Journal of Physiology. Regulatory, Integrative and Comparative Physiology* 282, R537–R545.
50. Holstege, G. (2005). Central nervous system control of ejaculation. *World Journal of Urology* 23, 109–114.
51. Holstege, G., Griffiths, D., de Wall, H., and Dalm, E. (1986). Anatomical and physiological observations on supraspinal control of bladder and urethral sphincter muscles in the cat. *Journal of Comparative Neurology* 250, 449–461.
52. Hornby, P. J. (2001). Receptors and transmission in the brain-gut axis. *II.* Excitatory amino acid receptors in the brain-gut axis. *American Journal of Physiology. Gastrointestinal and Liver Physiology* 280, G1055–G1060.
53. Hyland, N. P., Abrahams, T. P., Fuchs, K., Burmeister, M. A., and Hornby, P. J. (2001). Organization and neurochemistry of vagal preganglionic neurons innervating the lower esophageal sphincter in ferrets. *Journal of Comparative Neurology* 430, 222–234.
54. Izzo, P. N., Deuchars, J., and Spyer, K. M. (1993). Localization of cardiac vagal preganglionic motoneurones in the rat: Immunocytochemical evidence of synaptic inputs containing 5-hydroxytryptamine. *Journal of Comparative Neurology* 327, 572–583.
55. Jiang, C., Fogel, R., and Zhang, X. (2003). Lateral hypothalamus modulates gut-sensitive neurons in the dorsal vagal complex. *Brain Research* 980, 31–47.
56. Johansson, O., Hokfelt, T., Pernow, B., Jeffcoate, S. L., White, N., Steinbusch, H. W., Verhofstad, A. A., Emson, P. C., and Spindel, E. (1981). Immunohistochemical support for three putative transmitters in one neuron: Coexistence of 5-hydroxytryptamine, substance P- and thyrotropin releasing hormone-like immunoreactivity in medullary neurons projecting to the spinal cord. *Neuroscience* 6, 1857–1881.
57. Jones, J. F., Wang, Y., and Jordan, D. (1995). Heart rate responses to selective stimulation of cardiac vagal C fibres in anaesthetized cats, rats and rabbits. *Journal of Physiology* 489, 203–214.
58. Jones, J. F., Wang, Y., and Jordan, D. (1998). Activity of C fibre cardiac vagal efferents in anaesthetized cats and rats. *Journal of Physiology* 507, 869–880.
59. Jordan, D. (2001). Central nervous pathways and control of the airways. *Respiratory Physiology* 125, 67–81.
60. Jordan, D. (2005). Autonomic control. In: *Encyclopedia of Life Sciences*, http://www.els.net [doi: DOI: 10.1038.npg.els.0000018]. London, U.K.: Nature Publishing Group.
61. Jordan, D. (2005). Vagal control of the heart: Central serotonergic (5-HT) mechanisms. *Experimental Physiology* 90, 175–181.
62. Jordan, D., and Spyer, K. M. (1987). Central neural mechanisms mediating respiratory-cardiovascular interactions. In E. W. Taylor (Ed.), *Neurobiology of the Cardiorespiratory System*, pp. 322–341. Manchester, U.K.: Manchester University Press.
63. Jordan, D., and Wang, Y. (1997). Involvement of GABAa receptors in the inhibition of dorsal preganglionic neurones by vagal afferents in anaesthetised rats: an *in vivo* intracellular study. *Journal of Physiology* 501 72P–73P.
64. Kellett, D. O., Ramage, A. G., and Jordan, D. (2005). Central 5-HT7 receptors are critical for reflex activation of cardiac vagal drive in anaesthetized rats. *Journal of Physiology* 563, 319–331.
65. Kellett, D. O., Stanford, S. C., Machado, B. H., Jordan, D., and Ramage, A. G. (2005). Effect of 5-HT depletion on cardiovascular vagal reflex sensitivity in awake and anesthetized rats. *Brain Research* 1054, 61–72.
66. Kohno, J., Shinoda, K., Kawai, Y., Peng, Y., Ono, K., and Shiotani, Y. (1988). Direct adrenergic inputs to sacral autonomic neurons: Using a double-immunostaining method at the light and electron microscopic levels. *Brain Research* 461, 158–162.
67. Krowicki, Z. K., Burmeister, M. A., Berthoud, H. R., Scullion, R. T., Fuchs, K., and Hornby, P. J. (2002). Orexins in rat dorsal motor nucleus of the vagus potently stimulate gastric motor function.

*American Journal of Physiology. Gastrointestinal and Liver Physiology* 283, G465–G472.

68. Krowicki, Z. K., and Hornby, P. J. (2000). Substance P in the dorsal motor nucleus of the vagus evokes gastric motor inhibition via neurokinin 1 receptor in rat. *Journal of Pharmacology and Experimental Therapeutics* 293, 214–221.
69. Krowicki, Z. K., Sharkey, K. A., Serron, S. C., Nathan, N. A., and Hornby, P. J. (1997). Distribution of nitric oxide synthase in rat dorsal vagal complex and effects of microinjection of nitric oxide compounds upon gastric motor function. *Journal of Comparative Neurology* 377, 49–69.
70. Ladic, L. A., and Buchan, A. M. (1996). Association of substance P and its receptor with efferent neurons projecting to the greater curvature of the rat stomach. *Journal of the Autonomic Nervous System* 58, 25–34.
71. Lewis, D. I. (1994). Dye-coupling between vagal motoneurones within the compact region of the adult rat nucleus ambiguus, in-vitro. *Journal of the Autonomic Nervous System* 47, 53–58.
72. Lewis, M. W., and Travagli, R. A. (2001). Effects of substance P on identified neurons of the rat dorsal motor nucleus of the vagus. *American Journal of Physiology. Gastrointestinal and Liver Physiology* 281, G164–G172.
73. Loewy, A. D., Franklin, M. F., and Haxhiu, M. A. (1994). CNS monoamine cell groups projecting to pancreatic vagal motor neurons: A transneuronal labeling study using pseudorabies virus. *Brain Research* 638, 248–260.
74. Loewy, A. D., and Spyer, K. M. (1990). Vagal preganglionic neurons. In A. D. Loewy and K. M. Spyer (Eds.), *Central Regulation of Autonomic Function*, pp. 533–538. New York: Oxford University Press.
75. Maqbool, A., Batten, T. F., and McWilliam, P. N. (1991). Ultrastructural relationships between GABAergic terminals and cardiac vagal preganglionic motoneurons and vagal afferents in the cat: A combined HRP tracing and immunogold labelling study. *European Journal of Neuroscience* 3, 501–513.
76. Marson, L., Cai, R., and Makhanova, N. (2003). Identification of spinal neurons involved in the urethrogenital reflex in the female rat. *Journal of Comparative Neurology* 462, 355–370.
77. Marson, L., and McKenna, K. E. (1990). The identification of a brainstem site controlling spinal sexual reflexes in male rats. *Brain Research* 515, 303–308.
78. Marson, L., and McKenna, K. E. (1992). A role for 5-hydroxytryptamine in descending inhibition of spinal sexual reflexes. *Experimental Brain Research* 88, 313–320.
79. Marson, L., and McKenna, K. E. (1994). Serotonergic neurotoxic lesions facilitate male sexual reflexes. *Pharmacology, Biochemistry and Behavior* 47, 883–888.
80. Marson, L., and McKenna, K. E. (1994). Stimulation of the hypothalamus initiates the urethrogenital reflex in male rats. *Brain Research* 638, 103–108.
81. Marson, L., and Murphy, A. Z. (2006). Identification of neural circuits involved in female genital responses in the rat: A dual virus and anterograde tracing study. *American Journal of Physiology. Regulatory, Integrative and Comparative Physiology* 291, R419–R428.
82. Marson, L., Platt, K. B., and McKenna, K. E. (1993). Central nervous system innervation of the penis as revealed by the transneuronal transport of pseudorabies virus. *Neuroscience* 55, 263–280.
83. Martinez, P., Rogers, R. C., Hermann, G. E., and Travagli, R. A. (2004). Norepinephrine effects on identified neurons of the rat dorsal motor nucleus of the vagus. *American Journal of Physiology. Gastrointestinal and Liver Physiology* 286, G333–G339.
84. Massari, V. J., Johnson, T. A., Gillis, R. A., and Gatti, P. J. (1996). What are the roles of substance P and neurokinin-1 receptors in the control of negative chronotropic or negative dromotropic vagal motoneurons? A physiological and ultrastructural analysis. *Brain Research* 715, 197–207.
85. Massari, V. J., Johnson, T. A., Llewellyn-Smith, I. J., and Gatti, P. J. (1994). Substance P nerve terminals synapse upon negative chronotropic vagal motoneurons. *Brain Research* 660, 275–287.
86. McAllen, R. M., and Spyer, K. M. (1978). The baroreceptor input to cardiac vagal motoneurones. *Journal of Physiology* 282, 365–374.
87. McAllen, R. M., and Spyer, K. M. (1978). Two types of vagal preganglionic motoneurones projecting to the heart and lungs. *Journal of Physiology* 282, 353–364.
88. McCann, M. J., and Rogers, R. C. (1990). Oxytocin excites gastric-related neurones in rat dorsal vagal complex. *Journal of Physiology* 428, 95–108.
89. McKenna, K. E. (2002). The neurophysiology of female sexual function. *World Journal of Urology* 20, 93–100.
90. McMahon, S. B., and Spillane, K. (1982). Brain stem influences on the parasympathetic supply to the urinary bladder of the cat. *Brain Research* 234, 237–249.
91. Mendelowitz, D. (2000). Superior laryngeal neurons directly excite cardiac vagal neurons within the nucleus ambiguus. *Brain Research Bulletin* 51, 135–138.

92. Miura, A., Kawatani, M., Maruyama, T., and De Groat, W. C. (2002). Effect of prostaglandins on parasympathetic neurons in the rat lumbosacral spinal cord. *NeuroReport* 13, 1557–1562.
93. Morgan, C., Nadelhaft, I., and De Groat, W. C. (1981). The distribution of visceral primary afferents from the pelvic nerve to Lissauer's tract and the spinal gray matter and its relationship to the sacral parasympathetic nucleus. *Journal of Comparative Neurology* 201, 415–440.
94. Morgan, C. W., De Groat, W. C., Felkins, L. A., and Zhang, S. J. (1993). Intracellular injection of neurobiotin or horseradish peroxidase reveals separate types of preganglionic neurons in the sacral parasympathetic nucleus of the cat. *Journal of Comparative Neurology* 331, 161–182.
95. Mussa, B. M., and Verberne, A. J. (2008). Activation of the dorsal vagal nucleus increases pancreatic exocrine secretion in the rat. *Neuroscience Letters* 433, 71–76.
96. Nadelhaft, I., De Groat, W. C., and Morgan, C. (1980). Location and morphology of parasympathetic preganglionic neurons in the sacral spinal cord of the cat revealed by retrograde axonal transport of horseradish peroxidase. *Journal of Comparative Neurology* 193, 265–281.
97. Nadelhaft, I., Miranda-Sousa, A. J., and Vera, P. L. (2002). Separate urinary bladder and prostate neurons in the central nervous system of the rat: Simultaneous labeling with two immunohistochemically distinguishable pseudorabies viruses. *BMC Neuroscience* 3, 8.
98. Nadelhaft, I., and Vera, P. L. (2001). Separate urinary bladder and external urethral sphincter neurons in the central nervous system of the rat: Simultaneous labeling with two immunohistochemically distinguishable pseudorabies viruses. *Brain Research* 903, 33–44.
99. Nadelhaft, I., Vera, P. L., Card, J. P., and Miselis, R. R. (1992). Central nervous system neurons labelled following the injection of pseudorabies virus into the rat urinary bladder. *Neuroscience Letters* 143, 271–274.
100. Neff, R. A., Humphrey, J., Mihalevich, M., and Mendelowitz, D. (1998). Nicotine enhances presynaptic and postsynaptic glutamatergic neurotransmission to activate cardiac parasympathetic neurons. *Circulation Research* 83, 1241–1247.
101. Neff, R. A., Mihalevich, M., and Mendelowitz, D. (1998). Stimulation of NTS activates NMDA and non-NMDA receptors in rat cardiac vagal neurons in the nucleus ambiguus. *Brain Research* 792, 277–282.
102. Neuhuber, W. L., and Sandoz, P. A. (1986). Vagal primary afferent terminals in the dorsal motor nucleus of the rat: are they making monosynaptic contacts on preganglionic efferent neurons? *Neuroscience Letters* 69, 126–130.
103. Panico, W. H., Cavuto, N. J., Kallimanis, G., Nguyen, C., Armstrong, D. M., Benjamin, S. B., Gillis, R. A., and Travagli, R. A. (1995). Functional evidence for the presence of nitric oxide synthase in the dorsal motor nucleus of the vagus. *Gastroenterology* 109, 1484–1491.
104. Peters, J. H., McDougall, S. J., Kellett, D. O., Jordan, D., Llewellyn-Smith, I. J., and Andresen, M. C. (2008). Oxytocin enhances cranial visceral afferent synaptic transmission to the solitary tract nucleus. *Journal of Neuroscience* 28, 11731–11740.
105. Ramage, A. G. (2006). The role of central 5-hydroxytryptamine (5-HT, serotonin) receptors in the control of micturition. *British Journal of Pharmacology* 147 Suppl 2, S120–S131.
106. Richter, D. W., and Spyer, K. M. (1990). Cardiorespiratory control. In D. W. Richter and K. M. Spyer (Eds.), *Central Regulation of Autonomic Functions*, pp. 189–207. New York: Oxford University Press.
107. Rinaman, L., Card, J. P., Schwaber, J. S., and Miselis, R. R. (1989). Ultrastructural demonstration of a gastric monosynaptic vagal circuit in the nucleus of the solitary tract in rat. *Journal of Neuroscience* 9, 1985–1996.
108. Rinaman, L., and Miselis, R. R. (1987). The organization of vagal innervation of rat pancreas using cholera toxin-horseradish peroxidase conjugate. *Journal of the Autonomic Nervous System* 21, 109–125.
109. Rogers, R. C., and Hermann, G. E. (1985). Dorsal medullary oxytocin, vasopressin, oxytocin antagonist, and TRH effects on gastric acid secretion and heart rate. *Peptides* 6, 1143–1148.
110. Rogers, R. C., and Hermann, G. E. (1987). Oxytocin, oxytocin antagonist, TRH., and hypothalamic paraventricular nucleus stimulation effects on gastric motility. *Peptides* 8, 505–513.
111. Rouzade-Dominguez, M. L., Pernar, L., Beck, S., and Valentino, R. J. (2003). Convergent responses of Barrington's nucleus neurons to pelvic visceral stimuli in the rat: A juxtacellular labelling study. *European Journal of Neuroscience* 18, 3325–3334.
112. Ryall, R. W., and De Groat, W. C. (1972). The microelectrophoretic administration of noradrenaline, 5-hydroxytryptamine, acetylcholine

and glycine to sacral parasympathetic preganglionic neurones. *Brain Research* 37, 345–347.

113. Sawchenko, P. E., and Swanson, L. W. (1982). Immunohistochemical identification of neurons in the paraventricular nucleus of the hypothalamus that project to the medulla or to the spinal cord in the rat. *Journal of Comparative Neurology* 205, 260–272.
114. Schroder, H. D., and Skagerberg, G. (1985). Catecholamine innervation of the caudal spinal cord in the rat. *Journal of Comparative Neurology* 242, 358–368.
115. Shibata, T., Watanabe, M., Ichikawa, R., Inoue, Y., and Koyanagi, T. (1999). Different expressions of alpha-amino-3-hydroxy-5-methyl-4-isoxazole propionic acid and N-methyl-D-aspartate receptor subunit mRNAs between visceromotor and somatomotor neurons of the rat lumbosacral spinal cord. *Journal of Comparative Neurology* 404, 172–182.
116. Siaud, P., Puech, R., Assenmacher, I., and Alonso, G. (1990). Adrenergic innervation of the dorsal vagal motor nucleus: Possible involvement in inhibitory control of gastric acid and pancreatic insulin secretion. *Cell and Tissue Research* 259, 535–542.
117. Siaud, P., Puech, R., Assenmacher, I., and Alonso, G. (1991). Microinjection of oxytocin into the dorsal vagal complex decreases pancreatic insulin secretion. *Brain Research* 546, 190–194.
118. Sie, J. A., Blok, B. F., de Weerd, H., and Holstege, G. (2001). Ultrastructural evidence for direct projections from the pontine micturition center to glycine-immunoreactive neurons in the sacral dorsal gray commissure in the cat. *Journal of Comparative Neurology* 429, 631–637.
119. Sivarao, D. V., Krowicki, Z. K., and Hornby, P. J. (1998). Role of GABAA receptors in rat hindbrain nuclei controlling gastric motor function. *Neurogastroenterology and Motility* 10, 305–313.
120. Standish, A., Enquist, L. W., Escardo, J. A., and Schwaber, J. S. (1995). Central neuronal circuit innervating the rat heart defined by transneuronal transport of pseudorabies virus. *Journal of Neuroscience* 15, 1998–2012.
121. Streefland, C., Maes, F. W., and Bohus, B. (1998). Autonomic brainstem projections to the pancreas: A retrograde transneuronal viral tracing study in the rat. *Journal of the Autonomic Nervous System* 74, 71–81.
122. Stuesse, S. L., and Fish, S. E. (1984). Projections to the cardioinhibitory region of the nucleus ambiguus of rat. *Journal of Comparative Neurology* 229, 271–278.
123. Taché, Y., Garrick, T., and Raybould, H. (1990). Central nervous system action of peptides to influence gastrointestinal motor function. *Gastroenterology* 98, 517–528.
124. Taché, Y., Yang, H., and Kaneko, H. (1995). Caudal raphé-dorsal vagal complex peptidergic projections: Role in gastric vagal control. *Peptides* 16, 431–435.
125. Tang, Y., Rampin, O., Calas, A., Facchinetti, P., and Giuliano, F. (1998). Oxytocinergic and serotonergic innervation of identified lumbosacral nuclei controlling penile erection in the male rat. *Neuroscience* 82, 241–254.
126. Taylor, E. W., Jordan, D., and Coote, J. H. (1999). Central control of the cardiovascular and respiratory systems and their interactions in vertebrates. *Physiological Reviews* 79, 855–916.
127. Thor, K. B., Nickolaus, S., and Helke, C. J. (1993). Autoradiographic localization of 5-hydroxytryptamine1A., 5-hydroxytryptamine1B and 5-hydroxytryptamine1C/2 binding sites in the rat spinal cord. *Neuroscience* 55, 235–252.
128. Travagli, R. A., and Gillis, R. A. (1995). Effects of 5-HT alone and its interaction with TRH on neurons in rat dorsal motor nucleus of the vagus. *American Journal of Physiology* 268, G292–G299.
129. Travagli, R. A., Gillis, R. A., Rossiter, C. D., and Vicini, S. (1991). Glutamate and GABA-mediated synaptic currents in neurons of the rat dorsal motor nucleus of the vagus. *American Journal of Physiology* 260, G531–G536.
130. Valentino, R. J., Kosboth, M., Colflesh, M., and Miselis, R. R. (2000). Transneuronal labeling from the rat distal colon: Anatomic evidence for regulation of distal colon function by a pontine corticotropin-releasing factor system. *Journal of Comparative Neurology* 417, 399–414.
131. Veronneau-Longueville, F., Rampin, O., Freund-Mercier, M. J., Tang, Y., Calas, A., Marson, L., McKenna, K. E., Stoeckel, M. E., Benoit, G., and Giuliano, F. (1999). Oxytocinergic innervation of autonomic nuclei controlling penile erection in the rat. *Neuroscience* 93, 1437–1447.
132. Vizzard, M. A., Erickson, V. L., Card, J. P., Roppolo, J. R., and De Groat, W. C. (1995). Transneuronal labeling of neurons in the adult rat brainstem and spinal cord after injection of pseudorabies virus into the urethra. *Journal of Comparative Neurology* 355, 629–640.
133. Wang, J., Irnaten, M., and Mendelowitz, D. (2001). Characteristics of spontaneous and evoked GABAergic synaptic currents in cardiac vagal neurons in rats. *Brain Research* 889, 78–83.

134. Wang, Y., and Ishizuka, K. I. J. D. (1997). Involvement of GABAa receptors in the inhibition of dorsal vagal preganglionic neurones (DVPNs) by vagal afferents in anaesthetised rats. *Journal of the Autonomic Nervous System* 65, 107.
135. Wang, Y., Jones, J. F., Jeggo, R. D., de Burgh, D. M., Jordan, D., and Ramage, A. G. (2000). Effect of pulmonary C-fibre afferent stimulation on cardiac vagal neurones in the nucleus ambiguus in anaesthetized cats. *Journal of Physiology* 526, 157–165.
136. Wang, Y., Jones, J. F., Ramage, A. G., and Jordan, D. (1995). Effects of 5-HT and 5-HT1A receptor agonists and antagonists on dorsal vagal preganglionic neurones in anaesthetized rats: An ionophoretic study. *British Journal of Pharmacology* 116, 2291–2297.
137. Wang, Y., and Ramage, A. G. (2001). The role of central 5-HT(1A) receptors in the control of B-fibre cardiac and bronchoconstrictor vagal preganglionic neurones in anaesthetized cats. *Journal of Physiology* 536, 753–767.
138. Wang, Y., Ramage, A. G., and Jordan, D. (1998). Presynaptic 5-HT3 receptors evoke an excitatory response in dorsal vagal preganglionic neurones in anaesthetized rats. *Journal of Physiology* 509, 683–694.
139. Westlund, K. N., Bowker, R. M., Ziegler, M. G., and Coulter, J. D. (1983). Noradrenergic projections to the spinal cord of the rat. *Brain Research* 263, 15–31.
140. Wu, W., Elde, R., and Wessendorf, M. W. (1993). Organization of the serotonergic innervation of spinal neurons in rats—III. Differential serotonergic innervation of somatic and parasympathetic preganglionic motoneurons as determined by patterns of co-existing peptides. *Neuroscience* 55, 223–233.
141. Yaici, E. D., Rampin, O., Tang, Y., Calas, A., Jestin, A., Leclerc, P., Benoit, G., and Giuliano, F. (2002). Catecholaminergic projections onto spinal neurons destined to the pelvis including the penis in rat. *International Journal of Impotence Research* 14, 151–166.

# 8

# Spinal Interneurons in the Control of Autonomic Function

SUSAN A. DEUCHARS

The spinal cord is more than a relay for transmission of information between the brain and periphery. It integrates, manipulates, and even generates neural activity using complex intrinsic neuronal circuits. The control of autonomic activity is a prime example since intrinsic spinal circuits are major determinants of sympathetic and parasympathetic outflow. Embedded within these spinal circuits are local interneurons. An *interneuron* is generally defined as a neuron that only synapses onto other neurons. In the central nervous system, interneurons are considered to be the neurons that have local rather than long-distance projections, although it is not always possible to rule out longer projections of these interneurons. Autonomic interneurons are often located in the spinal cord, where they innervate autonomic preganglionic neurons to influence their activity. They therefore have the capacity to dictate the final levels of excitability of preganglionic neurons that are in circuits innervating peripheral targets. Considering the importance of the autonomic nervous system in maintaining homeostasis, our understanding of spinal autonomic circuitry, particularly the role of interneurons, is far from complete. This chapter will examine the role of *local* interneurons in sympathetic and parasympathetic control.

## INTERNEURONS INVOLVED IN SYMPATHETIC CONTROL

The investigation of interneurons in specific circuits involved in sympathetic control has been difficult since there are problems associated with identifying these neurons and determining their innervation targets. However, current evidence indicates that interneurons form components of descending and ascending (afferent) circuitry and may contribute extensively to the generation of sympathetic outflow.

There is no doubt that interneurons involved in sympathetic control are numerous and widespread. The locations in the spinal cord of interneurons involved in sympathetic control have been revealed with a series of elegant experiments using viral tracers, which cross the synapses between sympathetic preganglionic neurons and interneurons. In the first of these studies, Strack and colleagues carried out an extensive analysis of sympathetic interneurons by injecting pseudorabies virus into a number of sympathetic ganglia and into the adrenal gland[94] and revealed interneurons in spinal cord laminae VII and X. Subsequently, injections into the superior cervical ganglion labeled interneurons principally in lamina V and the dorsolateral region of lamina VII, ipsilateral to and at the same segmental levels as the labeled sympathetic preganglionic neurons[15]. Similar labeling patterns occur after injection of virus into different end organs, including the adrenal medulla[39], kidney[98] and stellate ganglion[38]; and additionally interneurons in the intermediolateral cell column itself are labeled (Figure 8–1). Furthermore, Deuchars and colleagues demonstrated that some transneuronally labeled interneurons in lamina X are inhibitory, as they contain markers for gamma amino butyric acid (GABA) synthesis[24]. Thus, presympathetic interneurons are dispersed throughout the dorsal spinal cord, predominantly in laminae V, VII, and X.

Physiological studies, rather than pinpointing the location of interneurons, provide evidence of their existence and insight into how and when they may be active. The occurrence of ongoing synaptic activity in sympathetic preganglionic neurons in spinal cord slices is due to spontaneously active local interneurons that synapse on to sympathetic preganglionic neurons, since other inputs are absent. In sympathetic preganglionic neurons, both excitatory postsynaptic potentials (EPSPs) and inhibitory postsynaptic potentials (IPSPs) are observed, and these are blocked by excitatory and inhibitory amino acid–receptor antagonists, and also by tetrodotoxin, which blocks synaptic activity[28,42,44,91]. It is striking that in the spinal cord slice, the proportions of EPSPs recorded in sympathetic preganglionic neurons are relatively low compared to sympathetic preganglionic neurons in the intact spinal cord *in vivo*[21]. This observation suggests that in reduced preparations, either excitatory interneurons are not present or their activity is driven by descending or afferent inputs. The latter appears to be true since stimulation of the dorsal roots elicits polysynaptic EPSPs in sympathetic preganglionic neurons (e.g., [88]), as does application of agonists that activate specific receptors (see below). What is also not proven is whether the inhibitory presympathetic interneurons are normally active in the intact preparation or whether they are subject to tonic descending inhibition that reduces their role under normal conditions.

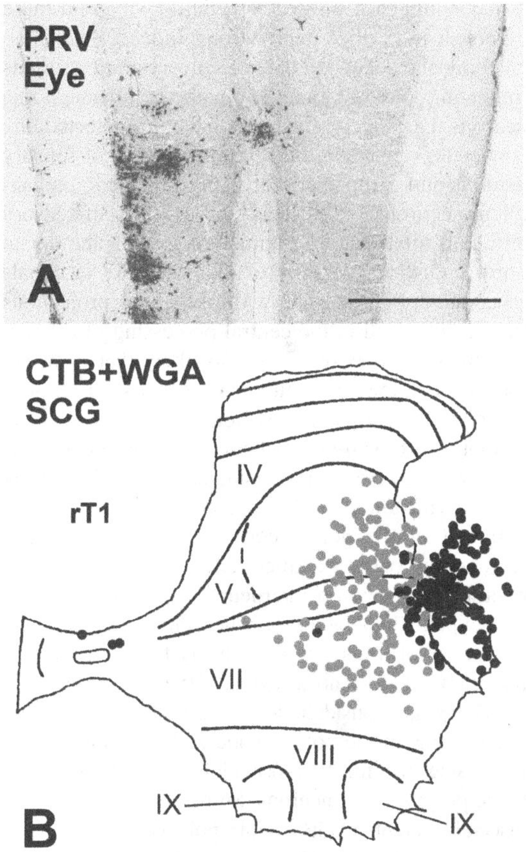


Figure 8–1 Transneuronal labelling of interneurons in the spinal cord. *A:* Light micrograph showing viral-labeled neurons (both sympathetic preganglionic neurons and interneurons) in the thoracic spinal cord (thoracic segments 1 and 2) after infection of the eye with pseudorabies virus (PRV). Scale bar, 1 mm. Reproduced from Strack and Loewy (1990)[93], with permission. *B:* Line drawing of the thoracic spinal cord showing the distribution of sympathetic preganglionic neurons (black circles) retrogradely labeled with cholera toxin B subunit (CTB) and interneurons (gray circles) transneuronally labeled with wheatgerm agglutinin (WGA). Tracers were injected into the superior cervical ganglion (SCG). rT1, rostral thoracic segment 1. IV–IX, spinal cord laminae. Modified from Cabot et al. (1994)[15], with permission.

Although interneurons in the spinal cord slice may not always be spontaneously firing, activation of specific receptors known to be involved in sympathetic control elicits indirect effects in sympathetic preganglionic neurons due to an action on antecedent interneurons. Some receptors, when activated, increase inhibitory synaptic activity. These include substance P[27,16], adrenaline[65], oxytocin and vasopressin[86], angiotensin II[43], and 5-hydoxytryptamine (5-HT)[44]. Activation of other receptors increases excitatory transmission via interneurons, including receptors for oxytocin and vasopressin[86], angiotensin II[43], and 5-HT[44]. Since the majority of these neuromodulators are known to be located in descending pathways, interneurons expressing receptors for these substances may be crucial links in particular reflex pathways that maintain homeostasis.

## Origin of Inputs to Spinal Sympathetic Interneurons

Proof that interneurons exist is one step in the search for how they fit into spinal cord circuitry controlling sympathetic outflow. These interneurons clearly project to sympathetic preganglionic neurons—but what controls *their* activity? The origin of inputs to interneurons is therefore of fundamental importance if we are to understand their role(s) in spinal autonomic circuitry.

### *Descending Inputs*

Major inputs from the brainstem and higher regions are crucial in maintaining sympathetic outflow, and many studies have provided evidence of direct inputs onto sympathetic preganglionic neurons. However, some of the descending inputs also impinge on interneurons antecedent to sympathetic preganglionic neurons. Stimulation of specific regions of the medulla[25,26] or the lateral funiculus, which contains descending fibers that innervate the IML[21], can evoke polysynaptic responses in sympathetic preganglionic neurons, indicating an intervening interneuron in this pathway. Indeed, it is possible to elicit polysynaptic responses in sympathetic preganglionic neurons by stimulating the lateral funiculus in a 300 μm spinal cord slice[13,22], indicating that some interneurons lie quite close to the sympathetic preganglionic neurons that they innervate. The majority of axonal boutons labeled anterogradely from the rostral ventrolateral medulla (RVLM) closely appose sympathetic preganglionic neurons[76]. However, appositions also occur on interneurons, and these may play a role in amplifying or modulating the response at a spinal level. This role is supported by the fact that stimulation of the lateral funiculus elicits monosynaptic responses in interneurons in the IML[13,22]. In contrast, anterogradely labeled inputs arriving via the corticospinal tract, although few in number (which may be due to the exceptional difficulties in labeling all corticospinal axons in studies that involve transneuronal tracing), make close appositions with more interneurons than sympathetic preganglionic neurons[76]. Furthermore, direct projections from the medial prefrontal cortex, which, when stimulated, decrease blood pressure and heart rate, are targeted to the central region of the spinal cord where there are few sympathetic preganglionic neurons[3]. Inhibitory interneurons have been proposed as the targets of these inputs, and GABAergic neurons in this region have recently been shown to innervate sympathetic preganglionic neurons[24].

Interneurons may also have a role in mediating inputs from the paraventricular nucleus (PVN) of the hypothalamus[94]. Although PVN neurons that contain oxytocin and vasopressin project to the spinal cord[109], few of these neurons are infected after injections of pseudorabies virus into the adrenal gland. Hence, it seems likely that these supraspinal inputs are directed predominantly to interneurons rather than sympathetic preganglionic neurons. In support of this hypothesis, electrophysiological studies have confirmed that vasopressin and oxytocin affect sympathetic preganglionic neurons both directly and indirectly[86].

The actual contribution of spinal interneurons to the bulbospinal control of sympathetic preganglionic neurons is unknown: but there are at least two possibilities. First, interneurons may help maintain and synchronize a particular input by innervating a number of sympathetic preganglionic neurons to amplify and prolong the effect of that input. Second, the extensive arborization of interneuronal dendrites suggests that both sensory afferents and descending inputs may converge onto a single interneuron. Filtering of sensory and descending information at the interneuronal level could shape the final firing patterns of sympathetic preganglionic neurons.

### *Afferent Inputs*

Activation of somatic and visceral afferent inputs has a major influence on sympathetic activity, and these inputs always utilize interneurons. Indeed, there is no anatomical evidence to date of sensory afferent inputs impinging directly onto sympathetic preganglionic neurons. Degeneration studies have not detected any connections between the central terminals of sensory neurons and sympathetic or parasympathetic preganglionic neurons[79,100]. Instead, the majority of sensory terminals are located in laminae I to V of the dorsal horn[100]. Obviously, many of these sensory terminals innervate spinal neurons with ascending projections that are involved in the central processing of afferent information. However, it is also likely that there are totally separate sets of interneurons that send collaterals to spinal sympathetic regions and are involved in mediating somato-sympathetic and viscero-sympathetic reflexes. Temperature changes also elicit strong somatosympathetic reflexes[36], and a pathway from lamina I of the dorsal horn to spinal sympathetic regions has been identified[19]. In lamina X, sensory boutons terminate on interneurons that may impinge on sympathetic preganglionic neurons[34], indicating the possibility of a disynaptic pathway for sensory input that goes via the central region of the spinal cord.

There is considerable functional evidence for interneurons in the polysynaptic pathways involved in processing of afferent information received by sympathetic preganglionic neurons. Stimulation of somatic or visceral afferents elicits mainly polysynaptic EPSPs in single sympathetic preganglionic neurons and occasional IPSPs[21]. In contrast, stimulation of the ulnar or sciatic nerve inhibits the activity of sympathetic preganglionic neurons, an effect that persists in cats after spinal cord transection[112]. Some presumptive interneurons in this study were also excited by afferent stimulation, whilst others were inhibited. The time course of the inhibitory effects is similar to that of the inhibition of sympathetic preganglionic neurons, suggesting disfacilitation of sympathetic preganglionic neurons through inhibition of excitatory interneurons. In the spinal cord slice or isolated spinal cord, stimulation of the dorsal roots elicits polysynaptic EPSPs[87] and IPSPs[28,91], or both[60], in sympathetic preganglionic neurons. Hence, both inhibitory (probably glycinergic) and excitatory glutamatergic interneurons are involved in conveying afferent information to sympathetic preganglionic neurons.

## Properties of Interneurons Involved in Sympathetic Control

Several heroic studies using extracellular recordings in animals with both intact and transected spinal cords have identified spinal interneurons that fire in correlation with sympathetic activity. In intact cats, interneurons in the IML with firing frequencies of up to 50 Hz exhibit firing that correlates with the cardiac cycle, implying a role in sympathetic control[5,30]. Indeed, the peak activity in the interneurons preceded that of sympathetic preganglionic neurons, reinforcing the idea that the interneurons were presympathetic[30]. These interneurons are reflexively inhibited by raising blood pressure and activated by stimulation of sympathoexcitatory regions in the medulla, suggesting that they play a role in sympathoexcitation. Some interneurons in the cat IML also have activity that is decreased by occlusion of the common carotid arteries[58] and correlates with the R-wave of the electrocardiogram. These interneurons are excited by stimulation of the depressor region of the nucleus of the solitary tract (NTS), suggesting that they have an inhibitory role. In rats, a population of interneurons in the IML with cardiac-related activity was also observed, and these neurons were inhibited by stimulation of the NTS, implicating a sympathoexcitatory role. Again, peak activity occurred in these neurons before that in sympathetic preganglionic neurons, indicating that these were presympathetic.

In rats with intact and transected spinal cords, interneurons in thoracic segment 10 exhibit firing linked to renal sympathetic nerve activity[17,63,97]. The firing of most of these interneurons is positively correlated to sympathetic activity and precedes the sympathetic peak (Figure 8–2A), suggesting that they excite sympathetic preganglionic neurons. There are also some interneurons with firing that is negatively correlated with sympathetic activity, indicating an inhibitory role. Both types of interneurons occur in the IML and laminae I–V and X of the spinal cord. Surprisingly, positively correlated interneurons are more numerous in spinalized rats than in those with intact spinal cords, and negatively correlated interneurons are scarcer. This change in the proportions of excitatory versus inhibitory interneurons may be due to removal of supraspinal inhibitory drive. Colorectal stimulation excites interneurons in the dorsal horn but inhibits interneurons in the IML, suggesting differences in function (Figure 8–2B). Interneurons in the IML show variable responses to noxious somatic stimulation. The extent and nature of their receptive fields are also varied and more complicated than those of dorsal horn interneurons[17].

In the spinal cord slice, interneurons in the IML fire at faster frequencies than do sympathetic preganglionic

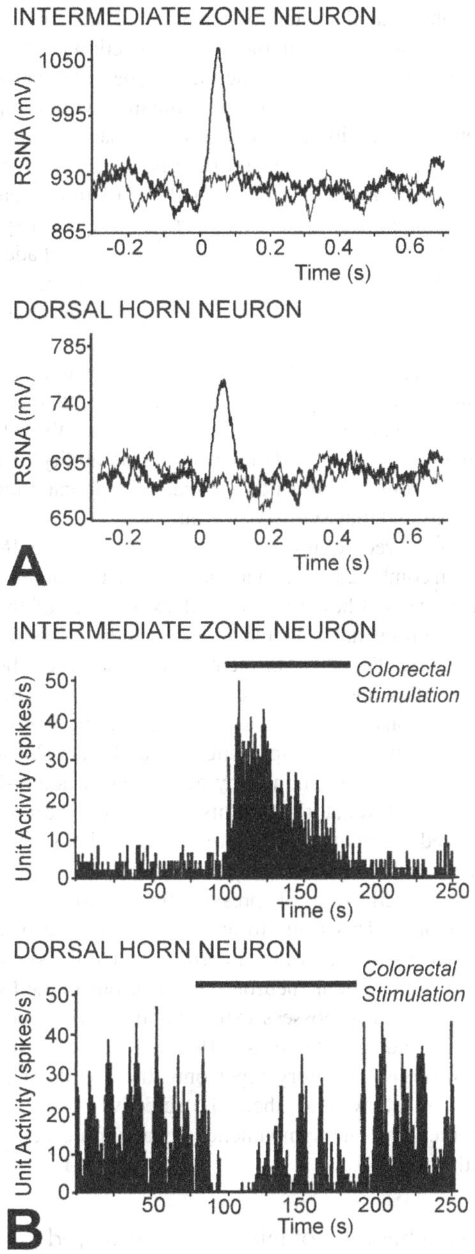


Figure 8–2 Properties of spinal autonomic interneurons in the rat. *A:* Spike-triggered averages of renal sympathetic nerve activity triggered by action potentials either from an interneuron in the intermediate zone (*top*) or from a dorsal horn neuron (*bottom*). The magnitude of correlation was significantly higher for interneurons in the intermediate zone. *B:* Responses of an interneuron in either the intermediate zone (*top*) or the dorsal horn (*bottom*) to colorectal distension. The different response patterns suggest that the two interneurons receive different synaptic inputs. Adapted from Chau et al. (2000)[17], with permission.

neurons[23], a characteristic also noted *in vivo* (see above). Interneurons in the IML have action potentials of shorter duration, smaller afterhyperpolarizations, and faster firing frequencies compared with sympathetic preganglionic neurons in the same region[23]. These electrophysiological differences may be due in part to the Kv3.1b-voltage gated potassium channel subunit, which is present in interneurons but not sympathetic preganglionic neurons[14,23], since blockade of this channel increases action potential duration and decreases firing frequencies. These interneurons have axons that ramify in the IML[23], and at the electron microscopic level, direct synaptic contacts onto sympathetic preganglionic neurons are observed (Figure 8–3). The challenge now is to determine how these fast firing characteristics are reflected in the ability of the interneurons to influence sympathetic preganglionic neurons and thus sympathetic outflow.

Direct recordings from interneurons in the IML region combined with pharmacological manipulations have revealed how the levels of excitability of these interneurons are affected by activation of specific receptors. These experiments have identified both similarities and differences between presympathetic interneurons and sympathetic preganglionic neurons. Interneurons, like sympathetic preganglionic neurons, are affected differentially by activation of adenosine receptors. Excitatory transmission to interneurons is reduced by activation of presynaptic adenosine A1 receptors[22] while inhibitory transmission is enhanced through activation of presynaptic adenosine A2A receptors[13]. This leads to an overall decrease in the level of excitability of the interneuron. Unlike sympathetic preganglionic neurons, interneurons in the IML do not seem to possess extrasynaptic GABA receptors[107], and thus there is little evidence of a tonic GABAergic inhibitory input onto these cells. These findings show that there is selective control of interneurons and sympathetic preganglionic neurons within the IML.

## Neurochemistry of Interneurons Involved in Sympathetic Control

There is little direct information regarding the neurochemistry of interneurons in the spinal cord that are involved in sympathetic control. This lack of data is probably due to technical difficulties associated with identification of presympathetic interneurons and subsequent immunohistochemical analysis.

The most comprehensive study of the neurochemistry of presympathetic interneurons comes from Jansen et al. (1995)[38], who showed that virally infected interneurons in laminae V and VII could contain substance P, enkephalin, and somatostatin, whilst cholecystokinin-8, corticotropin-releasing factor, and vasoactive intestinal peptide were absent. Many axon terminals in the dorsal horn that do not arise from primary afferents contain substance P and are also immunoreactive for vesicular glutamate transporter 2[101], so glutamate and substance P may coexist in these interneurons. In spinal cord slices, much of the ongoing inhibitory activity in sympathetic preganglionic neurons is glycinergic, and IPSPs evoked by stimulation of the dorsal roots are glycinergic[28,42,91]. However, it is also possible to record ongoing GABAergic IPSPs in sympathetic preganglionic neurons in the spinal cord slice, and glutamate administration in lamina X elicits GABAergic IPSPs (Figure 8–4). GABAergic interneurons in this region are transneuronally labeled following injections of pseudorabies virus into the adrenal gland[24]. These GABAergic interneurons may form an important component of descending pathways such as that from the medial prefrontal cortex (see above) or the A5 region of the pons, since intrathecal injections of bicuculline reduce the depressor response to A5 stimulation[33]. In addition, small enkephalin-containing interneurons are present in lamina X[45]. Since enkephalin often co-exists with GABA in the dorsal horn[102], enkephalin may be present in the GABAergic neurons in lamina X that innervate sympathetic preganglionic neurons.

Neuropeptide Y-containing interneurons are found in the vicinity of spinal autonomic regions such as laminae V and VII, in close proximity to sympathetic preganglionic neurons[64]. Because most neuropeptide Y-containing axons in the dorsal horn also express GABA[80], these interneurons may have an inhibitory role. Cholinergic interneurons situated in laminae VII and X[4] may also play an important role in sympathetic control. There is little evidence for a supraspinal cholinergic input onto sympathetic preganglionic neurons[89]. Nevertheless, these neurons are heavily influenced by activation of cholinoceptors[12,18,31], indicating a local source of inputs.

## Role of Sympathetic Interneurons after Spinal Cord Injury

Spinal cord transection results in gross changes in autonomic function. Many people with spinal cord injuries suffer from hypotension associated with orthostatic intolerance, while another major problem is autonomic dysreflexia, a condition where innocuous or noxious sensory stimulation below the lesion causes large increases in sympathetic activity and blood pressure[37,40,57]. Changes in the role(s) of interneurons are highly likely to underlie these conditions, since both excitatory and inhibitory supraspinal input is lost and only spinal circuits remain. Chronic transection

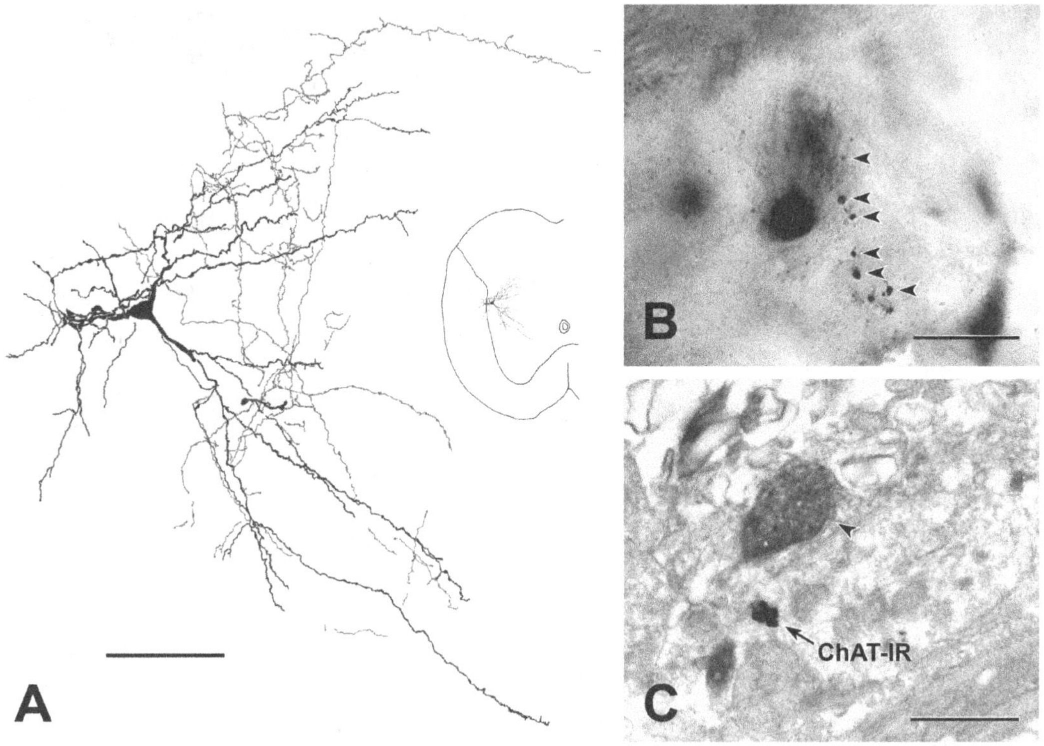


Figure 8–3 Morphology of autonomic interneurons in the IML. *A:* Drawing of an interneuron that was filled with neurobiotin during recording and electrophysiological characterization. The inset shows the location of the interneuron in the slice, which was taken from the upper thoracic cord of a neonatal rat. The cell body and dendrites are shown in black; the axon is in grey. Note the extensive arborization of the axon within the spinal cord. Scale bar, 50 μm. Reproduced from Deuchars et al. (2001)[23]. *B:* A high magnification light micrograph showing the axon of an interneuron in the IML that was filled with neurobiotin. *Arrowheads* point to boutons. To label sympathetic preganglionic neurons, the tissue was also processed to reveal immunoreactivity for choline acetyltransferase (ChAT-IR) using a silver intensified immunogold pre-embedding labeling procedure. Scale bar, 10 μm. *C:* At the electron microscopic level, a neurobiotin-labeled interneuronal terminal forms a synapse (arrowhead) on a ChAT-immunoreactive dendrite. Scale bar, 500 nm. *B* and *C* show unpublished data from Deuchars, Brooke, Frater, and Deuchars.

leads to plastic changes in the spinal cord, which may include changes in the numbers, activity, and patterns of innervation of interneurons.

In the short term, as little as two and a half hours after spinal cord transection in rats, there is a vast increase in numbers of neurons that are immunoreactive for Fos, the protein product of the immediate early gene *c-fos*, which is a marker of neuronal activation. These Fos-immunoreactive neurons lie in laminae known to contain sympathetic interneurons, and the increase in the number of Fos-positive neurons may reflect increases in their activity due to loss of inhibitory supraspinal inputs[84]. Moreover, the proportion of interneurons with firing patterns that correlate with renal sympathetic nerve activity is higher after acute transection than in the intact cord[63]. This immediate change in activity may be the cause of exaggerated reflexes observed shortly after spinal cord injury.

Changes in numbers and connectivity of interneurons may underlie longer-term effects of spinal lesions. At 14 days post-transection, a number of interneurons in the intermediate gray matter and in the IML caudal to the lesion were immunoreactive for the growth-associated protein 43, which is a marker for reactive sprouting; and at 30 days, the number of immunoreactive somata had increased further (Figure 8–5)[108]. At this stage, afferent sprouting also occurred in regions where interneurons expressing growth-associated protein 43 are located[110], perhaps due to formation of new circuits involving somatic afferents and interneurons involved in sympathetic control. One month after transection, the responses of interneurons to noxious and innocuous

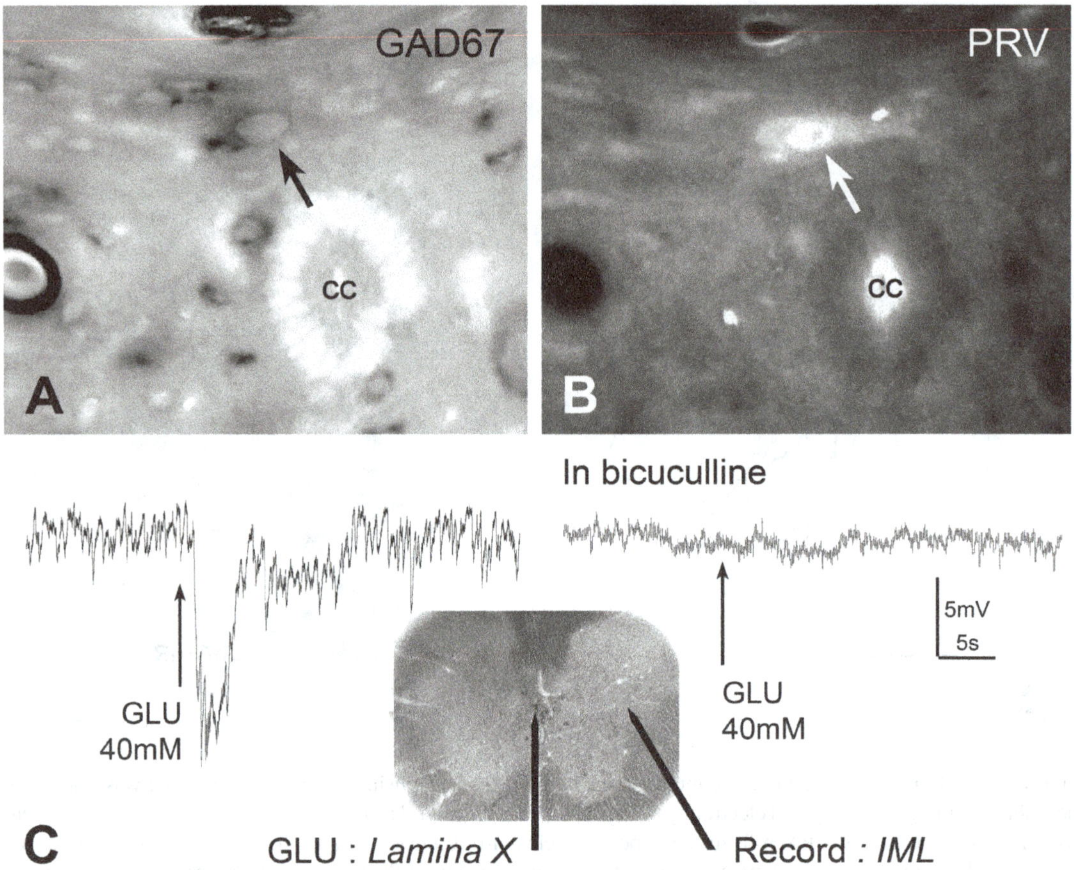


Figure 8–4 GABAergic interneurons innervate sympathetic preganglionic neurons. *A:* Light micrographs of the same spinal cord section showing (*A*) the presence of glutamate decarboxylase (GAD-67) mRNA in a lamina X interneuron that was also (*B*) transneuronally labeled with pseudorabies virus (PRV) after injection of the virus into the medulla of the adrenal gland. *C:* The trace on the left shows the hyperpolarizing response of a sympathetic preganglionic neuron to microinjection of glutamate (GLU) into lamina X which activates the GABAergic interneurons in this lamina. The trace on the right shows that the hyperpolarizing response in this sympathetic preganglionic neuron to glutamate microinjection is antagonized by bicuculline. *Inset,* The spinal cord slice showing the position of the recording electrode in a sympathetic preganglionic neuron in the intermediolateral cell column (IML) and the glutamate-filled microelectrode in lamina X. Reproduced from Deuchars et al. (2005)[24], with permission.

stimulation were greatly exaggerated, even compared to the acutely transected state (Figure 8–5B)[40], so these new circuits may be responsible for the change in the magnitude of sympathetic responses. Injury-induced reorganization of circuits and enhancement of responses may account for the onset of autonomic dysreflexia and episodic hypertension, which takes weeks to months to develop in humans and would therefore reflect long-term changes in spinal cord circuitry rather than just loss of inhibition. Interestingly, the proportion of inhibitory synapses onto sympathetic preganglionic neurons increases compared to excitatory inputs[46] and this may contribute to the hypotension. In cats, some inhibitory reflexes to visceral stimuli never recover from spinalization, which suggests that these circuits are somehow lost or changed to become excitatory in nature[37].

## INTERNEURONS INVOLVED IN PARASYMPATHETIC CONTROL

The major characteristic of the sacral parasympathetic outflow is that there is no overlap in the parasympathetic preganglionic neurons innervating specific end

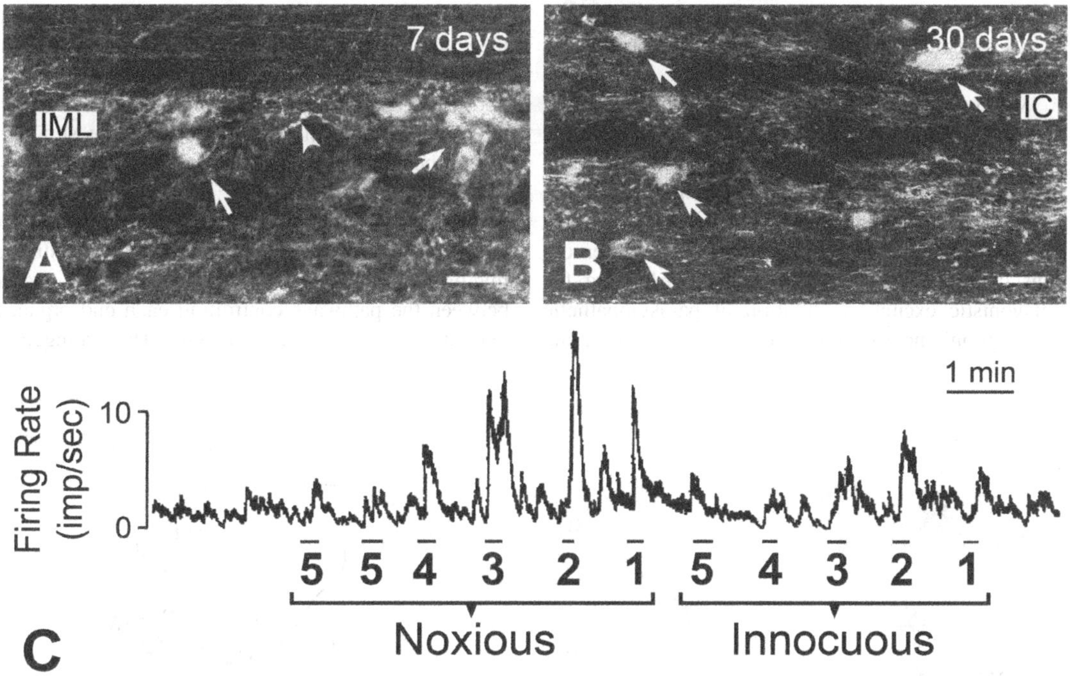


Figure 8–5 Spinal cord transection increases the number of GAP-43 immunoreactive neurons below the lesion and causes exaggerated sympathetic responses. Fluorescence micrographs of horizontal spinal cord sections with occasional neurons containing immunoreactivity for growth associated protein 43 (*arrows*) at 7 days after a complete spinal cord transection (*A*) and many more immunoreactive neurons at 30 days post-lesion (*B*). Scale bars, 50 μm. Modified from Weaver et al. (1997)[108], with permission. *C:* Responses of a sympathetic-correlated interneuron to noxious and innocuous cutaneous stimulation after an acute spinal transection, showing exaggerated response to these manipulations. Reproduced from Krassioukov et al. (2002)[40], with permission.

organs, so that a parasympathetic preganglionic neuron innervating the bladder will not also innervate the bowel. In most species, the anatomy of the parasympathetic outflow reflects this specificity, with parasympathetic preganglionic neurons terminating in ganglia near to, or within, the target organs. In rats and mice, however, parasympathetic post-ganglionic neurons are collected together into the major pelvic ganglion, which is unusual because it also contain sympathetic post-ganglionic neurons. Regardless of the location of parasympathetic post-ganglionic neurons, there is a precise orchestration of reflex function between the different end organs, and here the contribution of interneurons is immense. For example, an interneuron activated by a stimulus, such as bladder contraction, may exert its influence by inhibiting parasympathetic preganglionic neurons involved in bowel contraction rather than having a direct effect on efferent activity to the bladder.

Interneurons in the sacral spinal cord play major roles in a number of reflexes, including micturition, defecation, and sexual function. Each group of interneurons will be considered separately.

## Interneurons Involved in the Micturition Reflex and Defecation

*Micturition* is the reflex that empties urine from the bladder whilst *defecation* involves emptying of waste products from the bowel. Control of bladder and bowel function is extremely complex, with both spinal and supraspinal reflexes involved in storage and voiding. Both functions involve integration of parasympathetic excitatory inputs and sympathetic inhibitory inputs to the bladder and colorectum and coordination with motor outflow, which is critical for the control of sphincters. These autonomic reflexes are normally under voluntary control involving supraspinal pathways that utilize interneurons to orchestrate the appropriate response at the level of the spinal cord. A number of purely spinal pathways also contribute to the storage and release of waste. Thus, the role of specific interneurons in integrating the series of complex events associated with smooth action of the bladder and bowel is vital.

Micturition and defecation involve distinct spatially segregated populations of sympathetic preganglionic neurons, parasympathetic preganglionic neurons, and afferent terminations. Many of the neurons lying between the parasympathetic preganglionic neurons and sympathetic preganglionic neurons are interneurons that may be critical links in coordinating the antagonistic excitation/inhibition of parasympathetic preganglionic neurons involved in the micturition and defecation reflexes. Injection of pseudorabies virus into the colon labels interneurons in the IML, dorsal commissure (dorsal lamina X), and throughout the dorsal horn at thoracic level 13 to lumbar level 1 and lumbar level 6 to sacral level 1 segments in regions similar to those labeled from the bladder. However, labeling from the colon[105], the bladder[51,70,71,73,96,106], or indeed from both[83] demonstrates that, although there are many interneurons involved in mediating reflex control of micturition and defecation, there is little overlap between the pathways controlling each end organ, at least at the spinal level (Figure 8–6). This arrangement

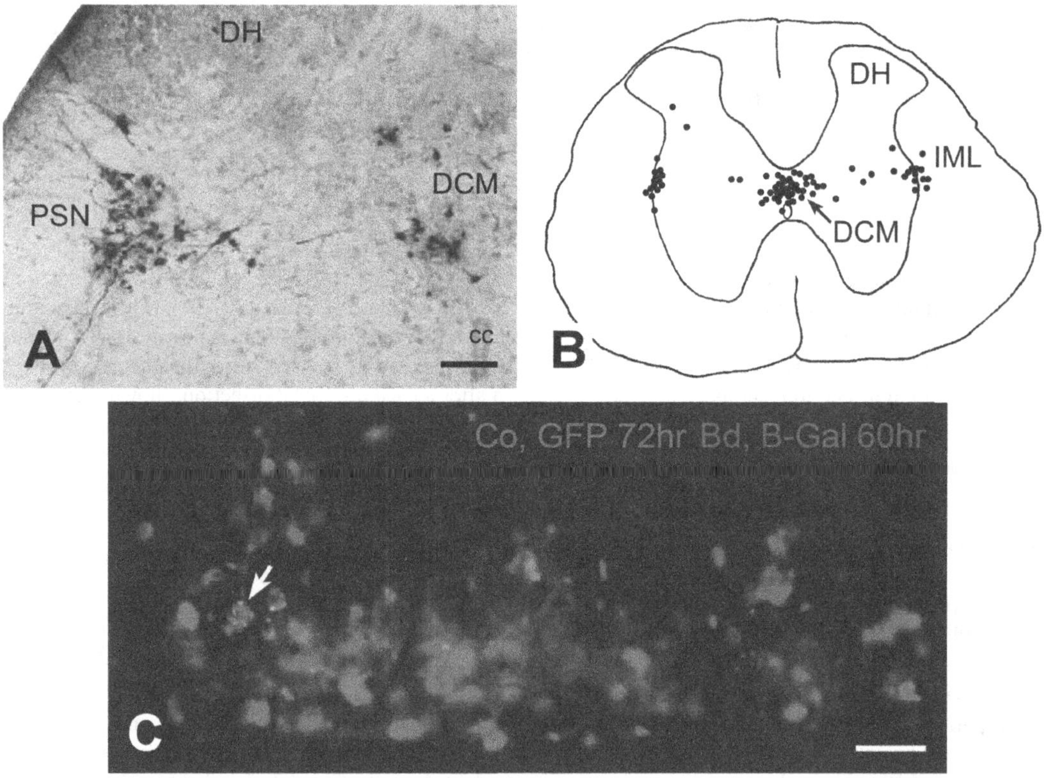


Figure 8–6 Comparison of the distribution of transneuronally labeled neurons after injection of pseudorabies virus into the urethra or bladder and colon. For a color version of Figure 8–6, see Color Plate 8–6 between pages 224 and 225. *A:* Light micrograph of transneuronally labeled neurons in the first sacral spinal segment after injection of pseudorabies virus into the colon. Scale bar, 150 μm. Modified from Vizzard et al. (2000)[105], with permission. cc, central canal; DCM, dorsal gray commissure; DH, dorsal horn; PSN, sacral parasympathetic nucleus. *B:* Line drawing illustrating the distribution of neurons in the first sacral spinal segment that were transneuronally labeled after virus injection into the urethra. DCM, dorsal gray commissure; DH, dorsal horn; IML, intermediolateral cell column;. Modified from Vizzard et al. (1995)[106], with permission. *C:* Injection of two different strains of pseudorabies virus into the bladder and colon results in rare double-labeled neurons (arrow) in the spinal cord. Bd, B-Gal 60H, Pseudorabies virus ß-galactosidase injected into bladder 60 hours prior to sacrifice; Co, GFP 72H, Pseudorabies virus green fluorescent protein injected into colon 72 hours prior to sacrifice. Scale bar, 30 μm. Reproduced from Rouzade Dominiguez et al. (2003)[83], with permission.

would prevent simultaneous excitation or inhibition of autonomic outflows by the activity of one interneuron.

Interneurons also appear to be the targets for sensory afferent input. Visceral afferents traveling via the pelvic nerve terminate in many regions, including the sacral parasympathetic nucleus; but afferents from the pudendal nerve[59,82,99] terminate more medially in laminae I–IV and dorsally in the dorsal commissure. Afferents travelling in the hypogastric nerve terminate in the lower lumbar regions of the spinal cord, mainly in the lateral parts of laminae I, V, and VII[68]. Thus, in the sacral cord, afferents generally do not terminate in regions containing parasympathetic preganglionic neurons and are therefore likely to target interneurons. Differences in the locations in which afferents terminate are likely to reflect the requirement to activate interneurons involved in specific components of different autonomic reflexes.

### *Interneurons in Spinal Pathways Controlling Bladder and Bowel Function*

Stimulation of bladder and urethral afferents induces Fos-immunoreactivity in the nuclei of activated interneurons involved in the micturition reflex, and these Fos-positive neurons occur in spinal cord laminae I, IV, V, and X[6–8]. Application of a chemical irritant to the bladder induces Fos expression in more neurons in the medial part of the dorsal horn, suggesting that different pathways are being activated[6]. The numbers and distribution of Fos-immunoreactive neurons are not affected by spinal cord transection, suggesting that these interneurons are involved in spinal reflex pathways. Colorectal distension in rats increases the number of Fos-positive neurons in laminae I–II, V–VII, and X of the lumbrosacral spinal cord, with the highest concentrations in lumbar level 6 and sacral level 1[6,103,114]. Since some of these labeled neurons may be interneurons involved in inhibiting one reflex while another reflex is active, it is impossible to segregate each reflex completely and study it in isolation. Hence, a series of sophisticated and complex experiments would be needed to identify an exact role for any single interneuron.

The actual spinal pathways involved in spinal reflex control of the bladder have been studied extensively (see Chapter 19). Transneuronal viral labeling and nerve lesions have identified a pathway in the pelvic nerve through which parasympathetic preganglionic neurons are first infected in the IML and then interneurons in the sixth lumbar to first sacral segments of the spinal cord. Afferent fibers that also travel in the pelvic nerve terminate close to these interneurons, which are located in the dorsal horn, dorsal commissure, and IML regions. This pathway may form the short spinal loop described from electrophysiological studies[49], which is observed in all spinalized rats and a smaller proportion of rats with intact cords. Spinal sympathetic pathways are more complex. Interneurons in the first and second lumbar segments form a local circuit at that level, while interneurons in lower lumbar and upper sacral levels may form part of a sacrolumbar intersegmental reflex arc involved in sympathetic control of the bladder. Thus, these pathways provide scope for specific control of interneurons that mediate different spinal components of the micturition reflex. Some of the interneurons in the sixth lumbar to first sacral segments may also be important for coordinating the antagonistic control of sympathetic and parasympathetic outflows.

Electrophysiological studies have identified sacral interneurons that are excited by stimulation of the pelvic nerve and to a lesser degree by stimulation of the hypogastric and lumbar colonic nerves[61]. Afferents from these nerves show a degree of convergence onto single interneurons, indicating that natural stimulation of either the bladder or the bowel can elicit both excitatory and inhibitory responses. De Groat and colleagues identified two common classes of interneurons[20]. The first class, including those excited by bladder distension and inhibited by distension of the colon, exhibit firing correlated with spontaneous bladder contractions. These interneurons are inhibited by stimulation of the reproductive organs, which also inhibits micturition. Since these interneurons exhibit varying levels of firing during bladder filling, they can be further subclassified. One subclass fires exclusively at the beginning of a bladder contraction, a pattern of activity similar to that of the parasympathetic preganglionic neurons. Hence, these interneurons may be involved in the descending excitatory pathway. The second main class are inhibited during spontaneous or evoked bladder contractions and excited by distension of the large intestine. These interneurons may be important in the inhibition of micturition during defecation. Both glycinergic and GABAergic interneurons may play a role in this inhibition, since in rats inhibition of the micturition reflex by rectal distension is reduced by intrathecal application of either strychnine or bicuculline and abolished by simultaneous application of these glycine- and GABA-receptor antagonists[66,67] Interestingly, at least a component of this inhibition may involve spinal circuits alone since similar effects are observed after spinal cord transection[66,67].

### *Role of Interneurons in Supraspinal Control of Bladder and Bowel Function*

Micturition also involves supraspinal circuits in which spinal interneurons play a part. Barrington's nucleus in the pons has a major influence on micturition.

Stimulation of this region directly excites parasympathetic preganglionic neurons controlling bladder contraction but also inhibits motor neurons innervating the external urethral sphincter muscles (see Chapter 19). Anterogradely labeled axons from Barrington's nucleus form close appositions with presumptive interneurons that lie dorsal to parasympathetic preganglionic neurons[111]. Stimulation of Barrington's nucleus also induces Fos expression in interneurons in similar regions of the spinal cord to those that show Fos-immunoreactivity after afferent stimulation[32], suggesting that interneurons receive convergent inputs from afferent and descending pathways that are integrated at the spinal level. Barrington's nucleus also has a role in colon function, since viral injection into the colon transneuronally labels populations of neurons in this region[104,105], and stimulation of this nucleus increases colonic intraluminal pressure[78]. What is unusual is the fact that dual transneuronal tracing reveals a proportion of neurons in Barrington's nucleus infected from both the colon and bladder[83]. Since in normal situations there is inverse control of these end organs, spinal interneurons may gate inputs from Barrington's nucleus to maintain this reciprocity[83].

Voiding of the bladder involves reciprocal contraction of the bladder and relaxation of the urethral sphincter due to simultaneous excitation of parasympathetic preganglionic neurons and inhibition of somatic motor neurons innervating the sphincter. Injections of different transneuronal viral tracers into the external urethral sphincter and the bladder do not result in double labeling of parasympathetic preganglionic neurons. The majority of interneurons are also singly labeled[72]. Thus, different groups of interneurons are activated to excite or inhibit parasympathetic preganglionic neurons and motor neurons to allow antagonistic responses. Blok et al. have described a group of GABAergic interneurons that receive input from Barrington's nucleus[10]. Since stimulation in this region decreases urethral pressure, these interneurons may inhibit motor neurons that control the sphincter[11]. A proportion of these interneurons may, in fact, contain both GABA and glycine[90] (Figure 8–7). A number of interneurons in the dorsal commissure, the IML, and the superficial dorsal horn can be labeled from viral injections into both the bladder and the sphincter[72]. Although the role of these interneurons is not clear, their existence highlights the complexity of the control that occurs at the level of the spinal cord to maintain continence.

Other pontine regions project directly to the spinal cord to inhibit micturition. These include the rostral pontine reticular formation and the subcoeruleus nucleus. These regions are transneuronally labeled following injections of virus into the bladder or urethra[73,96,106]. Stimulation of the rostral pontine reticular formation may inhibit bladder contraction by activating glycinergic spinal interneurons, since glutamate and glycine increase in the spinal cord after activation of this region[74]. The subcoeruleus nucleus (but not the rostral pontine reticular formation) may be vital for inhibiting bladder contraction during penile erection, since stimulation of this nucleus causes simultaneous increases in intracavernous pressure and inhibition of spontaneous bladder contractions[95]. Transection of the spinal cord abolishes bladder contractions and induces spontaneous increases in intracavernous pressure, suggesting that inhibition of penile erection is under tonic descending inhibitory control.

Other regions, such as the raphé nuclei that send serotonergic projections to the spinal cord, may also be important in bladder control. Electrical stimulation of raphé nuclei inhibits bladder contraction[62], so this region may be involved in urine storage. Stimulation of the raphé nuclei also causes penile contraction[48]. The bladder is inhibited when intracavernous pressure increases as a result of raphé stimulation[95], again suggesting reciprocal inhibition. These supraspinal pathways are likely to recruit spinal interneurons to coordinate such activity.

## INTERNEURONS INVOLVED IN SEXUAL REFLEXES

Like the bladder, the reproductive organs of both males and females are innervated by both sympathetic and parasympathetic branches of the autonomic nervous system and by somatic nerves. Sexual reflexes are complicated and involve a number of organs and phases that are described in detail in Chapter 20. Since this cycle needs precise synchronization of the autonomic and motor outflows and concomitant inhibition of bladder and lower bowel, the role of interneurons in coordinating sexual responses is crucial.

Injections of transneuronal viral tracers into the bulbospongiosus and ischiocavernosus muscles of the penis[55,113] or the corpus cavernosus[56] in male rats, or into the clitoris[50] or uterine cervix[77] in female rats, label many interneurons in the lateral horn and in lamina X in the thirteenth thoracic to second lumbar and in the sixth lumbar to first sacral spinal segments. Surprisingly, few interneurons are labeled in the dorsal or ventral horns, unlike the labeling pattern from the bladder and bowel. Interneurons labeled from the prostate are located mainly in the dorsal gray commissure and the IML[53,75], both ipsilateral and contralateral to the injection site, suggesting that control of the two prostate glands is achieved by activation of interneurons with axons that cross in the spinal cord.

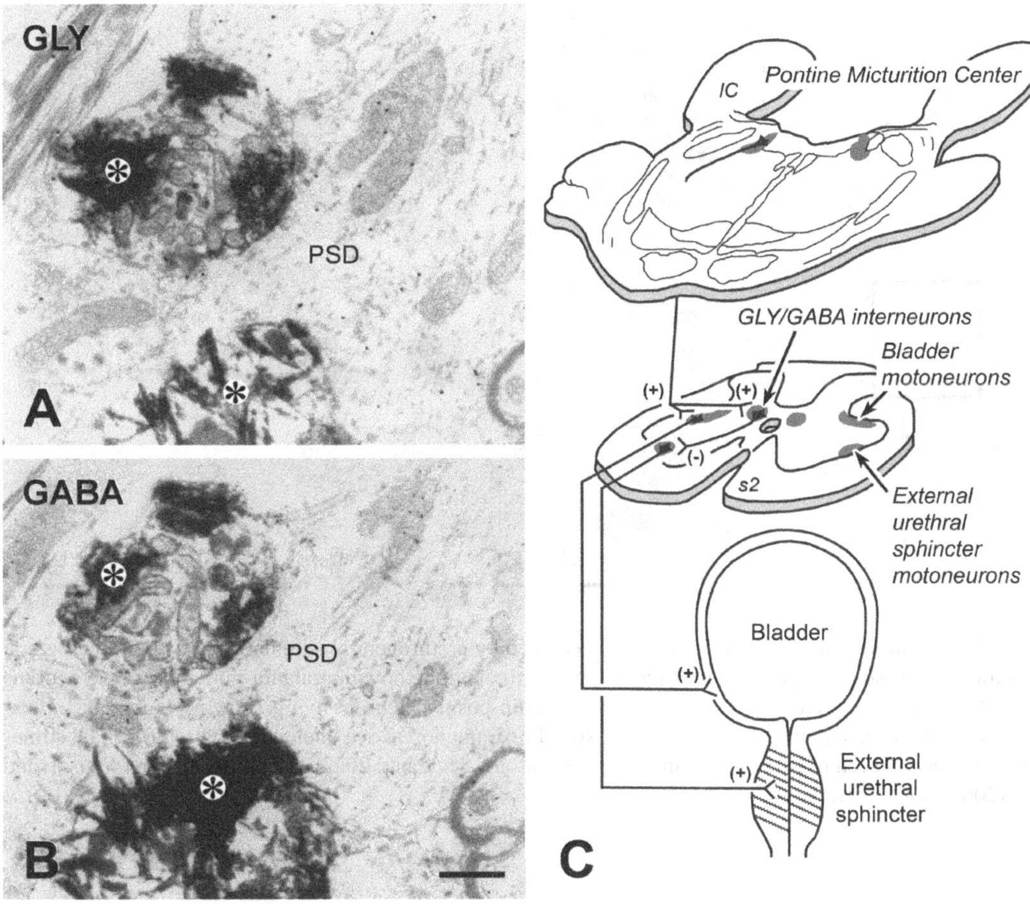


Figure 8–7 Activation of the pontine micturition center (which includes Barrington's nucleus) activates GABA/glycinergic interneurons that inhibit sphincter motor neurons. Electron micrographs of adjacent ultrathin sections of spinal cord showing that terminals anterogradely labeled after injections into the pontine micturition center (including Barrington's nucleus; *asterisks*) contact a dendrite that is immunoreactive for both GABA (*A*) and glycine (GLY, *B*). Scale bar, 500 nm. *C:* Line diagram showing the pathway from the pontine micturition center (including Barrington's nucleus) through these GLY/GABA interneurons in the spinal cord to the external urethral sphincter. (+), excitatory connection; (–), inhibitory connection. Modified from Sie et al. (2001)[90], with permission.

Injections of two different transneuronal tracers into the prostate and bladder label separate groups of preganglionic neurons[69], and there is a degree of segregation of interneurons. However, there is a small but significant number of doubly infected interneurons in the IML region of upper lumbar spinal cord and in the parasympathetic nucleus and dorsal gray commissure in lumbar segment 6 and sacral segment 1. Although the role of these double-labeled interneurons is unclear, they are likely to be activated only in exceptional circumstances.

### Functional Evidence

Stimulation of the pudendal and perineal nerves elicits field potentials in regions of the spinal cord containing interneurons, including laminae V, VI, and X in sacral spinal segments 1–3[29]. In both male and female rats, stimulating genital afferents or the urethra induces Fos-immunoreactivity in spinal cord regions, including the medial dorsal horn, dorsal gray commissure, and IML (Figure 8–8; [9,52,54,81]). Although these studies cannot determine the likelihood of information converging onto one interneuron,

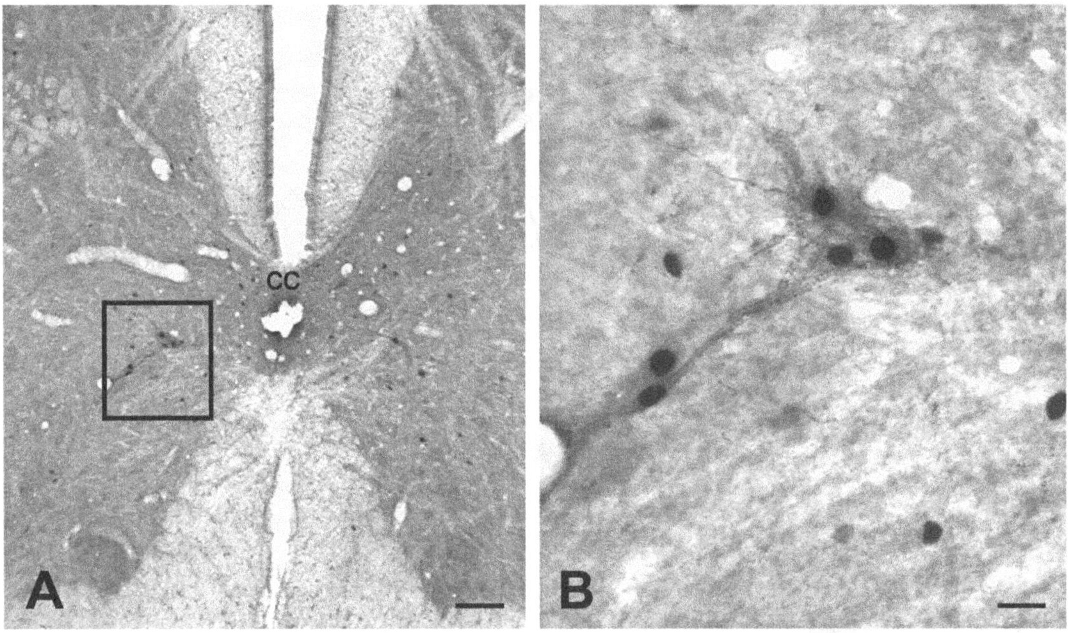


Figure 8–8 Galanin-immunoreactive neurons are activated by urethrogenital stimulation. *A:* Light micrograph of the third lumbar spinal segment after urethrogenital stimulation showing galanin-immunoreactive neurons lateral to the central canal. The *box* drawn around the galanin-positive neurons in *A* is shown at higher magnification in *B*. cc, central canal. Scale bar, 100 μm. *B:* Now, Fos-immunoreactive nuclei due to urethrogenital stimulation can be clearly seen in galanin-immunoreactive neurons. Scale bar, 20 μm. Reproduced from Marson and Gravitt (2004)[54], with permission.

single-cell recordings in cats have shown that stimulation of the perineum or pelvic viscera activates neurons in lamina X. Some of these neurons have local axon arborizations[35] and receive convergent information from somatic and visceral afferents from both sides of the body. These observations indicate a high degree of complex coordination through these interneurons.

These studies and others suggest that much of the circuitry controlling sexual activity is at the spinal level. Inputs from sensory receptors elicit spinal reflex activity, which is influenced by supraspinal excitation and inhibition. The nucleus paragigantocellularis projects not only to motor neurons but also to interneurons[52]. Lesions of this region allow the coitus reflex to occur after urethral distension, indicating a robust inhibitory control from this region in intact rats. During sexual activity, simultaneous sensory activation of the sex organs decreases this inhibitory input, disinhibiting interneurons so that sexual reflexes can occur. Thus, interneurons also provide an important integration center for control of sexual reflexes.

## GENERAL PROPERTIES AND NEUROCHEMISTRY OF INTERNEURONS IN PARASYMPATHETIC CONTROL OF UNSPECIFIED FUNCTIONS

Although mention has been made of the role of specific spinal interneurons in micturition, defecation, and reproductive reflexes, many studies have looked more generally at the properties of sacral interneurons without focus on their possible function.

Araki and de Groat classified responses of parasympathetic preganglionic neurons to extracellular stimulation of interneurons in specific regions of the sacral spinal cord[1,2]. By labeling parasympathetic preganglionic neurons with fluorescent tracer applied to the cut pelvic nerve, it was possible to record from single parasympathetic preganglionic neurons and stimulate a single unlabeled interneuron that lay within 100 μm of the recorded neurons. The postsynaptic responses were monosynaptic and appeared unitary. The nature of the excitatory response, such as synaptic efficacy (see Figure 8–9), was dependent on whether the stimulating site was dorsal or medial to the recorded preganglionic neuron. The locations of dorsal interneurons corresponded well with the termination sites of primary afferent inputs to the sacral spinal cord, indicating a possible role for the interneurons in specific spinal parasympathetic reflexes. The main site of interneurons that elicited inhibitory responses was dorsomedial to parasympathetic preganglionic neurons[1,59,92].

### Excitatory Interneurons

Araki and de Groat[2] provide clear evidence that glutamatergic interneurons in both dorsal and medial regions monosynaptically innervate parasympathetic preganglionic neurons. These inputs are mediated by both *N*-methyl-D-aspartate (NMDA) and non-NMDA receptors (Figure 8–9). Many substance P-immunoreactive neurons that show Fos-immunoreactivity following irritation of the bladder are located in and around the sacral parasympathetic nucleus, which contains the cell bodies of parasympathetic preganglionic neurons[47]. Although the Fos-positive neurons were not proved unequivocally to be innervating parasympathetic preganglionic neurons, they are likely to form a subset of the excitatory interneurons that are known to influence the activity of parasympathetic preganglionic neurons. The substance P-immunoreactive neurons may also contain and release glutamate and play an important role in mediating afferent inputs. Many other neuropeptide transmitters occur in interneurons in regions of the sacral spinal cord that are involved in parasympathetic control[85]. These peptides include enkephalin, dynorphin, somatostatin, cholecystokinin, galanin, and vasoactive intestinal peptide. Urethrogenital stimulation increases Fos-immunoreactivity in galanin-immunoreactive interneurons, implicating this neuropeptide in the control of sexual reflexes [54] (Figure 8–8).

### Inhibitory Interneurons

IPSCs elicited by stimulation of interneurons mediodorsal to parasympathetic preganglionic neurons[1] are partially blocked by strychnine and abolished by further applications of bicuculline. This finding suggests that either more than one inhibitory interneuron was being activated or that GABA and glycine are co-localized in the same interneuron. Inhibitory interneurons are also likely to contain at least some of the neuropeptides mentioned above, although double labeling to confirm this has not yet been performed. Neuropeptide Y is often expressed in GABAergic interneurons, and high numbers of interneurons expressing mRNA for neuropeptide Y are located dorsal to the central canal in the sacral spinal cord[64]. This observation suggests a role for neuropeptide Y-expressing interneurons in parasympathetic control, but the precise function of this subgroup of interneurons is not known.

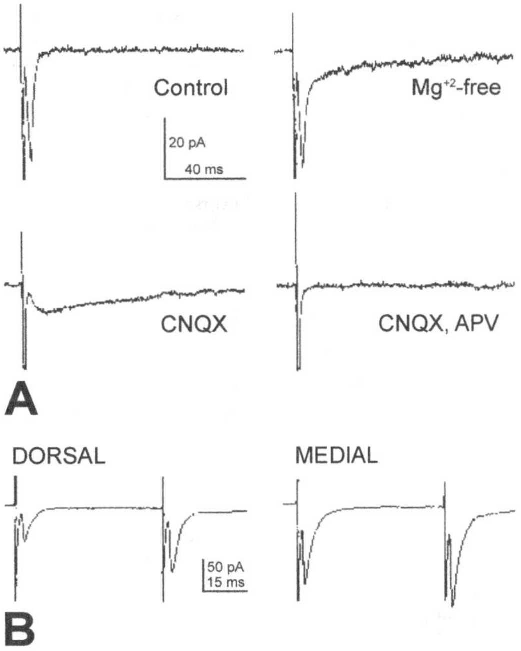


Figure 8–9 Responses of parasympathetic preganglionic neurons to stimulation of adjacent interneurons. *A:* Excitatory postsynaptic currents (EPSCs) elicited in a parasympathetic preganglionic neuron in response to stimulation of an interneuron in the vicinity of the recording site. EPSCs are reduced by the non-NMDA antagonist, 6-cyano-7-nitroquinoxaline-2,3-dione (CNQX) in control conditions. In $Mg^{2+}$ free solution, a later component is unmasked that is reduced in amplitude by the NMDA receptor antagonist, 2-amino-5-phosphonovaleric acid (APV). *B:* Responses of a single parasympathetic preganglionic neuron to stimulation of interneurons in two different regions, dorsal and medial to the recording site. The paired pulse ratio of the EPSCs elicited from the two regions differs, suggesting varying synaptic efficacies. Reproduced from Araki and de Groat (1996)[2], with permission.

## CONCLUDING REMARKS

This chapter has reviewed the existing evidence for interneurons as crucial components of the spinal cord circuitry involved in autonomic control. Table 8–1 and Figure 8–10 summarize the known similarities and

Table 8–1. Comparison of Properties of Spinal Interneurons Involved in Controlling Sympathetic and Parasympathetic Outflow

| Property | Sympathetic Interneurons | Parasympathetic Interneurons |
|---|---|---|
| **Descending inputs** | yes | yes |
| **Afferent inputs** | yes | yes |
| **Neurochemistry** | Diverse<br>*Correlation with function unknown* | Diverse<br>*May be some functional correlation; e.g., galanin involved in sexual reflexes* |
| **Function** | Not definitely known.<br>*May serve more than one function* | Normally limited to one function; e.g., bladder control |
| **Inhibitory interneurons?** | yes | yes |
| **Excitatory interneurons?** | yes | yes |
| **Location** | Laminae V, VII, X, IML | Bladder and bowel— Laminae I–II, V–VII, X, IML<br>Sexual organs— Less widespread, more in lamina X and IML |
| **Ongoing Activity** | Correlated with sympathetic activity; Can be correlated with cardiac rhythm | Wide range of spike firing frequencies |
| **Respond to Noxious Stimulation** | yes | yes |

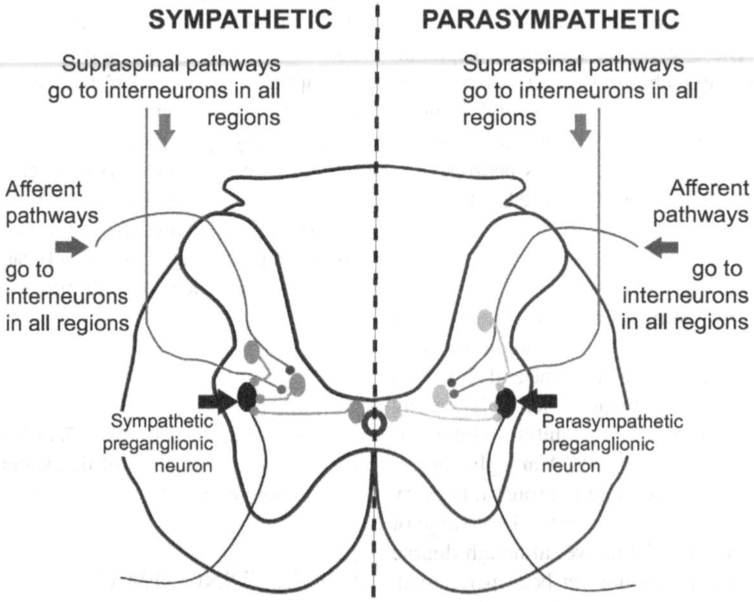


Figure 8–10 Locations and inputs to sympathetic and parasympathetic interneurons. The diagram shows some (but not all) of the locations of sympathetic and parasympathetic interneurons and their innervation by afferent and descending pathways. For simplicity, inputs to all interneurons have not been shown. However, interneurons in each location are likely to receive afferent and descending inputs.

differences between spinal interneurons involved in sympathetic and parasympathetic control. Nevertheless, there is still much to be learned about both groups of interneurons. Spinal autonomic interneurons integrate information and help coordinate the precise and complex control of autonomic outflow to many end organs. Indeed, the impact of autonomic interneurons in both transected and intact spinal systems is yet to be fully appreciated and should form the basis for many future studies.

On that note, it is important that future studies should not infer that so-called autonomic interneurons only play a role in control of autonomic outflow, since there may be integration involving other motor outflows. Such integration occurs in the pedunculopontine tegmental nucleus and lateral hypothalamus[38,41], so why not at the level of the spinal cord? The extensive dendritic arborizations of spinal autonomic interneurons may reflect the presence of a plethora of inputs from a variety of sources onto one neuron. Such a diversity of input would allow a spinal interneuron to play a more global regulatory role. Some spinal interneurons may also be vital in orchestrating autonomic components of responses to, for example, pain, and so may have roles in addition to those mediating conventional autonomic reflexes. Much still needs to be learned before we fully understand how spinal interneurons participate in the many circuits that control overall autonomic outflow. A major aim of this chapter is to inspire further work to increase that understanding.

ACKNOWLEDGEMENTS I would like to thank Jim Deuchars for his critical input to this chapter, and to all the people, past and present, who have contributed to our research on interneurons. The generous support of the British Heart Foundation and The Wellcome Trust is gratefully acknowledged.

## References

1. Araki, I. (1994). Inhibitory postsynaptic currents and the effects of GABA on visually identified sacral parasympathetic preganglionic neurons in neonatal rats. *Journal of Neurophysiology* 72, 2903–2910.
2. Araki, I., and de Groat, W. C. (1996). Unitary excitatory synaptic currents in preganglionic neurons mediated by two distinct groups of interneurons in neonatal rat sacral parasympathetic nucleus. *Journal of Neurophysiology* 76, 215–226.
3. Bacon, S. J., and Smith, A. D. (1993). A monosynaptic pathway from an identified vasomotor centre in the medial prefrontal cortex to an autonomic area in the thoracic spinal cord. *Neuroscience* 54, 719–728.
4. Barber, R. P., Phelps, P. E., Houser, C. R., Crawford, G. D., Salvaterra, P. M., and Vaughn, J. E. (1984). The morphology and distribution of neurons containing choline acetyltransferase in the adult rat spinal cord: An immunocytochemical study. *The Journal of Comparative Neurology* 229, 329–346.
5. Barman, S. M., and Gebber, G. L. (1984). Spinal interneurons with sympathetic nerve-related activity. *American Journal of Physiology* 247, R761–R767.
6. Birder, L. A., and de Groat, W. C. (1993). Induction of c-Fos expression in spinal neurons by nociceptive and nonnociceptive stimulation of LUT. *American Journal of Physiology* 265, R326–R333.
7. Birder, L. A., and de Groat, W. C. (1992). Increased c-Fos expression in spinal neurons after irritation of the lower urinary tract in the rat. *The Journal of Neuroscience* 12, 4878–4889.
8. Birder, L. A., Roppolo, J. R., Erickson, V. L., and de Groat, W. C. (1999). Increased c-Fos expression in spinal lumbosacral projection neurons and preganglionic neurons after irritation of the lower urinary tract in the rat. *Brain Research* 834, 55–65.
9. Birder, L. A., Roppolo, J. R., Iadarola, M. J., and de Groat, W. C. (1991). Electrical stimulation of visceral afferent pathways in the pelvic nerve increases c-Fos in the rat lumbosacral spinal cord. *Neuroscience Letters* 129, 193–196.
10. Blok, B. F., de Weerd, H., and Holstege, G. (1997). The pontine micturition center projects to sacral cord GABA immunoreactive neurons in the cat. *Neuroscience Letters* 233, 109–112.
11. Blok, B. F., van Maarseveen, J. T., and Holstege, G. (1998). Electrical stimulation of the sacral dorsal gray commissure evokes relaxation of the external urethral sphincter in the cat. *Neuroscience Letters* 249, 68–70.
12. Bordey, A., Feltz, P., and Trouslard, J. (1996). Nicotinic actions on neurones of the central autonomic area in rat spinal cord slices. *Journal of Physiology* 497, 175–187.
13. Brooke, R. E., Deuchars, J., and Deuchars, S. A. (2004). Input-specific modulation of neurotransmitter release in the lateral horn of the spinal cord via adenosine receptors. *Journal of Neuroscience* 24, 127–137.
14. Brooke, R. E., Pyner, S., McLeish, P., Buchan, S., Deuchars, J., and Deuchars, S. A. (2002). Spinal cord interneurones labelled transneuronally from the adrenal gland by a GFP-herpes virus construct contain the potassium channel subunit Kv3.1b. *Autonomic Neuroscience: Basic and Clinical* 98, 45–50.

15. Cabot, J. B., Alessi, V., Carroll, J., and Ligorio, M. (1994). Spinal cord lamina V and lamina VII interneuronal projections to sympathetic preganglionic neurons. *Journal of Comparative Neurology* 347, 515–530.
16. Cammack, C., and Logan, S. D. (1996). Excitation of rat sympathetic preganglionic neurones by selective activation of the NK1 receptor. *Journal of the Autonomic Nervous System* 57, 87–92.
17. Chau, D., Johns, D. G., and Schramm, L. P. (2000). Ongoing and stimulus-evoked activity of sympathetically correlated neurons in the intermediate zone and dorsal horn of acutely spinalized rats. *Journal of Neurophysiology* 83, 2699–2707.
18. Chen, H. K., and Su, C. K. (2006). Endogenous activation of nicotinic receptors underlies sympathetic tone generation in neonatal rat spinal cord in vitro. *Neuropharmacology* 51, 1120–1128.
19. Craig, A. D. (1993). Propriospinal input to thoracolumbar sympathetic nuclei from cervical and lumbar lamina I neurons in the cat and the monkey. *Journal of Comparative Neurology* 331, 517–530.
20. De Groat, W. C., Nadelhaft, I., Milne, R. J., Booth, A. M., Morgan, C., and Thor, K. (1981). Organization of the sacral parasympathetic reflex pathways to the urinary bladder and large intestine. *Journal of the Autonomic Nervous System* 3, 135–160.
21. Dembowsky, K., Czachurski, J., and Seller, H. (1985). An intracellular study of the synaptic input to sympathetic preganglionic neurones of the third thoracic segment of the cat. *Journal of the Autonomic Nervous System* 13, 201–244.
22. Deuchars, S. A., Brooke, R. E., and Deuchars, J. (2001). Adenosine A1 receptors reduce release from excitatory but not inhibitory synaptic inputs onto lateral horn neurons. *Journal of Neuroscience* 21, 6308–6320.
23. Deuchars, S. A., Brooke, R. E., Frater, B., and Deuchars, J. (2001). Properties of interneurones in the intermediolateral cell column of the rat spinal cord: Role of the potassium channel subunit Kv3.1. *Neuroscience* 106, 433–446.
24. Deuchars, S. A., Milligan, C. J., Stornetta, R. L., and Deuchars, J. (2005). GABAergic neurons in the central region of the spinal cord: A novel substrate for sympathetic inhibition. *Journal of Neuroscience* 25, 1063–1070.
25. Deuchars, S. A., Morrison, S. F., and Gilbey, M. P. (1995). Medullary-evoked EPSPs in neonatal rat sympathetic preganglionic neurones in vitro. *Journal of Physiology* 487, 453–463.
26. Deuchars, S. A., Spyer, K. M., Brooks, P. A., and Gilbey, M. P. (1995). A study of sympathetic preganglionic neuronal activity in a neonatal rat brainstem-spinal cord preparation. *Journal of the Autonomic Nervous System* 52, 51–63.
27. Dun, N. J., and Mo, N. (1988). In vitro effects of substance P on neonatal rat sympathetic preganglionic neurones. *Journal of Physiology* 399, 321–333.
28. Dun, N. J., and Mo, N. (1989). Inhibitory postsynaptic potentials in neonatal rat sympathetic preganglionic neurones in vitro. *Journal of Physiology* 410, 267–281.
29. Fedirchuk, B., Song, L., Downie, J. W., and Shefchyk, S. J. (1992). Spinal distribution of extracellular field potentials generated by electrical stimulation of pudendal and perineal afferents in the cat. *Experimental Brain Research* 89, 517–520.
30. Gebber, G. L., and McCall, R. B. (1976). Identification and discharge patterns of spinal sympathetic interneurons. *American Journal of Physiology* 231, 722–733.
31. Gibson, I. C., and Logan, S. D. (1995). Effects of muscarinic receptor stimulation of sympathetic preganglionic neurones of neonatal rat spinal cord in vitro. *Neuropharmacology* 34, 309–318.
32. Grill, W. M., Wang, B., Hadziefendic, S., and Haxhiu, M. A. (1998). Identification of the spinal neural network involved in coordination of micturition in the male cat. *Brain Research* 796, 150–160.
33. Hara, K., Miyawaki, T., Minson, J., Arnolda, L., Llewellyn-Smith, I., Chalmers, J., and Pilowsky, P. (1997). Role of spinal GABA receptors in depressor responses to chemical stimulation of the A5 area in normal and hypertensive rats. *Journal of the Autonomic Nervous System* 66, 53–61.
34. Hofstetter, C. P., Card, J. P., and Olson, L. (2005). A spinal cord pathway connecting primary afferents to the segmental sympathetic outflow system. *Experimental Neurology* 194, 128–138.
35. Honda, C. N. (1985). Visceral and somatic afferent convergence onto neurons near the central canal in the sacral spinal cord of the cat. *Journal of Neurophysiology* 53, 1059–1078.
36. Janig, W. (1988). Pre- and postganglionic vasoconstrictor neurons: Differentiation, types, and discharge properties. *Annual Review of Physiology* 50, 525–539.
37. Janig, W., and Spilok, N. (1978). Functional organization of the sympathetic innervation supplying the hairless skin of the hindpaws in chronic spinal cats. *Pflugers Archives* 377, 25–31.
38. Jansen, A. S., Wessendorf, M. W., and Loewy, A. D. (1995). Transneuronal labeling of CNS neuropeptide and monoamine neurons after pseudorabies

virus injections into the stellate ganglion. *Brain Research* 683, 1–24.

39. Joshi, S., Levatte, M. A., Dekaban, G. A., and Weaver, L. C. (1995). Identification of spinal interneurons antecedent to adrenal sympathetic preganglionic neurons using trans-synaptic transport of herpes simplex virus type 1. *Neuroscience* 65, 893–903.
40. Krassioukov, A. V., Johns, D. G., and Schramm, L. P. (2002). Sensitivity of sympathetically correlated spinal interneurons, renal sympathetic nerve activity, and arterial pressure to somatic and visceral stimuli after chronic spinal injury. *Journal of Neurotrauma* 19, 1521–1529.
41. Krout, K. E., Mettenleiter, T. C., and Loewy, A. D. (2003). Single CNS neurons link both central motor and cardiosympathetic systems: A double-virus tracing study. *Neuroscience* 118, 853–866.
42. Krupp, J., and Feltz, P. (1993). Synaptic- and agonist-induced chloride currents in neonatal rat sympathetic preganglionic neurones in vitro. *Journal of Physiology* 471, 729–748.
43. Lewis, D. I., and Coote, J. H. (1993). Angiotensin II in the spinal cord of the rat and its sympatho-excitatory effects. *Brain Research* 614, 1–9.
44. Lewis, D. I., Sermasi, E., and Coote, J. H. (1993). Excitatory and indirect inhibitory actions of 5-hydroxytryptamine on sympathetic preganglionic neurones in the neonate rat spinal cord in vitro. *Brain Research* 610, 267–275.
45. Llewellyn-Smith, I. J., Dicarlo, S. E., Collins, H. L., and Keast, J. R. (2005). Enkephalin-immunoreactive interneurons extensively innervate sympathetic preganglionic neurons regulating the pelvic viscera. *Journal of Comparative Neurology* 488, 278–289.
46. Llewellyn-Smith, I. J., and Weaver, L. C. (2001). Changes in synaptic inputs to sympathetic preganglionic neurons after spinal cord injury. *Journal of Comparative Neurology* 435, 226–240.
47. Lu, Y., Jin, S. X., Xu, T. L., Qin, B. Z., Li, J. S., Ding, Y. Q., Shigemoto, R., and Mizuno, N. (1995). Expression of c-Fos protein in substance P receptor-like immunoreactive neurons in response to noxious stimuli on the urinary bladder: An observation in the lumbosacral cord segments of the rat. *Neuroscience Letters* 198, 139–142.
48. Maeda, N., Matsuoka, N., and Yamaguchi, I. (1994). Role of the dopaminergic, serotonergic and cholinergic link in the expression of penile erection in rats. *Japanese Journal of Pharmacology* 66, 59–66.
49. Mallory, B., Steers, W. D., and de Groat, W. C. (1989). Electrophysiological study of micturition reflexes in rats. *American Journal of Physiology* 257, R410–R421.
50. Marson, L. (1995). Central nervous system neurons identified after injection of pseudorabies virus into the rat clitoris. *Neuroscience Letters* 190, 41–44.
51. Marson, L. (1997). Identification of central nervous system neurons that innervate the bladder body, bladder base, or external urethral sphincter of female rats: A transneuronal tracing study using pseudorabies virus. *Journal of Comparative Neurology* 389, 584–602.
52. Marson, L., Cai, R., and Makhanova, N. (2003). Identification of spinal neurons involved in the urethrogenital reflex in the female rat. *Journal of Comparative Neurology* 462, 355–370.
53. Marson, L., and Carson, C. C. (1999). Central nervous system innervation of the penis, prostate, and perineal muscles: A transneuronal tracing study. *Molecular Urology* 3, 43–50.
54. Marson, L., and Gravitt, K. (2004). Spinal neurons activated with the urethrogenital reflex in the male rat. *Brain Research* 1026, 108–115.
55. Marson, L., and McKenna, K. E. (1996). CNS cell groups involved in the control of the ischiocavernosus and bulbospongiosus muscles: A transneuronal tracing study using pseudorabies virus. *Journal of Comparative Neurology* 374, 161–179.
56. Marson, L., Platt, K. B., and McKenna, K. E. (1993). Central nervous system innervation of the penis as revealed by the transneuronal transport of pseudorabies virus. *Neuroscience* 55, 263–280.
57. Mathias, C. J., and Frankel, H. L. (1983). Clinical manifestations of malfunctioning sympathetic mechanisms in tetraplegia. *Journal of the Autonomic Nervous System* 7, 303–312.
58. McCall, R. B., Gebber, G. L., and Barman, S. M. (1977). Spinal interneurons in the baroreceptor reflex arc. *American Journal of Physiology* 232, H657–H665.
59. McKenna, K. E., and Nadelhaft, I. (1986). The organization of the pudendal nerve in the male and female rat. *Journal of Comparative Neurology* 248, 532–549.
60. McKenna, K. E., and Schramm, L. P. (1983). Sympathetic preganglionic neurons in the isolated spinal cord of the neonatal rat. *Brain Research* 269, 201–210.
61. McMahon, S. B., and Morrison, J. F. (1982). Two group of spinal interneurones that respond to stimulation of the abdominal viscera of the cat. *Journal of Physiology* 322, 21–34.
62. McMahon, S. B., and Spillane, K. (1982). Brain stem influences on the parasympathetic supply to the urinary bladder of the cat. *Brain Research* 234, 237–249.

63. Miller, C. O., Johns, D. G., and Schramm, L. P. (2001). Spinal interneurons play a minor role in generating ongoing renal sympathetic nerve activity in spinally intact rats. *Brain Research* 918, 101–106.
64. Minson, J. B., Llewellyn-Smith, I. J., and Arnolda, L. F. (2001). Neuropeptide Y mRNA expression in interneurons in rat spinal cord. *Autonomic Neuroscience: Basic and Clinical* 93, 14–20.
65. Miyazaki, T., Coote, J. H., and Dun, N. J. (1989). Excitatory and inhibitory effects of epinephrine on neonatal rat sympathetic preganglionic neurons in vitro. *Brain Research* 497, 108–116.
66. Miyazato, M., Sugaya, K., Nishijima, S., Ashitomi, K., Ohyama, C., and Ogawa, Y. (2004). Rectal distention inhibits bladder activity via glycinergic and GABAergic mechanisms in rats. *Journal of Urology* 171, 1353–1356.
67. Miyazato, M., Sugaya, K., Nishijima, S., Morozumi, M., Ohyama, C., and Ogawa, Y. (2005). Rectal distention inhibits the spinal micturition reflex via glycinergic or GABAergic mechanisms in rats with spinal cord injury. *Urology International* 74, 160–165.
68. Morgan, C., de Groat, W. C., and Nadelhaft, I. (1986). The spinal distribution of sympathetic preganglionic and visceral primary afferent neurons that send axons into the hypogastric nerves of the cat. *Journal of Comparative Neurology* 243, 23–40.
69. Nadelhaft, I., Miranda-Sousa, A. J., and Vera, P. L. (2002). Separate urinary bladder and prostate neurons in the central nervous system of the rat: Simultaneous labeling with two immunohistochemically distinguishable pseudorabies viruses. *BioMed Central Neuroscience* 3, 8.
70. Nadelhaft, I., and Vera, P. L. (1995). Central nervous system neurons infected by pseudorabies virus injected into the rat urinary bladder following unilateral transection of the pelvic nerve. *Journal of Comparative Neurology* 359, 443–456.
71. Nadelhaft, I., and Vera, P. L. (1996). Neurons in the rat brain and spinal cord labeled after pseudorabies virus injected into the external urethral sphincter. *Journal of Comparative Neurology* 375, 502–517.
72. Nadelhaft, I., and Vera, P. L. (2001). Separate urinary bladder and external urethral sphincter neurons in the central nervous system of the rat: Simultaneous labeling with two immunohistochemically distinguishable pseudorabies viruses. *Brain Research* 903, 33–44.
73. Nadelhaft, I., Vera, P. L., Card, J. P., and Miselis, R. R. (1992). Central nervous system neurons labelled following the injection of pseudorabies virus into the rat urinary bladder. *Neuroscience Letters* 143, 271–274.
74. Nishijima, S., Sugaya, K., Miyazato, M., Shimabukuro, S., Morozumi, M., and Ogawa, Y. (2005). Activation of the rostral pontine reticular formation increases the spinal glycine level and inhibits bladder contraction in rats. *Journal of Urology* 173, 1812–1816.
75. Orr, R., and Marson, L. (1998). Identification of CNS neurons innervating the rat prostate: A transneuronal tracing study using pseudorabies virus. *Journal of the Autonomic Nervous System* 72, 4–15.
76. Pan, B., Kim, E. J., and Schramm, L. P. (2005). Increased close appositions between corticospinal tract axons and spinal sympathetic neurons after spinal cord injury in rats. *Journal of Neurotrauma* 22, 1399–1410.
77. Papka, R. E., Williams, S., Miller, K. E., Copelin, T., and Puri, P. (1998). CNS location of uterine-related neurons revealed by trans-synaptic tracing with pseudorabies virus and their relation to estrogen receptor-immunoreactive neurons. *Neuroscience* 84, 935–952.
78. Pavcovich, L. A., Yang, M., Miselis, R. R., and Valentino, R. J. (1998). Novel role for the pontine micturition center, Barrington's nucleus: Evidence for coordination of colonic and forebrain activity. *Brain Research* 784, 355–361.
79. Petras, J. M., and Cummings, J. F. (1972). Autonomic neurons in the spinal cord of the rhesus monkey: A correlation of the findings of cytoarchitectonics and sympathectomy with fiber degeneration following dorsal rhizotomy. *Journal of Comparative Neurology* 146, 189–218.
80. Polgar, E., Shehab, S. A., Watt, C., and Todd, A. J. (1999). GABAergic neurons that contain neuropeptide Y selectively target cells with the neurokinin 1 receptor in laminae III and IV of the rat spinal cord. *Journal of Neuroscience* 19, 2637–2646.
81. Rampin, O., Gougis, S., Giuliano, F., and Rousseau, J. P. (1997). Spinal Fos labeling and penile erection elicited by stimulation of dorsal nerve of the rat penis. *American Journal of Physiology* 272, R1425–R1431.
82. Roppolo, J. R., Nadelhaft, I., and de Groat, W. C. (1985). The organization of pudendal motoneurons and primary afferent projections in the spinal cord of the rhesus monkey revealed by horseradish peroxidase. *Journal of Comparative Neurology* 234, 475–488.
83. Rouzade-Dominguez, M. L., Miselis, R., and Valentino, R. J. (2003). Central representation of bladder and colon revealed by dual transsynaptic

tracing in the rat: Substrates for pelvic visceral coordination. *European Journal of Neuroscience* 18, 3311–3324.

84. Ruggiero, D. A., Anwar, M., Kim, J., Sica, A. L., Gootman, N., and Gootman, P. M. (1997). Induction of c-Fos gene expression by spinal cord transection in the rat. *Brain Research* 763, 21–29.
85. Sasek, C. A., Seybold, V. S., and Elde, R. P. (1984). The immunohistochemical localization of nine peptides in the sacral parasympathetic nucleus and the dorsal gray commissure in rat spinal cord. *Neuroscience* 12, 855–873.
86. Sermasi, E., and Coote, J. H. (1994). Oxytocin acts at V1 receptors to excite sympathetic preganglionic neurones in neonate rat spinal cord in vitro. *Brain Research* 647, 323–332.
87. Shen, E., and Dun, N. J. (1990). Neonate rat sympathetic preganglionic neurons intracellularly labelled with lucifer yellow in thin spinal cord slices. *Journal of the Autonomic Nervous System* 29, 247–254.
88. Shen, E., Mo, N., and Dun, N. J. (1990). APV-sensitive dorsal root afferent transmission to neonate rat sympathetic preganglionic neurons in vitro. *Journal of Neurophysiology* 64, 991–999.
89. Sherriff, F. E., Henderson, Z., and Morrison, J. F. (1991). Further evidence for the absence of a descending cholinergic projection from the brainstem to the spinal cord in the rat. *Neuroscience Letters* 128, 52–56.
90. Sie, J. A., Blok, B. F., de Weerd, H., and Holstege, G. (2001). Ultrastructural evidence for direct projections from the pontine micturition center to glycine-immunoreactive neurons in the sacral dorsal gray commissure in the cat. *Journal of Comparative Neurology* 429, 631–637.
91. Spanswick, D., Pickering, A. E., Gibson, I. C., and Logan, S. D. (1994). Inhibition of sympathetic preganglionic neurons by spinal glycinergic interneurons. *Neuroscience* 62, 205–216.
92. Steers, W. D., Ciambotti, J., Etzel, B., Erdman, S., and de Groat, W. C. (1991). Alterations in afferent pathways from the urinary bladder of the rat in response to partial urethral obstruction. *Journal of Comparative Neurology* 310, 401–410.
93. Strack, A. M., and Loewy, A. D. (1990). Pseudorabies virus: A highly specific transneuronal cell body marker in the sympathetic nervous system. *Journal of Neuroscience* 10, 2139–2147.
94. Strack, A. M., Sawyer, W. B., Platt, K. B., and Loewy, A. D. (1989). CNS cell groups regulating the sympathetic outflow to adrenal gland as revealed by transneuronal cell body labeling with pseudorabies virus. *Brain Research* 491, 274–296.
95. Sugaya, K., Ogawa, Y., Hatano, T., Koyama, Y., Miyazato, T., and Oda, M. (1998). Evidence for involvement of the subcoeruleus nucleus and nucleus raphé magnus in urine storage and penile erection in decerebrate rats. *Journal of Urology* 159, 2172–2176.
96. Sugaya, K., Roppolo, J. R., Yoshimura, N., Card, J. P., and de Groat, W. C. (1997). The central neural pathways involved in micturition in the neonatal rat as revealed by the injection of pseudorabies virus into the urinary bladder. *Neuroscience Letters* 223, 197–200.
97. Tang, X., Neckel, N. D., and Schramm, L. P. (2003). Locations and morphologies of sympathetically correlated neurons in the T(10) spinal segment of the rat. *Brain Research* 976, 185–193.
98. Tang, X., Neckel, N. D., and Schramm, L. P. (2004). Spinal interneurons infected by renal injection of pseudorabies virus in the rat. *Brain Research* 1004, 1–7.
99. Thor, K. B., Morgan, C., Nadelhaft, I., Houston, M., and de Groat, W. C. (1989). Organization of afferent and efferent pathways in the pudendal nerve of the female cat. *Journal of Comparative Neurology* 288, 263–279.
100. Todd, A. J. (2002). Anatomy of primary afferents and projection neurones in the rat spinal dorsal horn with particular emphasis on substance P and the neurokinin 1 receptor. *Experimental Physiology* 87, 245–249.
101. Todd, A. J., Hughes, D. I., Polgar, E., Nagy, G. G., Mackie, M., Ottersen, O. P., and Maxwell, D. J. (2003). The expression of vesicular glutamate transporters VGLUT1 and VGLUT2 in neurochemically defined axonal populations in the rat spinal cord with emphasis on the dorsal horn. *European Journal of Neuroscience* 17, 13–27.
102. Todd, A. J., Spike, R. C., Russell, G., and Johnston, H. M. (1992). Immunohistochemical evidence that Met-enkephalin and GABA coexist in some neurones in rat dorsal horn. *Brain Research* 584, 149–156.
103. Traub, R. J., Pechman, P., Iadarola, M. J., and Gebhart, G. F. (1992). Fos-like proteins in the lumbosacral spinal cord following noxious and non-noxious colorectal distention in the rat. *Pain* 49, 393–403.
104. Valentino, R. J., Kosboth, M., Colflesh, M., and Miselis, R. R. (2000). Transneuronal labeling from the rat distal colon: Anatomic evidence for regulation of distal colon function by a pontine corticotropin-releasing factor system. *Journal of Comparative Neurology* 417, 399–414.

105. Vizzard, M. A., Brisson, M., and de Groat, W. C. (2000). Transneuronal labeling of neurons in the adult rat central nervous system following inoculation of pseudorabies virus into the colon. *Cell and Tissue Research* 299, 9–26.
106. Vizzard, M. A., Erickson, V. L., Card, J. P., Roppolo, J. R., and de Groat, W. C. (1995). Transneuronal labeling of neurons in the adult rat brainstem and spinal cord after injection of pseudorabies virus into the urethra. *Journal of Comparative Neurology* 355, 629–640.
107. Wang, L., Spary, E., Deuchars, J., and Deuchars, S. A. (2008). Tonic GABAergic inhibition of sympathetic preganglionic neurons: A novel substrate for sympathetic control. *Journal of Neuroscience* 28, 12445–12452.
108. Weaver, L. C., Cassam, A. K., Krassioukov, A. V., and Llewellyn-Smith, I. J. (1997). Changes in immunoreactivity for growth associated protein-43 suggest reorganization of synapses on spinal sympathetic neurons after cord transection. *Neuroscience* 81, 535–551.
109. White, J. D., Krause, J. E., and McKelvy, J. F. (1986). In vivo biosynthesis and transport of oxytocin, vasopressin and neurophysin from the hypothalamus to the spinal cord. *Neuroscience* 17, 133–140.
110. Wong, S. T., Atkinson, B. A., and Weaver, L. C. (2000). Confocal microscopic analysis reveals sprouting of primary afferent fibres in rat dorsal horn after spinal cord injury. *Neuroscience Letters* 296, 65–68.
111. Wu, X., and Xiao, C. (2005). Morphologic relationship between the pontine micturition center and the sympathetic center in the spinal cord of the rat. *Journal of Huazhong University of Science and Technology. Medical Sciences* 25, 313–316.
112. Wyszogrodski, I., and Polosa, C. (1973). The inhibition of sympathetic preganglionic neurons by somatic afferents. *Canadian Journal of Physiology and Pharmacology* 51, 29–38.
113. Xu, C., Yaici, E. D., Conrath, M., Blanchard, P., Leclerc, P., Benoit, G., Verge, D., and Giuliano, F. (2005). Galanin and neurokinin-1 receptor immunoreactivity spinal neurons controlling the prostate and the bulbospongiosus muscle identified by transsynaptic labeling in the rat. *Neuroscience* 134, 1325–1341.
114. Zhai, Q. Z., and Traub, R. J. (1999). The NMDA receptor antagonist MK-801 attenuates c-Fos expression in the lumbosacral spinal cord following repetitive noxious and non-noxious colorectal distention. *Pain* 83, 321–329.

# 9

# Regulation of Autonomic Function by Visceral and Somatic Afferents

JOHN C. LONGHURST

The autonomic nervous system provides tonic and phasic regulation of the function of effector organs, including, among others, the cardiovascular, gastrointestinal and respiratory systems[71]. While the ongoing 2 Hz to 6 Hz rhythm of the sympathetic vasomotor outflow contributes to cardiovascular function under basal conditions by maintaining cardiac output, regional blood flow, and blood pressure[5,35], the superimposition of neural reflex control allows both immediate and long-term responses to perturbations in normal bodily homeostasis. Reflex regulation consists of an afferent or sensory arm, integration within the central nervous system, (CNS) and ultimately an efferent or autonomic motor limb that modifies the function of effector organs. Of the many examples of reflex autonomic regulation, this chapter focuses on three physiological or pathophysiological conditions: one that involves visceral afferents, one that involves somatic afferents, and a third in which somatic and visceral afferents interact. Sensory stimulation during ischemia exemplifies the stimulus to visceral afferents; muscle contraction due to exercise is the stimulus to somatic afferents. Acupuncture is a somatic stimulus that produces profound interaction between somatic and evoked visceral afferent input in the hypothalamic, midbrain, and medullary brainstem regions that regulate sympathetic outflow.

## VISCERAL AND SOMATIC AFFERENT INPUTS

Langley noted in 1921 that autonomic nerves coexist with the axons of sensory neurons in peripheral nerve bundles[57], leading to the commonly used designations *sympathetic* or *parasympathetic afferents*. Since information coming from sympathetic afferents ascends through the spinal cord, the term *spinal afferents* is preferred by some neuroscientists. Both terms identify the initial limb of a reflex pathway that ultimately regulates autonomic outflow. However, the term "spinal afferents" does not provide any useful distinction between sympathetic afferents and other afferents, such as proprioceptors, that travel in somatic motor nerves. Consequently, in this chapter, afferents that travel in sympathetic nerve bundles will be referred to as "sympathetic afferents."

Langley and Anderson[58] originally estimated that the ratio of efferent to afferent fibers in the hypogastric and splanchnic nerves was 10:1. However, more recent evidence from electron microscopy and tract tracing methods to identify the smallest afferent fibers demonstrates that the ratios are variable, ranging from 8:2 (efferents to afferents) in sympathetic nerves that provide spinal input through thoracic, splanchnic, and colonic nerves[51]; and 2:8 to 1:1 in parasympathetic nerves, such as the vagus and pelvic nerves, respectively[3]. Many more unmyelinated than myelinated sensory axons (90% vs. 10%) are present in visceral sympathetic and parasympathetic nerves[8,56]. Somatic nerves also contain many unmyelinated fibers, especially the more distal nerves. The ratio of motor to sensory fibers in the triceps surae nerve is approximately 3:2[82]. Both myelinated and unmyelinated visceral and somatic afferent fibers, called types Aδ- and C-fibers (visceral) or Groups III and IV fibers (somatic), form the afferent limb of autonomic reflex arcs[52,74]. Since Aδ and Group III fibers are finely myelinated, they conduct more rapidly than unmyelinated type C and Group IV fibers, at conduction velocities, for example in cats, at 2.5 to 30 m/s and <2.5 m/s, respectively[2].

Stimulation of sympathetic afferents, including those innervating both somatic and visceral organs, commonly leads to excitatory sympathetic motor responses. These responses are manifested as increases in blood pressure, heart rate or myocardial contractility, regional vasoconstriction, rapid breathing ("tachypnea"), and tracheal relaxation[4,50,55,67-69,88,99,104] (Figure 9–1). Conversely, activation of vagal afferents from visceral organs, such as the heart, typically leads to inhibitory reflex sympathetic responses, consisting of bradycardia and decreases in blood pressure and myocardial contractility[50] (Figure 9–1).

## AUTONOMIC REFLEXES EVOKED BY VISCERAL AFFERENTS

Chemosensitive sympathetic Aδ- and C-fiber afferent axons innervating a number of abdominal and thoracic visceral organs, including the stomach, pancreas, intestine, liver, gallbladder, and heart, respond to exogenous and endogenous chemicals, particularly when they are applied to the serosal or epicardial surfaces[68,70,71,76,103]. Likewise, mechanical stimulation to an extent that might occur during and following food ingestion activates sympathetic afferent terminals in some hollow organs, like the stomach and intestine, but not the gallbladder[68,73,88] at least within the physiological range of tension development.

### Spatial and Temporal Summation

Stimulation of chemo- and mechanosensitive sympathetic afferents in a dose-dependent manner causes sympathoexcitation and reflex activation of the cardiovascular system. As electrical stimulation of the splanchnic nerve demonstrates, both summation of activity of greater numbers of Aδ- and C-fiber afferents (spatial summation) and summation of activity of Aδ- and C-fibers firing with greater frequency (temporal summation) contribute to the magnitude of the reflex excitatory cardiovascular response[92]. However, it has not been possible to identify individual

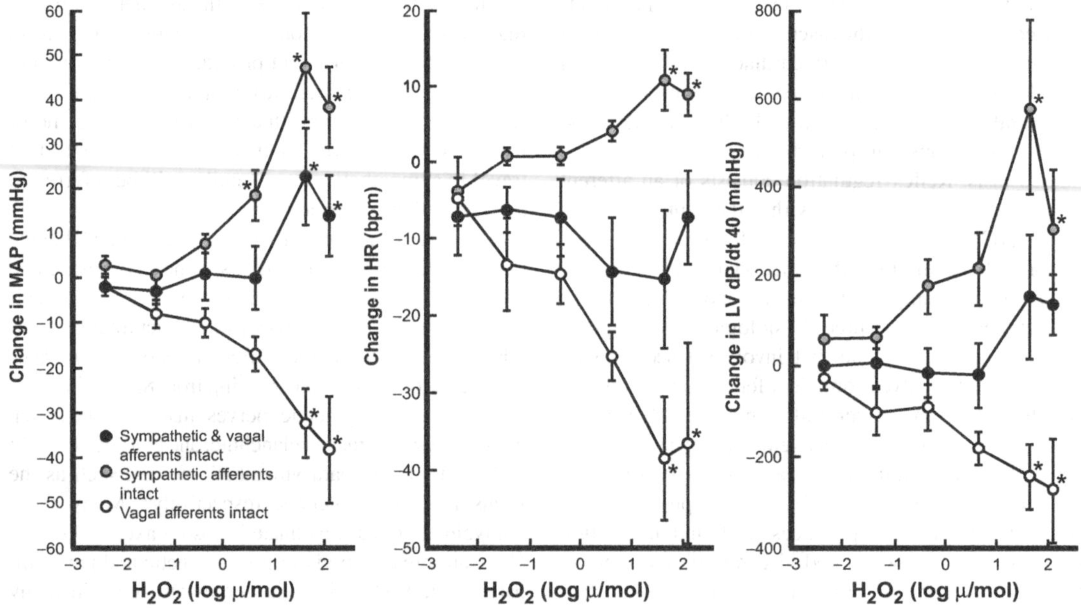


Figure 9–1 Cardiovascular responses to chemical stimulation of sympathetic and parasympathetic cardiac afferents. Dose-dependent changes in mean arterial pressure (MAP), heart rate (HR), and left ventricular dP/dt at 40 mmHg developed pressure (LV $dP/dt_{40}$) following application of increasing concentrations of hydrogen peroxide ($H_2O_2$) to the anterior surface of the ventricle in intact (vagal and sympathetic cardiac afferents intact, n = 8), bilateral cervical vagotomized (sympathetic afferents intact, n = 6), or bilateral $T_1$-$T_4$ ganglionectomized (vagal afferents intact, n = 6) cats. *Closed circles* and *brackets* represent means and standard errors, respectively. *, significantly different from saline control, $P < 0.05$. Modified from Huang et al. (1995) [50], with permission.

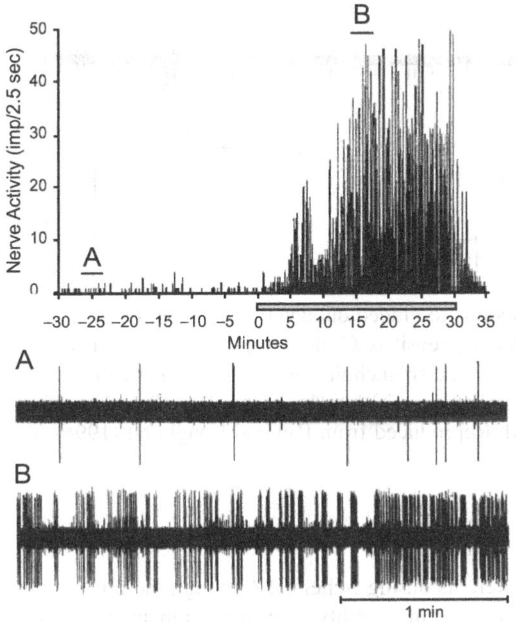


Figure 9–2 Afferent activity during ischemia and reperfusion of the pancreas. The top trace shows activity in an afferent ending in the pancreas during a 30-minute control period before ischemia, 30 minutes of ischemia (*gray bar*), and 5 minutes of reperfusion. The conduction velocity of the afferent was 0.30 m/sec. Panels *A* and *B* are representative traces showing C-fiber afferent activity at times indicated by the bars labeled *A* and *B* above the top trace. Reproduced from Pan et al. (1997)[97], with permission.

contributions from myelinated and unmyelinated fibers to the magnitude of the reflex response[92].

## Responses of Visceral Afferents to Ischemia

Sympathetic afferents innervating abdominal and thoracic viscera respond to brief, and even more strongly to prolonged, ischemia[49,68] (Figure 9–2). Stimulation of abdominal and thoracic sympathetic afferents increases blood pressure and myocardial contractility[48] through reflex mechanisms involving the sympathoadrenal system[69] (Figure 9–3). The magnitude of activation of C-fiber afferents depends on the duration of ischemia. Over a 30-minute period of prolonged ischemia, more afferents are recruited, and each afferent progressively responds more strongly. Hence, the spatial and temporal characteristics of the C-fiber discharge encode the afferent signal that largely determines the magnitude of the reflex increase in arterial blood pressure. Compared to C-fiber afferents that are not sensitive to ischemia, ischemically sensitive sympathetic afferents that innervate the gastrointestinal tract in cats have significantly higher thresholds to mechanical distension, suggesting that endings of these sensory nerves function as nociceptors[89] (Figure 9–4). These data support the argument of Cervero and Foreman[7] that a specific category of afferents transduces signals associated with pain, and refute the so-called intensity theory[51,80]. This theory proposes that all sensory fibers are potentially capable of transducing both nociceptive and non-nociceptive signals, with noxious stimuli producing high frequencies of discharge, and innocuous stimuli producing smaller responses. Both mechanical and chemical stimuli, as well as ischemia, have been used to test hypotheses of receptor specificity.

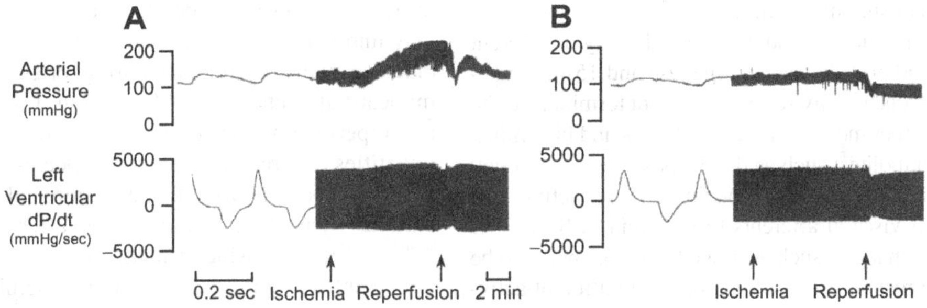


Figure 9–3 Cardiovascular responses to abdominal ischemia. Cardiovascular responses evoked by abdominal ischemia before (*A*) and after (*B*) in a cat. Before the experiment, the celiac and superior mesenteric ganglia were removed. To prevent passive shifts in blood volume during mesenteric arterial occlusion, an arterial autoperfusion circuit that kept venous return constant was used. Reproduced from Huang and Longhurst (1994), with permission[48].

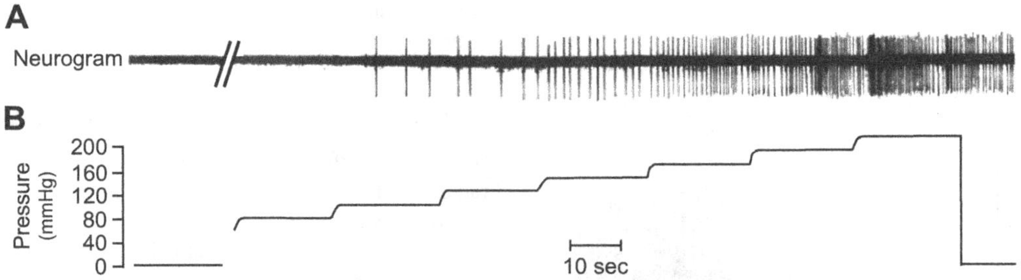


Figure 9–4 An ischemically sensitive C-fiber afferent responds to graded duodenal distension. Graded distension of the duodenum (*B*) evoked activity (*A*) of an ischemically sensitive C-fiber afferent (conduction velocity, 0̃.45 m/sec). Discharge activity of this fiber was recorded from the splanchnic nerve and began at a threshold of 75 mmHg. The pressure required to distend the balloon ex vivo was 20 mmHg–25 mmHg. Note that afferent discharge activity continued after the balloon was deflated. Reproduced from Pan and Longhurst (1996), with permission[89].

## Effective Stimuli for Visceral Afferents

Ischemia and reperfusion produce a number of metabolic changes, increasing the local concentration of chemical metabolites that activate or sensitize Aδ- and C-fiber afferent endings in the abdominal viscera to the action of other stimuli, leading to large reflex cardiovascular responses. These chemical stimuli include profound hypoxia[72], lactic acid[101], cyclooxygenase products (e.g., prostaglandin $E_2$[68]), 15-lipoxygenase products (e.g., [8*R*,15*S*]-dihydroxyeica[5*E*-9,11,13*Z*] tetranenoic acid[94]), bradykinin[68,70,71,74,88,95] histamine[28,32], serotonin (5-hydroxytryptamine)[27], and reactive oxygen species, particularly hydroxyl radicals[100,102] (Figure 9–5). Many metabolic factors activate specific receptors on afferent terminals in the abdominal viscera to produce reflex responses. These receptors include bradykinin$_2$ ($BK_2$), histamine$_1$ ($H_1$), and 5-$HT_3$ receptor subtypes, which activate specific signaling pathways through second messenger systems, including protein kinase C and cyclic adenosine monophosphate[9,27,32,37,39]. Some metabolic factors, such as bradykinin, act directly on afferent endings. Others, like cyclooxygenase and 15-lipoxygenase products, mainly sensitize afferent terminals to the action of other mediators, such as kinins and histamine. Other metabolites, such as the 5-lipoxygenase product, leukotriene $B_4$, modulate or inhibit the activity of abdominal visceral afferents to ischemia[94] . Still other metabolic changes, such as tissue hypoxia, appear to be indirectly responsible for the increase in afferent activity during ischemia since there is a substantial lag between the decrease in tissue $pO_2$ and the observed increases in sympathetic afferent activity[25].

Despite changes in gastrointestinal motility[13,14], mechanosensitive receptors do not appear to play a role in activation of the terminals of sympathetic afferents during ischemia. Although there is an initial increase in motility, the predominant response is smooth muscle relaxation[93].

## Afferent and Reflex Responses to Myocardial Ischemia

Cardiac sympathetic afferents play an important role in mediating responses to pain and produce excitatory cardiovascular reflex responses even during relatively brief ischemia[21,65,81,123,124]. It is not possible to study prolonged myocardial ischemia, because infarction begins to occur within 10 to 15 minutes after initiating coronary artery occlusion. The responses of cardiac sympathetic afferents during myocardial ischemia show many similarities to abdominal sympathetic afferents, but there are also some differences and new mechanisms. Lactic acid (protons), bradykinin, histamine, and 5-HT, the latter three acting through specific receptor mechanisms, play important roles in activating the terminals of cardiac sympathetic afferents during brief (5 minutes) myocardial ischemia[26,76,116]. During both ischemia and reperfusion, purine metabolism forms sufficient quantities of reactive oxygen species, especially hydroxyl radicals, to activate ischemically sensitive cardiac sympathetic and vagal afferent endings [49,50,76,114,121]. Adenosine, a metabolite of adenosine-5' -triphosphate, is produced during ischemia and activates the axons of cardiac sympathetic afferents when given exogenously[17]. However, single-unit recordings of afferents in cats indicate that adenosine does not contribute to the enhanced activity during brief ischemia[91]. The differing conclusions about the role of adenosine in these studies may be related to

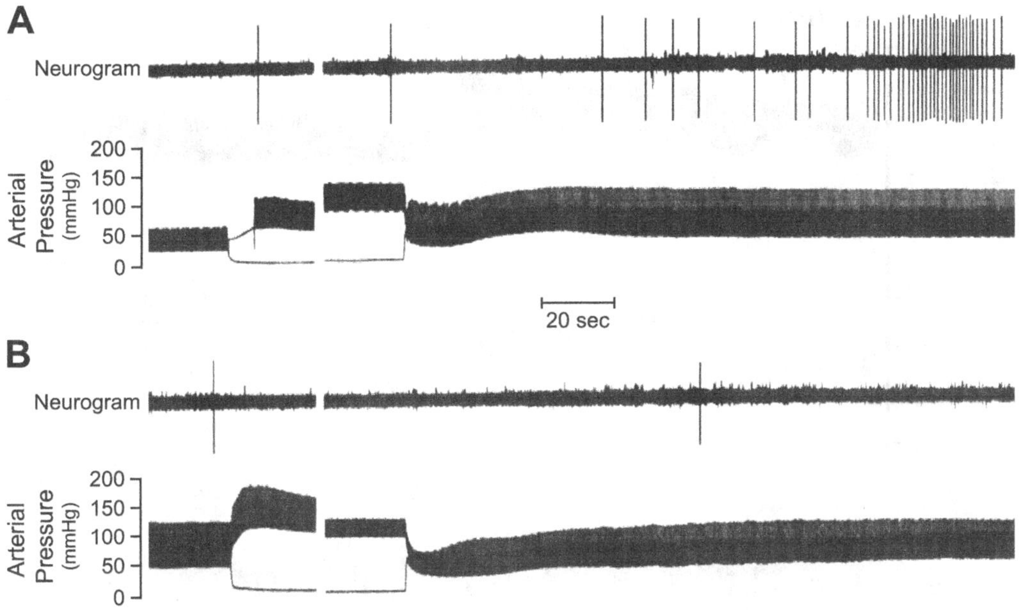


Figure 9–5 A C-fiber afferent that innervates the gallbladder responds to ischemia and reperfusion. Representative traces from a reperfusion-sensitive C-fiber afferent innervating the gallbladder (conduction velocity, 0.64 m/sec). Phasic pressure during ischemia was measured in the thoracic aorta, proximal to the occlusion cuff, and in the femoral artery, distal to the occlusion cuff. *A:* Reperfusion increased baseline activity from 0.02 to 0.68 imp/sec during reperfusion after an onset latency of 70 sec. *B:* Dimethylthiourea (10 mg/kg), an oxygen-derived free radical scavenger, abolished this reperfusion-induced increase in activity during a second episode of ischemia-reperfusion. Reproduced from Stahl et al. (1993), with permission[102].

species-specific responses or to the non-physiological (pharmacological) concentrations of adenosine administered exogenously.

Platelets are activated during brief ischemia and release a number of products, including histamine, 5-HT, and thromboxane $A_2$ (Figure 9–6), that subsequently lead to stimulation of sympathetic afferent terminals in the ventricle as well as sympathoexcitatory responses[23,24].

Important interactions occur between some of these metabolic factors. For example, bradykinin leads to the release of cyclooxygenase products that sensitize sensory nerves to the action of bradykinin and histamine[30,116]. Conversely, histamine inhibits the response to bradykinin[30]. The net result of these interactions, which normally occur during ischemia, is an enhanced response that is slightly less than a simple summation of the responses to the two mediators individually (Figure 9–7A). Another type of interaction occurs between bradykinin and thromboxane $A_2$. Both mediators sensitize the response of the other metabolite, resulting in synergistic afferent and reflex interactions when they are present together (Figure 9–7B)[31].

## Central Pathways that Process Information from Visceral Sympathetic Afferents

Once sensory information from the viscera enters the dorsal horn of the lumbar and thoracic spinal cord, it ascends through the spinothalamic, spinoreticular, spinomesencephalic, spinosolitary, and possibly other pathways to supraspinal nuclei involved in perception and autonomic regulation[7,125].

Until recently, relatively scant information was available on the supraspinal pathways and nuclei (other than the thalamus) involved in processing input from sympathetic afferents[7]. Recent studies employing Fos, the protein product of the immediate early gene *c-fos*, which is synthesized when neurons are activated, demonstrate that neurons in the hypothalamus[47], midbrain[38], pons[38], and medulla oblongata[46] receive input from chemosensitive cardiac sympathetic afferents. Double antibody labeling experiments have allowed identification of the neuronal phenotypes in these regions that are stimulated by the cardiac inputs.

Neurons in the arcuate nucleus in the ventral hypothalamus, the dorsal hypothalamic area, the paraventricular hypothalamus, and the periventricular

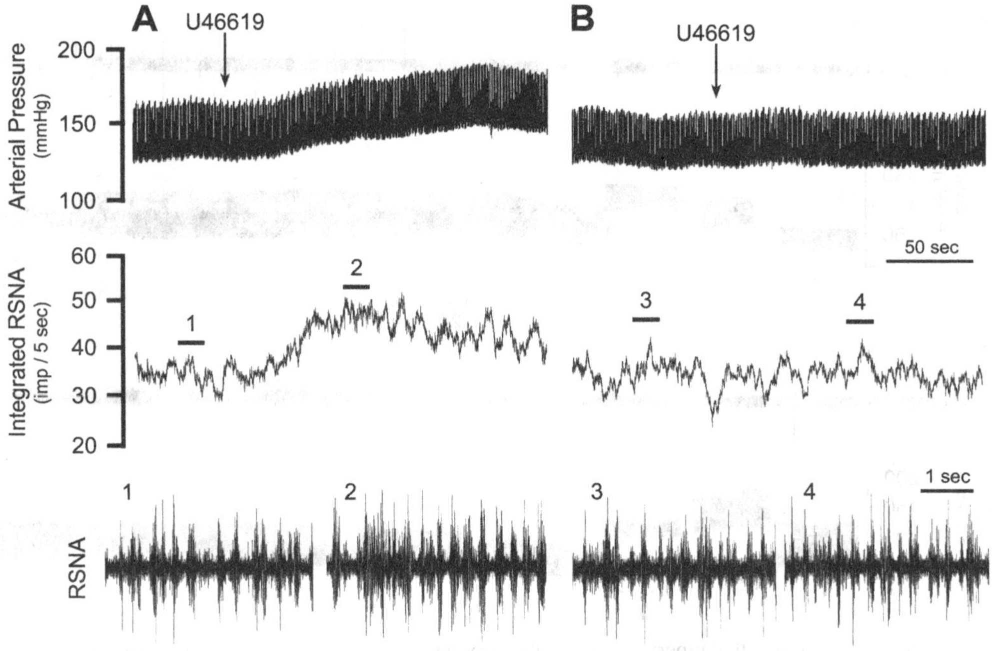


Figure 9–6 Cardiac-cardiovascular reflex responses to thromboxane. *A:* Responses of renal sympathetic nerve activity (RSNA), integrated RSNA and arterial pressure to stimulation of the anterior surface of the left ventricle with the stable thromboxane analogue U46619 (10 μg). *B:* Application of a local anesthetic (2% procaine) to the surface of the ventricle inhibited the response to subsequent application of U46619. Reproduced from Fu and Longhurst (2008), with permission[29].

hypothalamus receive input from cardiac sympathetic afferents[47]. Co-localization of nitric oxide synthase-immunoreactivity in Fos-containing neurons occurs in the paraventricular nucleus but not in other hypothalamic nuclei. The caudal and intermediate regions of the midbrain periaqueductal gray (PAG), including both the sympathoexcitatory dorsal and lateral PAG and the sympathoinhibitory ventrolateral PAG, also receive cardiac sympathetic afferent input[38].

In the pons, stimulation of cardiac sympathetic afferents increases Fos-immunoreactivity in the external lateral subnucleus of the parabrachial nucleus, the Kölliker-Fuse nucleus, and the dorsal and more ventral alpha regions of the locus coeruleus[38]. The external lateral parabrachial nucleus, responsible for sympathoexcitatory responses[10], may play a role in processing excitatory reflexes from the heart. The Kölliker-Fuse nucleus, as part of the parabrachial nucleus in the rostral lateral pons, is a major source of descending projections from the parabrachial complex to the nucleus of the solitary tract (NTS) and the ventrolateral medulla in the brainstem[34]. The locus coeruleus receives input from sympathetic afferents innervating the abdominal viscera and from vagal afferents[18,22,85]. There is little cardiac sympathetic afferent input to the A5 cell group in the ventrolateral pons or the central or ventrolateral subnuclei of the parabrachial nucleus. Furthermore, catecholaminergic neurons (identified by immunoreactivity for the catecholamine synthetic enzyme tyrosine hydroxylase) in the locus coeruleus (A6 area), Kölliker-Fuse (A7 area) or the external lateral parabrachial nuclei do not express *c-fos* following cardiac sympathetic afferent stimulation.

In the medulla, cardiac sympathetic afferent input occurs in the NTS, specifically in the caudal and intermediate regions; the ventrolateral medulla, including both the rostral and caudal regions; the lateral tegmental field, in the intermediate and rostral regions; and the vestibular nucleus, but not in the area postrema[46]. Although noradrenergic A1 neurons in the caudal ventrolateral medulla (CVLM) and C1 adrenergic neurons in the rostral ventrolateral medulla (RVLM) receive cardiac sympathetic afferent input, the A2 and C2 cell groups of the NTS[46] do not. After stimulation of cardiac sympathetic afferent input, neurons double

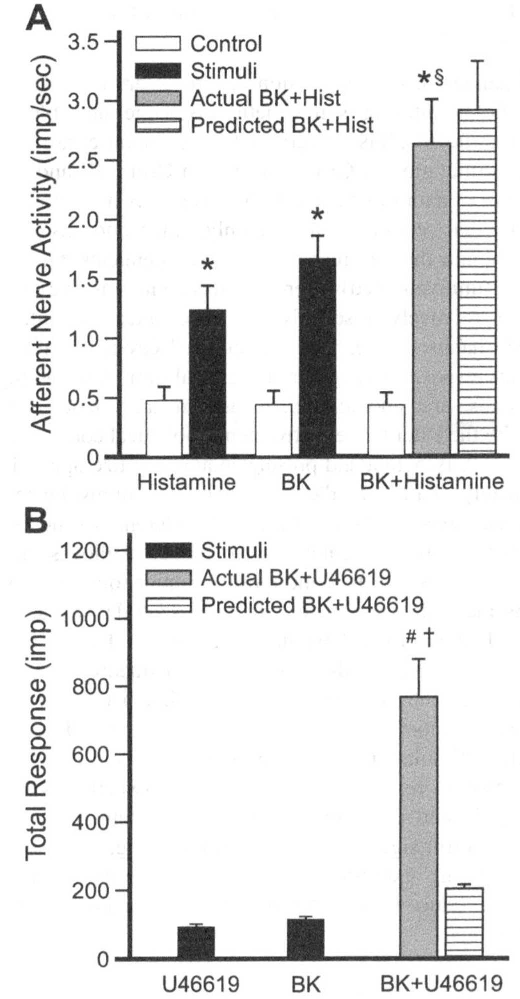


Figure 9–7 Effects of histamine on the activity of cardiac afferents during ischemia. *A:* Response of ischemically sensitive cardiac afferents to injection of histamine (hist, 1 mM, n = 9), bradykinin (BK, 1 μg, n = 7) and BK plus histamine (n = 16) into the left atrium. *Columns* and *error bars* represent means ± standard error of the mean. * $P < 0.05$ compared with control. § $P < 0.05$ compared with either BK or histamine. *B:* Responses of another group of 15 cardiac ischemically sensitive afferents to injection of thromboxane $A_2$ mimetic, U46619 (5 μg), BK (1 μg), and BK+U46619 into the left atrium. Reproduced from Fu et al. (2005 and 2010), with permission[26,31].

labeled for nitric oxide synthase and Fos occur in the NTS, the RVLM and CVLM, the lateral tegmental field, the locus coeruleus, and the parabrachial nucleus, suggesting that nitric oxide serves as a neurotransmitter or a neuromodulator in cardiac sympathoexcitatory reflexes[40] (see below).

## Central Mechanisms of Processing Visceral Afferent Information

Although activation of cardiac sympathetic afferents causes sympathoexcitatory reflex responses, and stimulation of cardiac vagal afferents leads to sympathoinhibition[50], combined stimulation, which occurs naturally, leads to an interactive response consisting of a small increase in blood pressure and sympathoexcitation[50] (Figure 9–1). One mechanism underlying this interaction may be occlusion in NTS neurons receiving input from both sympathetic and vagal cardiac afferents[115]. Occlusion is manifested as relative inhibition of NTS discharge when activity is evoked by simultaneous stimulation of cardiac vagal and sympathetic afferents compared to responses evoked by stimulation of the individual afferent pathways. Other CNS nuclei also may participate in the interactions between cardiac sympathetic and cardiac vagal afferents.

Recent studies have begun to identify central processing mechanisms of cardiovascular reflex responses to stimulation of abdominal and thoracic visceral afferents. Since it is well known that sympathetic afferent information ascends through the spinal cord[7], neurotransmitter systems in the spinal cord and supraspinal centers have been examined. For example, glutamate, operating through spinal ionotropic *N*-methyl-D-aspartate (NMDA) and non-NMDA (α-amino-3-hydroxy-5-methylisoxazole-4-propionate [AMPA]) receptors participate in spinal transmission of excitatory reflex blood pressure responses to mesenteric ischemia[36]. The tachykinin substance P, acting on neurokinin-1 receptors, likewise contributes to the ascending spinal limb of the sympathoexcitatory cardiovascular reflex responses to stimulation of chemosensitive receptors in the gallbladder[90]. The roles of other candidate neurotransmitters/neuromodulators, such as somatostatin, calcitonin gene-related peptide, and opioids, that may assist in spinal transmission of visceral autonomic responses remain to be identified.

Thoracic and abdominal afferents are capable of regulating sympathetic outflow through their actions in the medulla, midbrain, and hypothalamus. Since visceral input to medullary neurons that participate in regulating presympathetic vasomotor neurons, such as those in the RVLM, is mainly excitatory, the role of neurotransmitters such as glutamate has been examined [41,43,133]. Vesicular glutamate transporter 3, which identifies cell bodies containing glutamate but also labels some central neurons that contain γ-amino butyric acid, (GABA) is present in many (75%–80%)

RVLM neurons activated during gallbladder distension or stimulation of cardiac sympathetic afferents with bradykinin[41]. Furthermore, extracellular glutamate, recovered by microdialysis, increases during stimulation of abdominal visceral afferents[133]. The actions of glutamate appear to be modified by some neurotransmitters, such as nitric oxide. However, nitric oxide appears to have a ubiquitous influence in the CNS, since activation of glutamate receptors leads to nitric oxide formation and release[109]. Nitric oxide modulates the action of excitatory amino acid receptors in the dorsal horn of the spinal cord by facilitation of NMDA receptor-mediated responses and inhibition of AMPA receptor-mediated responses[6]. Nitric oxide in the RVLM interacts with both inhibitory (e.g., GABA) and excitatory (e.g., glutamate) neurotransmitters and may cause either inhibitory or excitatory cardiovascular responses[12,120]. Nitric oxide donors in rat RVLM can either decrease or increase baseline blood pressure in the absence of any reflex, depending upon the dose[84]. Systemic antagonism of nitric oxide synthase isoforms suggests that the composite response to nitric oxide in the brain, particularly that derived from neuronal nitric oxide synthase, facilitates cardiac visceral autonomic responses, while endothelial nitric oxide synthase in peripheral blood vessels modulates sympathoexcitatory reflexes[117]. Neuronal nitric oxide synthase, but not the other nitric oxide synthase isoforms (i.e., inducible and endothelial) in the RVLM, is responsible for processing visceral sympathoexcitatory reflexes[45].

## AUTONOMIC REFLEXES FROM SOMATIC AFFERENTS

### Origins of the Cardiovascular Response to Exercise

Somatic sensory nerves relay information to the CNS from skin, muscle, bone, and tendon. One of the better-characterized somatic-autonomic reflexes originates from skeletal muscle during exercise and is called the *exercise pressor reflex*. During exercise and muscle contraction, there are large alterations in cardio-respiratory function mediated by increased sympathetic and decreased parasympathetic outflow[75,87]. These include increases in blood pressure, regional vascular resistance, heart rate, myocardial contractility, cardiac output, respiration, and tracheal relaxation[4,67]. These responses form a feed-forward mechanism called "central command," originating, in part, from neurons in the hypothalamus and midbrain[19,122] and from an "exercise pressor reflex" originating in contracting skeletal muscle[53].

### Stimuli That are Effective for Activating Somatic Afferents

Changes in muscle tension or stretch are capable of reflexly altering sympathetic discharge and blood pressure[53,104]. It is not certain if these responses are due to stimulation of Group III or both Group III and IV sensory axons in muscle. Group III (finely myelinated) afferent endings are mainly mechanosensitive, although they do respond to some chemicals. Group IV (unmyelinated) afferents are chemosensitive and are relatively insensitive to mechanical stimuli[54]. Mechanosensitive, finely myelinated Group III afferents respond to a number of chemical stimuli, including kinins, arachidonic acid, potassium, and lactic acid, with the latter two effective at physiological concentrations[53]. Ischemia and prostaglandins sensitize approximately half of the terminals of unmyelinated chemosensitive Group IV muscle afferents to muscle contraction[53]. Ischemia also potentiates cardiovascular reflex responses to static muscle contraction, possibly by increasing production of carbon dioxide and lactic acid and further lowering tissue pH[106]. Kinins and prostaglandins produced locally in contracting skeletal muscle contribute to sensory stimulation that ultimately leads to reflex sympathoexcitation[53,96,98,105,107,108]. In general, stimulation of muscle afferents during exercise probably represents a mismatch between oxygen supply and consumption, which constitutes a metabolic error signal. When the mismatch is greater, such as during exercise or ischemia, more metabolites are produced and act together to stimulate sensory endings.

### Spinal Mechanisms of Somatic Afferent Neurotransmission

Somatic afferents convey information to the CNS through most or all of the same spinal cord pathways and neurotransmitter systems as visceral sympathetic afferents. Thus, in the dorsal horn of the spinal cord, glutamate[1,53] acts as an excitatory neurotransmitter, while substance P and neurokinin A and B function as neuromodulators. Both substance P and calcitonin gene-related peptide coexist with glutamate in spinal terminals of presumed Group III and IV axons and enhance the evoked release of glutamate[53].

Glutamate, operating through both NMDA and non-NMDA ionotropic receptors, contributes to spinal transmission of sensory input relating to static muscle contraction[1,53] that leads to blood pressure responses; as does substance P acting at neurokinin-1, but not neurokinin-2 or neurokinin-3, receptors[53]. There also is evidence for the participation of somatostatin[53]. Conversely, blockade of the actions of norepinephrine, opioids, and serotonin in the spinal cord does not alter the reflex responses to muscle contraction[53].

### Supraspinal Centers Processing Somatic Afferent Information

Medullary, midbrain, and hypothalamic regions, including the RVLM and CVLM, nucleus ambiguus, dorsal PAG, posterior hypothalamus, and supraoptic nucleus, among others, probably contribute to processing of somatic afferent input during muscle contraction[53] (Figure 9–8). Many neurons in these regions receive convergent input from both somatic and visceral afferents, suggesting the potential for interactions between these two systems, as described below.

## INTERACTION OF VISCERAL AND SOMATIC AFFERENT INPUT IN CARDIOVASCULAR REGULATION

### Importance of the Modality of Afferent Stimulation

Interactions between visceral and somatic afferents have profound autonomic and cardiovascular consequences. In fact, these interactions appear to form the basis for the autonomic influence of acupuncture, a therapy that has been applied clinically for over 3,000 years[66]. Thirty minutes of electrical stimulation of somatic sensory nerves at low frequency and low intensity (bilateral median nerves at 2 Hz–4 Hz, 1 mA–2 mA, 0.5 ms)—i.e., at a level that is just at the threshold for activation of the myelinated motor fibers to muscle—causes little or no change in baseline blood pressure in normotensive people or animals[59]. However, the same stimulus paradigm leads to an approximately 40% decrease in the magnitude of visceral sympathoexcitatory reflex blood pressure responses, for example, in response to stimulation of gallbladder afferents with bradykinin or during gastric distension[60,61]. The influence of low-level somatic afferent stimulation on excitatory blood pressure reflexes is prolonged, lasting for over an hour after termination of somatic nerve stimulation in anesthetized animals (Figure 9–9B) and for up to 12 hours in conscious animals with genetically elevated blood pressures[126]. Mechanical stimulation caused by needles inserted into the median nerves or by transcutaneous magnetic simulation of the median nerve produce similar responses to low-level electrical stimulation because somatic sensory fibers are similarly stimulated[128,131]. Group III and Group IV fibers both contribute to the somatic-visceral reflex modulation[61,118]. Also, low-frequency stimulation is much more effective than high-frequency stimulation. Little somatic modulation of the visceral autonomic reflex blood pressure response is noted above 20 Hz, mainly because higher frequencies of stimulation do not effectively entrain somatic afferents[128]. Deeper somatic neural pathways supplying muscle, bone, and joints are more effective in reducing visceral sympathoexcitatory responses than stimulation of superficial (cutaneous) nerves[61,112,128].

### Opioid and Opioid-like Neuromodulation

Both spinal and supraspinal regions contribute to the modulatory influence of somatic afferents on the sympathoexcitatory cardiovascular reflex evoked by visceral afferent stimulation. Several neurotransmitter systems mediate this interaction. Opioids, in particular, seem to be important at spinal and supraspinal levels because naloxone, a nonselective antagonist of opioid receptors, or selective opioid receptor blockade administered intravenously directly into regions such as the RVLM or intrathecally onto the spinal cord, rapidly reverses the effects of visceral-somatic interaction[11,62,111,130,131] (Figure 9–9A). The relative importance of different opioid receptors and the corresponding endogenous opioid ligands vary between different regions. In the spinal cord, intrathecal administration of δ- and κ-opioid receptor antagonists effectively inhibits the influence of somatic afferent stimulation on visceral sympathoexcitatory reflexes, suggesting that enkephalins and dynorphin participate as neuromodulators in this response[131]. In the medulla, μ- and δ-opioid antagonists are most effective at reversing the influence of prolonged, low-level stimulation of somatic nerves on visceral afferent cardiovascular reflexes, indicating that β-endorphin, endomorphin, and enkephalins probably are the relevant endogenous ligands in this region[62]. In addition, nociceptin in the RVLM and in the dorsal horn and intermediolateral cell column of the spinal cord facilitates somatic nerve-induced inhibition of the blood pressure response to gastric distension through an opioid independent mechanism involving nociceptin/orphanin FQ peptide receptors[16].

### Rostral Ventrolateral Medulla

Presympathetic neurons in the RVLM receive input from both somatic and visceral afferents and play a vital role in the central processing that prolongs the inhibition of viscerally evoked activity by somatic input[111-113,132]. The immediate response of RVLM neurons to simultaneous input from somatic and visceral afferents is neural occlusion, which is a short-lived inhibitory response lasting for seconds or minutes[111]. More prolonged inhibition of excitation evoked by

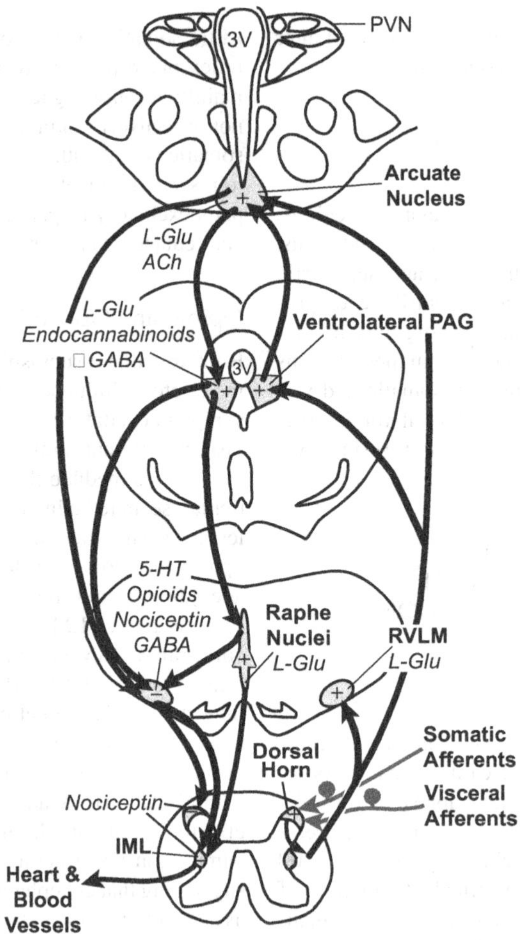


Figure 9–8 Central Interactions between visceral and somatic afferents. Afferents convey visceral and somatic sensory information to the dorsal horn of the spinal cord. For convenience, excitatory ascending pathways are shown on the *right* while excitatory and inhibitory descending pathways are displayed on the *left*. Afferent information ascends through spinal-CNS pathways to the arcuate nucleus in the ventral hypothalamus, the ventrolateral PAG in the midbrain and the RVLM. Input at all three sites is excitatory and results in visceral-somatic interactions in the RVLM that, in the short-term, are occlusive in nature since simultaneous stimulation of the two afferent systems reduces the response of neurons receiving convergent input compared to responses evoked separately by each input[111]. Prolonged (30-minute) low frequency (2–6 Hz) somatic stimulation activates a long-loop pathway that includes the arcuate nucleus and ventrolateral PAG[64]. There are reciprocal excitatory projections between the arcuate nucleus and the ventrolateral PAG that serve to enhance and prolong the increased activity during somatic afferent stimulation. An inhibitory projection from the PAG reduces excitation of premotor RVLM neurons that is caused by visceral afferent activation, ultimately reducing sympathetic outflow to the heart and vasculature[113]. An alternative pathway from the ventrolateral PAG projects to the raphé nuclei in the midline medulla, particularly the nucleus raphé pallidus[44]. Inhibitory 5-HT[83] and/or opioid[44] projections from the raphé nuclei to premotor neurons in the RVLM regulate sympathetic outflow. The raphé nuclei also may project directly to the intermediolateral region of the spinal cord. Modulation of visceral-induced activation of sympathoexcitatory premotor RVLM neurons during prolonged somatic stimulation involves opioid and opioid-like (nociceptin) neurotransmitters, as well as $\gamma$-amino butyric acid (GABA)[16,110]. Glutamate and acetylcholine (ACh) in the arcuate and glutamate in the ventrolateral PAG and RVLM mediate excitation while endocannabinoids in the PAG presynaptically inhibit the release of GABA leading to disinhibition of activity in the ventrolateral PAG [33,119]. A long projection from the arcuate nucleus supplies endorphins to the RVLM, while enkephalins are produced locally in this medullary region[42,63]. Nociceptin acting in the dorsal horn and IML of the spinal cord during prolonged somatic afferent stimulation also modulates sympathoexcitatory reflex activation during visceral afferent stimulation [129].

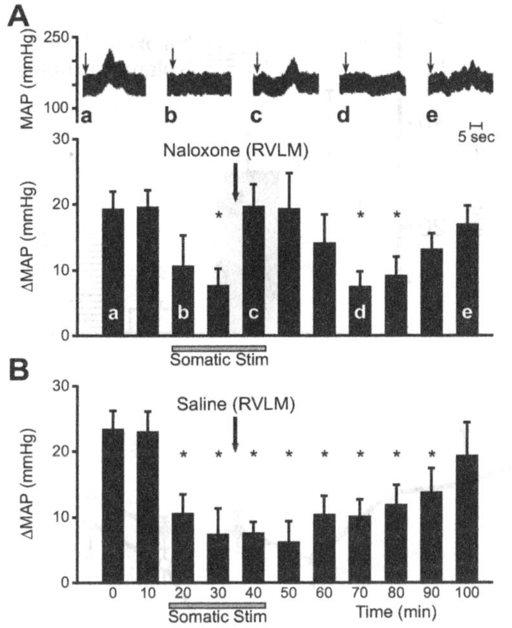


Figure 9–9 Naloxone in RVLM restores somatic stimulation-induced decreases in arterial pressure during repeated distension of the stomach. Stomachs of rats (n=12) were distended with 5–10 ml of air. In *B* and *C:* somatic nerves were stimulated bilaterally (1–2 mA, 2 Hz) with percutaneous needles inserted in median nerve for 30 minutes in both groups to simulate low frequency electroacupuncture. *A, top panel,* Mean arterial pressure (MAP) recorded in one rat. *Small arrows,* onset of distension of stomach. Traces a–e were recorded at times a–e in A, *lower panel.* a, Control; b, 10 minutes after initiating somatic nerve stimulation (Somatic Stim); c, after microinjection of naloxone into the RVLM; d, 30 minutes after cessation of somatic stimulation; e, 60 minutes after cessation of stimulation. *A, bottom panel,* Effects of microinjection of naloxone (0.1 mM, 100 nl) into the RVLM (n=6). *B:* Effects of microinjection of saline vehicle (0.9%, 100 nl) into the RVLM (n=6). Note that unilateral microinjection of naloxone into the RVLM transiently reversed the somatic stimulation related decrease in blood pressure elevation induced by gastric distension. * $P < 0.05$. Reproduced from Li et al. (2002), with permission[61].

stimulation of visceral afferents begins to occur after 10 to 15 minutes of a 30-minute period of somatic afferent stimulation, is both opioid and non-opioid dependent, and frequently lasts for over 90 minutes[16,111] (Figure 9–10). This prolonged modulation depends on a long-loop pathway that involves at least the arcuate nucleus in the ventral hypothalamus, the caudal midbrain ventrolateral PAG, and the midline raphé nuclei in the medulla (see below).

### Long-Loop Pathways in Visceral–Somatic Interactions

The arcuate nucleus is important for interactions between visceral and somatic input because this region links a number of functions, including pain and emotion. Along with the RVLM[42], this ventral hypothalamic region is a major site of synthesis of opioid peptides[15,86]. Many arcuate neurons receive input from visceral and somatic afferents[64]. There is an excitatory projection from the arcuate nucleus to the ventrolateral PAG, which is part of a non-nociceptive region that provides descending cardiovascular inhibition[77-79]. Depolarization blockade of the arcuate nucleus with kainic acid reverses the prolonged inhibition of visceral sympathoexcitatory reflexes induced by stimulation of somatic afferents[64]. The ventrolateral PAG, in turn, provides direct and indirect inhibitory projections to presympathetic neurons in the RVLM[113]. In addition, there is a reciprocal excitatory interaction between the ventrolateral PAG and the arcuate nucleus that reinforces somatic activation of both nuclei. Glutamate and GABA participate in the long-loop mediated inhibition of visceral sympathoexcitatory reflexes during somatic afferent stimulation, and endocannabinoids through a CB1 receptor mechanism reduce GABA release to cause disinhibition of ventrolateral PAG neurons[33,119]. Also, there is a direct opioid projection from the arcuate nucleus to the RVLM that provides endorphins to this region of the hindbrain[63]. The inhibitory projection from the ventrolateral PAG to the RVLM ultimately modulates sympathetic outflow and cardiovascular reflexes induced by stimulation of visceral afferents. Thus, like prolonged somatic afferent stimulation, repetitive chemical activation of neurons in the ventrolateral PAG leads to prolonged inhibition of increases in blood pressure caused by stimulating visceral afferents. Furthermore, depolarization blockade of neuronal activity in the arcuate nucleus or the ventrolateral PAG rapidly reverses the prolonged inhibition related to somatic afferent stimulation. The pathway from the ventrolateral PAG to the RVLM may be direct[20] or indirect, the latter involving midline raphé nuclei, especially enkephalinergic and serotonergic cells in the nucleus raphé pallidus[44,127].

## SUMMARY

Visceral afferents provide important signals to the CNS. These signals are initiated by activation of both chemo- and mechanosensitive sensory axons, with subsequent transmission through spinal pathways. These sensory neurons respond to nociceptive and non-nociceptive stimuli, with nociceptive input conveyed through a

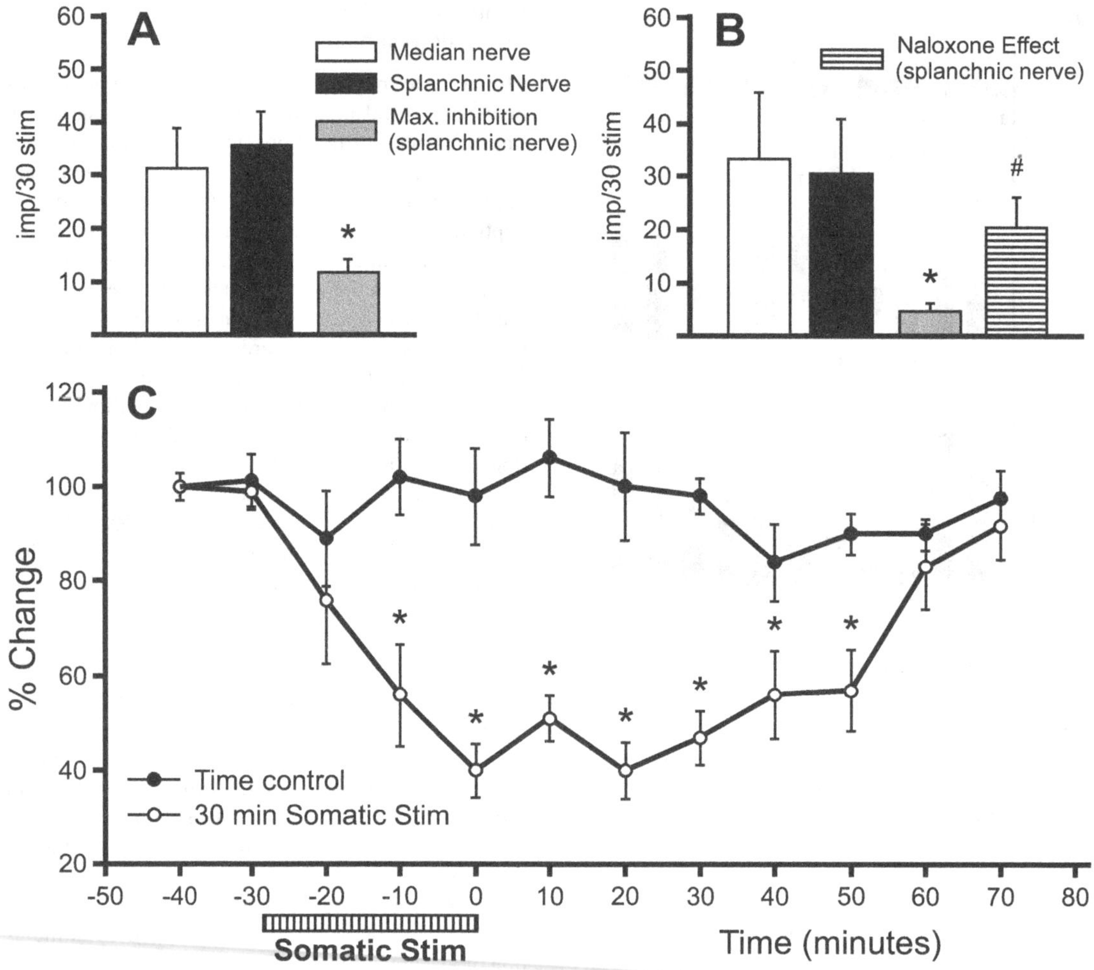


Figure 9–10 Somatic nerve stimulation during electroacupuncture affects the activity of RVLM neurons caused by stimulating sympathetic afferents. *A:* Effects of bilateral stimulation of a somatic nerve (median nerve) on the responses of 17 RVLM neurons to splanchnic nerve stimulation. Stimulating somatic afferents for 30 minutes inhibited the response (*) of the RVLM neurons that was evoked by visceral afferent stimulation. *B:* Five of the 17 RVLM neurons in A received naloxone by iontophoresis. Naloxone reversed the inhibition of RVLM neuronal activity due to repeated somatic afferent stimulation. *C:* Splanchnic nerve stimulation in the absence of somatic stimulation consistently increased the activity of 7 RVLM neurons (*filled circles*) , similar to responses during control stimulation at -40 minutes. Conversely, repeated stimulation of a somatic nerve (*open circles*) for 30 minutes significantly inhibited (*) the response of 5 of these RVLM neurons to splanchnic nerve stimulation. This effect lasted for 50 minutes after cessation of the somatic nerve stimulation. Two neurons demonstrated inhibition for up to 110 minutes. Reproduced from Tjen-A-Looi et al. (2003), with permission[111].

subset of Aδ- and C-fibers that respond to events like ischemia and inflammation. Ischemia and reperfusion alter the concentrations of a number of metabolites in the interstitial space, responses that activate sensory terminals responding to the different metabolites. This multifactorial signaling process leads to spatial and temporal recruitment as afferents are activated. Neurons in the hypothalamus, midbrain, and medulla process information received from visceral sensory fibers and are ultimately responsible for evoking changes in autonomic outflow that profoundly influence cardiovascular and respiratory function. Afferents that travel in sympathetic nerves and rely on spinal pathways to convey information to the brain (i.e., sympathetic afferents) primarily transmit sensory information from the abdominal region that influence cardiovascular function. Sensory information from the heart is transmitted to autonomic centers in the brain by both sympathetic and vagal afferents. These two cardiac afferent systems lead to directionally opposite autonomic responses that, when processed through the NTS, yield a small excitatory response as a result of neural occlusive interaction.

Somatic afferents that convey information through essentially the same spinal pathways as visceral afferents provide a feedback mechanism that, along with central command, alters autonomic outflow to optimize blood pressure and the distribution of cardiac output during exercise. The terminals of muscle afferents probably perceive chemical events associated with muscle contractions as an error signal (i.e., as a signal of an imbalance between oxygen supply and demand). These metabolite-evoked signals, along with signals caused by mechanical stimuli, activate spinal and supraspinal regions concerned with cardiovascular autonomic regulation.

Recent studies have highlighted neuronal interactions in the hypothalamus, midbrain, and medulla during simultaneous stimulation of visceral and somatic afferent pathways; for example, during acupuncture. Under basal or normotensive conditions, low-frequency, low-intensity activation of somatic afferents does not alter sympathetic outflow or blood pressure. However, under conditions in which the sympathetic nervous system is activated, such somatic stimulation profoundly modulates sympathetic outflow, resulting in sympathoinhibition. This sympathoinhibition occurs because long-loop pathways in the arcuate nucleus, PAG, and possibly other regions of the brain are activated, leading to both opioid and non-opioid modulation of excitatory neurotransmitters like glutamate. Among the many interesting unresolved questions in this research areas are:

1. Do other centers such as the midline medullary raphé nuclei participate in this long-loop pathway? Preliminary studies suggest that these nuclei may play an important role.
2. What mechanism(s) underlie the prolonged inhibition that a brief period of somatic stimulation exerts on sympathetic overactivity?
3. What interactions occur between spinal and supraspinal centers when somatic and visceral sensory input interact to influence autonomic function?
4. What long-term molecular messages are evoked by repetitive activation of somatic afferents during clinical procedures, such as acupuncture?

ACKNOWLEDGEMENTS This work has been supported by grants from the National Heart, Lung and Blood Institute of the National Institutes of Health, most recently including HL-66217, HL-63313 and HL-72125. This work was made possible by the hard work of many contributors over the last three decades. Special thanks are extended to Michelle Dang and Stephanie Tjen-A-Looi, who assisted in preparation of this chapter.

## References

1. Adreani, C. M., Hill, J. M., and Kaufman, M. P. (1996). Intrathecal blockade of both NMDA and non-NMDA receptors attenuates the exercise pressor reflex in cats. *Journal of Applied Physiology* 80, 315–322.
2. Andres, K. H., and von During, M. (1985). Sensory innervation of the Achilles tendon by group III and IV afferent fibers. *Anatomia Histologia Embryologia* 172, 145–156.
3. Andrews, P. L. R. (1986). Vagal afferent innervation of the gastrointestinal tract. In F. Cervero and J. F. B. Morrison (Eds.), *Visceral Sensation. Progress in Brain Research*, vol. 67, pp. 65–86. Amsterdam, Netherlands: Elsevier.
4. Aung-Din R., Mitchell J., and Longhurst, J. (1981). Reflex alpha-adrenergic coronary vasoconstriction during hindlimb static exercise in dogs. *Circulation Research* 48, 502–509.
5. Barman, S. M., and Gebber, G. L. (2000). "Rapid" rhythmic discharges of sympathetic nerves: Sources, mechanisms of generation, and physiological relevance. *Journal of Biological Rhythms* 15, 365–379.
6. Budai D., Wilcox, G. L., and Larson, A. A. (1995). Effects of nitric oxide availabilty on responses of spinal wide dynamic range neurons to excitatory amino acids. *European Journal of Pharmacology* 278, 39–47.
7. Cervero, F., and Foreman, R. (1990). Sensory innervation of the viscera. In A. D. Loewy and K. M. Spyer (Eds.), *Central Regulation of Autonomic Functions*, pp. 104–125. New York: Oxford University Press.
8. Cervero, F., and Sharkey, K. (1988). An electrophysiological and anatomical study of intestinal afferent fibres in the rat. *Journal of Physiology* 401, 361–380.
9. Chahal, P. S., Rendig, S. V., and Longhurst, J. C. (1998). Bradykinin $BK_2$–receptors contribute to reflex cardiovascular responses during brief abdominal ischemia. *American Journal of Physiology* 274, H308–H313.
10. Chamberlin, N., and Saper, C. (1992). Topographic organization of cardiovascular responses to electrical and glutamate microstimulation of the parabrachial nucleus in the rat. *Journal of Comparative Neurology* 326, 245–262.

11. Chao, D. M., Shen, L. L., Tjen-A-Looi S., Pitsillides, K. F., Li, P., and Longhurst, J. C. (1999). Naloxone reverses inhibitory effect of electroacupuncture on sympathetic cardiovascular reflex responses. *American Journal of Physiology* 276, H2127–H2134.
12. Chen, S. Y., Mao, S. P., and Chai, C. Y. (2001). Role of nitric oxide on pressor mechanisms within the dorsomedial and rostral ventrolateral medulla in anaesthetized cats. *Clinical and Experimental Pharmacology and Physiology* 28, 155–163.
13. Chou, C. C. (1989). Gastrointestinal circulation and motor function. In S. G. Schultz and J. D. Wood (Eds.), *Handbook of Physiology. Section 6: The Gastrointestinal System, vol. i, pt. 2*, pp. 1475–1518. Bethesda, MD: American Physiological Society.
14. Chou, C. C., and Gallavan, R. H. (1982). Blood flow and intestinal motility. *Federation Proceedings* 41, 2090–2095.
15. Chronwall, B. (1985). Anatomy and physiology of the neuroendocrine arcuate nucleus. *Peptides* 6, 1–11.
16. Crisostomo, M., Li, P., Tjen-A-Looi, S. C., and Longhurst, J. C. (2005). Nociceptin in rVLM mediates electroacupuncture inhibition of cardiovascular reflex excitatory response in rats. *Journal of Applied Physiology* 98, 2056–2063.
17. Dibner-Dunlap, M. E., Kinugawa, T., and Thames, M. D. (1993). Activation of cardiac sympathetic afferents: Effects of exogenous adenosine and adenosine analogues. *American Journal of Physiology* 265, H395–H400.
18. Elam, M., Svensson, T., and Thoren, T. (1985). Differentiated cardiovascular afferent regulation of locus coeruleus neurons and sympathetic nerves. *Brain Research* 358, 77–88.
19. Eldridge, F. L., Millhorn, D. E., and Waldrop, T. G. (1981). Exercise hyperpnea and locomotion: Parallel activation from the hypothalamus. *Science* 211, 844–864.
20. Farkas, E., Jansen, A. S. P., and Loewy, A. D. (1998). Periaqueductal gray matter input to cardiac-related sympathetic premotor neurons. *Brain Research* 792, 179–192.
21. Figueras, J., and Cinca, J. (1981). Acute arterial hypertension during spontaneous angina in patients with fixed coronary stenosis and exertional angina: An associated rather than a triggering phenomenon. *Circulation* 64, 60–68.
22. Foote, S., Bloom, F., and Aston-Jones, G. (1983). Nucleus locus ceruleus: New evidence of anatomical and physiological specificity. *Physiological Reviews* 63, 844–914.
23. Fu, L.-W., and Longhurst, J. C. (2002). Activated platelets contribute to stimulation of cardiac afferents during ischaemia in cats: Role of 5-$HT_3$ receptors. *Journal of Physiology* 544, 897–912.
24. Fu, L.-W., and Longhurst, J. C. (2002). Role of activated platelets in excitation of cardiac afferents during myocardial ischemia in cats. *American Journal of Physiology. Heart and Circulatory Physiology* 282, H100–H109.
25. Fu, L.-W., Pan H.-L., Pitsillides, K., and Longhurst, J. (1996). Hypoxia does not directly stimulate ischemically sensitive abdominal visceral afferents during ischemia. *American Journal of Physiology* 271, H261–H266.
26. Fu, L.-W., Schunack, W., and Longhurst, J. C. (2005). Histamine contributes to ischemia-related activation of cardiac spinal afferents: Role of $H_1$ receptors and PKC. *Journal of Neurophysiology* 93, 713–722.
27. Fu, L.-W., and Longhurst, J. (1998). Role of 5-$HT_3$ receptors in activation of abdominal sympathetic C-fibre afferents during ischemia in cats. *Journal of Physiology* 509, 729–740.
28. Fu, L.-W., Pan, H.-L., and Longhurst, J. C. (1997). Endogenous histamine stimulates ischemically sensitive abdominal visceral afferents through $H_1$ receptors. *American Journal of Physiology* 273, H2726–H2737.
29. Fu, L.-W., Phan, A., and Longhurst, J. C. (2008). Myocardial ischemia-mediated excitatory reflexes: A new function for thromboxane $A_2$? *American Journal of Physiology. Heart and Circulatory Physiology* 295, H2530–H2540.
30. Fu, L.-W., and Longhurst, J. C. (2005). Interactions between histamine and bradykinin in stimulation of ischaemically sensitive cardiac afferents in felines. *Journal of Physiology* 565, 1007–1017.
31. Fu, L.-W., and Longhurst, J. C. (2010). Bradykinin and thromboxane $A_2$ reciprocally interact to synergistically stimulate cardiac spinal afferents during myocardial ischemia. *Amerian Journal of Physiology. Heart and Circulatory Physiology* 298, H235–H244.
32. Fu, L.-W., O'Neill, C. A., and Longhurst, J. C. (1997). Increased histamine and 5-HT in portal vein plasma and mesenteric lymph during brief ischemia and reperfusion. *American Journal of Physiology* 273, H1135–H1141.
33. Fu,L.,andLonghurst,C.(2009).Electroacupuncture modulates vlPAG release of GABA through presynaptic cannabinoid $CB_1$ receptor. *Journal of Applied Physiology* 106, 1800–1809.
34. Fulwiler, C., and Saper, C. (1984). Subnuclear organization of the efferent connections of the parabrachial nucleus in the rat. *Brain Research* 319, 229–259.

35. Gebber, G. (1990). Central determinants of sympathetic nerve discharge. In A. D. Loewy and K. M. Spyer (Eds.), *Central Regulation of Autonomic Functions*, pp. 126–144. New York: Oxford University Press.
36. Gee, S., Tjen-A-Looi, S., Hill, J., Chahal, P., and Longhurst, J. (2002). Role of spinal NMDA and non-NMDA receptors in the pressor reflex response to abdominal ischemia. *American Journal of Physiology. Regulatory, Integrative and Comparative Physiology* 282, R850–R857.
37. Guo Z.-L., Fu, L.-W., Symons, J., and Longhurst, J. (1998). Signal transduction in activation of ischemically sensitive abdominal visceral afferents: Role of PKC. *American Journal of Physiology* 275, H1024–H1031.
38. Guo Z.-L., Li, P., and Longhurst, J. (2002). Central pathways in the pons and midbrain involved in cardiac sympathoexcitatory reflexes in cats. *Neuroscience* 113, 433–444.
39. Guo Z.-L., and Longhurst, J. (2000). Role of cAMP in activation of ischemically sensitive abdominal visceral afferents. *American Journal of Physiology. Heart and Circulatory Physiology* 278, H843–H852.
40. Guo Z.-L., and Longhurst, J. (2003). Activation of nitric oxide-producing neurons in the brain stem during cardiac sympathoexcitatory reflexes in the cat. *Neuroscience* 116, 167–178.
41. Guo Z.-L., and Longhurst, J. (2006). Responses of neurons containing VGLUT3/nNOS-cGMP in the rVLM to cardiac stimulation. *NeuroReport* 17, 255–259.
42. Guo Z.-L., Moazzami, A., and Longhurst, J. (2004). Electroacupuncture induces c-Fos expression in the rostral ventrolateral medulla and periaqueductal gray in cats: Relation to opioid containing neurons. *Brain Research* 1030, 103–115.
43. Guo Z.-L., Moazzami, A., and Longhurst, J. (2005). Stimulation of cardiac sympathetic afferent activates glutamatergic neurons in the parabrachial nucleus: Relation to neurons containing nNOS. *Brain Research* 1053, 36–48.
44. Guo Z.-L., Moazzami, A., Tjen-A-Looi, S., and Longhurst, J. (2008). Responses of opioid and serotonin containing medullary raphe neurons to electroacupuncture. *Brain Research* 1229, 125–136.
45. Guo, Z. L., Tjen-A-Looi, S. C., Fu, L. W., and Longhurst, J. C. (2009). Nitric oxide in rostral ventrolateral medulla regulates cardiac-sympathetic reflexes: Role of synthase isoforms. *American Journal of Physiology. Heart and Circulatory Physiology* 297, H1479–H1486.
46. Guo, Z., Lai, H., and Longhurst, J. (2002). Medullary pathways involved in cardiac sympathoexcitatory reflexes in the cat. *Brain Research* 925, 55–66.
47. Guo, Z., and Moazzami, A. (2004). Involvement of nuclei in the hypothalamus in cardiac sympathoexcitatory reflexes in cats. *Brain Research* 1006, 36–48.
48. Huang, H.-S., and Longhurst, J. (1994). Cardiovascular reflexes during abdominal ischemia in cats. *American Journal of Physiology* 267, R97–R106.
49. Huang, H.-S., Pan, H.-L., Stahl, G., and Longhurst, J. (1995). Ischemia- and reperfusion-sensitive cardiac sympathetic afferents: Influence of $H_2O_2$ and hydroxyl radicals. *American Journal of Physiology* 269, H888–H901.
50. Huang, H.-S., Stahl, G., and Longhurst, J. (1995). Cardiac-cardiovascular reflexes induced by hydrogen peroxide in cats. *American Journal of Physiology* 268, H2114–H2124.
51. Janig, W., and Morrison, J. F. B. (1986). Functional properties of spinal visceral afferents supplying abdominal and pelvic organs with special emphasis on visceral nociception. In F. Cervero and J. F. B. Morrison (Eds.), *Visceral Sensation. Progress in Brain Research*, pp. 87–114. Amsterdam, Netherlands: Elsevier.
52. Kaufman, M. P., Iwamoto, G. A., Longhurst, J. C., and Mitchell, J. H. (1982). Effects of capsaicin and bradykinin on afferent fibers with endings in skeletal muscle. *Circulation Research* 50, 133–139.
53. Kaufman, M., and Forster, H. (1996). Reflexes controlling circulatory, ventilatory and airway responses to exercise. In L. B. Rowell and J. T. Shepherd (Eds.), *Handbook of Physiology, Section 12, Exercise: Regulation and Integration of Multiple Systems*, pp. 381–447. New York: Oxford University Press.
54. Kaufman, M., Longhurst, J., Rybicki, K., Wallach, J., and Mitchell, J. (1983). Effects of static muscular contraction on impulse activity of group III and IV afferents in cats. *Journal of Applied Physiology* 55, 105–112.
55. Kaufman, M., Ordway, G. A., Longhurst, J., and Mitchell, J. (1982). Reflex relaxation of tracheal smooth muscle by thin-fiber muscle afferents in dogs. *American Journal of Physiology* 243, R383–R388.
56. Kuo, D., Yang, G., Yamasaki, D., and Krauthamer, G. (1982). A wide field electron microscopic analysis of the fiber constituents of the major splanchnic nerve in the cat. *Journal of Comparative Neurology* 210, 49–58.
57. Langley, J. N. (1921). *The Autonomic Nervous System*, Cambridge, England: Heffer & Sons.
58. Langley, J., and Anderson, H. (1894). The constituents of the hypogastric nerves. *Journal of Physiology* 17, 177–191.
59. Li, P., Ayannusi, O., Reed, C., and Longhurst, J. (2004). Inhibitory effect of electroacupuncture

(EA) on the pressor response induced by exercise stress. *Clinical Autonomic Research* 14, 182–188.

60. Li, P., Pitsillides, K., Rendig, S., Pan, H.-L., and Longhurst, J. (1998). Reversal of reflex-induced myocardial ischemia by median nerve stimulation: A feline model of electroacupuncture. *Circulation* 97, 1186–1194.
61. Li, P., Rowshan, K., Crisostomo, M., Tjen-A-Looi, S., and Longhurst, J. (2002). Effect of electroacupuncture on pressor reflex during gastric distention. *American Journal of Physiology. Regulatory, Integrative and Comparative Physiology* 283, R1335–R1345.
62. Li, P., Tjen-A-Looi, S., and Longhurst, J. (2001). Rostral ventrolateral medullary opioid receptor subtypes in the inhibitory effect of electroacupuncture on reflex autonomic response in cats. *Autonomic Neuroscience* 89, 38–47.
63. Li, P., Tjen-A-Looi, S., Guo, Z., Fu, L.-W., and Longhurst, J. C. (2009). Long-loop pathways in cardiovascular electroacupuncture responses. *Journal of Applied Physiology* 106, 620–630.
64. Li, P., Tjen-A-Looi, S., and Longhurst, J. (2006). Excitatory projections from arcuate nucleus to ventrolateral periaqueductal gray in electroacupuncture inhibition of cardiovascular reflexes. *American Journal of Physiology. Heart and Circulatory Physiology* 209, H2535–H2542.
65. Lombardi, F., Casalone, C., Bella, P. D., Malfatto, G., Pagani, M., and Malliani, A. (1984). Global versus regional myocardial ischaemia: Differences in cardiovascular and sympathetic responses in cats. *Cardiovascular Research* 18, 14–23.
66. Longhurst JC. (2002). Central and peripheral neural mechanisms of acupuncture in myocardial ischemia. In A. Sato, P. Li, and J. L. Campbell (Eds.), *Acupuncture: Is There a Physiological Basis?* pp. 79–87. New York: Elsevier Science.
67. Longhurst, J. C. (1984). Static contraction of hindlimb muscles in cats reflexly relaxes tracheal smooth muscle. *Journal of Applied Physiology* 57, 380–387.
68. Longhurst, J. C. (1995). Chemosensitive abdominal visceral afferents. In G. F. Gebhart (Ed.), *Proceedings: Visceral Pain Symposium*, pp. 99–132. Seattle, WA: IASP Press.
69. Longhurst, J. C., and Ibarra, J. (1982). Sympathoadrenal mechanisms in hemodynamic responses to gastric distention in cats. *American Journal of Physiology* 243, H748–H753.
70. Longhurst, J. (1991). Reflex effects from abdominal visceral afferents. In I. H. Zucker and J. P. Gillmore (Eds.), *Reflex Control of the Circulation*, pp. 551–577. Caldwell, NJ: Telford Press.
71. Longhurst, J. (2008). Neural regulation of the cardiovascular system. In L. R. Squire, F. E. Bloom, S. K. McConnel, J. L. Roberts, N. C. Spitzer, and M. J. Zigmond (Eds.), *Fundamental Neuroscience, 2nd ed.*, pp. 935–966.San Diego, CA: Academic Press.
72. Longhurst, J., and Dittman, L. (1987). Hypoxia, bradykinin, and prostaglandins stimulate ischemically sensitive visceral afferents. *American Journal of Physiology* 253, H556–H567.
73. Longhurst, J., and Ibarra, J. (1984). Reflex regional vascular responses during passive gastric distension in cats. *American Journal of Physiology* 247, R257–R265.
74. Longhurst, J., Kaufman, M., Ordway, G., and Musch, T. (1984). Effects of bradykinin and capsaicin on endings of afferent fibers from abdominal visceral organs. *American Journal of Physiology* 247, R552–R559.
75. Longhurst, J., and Mitchell, J. (1983). Does endurance training benefit the cardiovascular system? *Journal of Cardiovascular Medicine* 8, 227–236.
76. Longhurst, J., Tjen-A-Looi, S., and Fu, L-W. (2001). Cardiac sympathetic afferent activation provoked by myocardial ischemia and reperfusion: Mechanisms and reflexes. *Annals of the New York Academy of Sciences* 940, 74–95.
77. Lovick, T. A. (1987). Cardiovascular control from neurones in the ventrolateral medulla. In E. W. Taylor (Ed.), *Neurobiology of the Cardiorespiratory System*, pp. 197–208. Manchester, UK: Manchester University Press.
78. Lovick, T. A. (1992). Inhibitory modulation of the cardiovascular defence response by the ventrolateral periaqueductal grey matter in rats. *Experimental Brain Research* 89, 133–139.
79. Lovick, T., and Li, P. (1989). Integrated function of neurones in the rostral ventrolateral medulla. *Progress in Brain Research* 81, 223–231.
80. Malliani, A., Lombardi, F., and Pagani, M. (1986). Sensory innervation of the heart. In F. Cervero and J. F. B. Morrison (Eds.), *Visceral Sensation. Progress in Brain Research, vol. 67*, pp. 39–48. Amsterdam, Netherlands: Elsevier.
81. Malliani, A. (1990). Cardiocardiac excitatory reflexes during myocardial ischemia. *Basic Research in Cardiology* 85, 243–252.
82. Mitchell, J. H., and Schmidt, R. F. (1994). Cardiovascular reflex control by afferent fibers from skeletal muscle receptors. In J. T. Shepherd and F. M. Abboud (Eds.), *Handbook of Physiology*, pp. 623–658. Baltimore, MD: Waverly Press.
83. Moazzami, A., Tjen-A-Looi, S. C., and Longhurst, J. C. (2010). Serotonergic projection from nucleus raphé pallidus to rostral ventrolateral medulla modulates cardiovascular reflex responses

during acupuncture. *Journal of Applied Physiology* 108, 1336–1346.
84. Morimoto, S., Sasaki, S., Miki, S., Kawa, T., Nakamura, K., Itoh, H., Nakata, T., Takeda, K., Nakagawa, M., and Fushiki, S. (2000). Nitric oxide is an excitatory modulator in the rostral ventrolateral medulla in rats. *American Journal of Hypertension* 13, 1125–1134.
85. Murphy, A. Z., Ennis, M., Shipley, M. T., and Behbehani, M. M. (1994). Directionally specific changes in arterial pressure induce differential patterns of fos expression in discrete areas of the rat brainstem: A double labeling study for Fos and catecholamines. *Journal of Comparative Neurology* 349, 36–50.
86. O'Donohue, T., and Dorsa, D. (1982). The opiomelanotropinergic neuronal and endocrine systems. *Peptides* 3, 353–395.
87. Ordway, G., Floyd, D., Longhurst, J., and Mitchell, J. (1984). Oxygen consumption and hemodynamic responses during graded treadmill exercise in the dog. *Journal of Applied Physiology* 57, 601–607.
88. Ordway, G., and Longhurst, J. (1983). Cardiovascular reflexes arising form the gallbladder of the cat: Effects of capsaicin, bradykinin and distension. *Circulation Research* 52, 26–35.
89. Pan, H.-L., and Longhurst, J. C. (1996). Ischaemia-sensitive sympathetic afferents innervating the gastrointestinal tract function as nociceptors in cats. *Journal of Physiology* 492, 841–850.
90. Pan H.-L., Bonham, A. C., and Longhurst, J. C. (1995). Role of spinal $NK_1$ receptors in cardiovascular responses to chemical stimulation of the gallbladder. *American Journal of Physiology* 268, H526–H534.
91. Pan, H.-L., and Longhurst, J. (1995). Lack of a role of adenosine in activation of ischemically sensitive cardiac sympathetic afferents in cats. *American Journal of Physiology* 269, H106–H113.
92. Pan, H.-L., Zeisse, Z. B., and Longhurst, J. (1996). Role of summation of afferent input in cardiovascular reflexes from splanchnic nerve stimulation. *American Journal of Physiology* 270, H849–H856.
93. Pan, H.-L., Zeisse, Z. B., and Longhurst, J. (1997). Mechanical stimulation is not responsible for activation of gastrointestinal afferents during ischemia. *American Journal of Physiology* 272, H99–H106.
94. Pan, H.-L., Longhurst, J. C., and Stahl, G. L. (1995). Differential effect of 5- and 15-lipoxygenase products on ischemically sensitive abdominal visceral afferents. *American Journal of Physiology* 269, H96–H105.
95. Pan, H.-L., Stahl, G. L., Rendig, S. V., Carretero, O. A., and Longhurst, J. C. (1994). Endogenous BK stimulates ischemically sensitive abdominal visceral C fiber afferents through kinin $B_2$ receptors. *American Journal of Physiology* 267, H2398–H2406.
96. Pan, H.-L., Stebbins, C. L., and Longhurst, J. C. (1993). Bradykinin contributes to the exercise pressor reflex: Mechanism of action. *Journal of Applied Physiology* 75, 2061–2068.
97. Pan, H.-L., Zeisse, Z. B., Pitsillides, K. F., and Longhurst, J. C. (1997). Spatiotemporal aspects of sympathetic C-fiber afferent activity in pressor reflex during abdominal ischemia. *American Journal of Physiology* 272, H1928–H1936.
98. Rotto, D., Schultz, H., Longhurst, J., and Kaufman, M. (1990). Sensitization of group III muscle afferents to static contraction by arachidonic acid metabolism. *Journal of Applied Physiology* 68, 861–867.
99. Rybicki, K., Longhurst, J., and Kaufman, M. (1983). Stimulation of splanchnic afferents reflexly relaxes tracheal smooth muscle in dogs. *Journal of Applied Physiology* 55, 427–432.
100. Stahl, G., Halliwell, B., and Longhurst, J. (1992). Hydrogen peroxide-induced cardiovascular reflexes: Role of hydroxyl radicals. *Circulation Research* 71, 295–302.
101. Stahl, G., and Longhurst, J. (1992). Ischemically sensitive visceral afferents: Importance of $H^+$ derived from lactic acid and hypercapnia. *American Journal of Physiology* 262, H748–H753.
102. Stahl, G., Pan, H.-L., and Longhurst, J. (1993). Activation of ischemia and reperfusion-sensitive abdominal visceral C fiber afferents: Role of hydrogen peroxide and hydroxyl radicals. *Circulation Research* 72, 1266–1275.
103. Staszewska-Woolley, J., and Woolley, G. (1989). Participation of the kallikrein-kinin-receptor system in reflexes arising from neural afferents in the dog epicardium. *Journal of Physiology* 419, 33–44.
104. Stebbins, C. L., Brown, B., Levin, D., and Longhurst, J. C. (1988). Reflex effect of skeletal muscle mechanoreceptor stimulation on the cardiovascular system. *Journal of Applied Physiology* 65, 1539–1547.
105. Stebbins, C. L., and Longhurst, J. C. (1986). Bradykinin in the reflex cardiovascular responses to static muscular contraction. *Journal of Applied Physiology* 61, 271–279.
106. Stebbins, C. L., and Longhurst, J. C. (1989). Potentiation of the exercise pressor reflex by muscle ischemia. *Journal of Applied Physiology* 66, 1046–1053.
107. Stebbins, C., Maruoka, Y., and Longhurst, J. (1986). Prostaglandins contribute to cardiovascular

reflexes evoked by static muscular contraction. *Circulation Research* 59, 645–654.

108. Symons, J., Theodossy, S., Longhurst, J., and Stebbins, C. (1991). Intramuscular accumulation of prostaglandins during static contraction of the cat triceps surae. *Journal of Applied Physiology* 71, 1837–1842.
109. Talman, W. T., Dragon, D. H., Ohta, H., and Lin, L. H. (2001). Nitroxidergic influences on cardiovascular control by NTS: A link with glutamate. *Annals of the New York Academy of Sciences* 940, 169–178.
110. Tjen-A-Looi, S. C., Li, P., and Longhurst, J. C. (2007). Role of medullary GABA, opioids, and nociceptin in prolonged inhibition of cardiovascular sympathoexcitatory reflexes during electroacupuncture in cats. *American Journal of Physiology. Heart and Circulatory Physiology* 293, H3627–H3635.
111. Tjen-A-Looi, S. C., Li, P., and Longhurst, J. C. (2003). Prolonged inhibition of rostral ventral lateral medullary premotor sympathetic neuron by electroacupuncture in cats. *Autonomic Neuroscience* 106, 119–131.
112. Tjen-A-Looi, S. C., Li, P., and Longhurst, J. C. (2004). Medullary substrate and differential cardiovascular response during stimulation of specific acupoints. *American Journal of Physiology. Regulatory, Integrative and Comparative Physiology* 287, R852–R862.
113. Tjen-A-Looi, S. C., Li, P., and Longhurst, J. C. (2006). Midbrain vlPAG inhibits rVLM cardiovascular sympathoexcitatory responses during acupuncture. *American Journal of Physiology. Heart and Circulatory Physiology* 209, H2543–H2553.
114. Tjen-A-Looi, S., Fu, L.-W.,and Longhurst, J. C. (2002). Xanthine oxidase, but not neutrophils, contribute to activation of cardiac sympathetic afferents during myocardial ischaemia in cats. *Journal of Physiology* 543, 327–336.
115. Tjen-A-Looi, S., Bonham, A., and Longhurst, J. (1997). Interactions between sympathetic and vagal cardiac afferents in nucleus tractus solitarii. *American Journal of Physiology* 272, H2843–H2851.
116. Tjen-A-Looi, S., Pan, H.-L., and Longhurst, J. C. (1998). Endogenous bradykinin activates ischaemically sensitive cardiac visceral afferents through kinin $B_2$ receptors in cats. *Journal of Physiology* 510, 633–641.
117. Tjen-A-Looi, S. C., Phan, N. T., and Longhurst, J. C. (2001). Nitric oxide modulates sympathoexcitatory cardiac-cardiovascular reflexes elicited by bradykinin. *American Journal of Physiology. Heart and Circulatory Physiology* 281, H2010–H2017.
118. Tjen-A-Looi, S., Fu, L.-W., Zhou, W., and Longhurst, J. C. (2005). Role of unmyelinated fibers in electroacupuncture cardiovascular responses. *Autonomic Neuroscience* 118, 43–50.
119. Tjen-A-Looi, S., Li, P., and Longhurst, J. C. (2009). Processing cardiovascular information in the vlPAG during electroacupuncture in rats: Roles of endocannabinoids and GABA. *Journal of Applied Physiology* 1793–1799.
120. Tseng, C. J., Liu, H. Y., Lin, H. C., Ger, L. P., Tung, C. S., and Yen, M. H. (1996). Cardiovascular effects of nitric oxide in the brain stem nuclei of rats. *Hypertension* 27, 36–42.
121. Ustinova, E., and Schultz, H. D. (1994). Activation of cardiac vagal afferents by oxygen-derived free radicals in rats. *Circulation Research* 74, 895–903.
122. Waldrop, T. G., Eldridge, F. L., Iwamoto, G. A., and Mitchell, J. H. (1996). Central neural control of respiration and circulation during exercise. In L. B. Rowell and J. T. Shepherd (Eds.), *Handbook of Physiology. Section 12, Exercise: Regulation and Integration of Multiple Systems*, pp. 333–380. New York: Oxford University Press.
123. White, J. C. (1957). Cardiac pain: Anatomic pathway and physiologic mechanisms. *Circulation* 16, 644–655.
124. White, J., Garny, W., and Atkins, J. (1933). Cardiac innervation. *Archives of Surgery* 26, 765–786.
125. Willis, W. D., Jr. (1985). *The Pain System—The Neural Basis of Nociceptive Transmission in the Mammalian Nervous System*, Basel, Switzerland: Karger.
126. Yao, T., Andersson, S., and Thoren, P. (1982). Long-lasting cardiovascular depressor response following sciatic stimulation in spontaneously hypertensive rats. Evidence for the involvement of central endorphin and serotonin systems. *Brain Research* 244, 295–303.
127. Zhang, Y. M., Li, P., and Lovick, T. A. (1994). Role of the nucleus raphé obscurus in the inhibition of rostral ventrolateral medullary neurones induced by stimulation in the ventrolateral periaqueductal grey matter of the rabbit. *Neuroscience Letters* 176, 231–234.
128. Zhou W., Fu, L. W., Tjen-A-Looi, S. C., Li, P., and Longhurst, J. C. (2005). Afferent mechanisms underlying stimulation modality-related modulation of acupuncture-related cardiovascular responses. *Journal of Applied Physiology* 98, 872–880.
129. Zhou, W., Mahajan, A., and Longhurst, J. C. (2009). Spinal nociceptin mediates electroacupuncture-related modulation of visceral sympathoexcitatory reflex responses in rats. *American Journal of Physiology. Heart and Circulatory Physiology* 297 H859–H865.

130. Zhou, W., Fu, L.-W.,Guo, Z., and Longhurst, J. (2007). Role of glutamate in rostral ventrolateral medulla in acupuncture-related modulation of visceral reflex sympathoexcitation. *American Journal of Physiology. Heart and Circulatory Physiology* 292, H1868–H1875.
131. Zhou, W., Hsiao, I., Lin, V., and Longhurst, J. (2006). Modulation of cardiovascular excitatory responses in rats by transcutaneous magnetic stimulation: Role of the spinal cord. *Journal of Applied Physiology* 100, 926–932.
132. Zhou, W., Tjen-A-Looi, S., and Longhurst, J. C. (2005). Brain stem mechanisms underlying acupuncture modality-related modulation of cardiovascular responses in rats. *Journal of Applied Physiology* 99, 851–860.
133. Zhou, W., Fu, L. W., Tjen-A-Looi, S. C., Guo, Z. L., and Longhurst, J. C. (2006). Role of glutamate in a visceral sympathoexcitatory reflex in rostral ventrolateral medulla of cats. *Amerian Journal of Physiology. Heart and circulatory physiology* 291, H1309–H1318.

10

# Cardiorespiratory Integration

PATRICE G. GUYENET

This chapter provides a brief overview of how the central nervous system coordinates respiration and circulation to achieve $pO_2$ and $pCO_2$ homeostasis and optimal tissue oxygenation. During physical exercise, for example, pulmonary ventilation rises to meet the challenge of increased oxygen consumption and metabolic production of $CO_2$. Exercise also causes a coordinated rise in cardiac output and arterial pressure and reapportions cardiac output in favor of the exercising muscles. Under other circumstances, the relationship between breathing and cardiovascular regulation obeys different rules. For example, in response to severe hypoxia, available oxygen must be sent to the brain and the heart preferentially. As a result, breathing increases to maximize oxygen intake, and there is a concomitant reduction in cardiac output and blood flow to non-essential tissues. During diving, breathing stops, the heart slows, arterial $pCO_2$ is permitted to rise above normal levels, and blood flow to muscles is reduced by neurogenic vasoconstriction, despite the increased metabolism required by the dive.

From these few examples, it is clear that the relationship between respiration and cardiovascular (i.e., sympathetic vasomotor and cardiovagal) autonomic outflow depends on behavior and environment, and thus regulation of the cardiovascular system requires presumably all levels of the neuraxis from spinal cord to cortex. The first part of this chapter focuses on the most basic CNS processes involved in matching circulation to respiration. These processes take place within a set of interconnected pontomedullary structures represented in Figure 10–1. The second part of the chapter provides a brief description of the changes in cardiovascular autonomic outflow that occur during exercise, hypoxia, and diving. Detailed information on the organization of the respiratory network is beyond the scope of this chapter, and can be found elsewhere[6,23-25,100]. Prior reviews and books on cardiopulmonary afferents and integrated cardiorespiratory reflexes provide a useful background[6,12,32,97,111,112,120,127].

## RESPIRATORY FLUCTUATIONS OF THE CARDIOVAGAL AND SYMPATHETIC VASOMOTOR OUTFLOWS

Heart rate and sympathetic vasomotor nerve activity fluctuate with respiration in all species examined (Figure 10–2; for reviews see [42,61]). The respiratory fluctuation of heart rate is called sinus arrhythmia. The fluctuations of sympathetic nerve activity and heart rate are classically attributed to the combined effect of "central coupling" and feedback from cardiopulmonary sensory afferents (Figure 10–3).

Central coupling refers to the fluctuations in sympathetic nerve activity and heart rate that are synchronized with phrenic nerve discharge in experimental preparations in which cardiopulmonary afferents have been cut or are not phasically active[69,91]. These residual respiratory fluctuations indicate that the neural networks generating sympathetic and cardiovagal outflows receive inputs from the network that generates the respiratory outflow. When cardiopulmonary afferents are intact, the respiratory patterns in sympathetic nerve activity are more complex because of

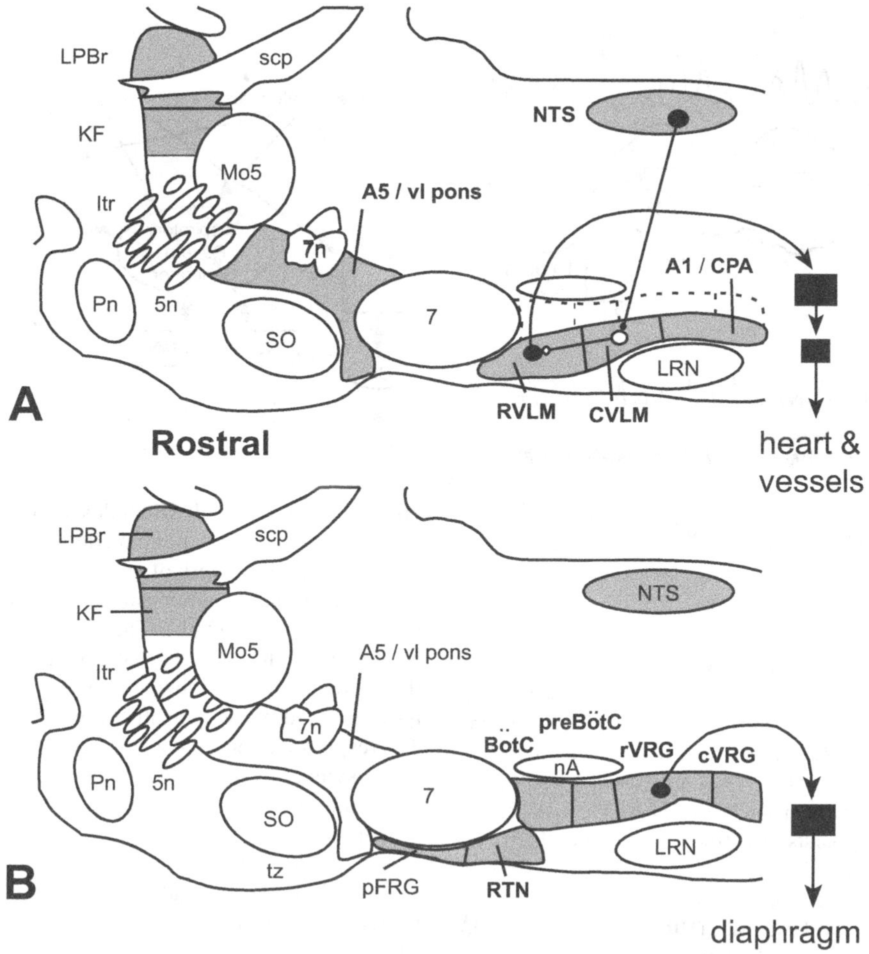


Figure 10–1 Main cardiorespiratory regions of the pons and medulla. On the basis of functional and anatomical criteria, cardiovascular physiologists have divided the ventrolateral medulla into three rostrocaudal regions, whereas respiratory physiologists divided the same area into four regions. *A:* The pontomedullary neurons that regulate the heart and vasomotor sympathetic outflow occur in a series of contiguous, reciprocally connected structures that extend from the spinomedullary junction to the dorsolateral pons. The parasagittal section in *A* (modified from Feldman and Del Negro (2006)[22], with permission) from a rat lies about 1.9 mm lateral to the midline. The core pathway of the baroreflex is drawn for orientation (*black circles*, glutamate transmission; *open circles*, GABA). *B:* The motor outflow to diaphragm and intercostals and airway respiratory muscles is generated within the same brain regions. The pre-Bötzinger region (pre-BötC) contains neurons that are essential to inspiratory rhythm generation[22]. Rhythmic respiratory-like activity survives in a coronal slice of the type depicted in Figure. 10.4. A1/CPA, region containing the A1 group of noradrenergic neurons also called "caudal pressor region"; A5/Vl pons, region of the ventrolateral pons containing the A5 group of noradrenergic neurons; BötC, Bötzinger region; CVLM, caudal ventrolateral medulla, here defined as the region that contains the major inhibitory relay of the sympathetic baroreflex; cVRG, caudal ventral respiratory group; Itr, inter-trigeminal region (not yet clearly identified as a region relevant to cardiovascular function); KF, Kölliker-Fuse nucleus; LPBr, lateral parabrachial region; LRN, lateral reticular nucleus; nA, nucleus ambiguus; NTS, nucleus of the solitary tract; Pn, pontine nuclei; RVLM, rostral ventrolateral medulla; RTN, retrotrapezoid nucleus (region containing central chemoreceptors in the adult[69]); pFRG, parafacial respiratory group (a poorly defined collection of neurons that may be important for respiratory rhythm generation at late gestational and early neonatal ages and are possibly selectively involved in generating expiratory activity[22]; the relationship between pfRG and RTN chemoreceptors is uncertain); rVRG, rostral ventral respiratory group; scp, superior cerebellar peduncle; SO, superior olive; tz, trapezoid nucleus; Mo5, trigeminal motor nucleus; 5n, trigeminal motor nerve; 7, facial motor nucleus; 7n, seventh nerve.

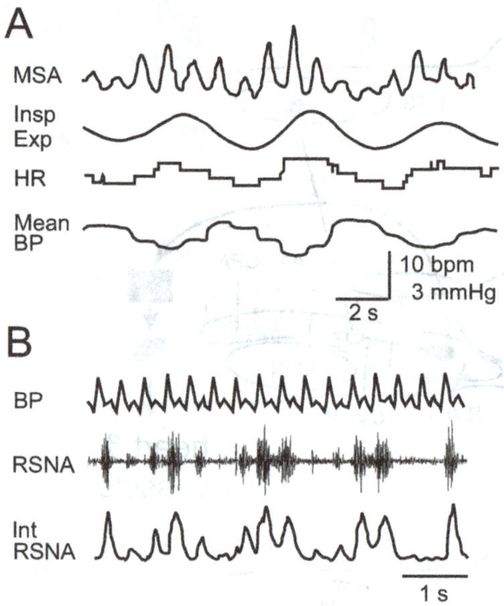


Figure 10–2 Respiratory fluctuations of heart rate and sympathetic nerve activity. *A:* Example of multi-unit sympathetic nerve activity from a fiber bundle that innervates skeletal muscle arteries (muscle sympathetic nerve activity [MSA]) in man. The recording is from the peroneal nerve of an awake subject (modified from Macefield and Wallin [1995][53], with permission). The bursts (rectified and smoothed) are synchronized with the pressure pulse (not illustrated). Their amplitude waxes and wanes with respiration (Insp/Exp). The heart rate (HR) also oscillates with respiration (sinus arrhythmia). *B:* Example of raw (30–2000 Hz; RSNA) and integrated (int RSNA) multi-unit sympathetic activity recorded from the renal nerve of an awake rabbit (reproduced from Malpas [1998][55], with permission). The sympathetic bursts occur in synchrony with the pulse. The amplitude of the bursts waxes and wanes at the frequency of respiration (about 1Hz), not recorded in this experiment. The integrated renal sympathetic nerve activity appears remarkably similar to the trace of human muscle SNA shown in *A*. BP, Blood pressure.

the superimposed influence of many sensory afferents from the thoracic region that also have respiration-related fluctuations in their discharge[42]. Such respiratory-modulated afferents include arterial baroreceptors, lung stretch receptors, cardiac receptors, low-pressure (volume) receptors, and joint and stretch receptors activated by the contraction of the diaphragm and intercostal muscles[42]. Detailed information regarding the properties of these various afferents can be

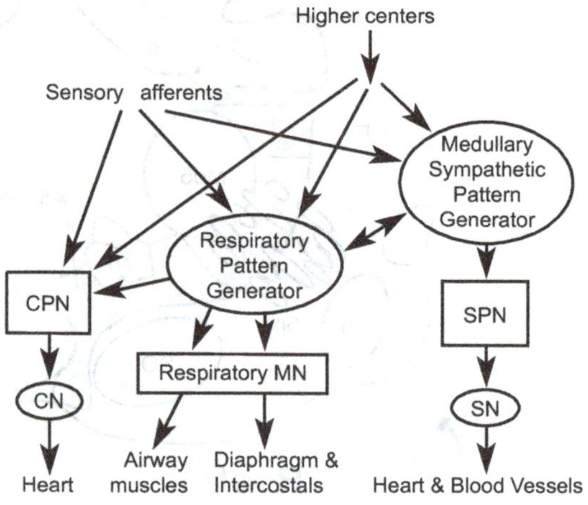


Figure 10–3 General principles of cardiorespiratory integration. The pontomedullary region contains a complex network of neurons that generate the various respiratory motor outflows (respiratory pattern generating network). The same general region also contains the network that generates the sympathetic vasomotor outflow grouped here under the term of "medullary sympathetic pattern generator". The respiratory pattern generating network and medullary sympathetic pattern generator interact at many levels and this interaction persists in the absence of sensory afferent input, a phenomenon called central coupling. Central coupling is believed to underlie the most basic level of adjustment of the circulation (cardiac output and arterial pressure) to breathing. The respiratory pattern generating network and medullary sympathetic pattern generator are controlled by the same set of sensory afferents, most prominently by cardiopulmonary afferents (e.g., baroreceptors, lung mechanoreceptors, chemoreceptors, etc.). These afferents usually influence the medullary sympathetic pattern generator both via the respiratory pattern generating network and independently of it. The respiratory pattern generating network and the medullary sympathetic pattern generator also receive input from higher centers, a process generally defined as "central command". Central command is essential for coordinating respiration and circulation during behavior, in particular during physical exercise. The cardiovagal outflow (CPN, cardiac parasympathetic preganglionic neurons; CN, cardiovagal parasympathetic motor neurons) is likewise subject to central command and to control by cardiopulmonary and other sensory afferents via the respiratory pattern generating network and independently of it. MN, motor neurons; SPN, sympathetic preganglionic neurons; SN, sympathetic post-ganglionic neurons.

found elsewhere[12,127]. These respiratory-modulated or respiratory-phasic afferents influence the autonomic outflows (cardiovagal and sympathetic) both through the respiratory network and via pathways that are independent of it (see below; and Figure 10–3).

### Sinus Arrhythmia

Sinus arrhythmia (Figure 10–2A) is due to respiration-synchronous fluctuations in the activity of cardiovagal motor neurons that innervate the sino-atrial node. Similar respiratory fluctuations presumably characterize the activity of vagal motor neurons supplying the atrioventricular node and the ventricles, but these fluctuations have no impact on the heart rate. The timing and the amplitude of sinus arrhythmia do not accurately reflect the timing and amplitude of the respiratory fluctuations in cardiovagal motoneuronal activity. Because muscarinic neuro-effector coupling at the sinus node is not instantaneous, the change in heart rate lags behind the change in motoneuronal activity, and its relative amplitude is dampened. These distortions increase at higher heart rates. The time constant of noradrenergic neuro-effector transmission in the sinus node is too long for the sympathetic innervation of the heart to influence heart rate on a beat-to-beat basis. The respiratory fluctuations in sympathetic nerve activity are thought to contribute little to sinus arrhythmia.

### Respiratory Fluctuations of Sympathetic Nerve Activity

The sympathetic nervous system regulates numerous physiological processes besides the circulation. In this chapter, sympathetic nerve activity refers to the activity of barosensitive efferents that innervate the heart, resistance vessels, the kidney (tubules, juxtaglomerular apparatus and blood vessels), the noradrenaline-releasing chromaffin cells in the medulla of the adrenal gland, and the large veins (for details, see[31]). These sympathetic efferents discharge in synchrony with the arterial pulse (Figure 10–2B) and can be completely silenced by even modest increases in arterial pressure via the arterial baroreflex. In concert with the parasympathetic innervation of the heart, barosensitive sympathetic efferents dominate short-term regulation of cardiac output and arterial pressure and are thus the most important partner of the respiratory system in maintaining blood gas homeostasis during exercise, short-term hypoxia, or diving[31]. Two other groups of sympathetic efferents also regulate the circulation. Cutaneous vasoconstrictor efferents are important in the context of thermoregulation and emotions; sympathetic efferents to adrenaline-secreting chromaffin cells play a role in the context of stress and exercise. Sympathetic preganglionic neurons that control adrenaline secretion are not influenced by baroreceptors, inhibited by cardiopulmonary receptors and activated by hypoxia. Cutaneous vasoconstrictor efferents are, at best, weakly affected by arterial baroreceptors. These efferents show respiratory modulation[42], but central mechanisms responsible for these respiratory fluctuations have not been investigated and therefore will not be dealt with further here.

Respiratory fluctuations of sympathetic nerve activity are observed in all mammalian species, including man, and are present both under anesthesia and in the awake state (Figure 10–2 A, B)[42,61]. Sympathetic postganglionic neurons show several respiratory-related patterns of activity[32,38,38]. These patterns are species-specific, vary according to the target tissue innervated by the sympathetic fibers, and depend on the type of cardiopulmonary afferents that are active at the time of measurement[2,42]. Synchronizing the discharge of barosensitive sympathetic efferents by baroreceptors and by respiration may facilitate neuro-effector coupling by promoting a bursting pattern of firing in postganglionic neurons[60,61].

## MECHANISMS OF CENTRAL COUPLING

As indicated above, "central coupling" denotes the fact that parasympathetic outflow to the heart and sympathetic vasomotor outflow still fluctuate in synchrony with the brainstem respiratory network when the brain no longer receives any cardiopulmonary afferent input. This section examines the mechanisms that underlie the synchronization of these autonomic outflows with the respiratory network.

### Synaptic Mechanisms Responsible for the Central Respiratory Modulation of Cardiovagal Preganglionic Neurons

In the absence of lung input, the discharge of cardiovagal parasympathetic preganglionic neurons reaches its nadir during central inspiration (as defined by phrenic nerve discharge). Its apex occurs during post-inspiration, and some intermediate level of activity is observed during late expiration[80,90,112]. This pattern is conserved across various mammalian species.

Sharp electrode intracellular recordings from two neurons in the cat *in vivo* and whole cell recordings in a rat brainstem slice that generates a respiratory-like activity (the neonate breathing slice) have revealed

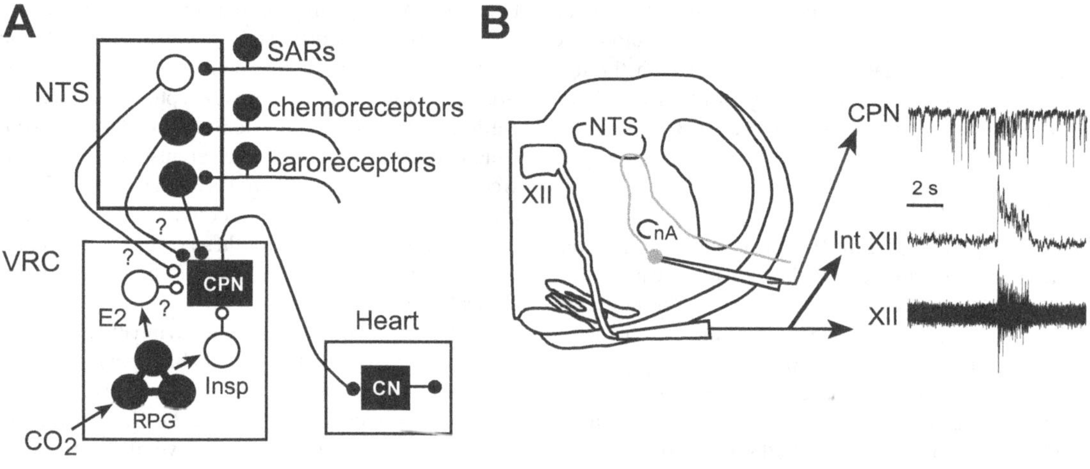


Figure 10–4 Respiratory control of cardiovagal preganglionic neurons. *A:* Cardiovagal parasympathetic preganglionic neurons (CPN) are continuously driven by arterial baroreceptors and also receive ill-defined tonic CNS inputs (not illustrated). Their respiratory modulation is due in large part to a periodic inhibition from the respiratory pattern generator (RPG) that is mediated by both GABA/glycine inspiratory-related neurons (Insp) and, possibly, by late-expiratory neurons (E2). The inspiratory and E2 inhibition of CPN contributes to sinus arrhythmia and causes the heart to accelerate during inspiration and late-expiration. The bradycardia associated with diving may rely on the same neural mechanism; i.e., the loss of the respiratory inhibition of CPNs. The primary bradycardia associated with protective cardiopulmonary reflexes (stimulation of the carotid body and cardiopulmonary C-fibers) could, in theory, rely on a direct excitatory input from NTS (represented in the figure) and on more indirect pathways through the RPG (not represented). The tachycardia associated with increased lung stretch activation could, also in theory, be caused by an inhibitory input from second-order NTS neurons that receive inputs from slowly adapting lung stretch receptors (SARs). *B:* Example of whole-cell patch recording (*right, top trace*) of a CPN (*gray*) in a thick slice of neonate rat medulla oblongata (unpublished illustration courtesy of Dr. D. Mendelowitz: see also [72]). CPNs were pre-labeled by administration of a fluorescent retrograde tracer in the pericardial sac and were identified several days later in the slice by their fluorescence. The slice retains core components of the respiratory network that are generating regular spontaneous oscillations. Rhythmic inspiratory activity was recorded from a rootlet of the hypoglossal (XII) nerve; middle and bottom traces show raw and integrated (Int) XII activities, respectively. A single CPN located in the loose formation of nucleus ambiguus (nA) is represented in the figure with its axon exiting from a ventral motor rootlet of the vagus nerve. Note the burst of GABAergic inhibitory post-synaptic currents in the CPN coincident with inspiration. VRC, ventral respiratory column.

some of the synaptic mechanisms that underlie the respiratory cyclic activity of cardiovagal preganglionic neurons (Figure 10–4)[28,80,112]. In both models, cardiovagal preganglionic neurons are actively inhibited during the inspiratory phase of the respiratory pattern generator[28,80]. In rat slices these inhibitory inputs have both a GABAergic and a glycinergic component[80]. Their differential sensitivity to nicotinic blockers suggests that GABA and glycine could be released by separate classes of neurons[80]. The Bötzinger region of the ventral respiratory column contains glycinergic neurons that are selectively active during central inspiration in slices[74] (Figure 10–4A). These neurons are a plausible source of inspiratory inhibition to the cardiovagal preganglionic neurons. Inspiratory-related inhibition is the only well-characterized respiratory input to cardiovagal preganglionic neurons. The mechanisms that underlie the fluctuations in their membrane potential during the post-inspiratory and late expiratory phases have not been determined precisely. The reduced discharge probability that occurs during the late expiratory phase may be due to an input from inhibitory expiratory augmenting neurons that are plentiful in the ventrolateral medulla[44]. The increased discharge probability of cardiovagal parasympathetic preganglionic neurons observed *in vivo* during the post-inspiratory period may reflect the relaxation of respiratory-related inhibition that occurs during both inspiration and late expiration (Figure 10–4A). The neurons may receive an excitatory drive during the post-inspiratory phase, but it is not present in slices, and its existence has not been conclusively demonstrated *in vivo*.

Since the strength of the inhibitory respiratory inputs to cardiovagal preganglionic neurons is proportional to the central inspiratory drive, central coupling should have the effect of increasing cardiac rate and output in proportion to breathing intensity, especially when the inspiratory drive is high, such as during exercise. However, in an awake and exercising mammal, cardiovagal tone could also be withdrawn by many other processes besides inhibition arising from the central respiratory network. These processes could include direct inhibition of the activity of cardiovagal preganglionic neurons by central command, inhibition by inputs from lung stretch afferents, or reductions in baroreceptor afferent input, which is probably one of the principal sources of excitatory drive to these preganglionic neurons *in vivo* (Figure 10–4). The relative importance of each of these mechanisms will have to be assessed in the future.

## Synaptic Mechanisms Responsible for the Central Respiratory Modulation of Barosensitive Sympathetic Efferents

Under anesthesia, and probably also in the awake state, barosensitive sympathetic preganglionic neurons derive a large portion of their excitatory input from bulbospinal neurons (adrenaline-synthesizing C1 neurons and non-adrenergic non-C1 neurons) located in the rostral ventrolateral medulla (RVLM) [31] (Figure 10–5). Subsets of RVLM neurons exert a variable influence over different vascular beds or the heart, an arrangement defined as organotopy. Although RVLM neurons have multiple respiration-independent sources of drive (see Chapter 5 or [31]), they retain a respiratory modulation even in the absence of cardiorespiratory afferent input. Hence this modulation is of central origin and is roughly proportional to the activity of the central respiratory pattern generator[38]. The respiratory patterns of activity found in RVLM neurons closely resemble those observed in individual barosensitive sympathetic efferents recorded under the same condition[31]. This similarity is the principal evidence that coupling between respiration and barosensitive sympathetic nerve activity occurs at the level of the RVLM or further upstream within the sympathetic network, rather than via direct inputs from the respiratory pattern generator to sympathetic preganglionic neurons (Figures 10.3 and 10.5).

Barosensitive neurons in the RVLM could, in theory, derive their central respiratory entrainment from both excitatory and inhibitory inputs. The best-documented source of respiratory modulated input to RVLM neurons is the γ-aminobutyric acid (GABA)-releasing neurons that relay the baroreflex. The cell bodies of these neurons are located in the ventrolateral medulla caudal to the sympathoexcitatory neurons (Figure 10–5; see Chapter 5)[62]. Most of these neurons in the caudal ventrolateral medulla (CVLM) reside slightly below the pre-Bötzinger complex and the immediately adjacent rostral ventral respiratory group (Figure 10–1)[105]. These two regions are core components of the network that generates the inspiratory motor outflow[23]. They are plausible sources of respiratory input to the CVLM neurons but there is currently no evidence to support this assertion except the argument of proximity. The respiratory modulation of CVLM neuronal activity probably accounts for the respiratory fluctuations in the strength of the baroreflex (Figure 10–5)[12,72] and could also explain the puzzling phase-shift between the respiratory fluctuation of baroreceptor afferents and that of sympathetic nerve activity seen in humans[27,59]. CVLM neurons have a variety of respiratory patterns[62]. Several of these patterns are the mirror image of those exhibited by RVLM sympathoexcitatory neurons. This finding suggests that clusters of sympathoexcitatory neurons in the RVLM may receive inputs from defined subgroups of CVLM neurons, perhaps indicating an extension of the organotopic organization found in the RVLM.

Evidence for other sources of respiratory modulated inhibitory input to RVLM neurons is less persuasive. The expiratory-incrementing (E2) neurons of the Bötzinger region[44] may be a source of late-expiratory inhibition to sympathetic nerve activity in rats, and some of these neurons appear to contact a subset of C1 neurons[116]. However, the Bötzinger E2 neurons identified so far are glycinergic[106], and strychnine administration into the RVLM does not change the respiratory modulation of sympathetic nerve activity[33]. Evidence for respiratory-modulated excitatory (glutamatergic) inputs to RVLM neurons is still weak because it relies on the effects produced by microinjection into the RVLM of drugs that change the operation of the entire respiratory network[33,70,71]. Accordingly, the hypothetical glutamatergic respiratory-modulated

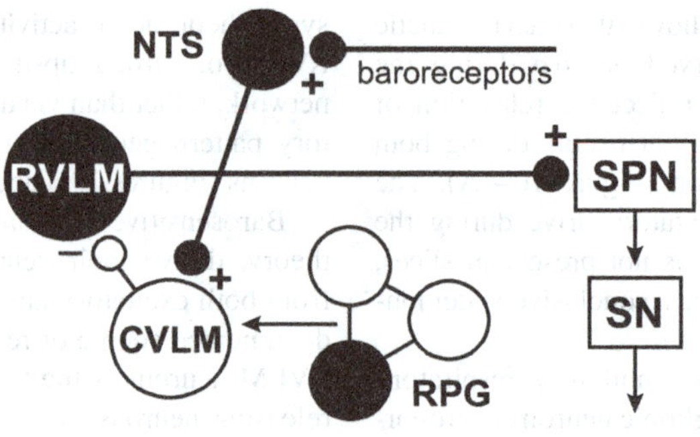


Figure 10–5 Central coupling between sympathetic vasomotor outflow and respiration. The respiratory modulation of individual sympathetic post-ganglionic barosensitive neurons (SN) shows striking similarities with that of subsets of barosensitive pre-sympathetic neurons of the ventrolateral medulla (RVLM)[35]. This similarity suggests that the respiratory centers influence the vaso- and cardiomotor sympathetic outflow, at least in part, via the sympathoexcitatory neurons of the RVLM. The respiratory modulation of RVLM neurons probably derives from respiratory fluctuations in the discharge of the GABAergic neurons of the CVLM that relay the arterial baroreflex[56] (for anatomical location of RVLM and CVLM neurons, *see also* Figure 10–1, panel A). It is not clear at the moment whether CVLM neurons receive excitatory, inhibitory or mixed inputs from the respiratory pattern generator (RPG). The scheme accounts well for the respiration-synchronous waxing and waning of the sympathetic discharge shown in Figure 10–2. NTS, nucleus of the solitary tract; SPN, sympathetic preganglionic neurons.

inputs to RVLM neurons, if they exist at all, could reside anywhere within the cardiorespiratory regions depicted in Figure 10–1.

Finally, several pathways that do not involve the RVLM have also been suggested as possible additional interfaces between the respiratory network and barosensitive sympathetic efferents. For example, the existence of direct or oligosynaptic inputs from bulbospinal inspiratory premotor neurons to sympathetic preganglionic neurons has been postulated to account for the respiratory modulation of barosensitive sympathetic efferents in species where this modulation is inspiratory (for references see [32]). However, there is still little anatomical support for such a pathway. Furthermore, the analogy between the respiratory pattern of sympathetic nerves and that of bulbospinal inspiratory neurons breaks down in species such as the rat and the rabbit, where the respiratory modulation of sympathetic nerve activity is not inspiratory but phase-spanning. In cats, the rostromedial medullary region contains bulbospinal neurons that may also regulate the discharge of barosensitive sympathetic efferents[4]. In theory, such neurons could also contribute to the respiratory fluctuations in sympathetic nerve activity because the raphé region contains many neurons with activity that shows respiratory modulation[56]. The caudal raphé of the rat contains bulbospinal neurons that are modestly inhibited by baroreceptor stimulation and are therefore also possibly "sympathoexcitatory"[92]. These neurons are more active during inspiration and could therefore contribute to the inspiratory modulation seen in some splanchnic nerve efferents. Under light anesthesia, the discharge of the pontine noradrenergic neurons of the A5 and A6 regions is entrained by the central respiratory network[34]. The barosensitive neurons of the RVLM innervate these noradrenergic neurons[7] and could be the source of their respiratory modulation, which, in turn, may further amplify the respiratory entrainment of sympathetic nerve activity mediated by the direct projection from RVLM to sympathetic preganglionic neurons.

In summary, the respiratory control of barosensitive sympathetic efferents operates at least in part via the barosensitive neurons of the RVLM, and the respiratory control of the latter neurons is best explained at present by respiratory fluctuations in the strength of their inhibitory input from the CVLM, as depicted in Figure 10–5. However, this interpretation rests on the results of experiments performed under anesthesia, primarily in rats. Additional mechanisms and pathways should not be discounted, but the level of evidence for these is weaker.

## CHEMORECEPTION AND CARDIORESPIRATORY INTEGRATION

An essential function of cardiorespiratory integration is to promote $pCO_2$ homeostasis by efficient removal of tissue $CO_2$. This section explores how barosensitive sympathetic efferents and the cardiovagal parasympathetic outflow are regulated by the activation of central and peripheral chemoreceptors.

### Central Chemoreceptors and Cardiorespiratory Integration

Sympathetic nerve activity is activated along with respiration by stimulating either central or peripheral chemoreceptors (Figure 10–6), and the effects of the two chemosensory inputs are at least additive and most probably supra-additive[5,36].

The way in which central chemoreceptors activate respiration and sympathetic nerve activity is related to the previously discussed issue of central coupling, because central coupling is primarily observed in anesthetized or reduced preparations in which the activity of the respiratory centers is driven by $CO_2$; i.e., by the activation of central chemoreceptors. However, several additional issues must be considered; namely, the nature of central chemoreceptors, whether the same, different, or overlapping chemoreceptors drive sympathetic nerve activity versus respiration and whether CNS acidification raises sympathetic nerve activity, not because, but in spite of the activation of the respiratory pattern generator.

Central chemosensitivity refers to the sensitivity of CNS neurons to local acidification, or to local increases in $pCO_2$, regardless of whether these neurons regulate the respiratory pattern generator, whereas the central chemoreflex is the network-dependent process by which these stimuli drive respiration and the autonomic outflows[25,35,94,103]. $pCO_2$ detection by central neurons is presumably in part a cell-autonomous property mediated by the effect of pH on ion channels and, perhaps, other forms of neuronal proton receptors[25,35,94,103]. Specialized glial cells also contribute to the response of central chemoreceptor neurons to $CO_2$[29], although the relative contribution of this paracrine component to overall central chemosensitivity is still to be defined. Until very recently, $CO_2$ was thought to modify neuronal activity exclusively by the proxy of pH changes (the reaction theory)[58]. This long-standing theory may have to be reconsidered, given recent evidence that molecular $CO_2$ directly affects the permeability of connexin hemichannels in glia causing the release of ATP[41]. CNS interstitial $pCO_2$ varies with the level of $CO_2$ in arterial blood and the local metabolic production of this gas by the brain. Therefore, interstitial pH and $pCO_2$ are also influenced by changes in cerebral blood flow[79].

Central chemoreception is incompletely understood both in cellular and in network terms. One view is that the central chemoreflex is a highly distributed (emergent) property of the respiratory network and results from the cumulative effects of pH on many, perhaps all, of its contributing neurons[25,47,77,94,96,103]. The existence of a distributed network of respiratory chemoreceptors is supported by two classes of evidence. First, brainstem neurons commonly respond to acidification *in vitro*[47]. Second, focal acidification of many segments of the medullary respiratory network *in vivo*, including the nucleus of the solitary tract (NTS), the ventral respiratory column from the rostral ventral respiratory group to the retrotrapezoid nucleus, and the raphé, increases the output of the respiratory network to some degree[25,78]. However, despite the widespread effect of pH on brainstem neurons, it is still highly probable that a few specialized clusters of neurons (*bona fide* chemoreceptors) have a dominant role in causing the extreme pH-sensitivity of the respiratory network[35]. The retrotrapezoid nucleus (Figure 10–6B), the raphé, the NTS, and regions of the ventral respiratory column caudal to the retrotrapezoid nucleus probably contain such specialized neurons[25,35,76,96]. The importance of these neurons may relate to the dynamic range of their discharge in response to changes in the pH of the extracellular fluid and/or to some particular combination of connectivity and transmitter effectiveness. There is no evidence yet that such neurons possess unique pH-sensitive ionic conductances. The probability that pH is sensed simultaneously at multiple sites within the lower brainstem, albeit with differing degrees of sensitivity, raises the possibility that several components of the central sympathetic network might also be part of what could be called a "central chemoreceptor complex". Because hypercapnia activates sympathetic nerve activity in bursts that are synchronized with the phrenic nerve, the classic interpretation is that CNS acidification is detected solely by respiratory neurons or by chemosensitive neurons antecedent to respiratory neurons, and that the activation of the respiratory network then produces the activation of the sympathetic vasomotor network[57,69]. However, sympathetic tone and the activity of RVLM neurons are still activated by hypercapnia after the respiratory network has been pharmacologically inactivated[73]. This activation does not appear to be a cell-autonomous property, however, because RVLM neurons do not respond to acidification in slices, at least not during the neonatal period[54]. Therefore $CO_2$ may activate RVLM neurons via brainstem chemosensitive interneurons that are not specifically devoted to respiratory control but multifunctional central chemoreceptors such as, perhaps, neurons in the retrotrapezoid nucleus[73,117] (Figure 10–6). Given this background, does central coupling (the periodic respiratory modulation of sympathetic nerve activity) have the effect of increasing or reducing sympathetic nerve activation caused by elevations in brain $pCO_2$? Contrary to expectation, reductions appear to be what occur, at least under anesthesia[73]. Hypercapnia elevates the activity of RVLM neurons by a mechanism that does not require an active respiratory pattern generator, and activation of the generator by $CO_2$ tends to

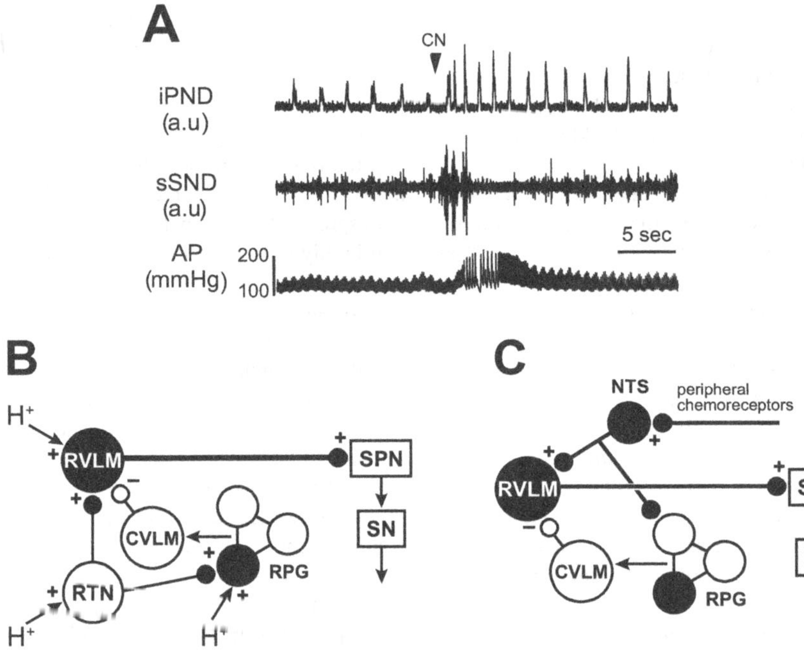


Figure 10–6 Sympathetic chemoreflexes. *A:* Brief carotid body stimulation with cyanide (CN) in a urethane-anesthetized rat increases phrenic nerve discharge (PND) and splanchnic sympathetic nerve discharge (sSND) and elevates arterial pressure (AP). The activation of the splanchnic nerve occurs in bursts that are synchronized with PND. Activation of central chemoreceptors by elevating end-expiratory $pCO_2$ in a rat subjected to denervation of peripheral chemoreceptors produces a similar albeit longer lasting respiratory-synchronous activation of the sympathetic outflow. *B:* Minimum circuitry that may underlie the sympathetic response to central chemoreceptors. CNS acidification caused by elevation in $pCO_2$ or by metabolic acidosis alters the activity of RVLM neurons via three classes of mechanisms whose relative importance is unclear. RVLM neurons may be detecting changes in the surrounding pH, directly or via glial cells. They may be activated by pH secondarily to the activation of bona fide ventral surface central chemoreceptors, possibly located in the retrotrapezoid nucleus (RTN)[69]. These two processes are independent of the effect of pH on the central pattern generator (RPG)[67]. The RPG is also vigorously activated by CNS acidification, either directly or via the bona fide central chemoreceptors. The RPG imposes a strong respiratory modulation to the CVLM GABAergic neurons which is relayed to the RVLM and ultimately causes the respiratory modulation of the sympathetic response to central chemoreceptor stimulation. *C:* Minimum circuitry that underlies the sympathetic response to peripheral chemoreceptor stimulation shown in panel A. The nucleus of the solitary tract (NTS) contains glutamatergic second-order neurons that drive the presympathetic neurons of the RVLM directly or at least independently of the respiratory pattern generator (RPG). The RPG-independent input to RVLM neurons is responsible for much of the increase in sympathetic outflow. RVLM neurons are also periodically inhibited by the RPG via CVLM neurons causing the respiratory modulation of the sympathetic response to peripheral chemoreceptor stimulation.

attenuate the overall rise in sympathetic nerve activity caused by hypercapnia[73]. This attenuation suggests that, under anesthesia, the respiratory entrainment of CVLM neurons could cause a global rise in their average level of discharge rather than an inhibition (Figure 10–6B). In addition, activation of the respiratory pattern generator may attenuate an excitatory chemoreceptor input to the RVLM, possibly from the retrotrapezoid nucleus.

## Peripheral Chemoreflex and Cardiorespiratory Adjustments to Hypoxia

Peripheral chemoreceptors detect hypoxia and also changes in arterial $pCO_2$, which they respond to with a faster time-constant than central chemoreceptors[77,110]. Hypoxic stimulation of the carotid bodies, if strong enough, is also a very powerful arousing stimulus. Peripheral chemoreceptor stimulation causes a primary, parasympathetically mediated bradycardia, which is secondarily offset by the activity of lung stretch receptors when ventilation increases. Peripheral chemoreceptor stimulation also activates most sympathetic barosensitive efferents, including those to the heart (Figure 10–6A)[85].

The presence of a vagally mediated primary bradycardia indicates that cardiovagal parasympathetic preganglionic neurons can be activated by peripheral chemoreceptor stimulation. This response may be triggered only by severe carotid body stimulation and is unlikely to be elicited by the modest physiological fluctuations in carotid body activity that regulate normoxic breathing. The mechanism assumed to underlie respiratory arrhythmia (increased inhibition of cardiovagal preganglionic neurons during inspiration and late expiration, Figure 10–4A) cannot be responsible for the hypoxia-induced bradycardia. Carotid body stimulation increases central inspiratory drive, which should inhibit cardiovagal preganglionic neurons and cause tachycardia, not bradycardia. The mechanism by which carotid body stimulation causes bradycardia must therefore be different and could conceivably involve a direct excitatory input from some of the second-order NTS neurons that are activated by carotid body stimulation (Figure 10–4). Indeed, a similar bradycardic response occurs after activation of many cardiopulmonary vagal C-fiber afferents, and all these stimuli appear to converge on a common set of NTS neurons that do not respond to cardiovascular and lung mechanoreceptors[87].

The activation of barosensitive sympathetic nerve activity caused by carotid body stimulation occurs in bursts synchronized to phrenic nerve discharge (Figure 10–6A). The same question arises as in the case of the effects of central chemoreceptor stimulation: does peripheral chemoreceptor stimulation raise sympathetic nerve activity because of (the usual interpretation) or in spite of this respiratory modulation? In any given species, the respiratory patterns of sympathetic nerve activity produced by carotid body stimulation are roughly the same as those elicited by central chemoreceptor stimulation. Hence, they presumably involve the same pathways, including the CVLM-RVLM connection (Figure 10–6C). Barosensitive neurons in the RVLM are no longer activated by carotid body stimulation after local blockade of glutamate receptors[114]. In contrast, after combined inhibition of the respiratory pattern generator and CVLM neurons, a very large activation persists, although RVLM activation and sympathetic nerve activation no longer occur in bursts[32]. This evidence suggests that during peripheral chemoreceptor stimulation, the respiratory fluctuations in the discharge of RVLM neurons are very likely to be relayed via the CVLM neurons (Figure 10–6C). As in the case of the central chemoreflex, this process is primarily responsible for the respiratory oscillations of sympathetic nerve activity and does not exert exclusive control over the rise in sympathetic nerve activity. The rise in sympathetic nerve activity elicited by carotid body stimulation is most likely due to an excitatory pathway from the carotid bodies to RVLM that bypasses the central respiratory pattern generator (Figure 10–6C). The pathway between chemoreceptors and RVLM may involve a single glutamatergic relay located in the commissural portion of the NTS[1,51,117]. These neurons probably contact the bulbospinal sympathoexcitatory neurons of the RVLM directly[1], although interneurons, such as the neurons in the retrotrapezoid nucleus[117], may also be part of the circuit. This scheme is compatible with results obtained in awake humans, where most of the response to chemoreceptor activation in muscle sympathetic nerve activity appears to be mediated independently of increased central respiratory motor output[14].

## Cardiorespiratory Integration During CNS Hypoxia

Under anesthesia, barosensitive sympathetic nerve activity is activated by ischemia or hypoxia even after denervation of the carotid chemoreceptors[106]. This response, the ischemic pressor response, is largely mediated by the activation of RVLM barosensitive neurons, including the C1 neurons. A related pathological response, the Cushing response[10], is triggered when blood flow to the brain is restricted by brain swelling. The acute hypoxic or ischemic activation of C1 neurons is not blocked by antagonists of ionotropic glutamate receptors and is mimicked by local application of cyanide[114]. Therefore, it is probably an intrinsic cellular response to hypoxia, although it could also be due to the release of some substance, conceivably ATP, from adjacent cells (glia, blood vessels, other neurons)[30]. Under anesthesia or in reduced preparations, hypoxia also reconfigures the activity of the respiratory network, resulting in gasping, which is associated with a decrease of synaptic inhibition and the emergence of pacemaker-like activity in the neurons of the pre-Bötzinger complex[84]. Hypoxia-induced gasping and hypoxic activation of RVLM neurons are almost certainly independent phenomena, because the hypoxic activation of RVLM neurons is tonic; i.e., it does not have a respiratory-like bursting pattern[114]. In short, under conditions of extreme CNS hypoxia, the brainstem mechanisms responsible for coordination between respiration and cardiovascular outflow break down, probably due to depression of the activity of as-yet-unspecified respiratory interneurons. Arterial pressure and ventilation are activated independently, presumably by hypoxia-induced changes in the intrinsic properties of RVLM and pre-Bötzinger neurons, respectively. These changes include an increase in persistent sodium current in neurons of the pre-Bötzinger complex and increases in calcium currents in the RVLM neurons[84,114,115].

Both gasping and the ischemic pressor response are obtained under artificial conditions and under hypoxic conditions that may be regarded as extreme. However, there is also evidence that brainstem $pO_2$ could be a physiological regulator of the cardiorespiratory network in the intact and unanesthetized state. The direct excitatory effect of hypoxia on this circuitry has been regarded by Reis and others as a potential homeostatic mechanism designed to maintain brain perfusion and oxygenation[95]. In essence, Reis' concept[95] is an elaboration of Cushing's 1901 "law of the brain"[11], which states that the brainstem regulates its perfusion at the expense of systemic blood pressure. The concept is not farfetched considering that even skeletal muscles trigger a pressor reflex (the exercise pressor reflex[45]) in response to ischemia. The concept is still currently invoked as a potential explanation for neurogenic essential hypertension[81] and derives some support from the fact that surgery designed to relieve pressure exerted on the medulla oblongata by a hypertrophied posterior cerebellar artery may reduce pressure in some forms of hypertension[55]. Another piece of supporting evidence is that relatively mild hypoxia stimulates breathing in unanesthetized dogs and goats, even when peripheral chemoreceptors are bypassed[10]. Because this response requires intact carotid chemoreceptors, the central stimulatory effect of hypoxia may act by potentiating a tonic excitatory input from peripheral chemoreceptors. The cellular mechanisms responsible for the central stimulatory effect of hypoxia on breathing and sympathetic tone are not well understood. Heme oxygenase II is constitutively expressed in the ventral respiratory column, and heme-oxygenase I is induced by hypoxia[63]. The C1 neurons express high levels of inducible factor 1-$\alpha$ and tyrosine-hydroxylase following hypoxia[83,98]. These enzymes are possibly involved in the acute and chronic stimulatory effects of hypoxia on cardiorespiratory function.

In summary, $pO_2$ may regulate cardiorespiratory circuitry by an action on the lower brainstem in addition to its better-known effects via peripheral chemoreceptors. The parallel with the regulation of the same circuitry by $pCO_2$ is noteworthy, but it should be stressed that the existence of physiologically relevant central oxygen receptors in the medulla oblongata is still somewhat controversial.

## REGULATION OF THE CIRCULATION BY LUNG AFFERENTS

Afferents from the lower respiratory tract trigger regulatory or defensive reflexes that have a prominent cardiac and sympathetic component[8,9]. Regulatory reflexes presumed to be triggered by slowly adapting lung stretch receptors will be considered first (for reviews, see [8,12,13,53,120]).

The effects of lung stretch afferents on autonomic outflow are complex, of variable magnitude depending on the species, and the underlying central circuitry is, in general, poorly understood. In anesthetized dogs, increasing pulmonary ventilation while maintaining arterial pressure and arterial $pCO_2$ constant reduces hindquarter vascular resistance, presumably by withdrawing sympathetic tone[13]. The sympathoinhibitory effect of lung inflation depends largely, though not completely, on central respiratory drive, since it is reduced but not eliminated by reducing central or peripheral chemoreceptor activity[2,13]. Furthermore, lung inflation may exert different effects on different types of sympathetic efferents[2]. Differential modulation of CVLM neurons by the respiratory pattern generator provides a possible explanation for the effects of lung inflation that depend on central respiratory drive. The respiratory pattern generator-independent portion of the sympathoinhibition caused by lung inflation is unexplained in network terms. Direct projections from the NTS "pump cells" (NTS neurons that receive direct input from the slowly adapting lung stretch receptors[53]) to either CVLM or RVLM neurons are a plausible but as-yet-untested mechanism. In man, most investigators agree that lung inflation is the most important factor that determines the within-breath respiratory fluctuations of sympathetic nerve activity[14,20]; but opinions differ as to the contribution to these fluctuations made by lung stretch afferents, baroreceptors (arterial or volume), and central coupling. At low tidal volume, within-breath fluctuations of sympathetic nerve activity do not appear related to the activity of lung or baroreceptor afferents and may be due to some form of central coupling[20,107]. At higher tidal volumes, the within-breath fluctuations of sympathetic nerve activity become larger. These fluctuations have been attributed to the activity of lung stretch receptors because they are attenuated in lung-transplant patients[107]. However, lung transplantation may also destroy other types of cardiopulmonary afferents (e.g., low-pressure baroreceptors from veins and the atrium) that may cause fluctuations in sympathetic nerve activity that relate to lung inflation. Curiously, the effect of lung inflation does not seem to depend on the intensity of the respiratory motor outflow[107]. These findings could be interpreted as evidence that, in awake humans, lung stretch afferents influence sympathetic nerve activity primarily via a pathway that is independent of the central respiratory drive. In short, the mechanism by which lung inflation controls sympathetic nerve activity remains uncertain at several levels. However, the central pathways that link lung mechanoreceptors to sympathetic nerve activity seem to include a respiratory pattern generator–dependent and a respiratory pattern generator–independent mechanism. The relative importance of these two mechanisms may depend on the species and/or on the state of vigilance (awake or anesthetized).

Lung inflation also causes cardiovagal inhibition, increasing the heart rate and contributing to sinus arrhythmia[8,9]. The cardiopulmonary afferents and central pathway responsible for this important phenomenon are undefined. Assuming that slowly adapting lung stretch receptors are the dominant input, one possibility is that cardiovagal preganglionic neurons might be directly targeted by the GABAergic pump cells of the ventrolateral NTS[53] (Figure 10–4).

Defensive cardiopulmonary reflexes caused by stimulation of bronchiopulmonary C-fibers are typically associated with a primary bradycardia and sympathoinhibition[8,12,120]. Judging from the Bezold-Jarisch reflex, a reflex triggered by the activation of axons that express 5-$HT_3$ receptors, a large component of the sympathoinhibition is independent of the activity of the respiratory pattern generator and relies on CVLM activation and downstream inhibition of RVLM neurons[121]. As mentioned previously, the cardiovagal activation caused by these stimuli is likewise probably independent of the respiratory pattern generator and could conceivably result from a direct excitatory input from the NTS (Figure 10–4A).

## THE NUCLEUS OF THE SOLITARY TRACT AND CARDIORESPIRATORY INTEGRATION

A large variety of sensory afferents (e.g., lung mechanoreceptors, arterial baroreceptors, atriovenous mechanoreceptors, subtypes of cardiopulmonary C-fibers, carotid body afferents, etc.) converge in the NTS and influence the activity of ventrolateral medullary and pontine neurons involved in respiratory and autonomic regulations[6,88]. Large populations of second-order NTS neurons receive inputs from a single or just a few types of cardiopulmonary afferents[3,15,51,53,86,88,89], and most of the NTS neurons that innervate the ventrolateral medulla are second-order neurons[3]. Hence, many ventrolateral medullary and pontine neurons receive and integrate sensory modality-specific inputs from the NTS (Figure 10–7).

For example, pump cells, the second-order neurons of slowly adapting lung stretch afferents, are not affected by baroreceptors, and these cells innervate vast tracts of the ventrolateral medulla and dorsal pons[53] (Figure 10–7). Commissural NTS neurons that respond to carotid body stimulation are generally insensitive to baroreceptor influences, and many also innervate the ventrolateral medulla[51]. Second-order baroreceptor neurons are also sensory-modality selective and generally innervate the ventrolateral medulla[15]. Reconstruction of second-order neurons (e.g., baroreceptive cells, pumps cells) usually reveals that these neurons also innervate the NTS, suggesting that they also function as interneurons within this structure[3,15,51,53,86,88,89] (Figure 10–7). Transmission between primary afferents and their second-order neurons is highly regulated (i.e., reduced, enhanced, or gated) by other brain structures, such as the spinal cord, medulla oblongata, pons, hypothalamus, or cortex (Figure 10–7). These regulations probably operate via direct inputs to the second-order neurons, via NTS interneurons, or by circulating factors acting via blood vessels[88,109] (Figure 10–7), and this presumably applies to all of the modality-specific inputs from NTS to the ventrolateral medulla. For example, information originating from arterial baroreceptors is modulated by hypothalamic and other inputs, which plays a central role in allowing blood pressure to rise

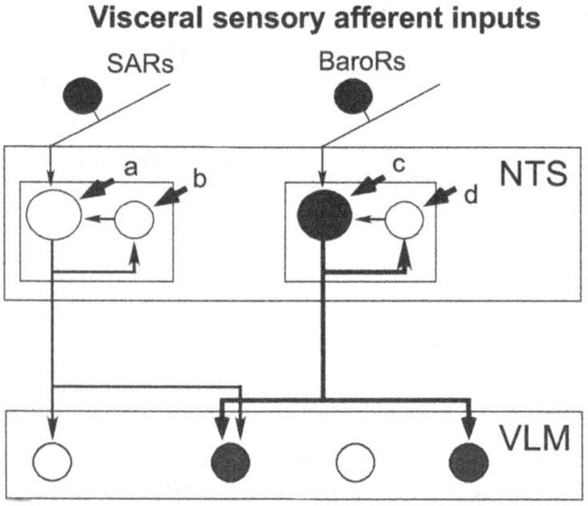


Figure 10–7 The nucleus of the solitary tract and cardiorespiratory integration. In this highly synthetic and somewhat speculative interpretation of the literature, the NTS is seen as consisting of modality-specific microcircuits that selectively process information from one or a small subset of visceral afferents. These microcircuits occupy spatially overlapping regions of the intermediate and caudal NTS. For simplicity, only two afferent modality-specific microcircuits (slowly adapting lung stretch receptors, SARs, baroreceptors, baroR) are represented in the scheme. The output of each microcircuit to the ventrolateral medulla is via second-order neurons that are either excitatory (baroreceptors), inhibitory (SARs), or perhaps both (SARs). These second-order neurons have extensive axonal collaterals within the NTS. These recurrent collaterals innervate interneurons that may, in turn, feedback onto the second-order neurons. Transmission between sensory afferents and second-order neurons is biased by inputs of somatosensory origin (e.g., nociceptive afferents, muscle metabotropic receptors) and from various cardiorespiratory regions within the brain (inputs symbolized by letters *a–d*). For example, inputs *c* and *d* might be responsible for the resetting of the baroreflex that allows blood pressure to rise during exercise. Inputs *a* and *b* may represent innervation from the respiratory pattern generator known to regulate pump cells in rats (SAR second-order neurons). Second-order neurons from the various modality-specific circuits differentially innervate ventrolateral medullary neurons that generate the respiratory and the cardiovascular autonomic outflows. The NTS has other output neurons (to the dorsal pons, periaqueductal gray matter, and hypothalamus) that are not represented.

during various behaviors[68] (Figure 10–7). Similarly, pump cells in rats are regulated by the respiratory network[53] (Figure 10–7), and somatic nociceptive stimulation or application of selected metabotropic receptor agonists to the NTS selectively attenuate the cardiac parasympathetic portion of the arterial baroreflex[90,109].

Other forms of integration also occur within the NTS. For example, the integrative properties of NTS efferents to the dorsolateral pons, periaqueductal gray (PAG), and hypothalamus are apparently different from that of the second-order neurons with ventrolateral medullary projection, since many of these output neurons are higher-order, rather than second-order, neurons[3].

In summary, information from various classes of cardiorespiratory afferents converges to only a limited degree on second-order NTS neurons, and these neurons may be viewed as the nodal points of modality-specific microcircuits (Figure 10–7). Because a very large proportion of these second-order neurons innervate the ventrolateral medulla and the pons, the bulk of the integration between various cardiopulmonary sensory modalities, which is essential to cardiorespiratory integration, probably occurs in these regions rather than in the NTS (Figure 10–7). However, for each sensory modality, information transfer through the NTS is differentially and highly regulated by inputs from the brain and spinal cord, and perhaps also by circulating factors such as angiotensin or by signals released by the vasculature within the NTS (Figure 10–7). These regulatory influences bias the strength of the inputs that individual ventrolateral medullary neurons receive from each type of cardiopulmonary afferent, and these regulations must contribute greatly to cardiorespiratory integration. Much less is known about how processing of afferent information in the NTS results in output to regions such as the central gray and the hypothalamus.

## CENTRAL AUTONOMIC NEURONS AS POTENTIAL SOURCES OF DRIVE TO THE RESPIRATORY NETWORK

Emerging evidence suggests that some of the tonic drives to respiratory neurons might be shared with or even originate from neurons that could be considered as core components of central autonomic circuitry (Figure 10–3).

### Brainstem Catecholamine Neurons

In certain preparations, A6 noradrenergic neurons of the locus coeruleus activate the respiratory rhythm generator[39], an observation that is generally consistent with the notion that A6 neurons exert a widespread facilitatory effect on somatomotor function. A5 neurons are viewed as core components of the brainstem autonomic circuitry[43], and their activation produces organ-specific changes in vascular conductance[40]. In addition to these cardiovascular changes, the A5 group appears to decrease the activity of the respiratory network, at least in neonatal *in vitro* preparations[39,52].

The catecholaminergic neurons of the ventrolateral medulla probably also regulate breathing, although the differential contribution of the noradrenergic A1 and adrenergic C1 groups has yet to be sorted out[126]. The C1 neurons are activated by all forms of physical and emotional stress[102], and many of these cells innervate regions that may be directly or indirectly involved in breathing[7].

### Serotonergic and Cholinergic Neurons

Cholinergic neurons modulate both respiration and sympathetic vasomotor efferents[99,108]. The pedunculopontine nucleus, which is thought to regulate sleep stages[125], is likely to provide a cholinergic input to both the respiratory and autonomic networks in the medulla. Cholinergic neurons also occur in the ventrolateral medulla and the NTS; but very little is known about these neurons. Brainstem serotonergic neurons also regulate both breathing and cardiovascular function[43,96].

### Neurons Involved in the Barorespiratory Reflex

The barorespiratory reflex is the little-studied inhibition of the respiratory outflow (typically phrenic nerve discharge) produced by activating arterial baroreceptors. A rise in arterial pressure could theoretically slow respiration by increasing brainstem perfusion and decreasing stimulation of central chemoreceptors. However, this explanation does not account for the fact that instantaneous respiratory inhibition is elicited by electrical stimulation of the aortic depressor nerve in rats[101] or by increasing arterial pressure selectively in the carotid sinus region, which was first described in dogs by Schmidt[104]. A short-latency slowing of phrenic nerve discharge is also observed in the rat working heart–brainstem preparation when perfusion pressure is increased[91], presumably stimulating baroreceptors. The central pathway of the barorespiratory reflex is unknown. A plausible but unproven mechanism could be a disfacilitation of the respiratory network by withdrawal of an excitatory drive from barosensitive RVLM neurons (for example, C1 neurons). Equally plausibly, the central respiratory network could be actively inhibited by the GABAergic baroactivated interneurons of the CVLM. The latter neurons are coextensive with the region of the ventral respiratory column containing the pre-Bötzinger neurons and the rostral ventral respiratory group and have axonal collaterals within that region[105].

## CARDIORESPIRATORY INTEGRATION DURING EXERCISE

Low to moderate exercise increases breathing, cardiac output, and arterial pressure without change in blood $pCO_2$ (isocapnia). More strenuous or prolonged exercise produces metabolic acidosis, which, in turn, causes further cardiovascular stimulation and an intense respiratory activation that leads to hypocapnia.

The cardiorespiratory adjustments to exercise are due to a mixture of central command and peripheral reflexes. The relative contribution of each mechanism depends greatly on the intensity of the exercise. The source of the hyperpnea and cardiovascular stimulation during exercise continues to generate vigorous controversy[122]. The reflex control hypothesis posits that cardiorespiratory stimulation results from the activation of sensory afferents after the onset of exercise[37,45]. The central command hypothesis holds that the brain generates efferent command signals that set the cardiorespiratory outflows to a level commensurate with the intensity of the exercise[21,122].

### Central Command

In decorticate or decerebrate cats, locomotor activity occurs spontaneously or can be elicited by electrical or chemical stimulation of specific brain regions (e.g., hypothalamic or mesencephalic "locomotor" regions). In a landmark series of studies, Eldridge and his collaborators[21,22] showed that this locomotor activity always occurred concurrently with an increase in respiration and arterial pressure, and that the magnitude of the cardiorespiratory changes was roughly proportional to the motor outflow to the muscles. The cardiorespiratory changes occurred without any significant lag time and could not have resulted from peripheral control, because they persisted during fictive locomotion (after muscle paralysis) and were independent of the integrity of the vagus nerves. Finally, the cardiorespiratory stimulation could not have been due to peripheral chemoreceptor activation since locomotion caused a mild hypocapnia. In recent years, the field of human exercise physiology has provided abundant evidence for a role of central command in the hyperpnea and cardiovascular stimulation of exercise. For example, a large component of the exercise pressor response is independent of the activity of motor neurons and of feedback from the exercising muscles[26]. Furthermore, imagined exercise in the absence of locomotion produces respiratory and heart rate changes that are reminiscent of those observed during real exercise, and these changes are correlated with the activation of specific areas of the cortex (supplemental motor area, premotor area, prefrontal cortex) and cerebellum[119]. The insular cortex is a likely relay for these autonomic effects since this region projects directly to the lateral hypothalamus, parabrachial nuclei, ventrolateral medulla, and NTS[123,124]. Work on the hypothalamic or mesencephalic locomotor regions has not kept pace with modern neurobiology, and the neurons that are engaged by stimulating these regions remain unidentified. The hypothalamic locomotor region may overlap with or be able to recruit the dorsomedial hypothalamic nucleus and/or perifornical region, which are sources of excitatory projections to the medulla oblongata, including the blood pressure–regulating neurons of the RVLM[16,65,66]. The dorsolateral pons may contribute to the synchronization between respiration and locomotion that is necessary for efficient breathing, especially in quadrupeds[46]. Based on retrograde trans-synaptic transport of the pseudorabies virus, brain structures such as the caudal and intermediate portions of the ventrolateral PAG appear connected oligosynaptically to both skeletal motor neurons and sympathetic preganglionic neurons[49]. In animals, these regions are involved in elaborating coping strategies to handle stressors that include changes in breathing[48]. Neurons located within the medullary ventral gigantocellular field establish mono- or oligosynaptic projections with both sympathetic preganglionic neurons and skeletal muscle motor neurons[50] and could conceivably contribute to the coordination between the skeletomotor and sympathetic outflows. The adjacent medullary raphé also contains bulbospinal and largely serotonergic neurons that may regulate gamma motoneuronal activity as well as the sympathetic outflow. However, these neurons probably intervene in the context of thermoregulation rather than exercise, generating heat via shivering or by raising the tone of postural muscles[118]. The same or neighboring cells control skin arterioles, thermogenic fat, or adrenaline release and not muscle resistance arterioles[75].

In summary, central command is almost certainly involved in the respiratory and circulatory correlates of exercise, but the central pathways need clarification.

### Peripheral Control

Reflexes initiated by muscle metaboreceptors contribute to the control of respiration and circulation during exercise[45]. These group III and IV afferents respond to the metabolic byproducts of exercise ($H^+$, lactate, ATP, prostaglandins, $K^+$), to muscle tension, and to temperature[37,45]. They may also respond to vessel distention, particularly at the level of muscle venules, suggesting that these afferents could monitor muscle blood flow by encoding the degree of recruitment of the muscle post-capillary network[37]. Thus, metabotropic group III and IV afferents have properties that are suitable to encode the overall metabolic activity of skeletal muscles during exercise.

The central pathways recruited by small-caliber muscle afferents to increase breathing and activate the circulation probably involve many brain structures, in particular the NTS and the ventrolateral medulla. The activation of second-order NTS neurons by baroreceptor afferents is attenuated by activation of muscle afferents. This resetting presumably contributes to the observed right shift of the baroreflex without change in gain that accompanies exercise[26,67,93]. The upward shift of the sympathetic nerve activity/arterial pressure relationship may involve a more direct influence of metabotropic muscle receptors on the ventrolateral medulla, perhaps via CVLM or RVLM neurons.

Reflexes from lung mechanoreceptors, described above, also contribute to cardiorespiratory adjustments during exercise. A primary contribution of peripheral chemoreceptors to exercise-induced hyperpnea has been excluded for very low levels of exercise because exercise is typically iso- or hypocapnic. However, during more intense exercise, carotid body activation by hypoxia and sensitization by potassium, metabolic acidosis, and catecholamines contributes considerably to exercise hyperpnea. The hypo- or isocapnic nature of exercise is classically interpreted as evidence that central chemoreceptors do not contribute to cardiorespiratory stimulation at the onset of exercise or during mild forms of exercise. However, this statement only means that, during exercise, the central chemoreceptors are not activated *by acidification*, at least not until metabolic acidosis sets in. These chemosensitive neurons could still be vigorously activated by central command during exercise, and therefore these cells could actually play a key role in cardiorespiratory stimulation. With more strenuous exercise, metabolic acidosis reduces brain pH despite the hypocapnia. Since central chemoreceptors are activated by metabolic acidosis[103], these neurons must contribute to further cardiorespiratory stimulation.

## CARDIORESPIRATORY INTEGRATION AND DIVING

The ability of mammals to dive for long periods requires the optimization of oxygen utilization. This is achieved by a cardiovascular adaptation known as the diving response, which is characterized by reduced

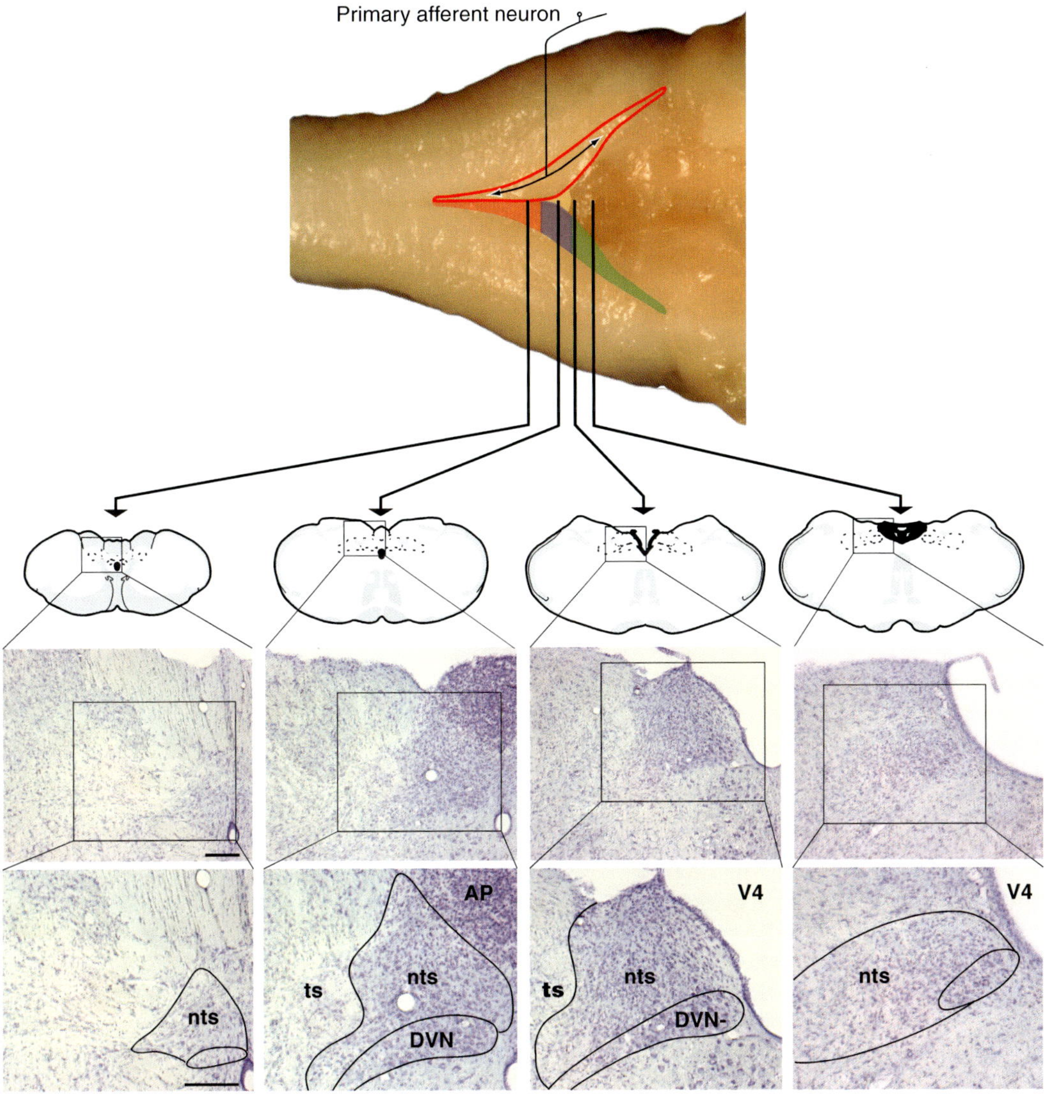


Figure 1–1 Organization of the nucleus of the solitary tract (NTS).See text discussion on page 6. The location of the NTS is mapped onto an image of the dorsal surface of the brainstem. NTS neurons are grouped into two long cell columns that fuse in the midline caudal to the area postrema (AP). The trajectory of primary sensory afferents that enter the NTS via the solitary tract is shown in the top column of the NTS. In the bottom column, the V-shaped structure of the NTS has been divided into three segments based on location relative to AP. The schematics above each column of micrographs show the location of the NTS in four coronal planes. The Nissl-stained photomicrographs below each schematic illustrate the cytoarchitecture of the boxed areas at intermediate and high magnification.AP, area postrema; DVN, dorsal vagal motor nucleus; ts, solitary tract; V4, fourth ventricle.

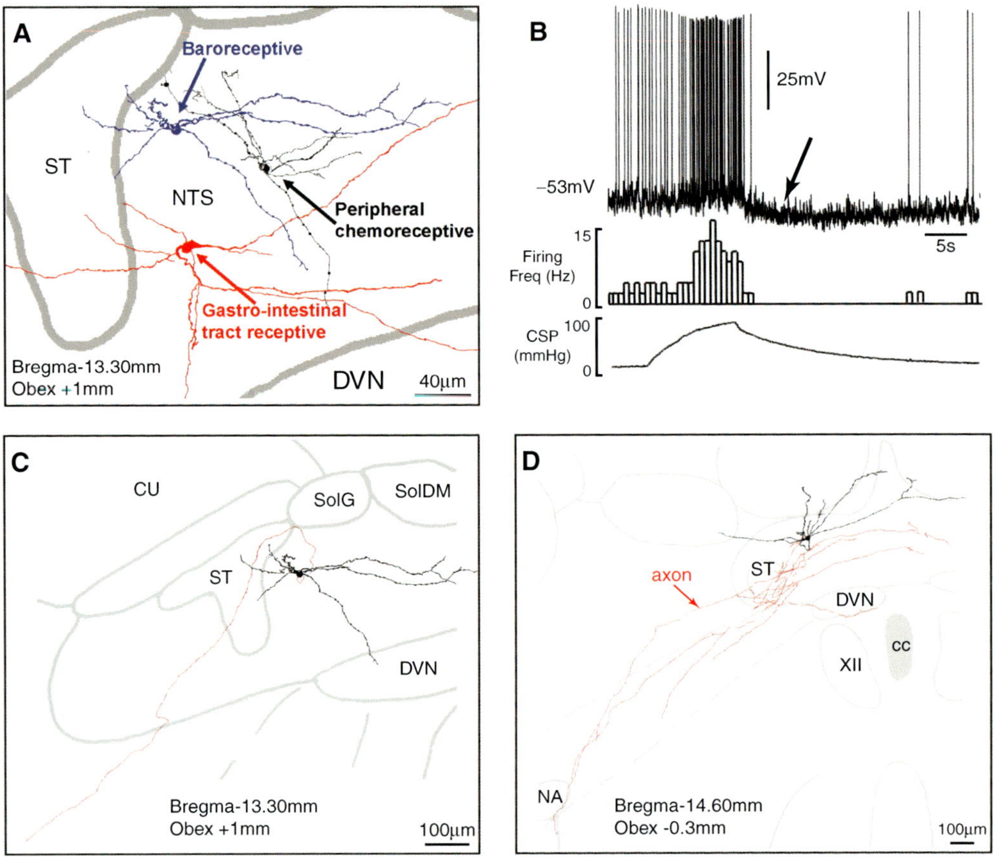


Figure 2–3 Morphological and electrophysiological properties of baroreceptive NTS neurons. See text discussion on page 26. *A*: Individual baroreceptive NTS neurons intermix with neurons belonging to other reflex circuits, suggesting that there is little or no "viscerotopic" organization within the NTS. Microinjection of a drug into the medial NTS would therefore activate many reflex circuits simultaneously, making it very difficult to identify which specific afferent pathway was activated. *B*: Whole-cell recording of a baroreceptive NTS neuron shows the firing frequency (Freq) response to raising carotid sinus pressure (CSP). Note the adaptive nature of the firing, with the peak response occurring before the maximal level of carotid sinus pressure (CSP), and the hyperpolarization following the stimulus (*arrow*). About 30% of baroreceptive NTS neurons exhibited these characteristics, indicating that powerful mechanisms regulate neuronal excitability. *C & D*: Two labeled baroreceptive NTS neurons that received constant short latency inputs after electrical stimulation of the solitary tract (ST). Most putative second-order baroreceptive neurons project out of the NTS towards the ventrolateral medulla (*C & D*), but some also have axons (*D, red*) that terminate within the NTS. Note the extent to which the dendrites (*black*) arborize ipsi- and contralaterally. CC, central canal; Cu, cuneate nucleus; DVN, dorsal vagal nucleus; Gn, gracile nucleus. Modified from Deuchars et al. (2000)[37] and Paton et al. (2000)[110], with permission.

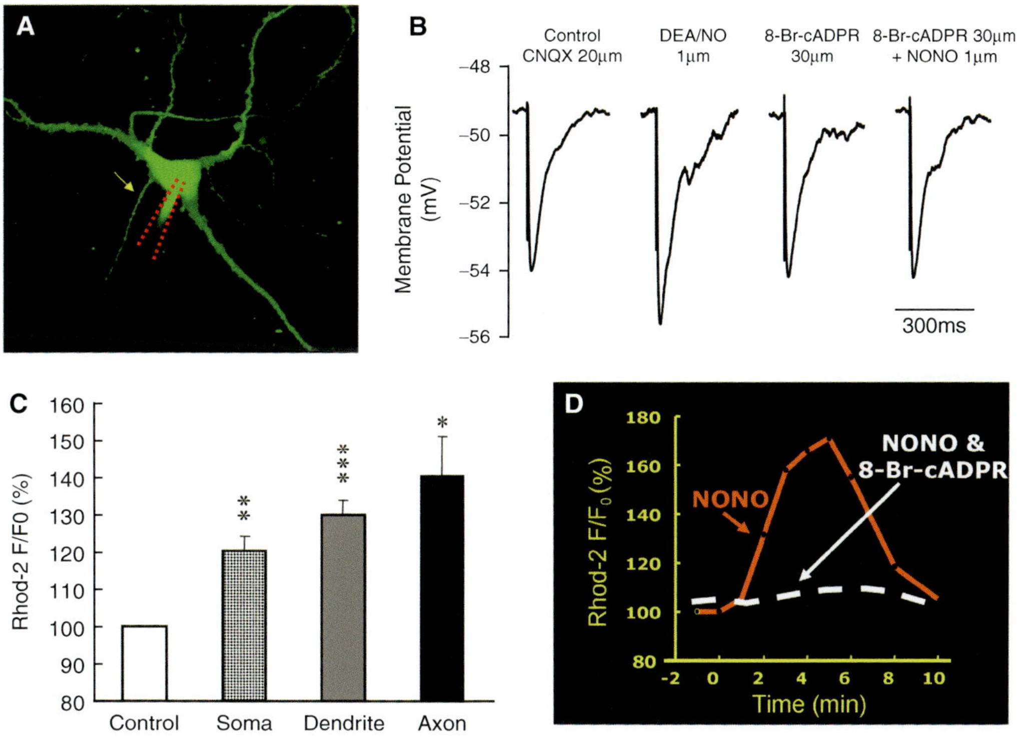


Figure 2–9 Nitric oxide effects on GABAergic transmission in the NTS. See text discussion on page 39. *A:* GABA-containing neuron in the NTS revealed using an adenovirus-expressing enhanced green fluorescent protein under the control of the GAD67 promoter. The dotted line indicates the position of the patch pipette. *B:* Electrically evoked monosynaptic IPSPs are augmented by the nitric oxide donor, diethylamine NONOate. This augmentation is prevented by selective antagonism of cyclic adenosine diphosphate ribose regulated ryanodine-sensitive intracellular calcium stores (cADPR) using 8-Br-cADPR. *C:* Measurements of intracellular calcium from different cellular compartments of GABAergic interneurons in the NTS when exposed to a nitric oxide donor. Neurons were loaded with a calcium-sensitive dye (Rhod-2) from the patch pipette. The most sensitive compartment was axonal. *D:* The rise in intracellular calcium recorded from a GABAergic interneuron when exposed to nitric oxide. Note that the response is abolished when 8-Br-cADPR blocks calcium release from cADPR-ryanodine sensitive intracellular stores. Data modified from Wang et al. (2006)[151], with permission.

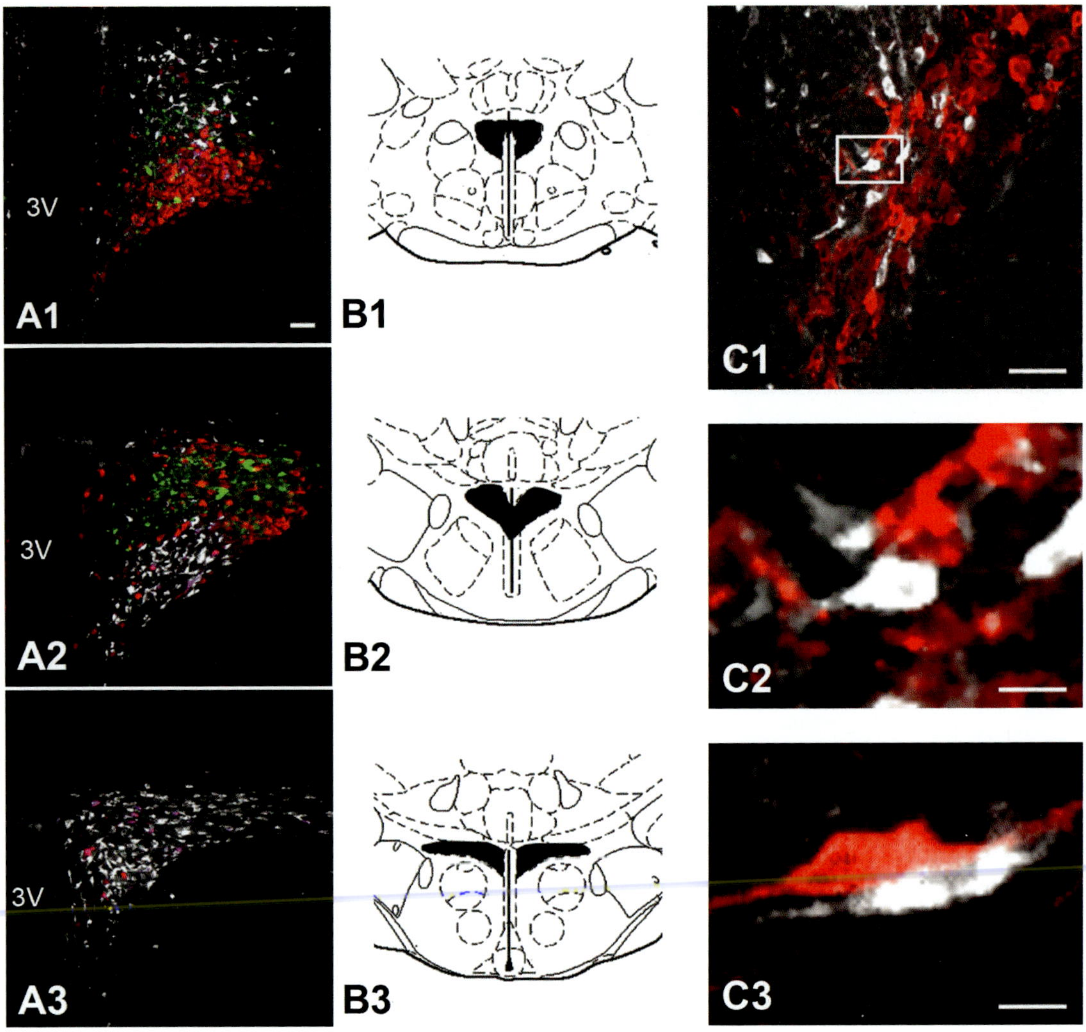


Figure 4–3 Cellular organization and heterogeneity within the PVN. See text discussion on page 66. *A*: Distributions within the PVN of PVN-preautonomic neurons retrogradely labeled from the RVLM (*white*), oxytocin-immunoreactive neurons (*red*) and vasopressin-immunoreactive neurons (*green*) at three rostrocaudal levels of the PVN (A1–A3). *B*: Brain maps (modified from Paxinos and Watson[84]) representing coronal sections at the level of the hypothalamus where the photomicrographs shown in A1–A3 were taken (B1, Bregma = -1.3; B2, Bregma = -1.80, B3, Bregma = -2.10). *C*: Close spatial relationship between oxytocin-immunoreactive magnocellular neurosecretory neurons (*red*) and PVN-preautonomic neurons retrogradely labeled from the RVLM (*white*). The image in C2 is a magnified view of the squared area in C1. 3V, third ventricle. Yellow- and purple-labeled cells in panels A1–A3 represent double-labeled oxytocin/vasopressin neurons (*yellow*) and double-labeled oxytocin/PVN-RVLM neurons, respectively. Bars: A, 100 μm; C1, 80 μm; C2–C3, 20 μm.

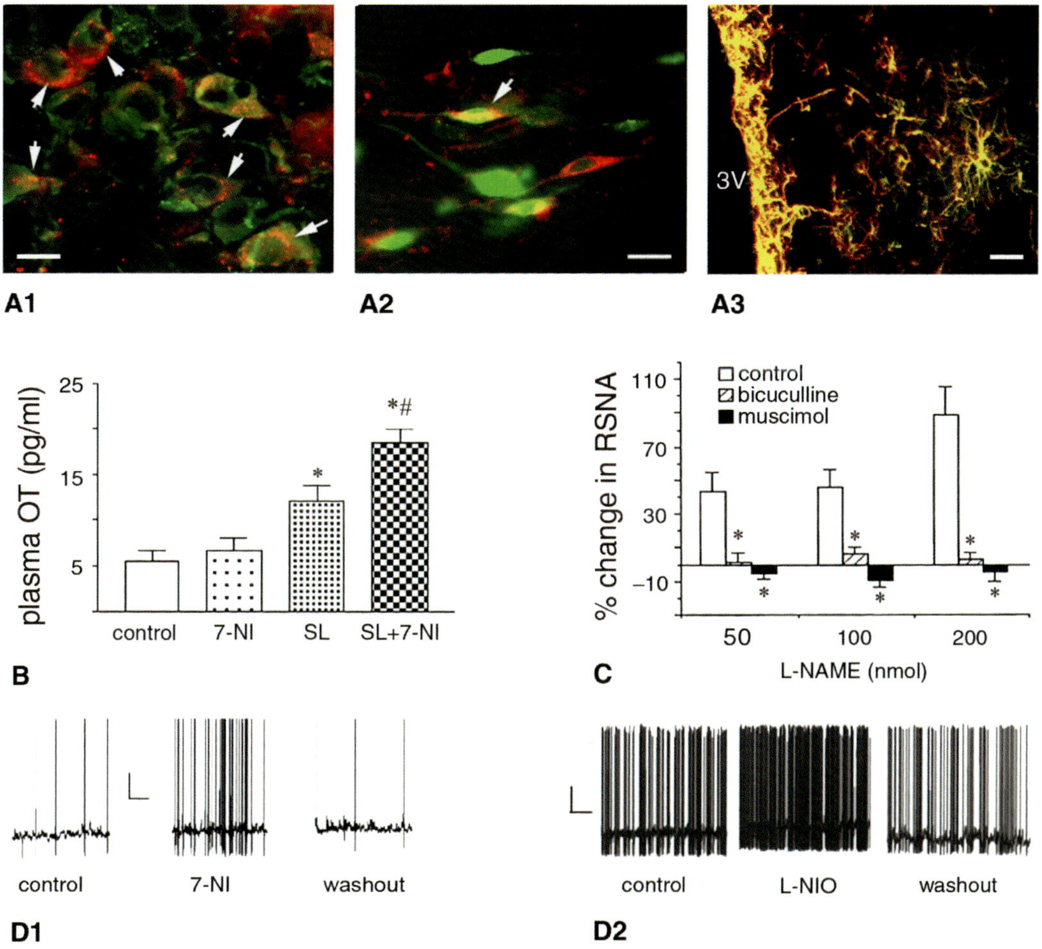


Figure 4–5 Nitric oxide modulatory actions on the autonomic and neuroendocrine PVN. See text discussion on page 69. *A:* Neuronal nitric oxide synthase immunoreactivity (*red*) in vasopressin-immunoreactive magnocellular neurosecretory neurons (*A1, green*) and in PVN-preautonomic neurons retrogradely labeled from the NTS (*A2, green*). Arrows, double-labeled neurons. *A3*: Double staining for glial fibrillary acidic protein (GFAP; *red*) and endothelial nitric oxide synthase (eNOS; *green*) in the PVN. There is a high degree of co-localization (*yellow*) of the two immunoreactivities. *B:* Effects of 7-nitroindazole (7-NI; 50 mg/kg), which blocks the activity of neuronal nitric oxide synthase, on plasma levels of oxytocin 24 hours after salt loading (SL). The increase in plasma oxytocin induced by SL is potentiated in the presence of 7-NI. *P< 0.05 compared with control; # P< 0.05 compared with SL group. *C:* Change in renal sympathetic nerve activity (RSNA) following microinjections of L-nitroarginine methyl ester (L-NAME), a non-specific antagonist of nitric oxide synthase, into the PVN in the absence or presence of the GABAA receptor antagonist, bicuculline, or agonist, muscimol, respectively. *P< 0.05 compared with control. *D:* Blockade of neuronal nitric oxide synthase (7-NI, 100 μM, *D1*) or endothelial nitric oxide synthase with *N*-iminoethyl-L-ornithine (L-NIO, 10 μM, *D2*), increases the firing of PVN-preautonomic neurons that project to the RVLM. Scale bars in *A1* and *A2:* 25 μm, Bar in A3: 70 μm. Vertical and horizontal bars in *D1* and *D2:* 20 mV and 2 s, and 20 mV and 10 s, respectively. *B1* reproduced from Ventura et al. (2005)[125], with permission. *C* reproduced from Zhang and Patel (1998)[133], with permission. *D1* modified from Li et al. (2003)[54], with permission.

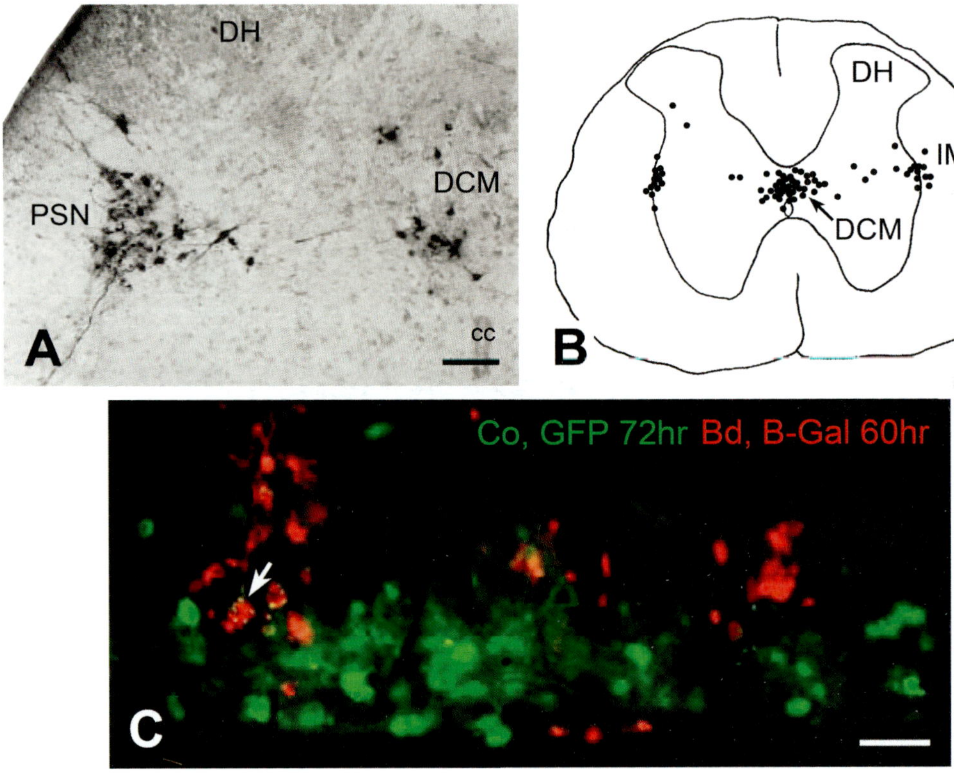


Figure 8–6 Comparison of the distribution of transneuronally labeled neurons after injection of pseudorabies virus into the urethra or bladder and colon. See text discussion on page 148. *A:* Light micrograph of transneuronally labeled neurons in the first sacral spinal segment after injection of pseudorabies virus into the colon. Scale bar, 150 μm. Modified from Vizzard et al. (2000)[105], with permission. cc, central canal; DCM, dorsal gray commissure; DH, dorsal horn; PSN, sacral parasympathetic nucleus. *B:* Line drawing illustrating the distribution of neurons in the first sacral spinal segment that were transneuronally labeled after virus injection into the urethra. DCM, dorsal gray commissure; DH, dorsal horn; IML, intermediolateral cell column;. Modified from Vizzard et al. (1995)[106], with permission. *C:* Injection of two different strains of pseudorabies virus into the bladder (red) and colon (green) results in rare double-labeled neurons (arrow) in the spinal cord. Bd, B-Gal 60H, Pseudorabies virus ß-galactosidase injected into bladder 60 hours prior to sacrifice; Co, GFP 72H, Pseudorabies virus green fluorescent protein injected into colon 72 hours prior to sacrifice. Scale bar, 30 μm. Reproduced from Rouzade Dominiguez et al. (2003)[83], with permission.

cardiac output and redirection of this output away from tissues with a capacity for anaerobic metabolism (skeletal muscles) towards tissues sensitive to hypoxia (brain and heart). The most characteristic cardiorespiratory changes associated with voluntary diving (apnea, parasympathetic bradycardia, glottal closure, and sympathetic vasoconstriction) can be triggered reflexively by immersion of the head in water or by the presence of water or irritants in the upper airways. This reflex occurs in both aquatic and non-aquatic species, including man. It can be elicited under anesthesia or in mid-collicular transected preparations by noxious stimulation of the nasal mucosa or by direct electrical stimulation of the ethmoidal nerve[19]. These findings suggest that the cardiopulmonary responses to diving are largely hardwired within the lower brainstem.

Ethmoidal nerve afferents project to the ventrolateral part of the spinal trigeminal nucleus that, in turn, innervates the caudal NTS, the ventrolateral medulla, and the ventrolateral parabrachial region, including the Kölliker-Fuse nucleus[82]. The medial NTS and the RVLM are both implicated in the sympathetic component of the response to nasal mucosa or ethmoidal nerve stimulation, but the dorsolateral pons is not[17,64]. The loss of inspiratory drive and the glottal closure have been attributed to the tonic activation of inhibitory post-inspiratory medullary interneurons[19]. The apnea requires glutamatergic activation of neurons located in the region of the Kölliker-Fuse nucleus[18], suggesting that pontine neurons could be driving the post-inspiratory interneurons of the ventrolateral medulla. A more direct pathway from the trigeminal nucleus to the ventrolateral medulla is also consistent with anatomical and physiological evidence[19]. In theory, the above-described mechanisms of sinus arrhythmia could be responsible for the bradycardia of the diving response. Specifically, the activation of cardiovagal motor neurons is plausibly due to disinhibition from respiratory neurons and, perhaps, concurrent excitation by post-inspiratory neurons. However, nasopharyngeal afferents could also activate cardiovagal motor neurons via excitatory inputs that are not rhythmically gated by the respiratory pattern generator. Surprisingly, the activity of the cardiac sympathetic nerve also appears to increase during the diving reflex[85]. Co-activation of the parasympathetic and sympathetic cardiac outflows is also elicited by hypoxic stimulation of peripheral chemoreceptors and may be needed to maintain ventricular ejection despite pronounced bradycardia and increased peripheral resistance[85]. Another interpretation is that the diving reflex, like hypoxia, is stressful, producing a more or less generalized sympathoactivation, including to the heart.

Trigeminal reflexes triggered by head immersion and nasal stimulation are viewed as actively inhibiting breathing, with trigeminal sensory afferents actively opposing the chemical drive of respiration via an increase in post-inspiratory neuronal activity. However, there is little evidence that this mechanism accounts for the cardiorespiratory adjustments elicited in deep-diving species. Computer simulation of diving behavior up to the estimated aerobic limit (18–25 minutes) in the Weddell seal indicates that the most effective means to prolong a dive would be an upward shift in central chemoreceptor threshold that would allow $pCO_2$ to accumulate well above normal levels, suppressing chemical drive and the urge to breathe during the dive[113].

## CONCLUSIONS

Cardiorespiratory integration occurs at many levels of the neuraxis and involves coordinated regulation of respiratory, cardiovagal, and sympathetic outflows. The coordination between respiration and the sympathetic vasomotor outflow is neither unidirectional nor hardwired. Many neurons within each of the two ventrolateral medullary networks (respiratory and autonomic) appear to be differentially and directly regulated by modality-specific oligosynaptic inputs from somatic and visceral sensory afferents (e.g., chemoreceptor, baroreceptor, lung mechanoreceptors, etc.). They are also differentially controlled by inputs from higher structures that are involved in the elaboration of behavior-specific cardiorespiratory patterns (e.g., cortex, hypothalamus, pons and PAG). The activity of cardiovagal premotor neuron, hence heart rate and atrioventricular nodal conduction, are clearly subject to control by the central respiratory generator, as revealed by the phenomenon of sinus arrhythmia. However, cardiovagal control is not exclusively influenced by the central respiratory network, as shown by the simple observation that this outflow either co-varies or responds in a manner opposite to the inspiratory drive, depending on the behavior or circumstance (cf. diving, hypoxia). Although increased inspiratory inhibition of cardiovagal motoneurons is likely to play some role in raising heart rate during exercise, the relative contribution of this mechanism versus respiratory-independent central command of cardiovagal activity remains to be determined. In general, much work remains to be done to identify both respiratory and non-respiratory neurons that innervate cardiovagal motoneurons.

One of the most significant new developments in understanding how the respiratory network modulates sympathetic vasomotor outflow has been the realization of the role played by disinhibition of the sympathoexcitatory RVLM neurons. Hence, the central respiratory network may regulate sympathetic outflow primarily by adjusting the degree of GABAergic inhibition that RVLM sympathoexcitatory neurons receive from the CVLM. Resting sympathetic vasomotor tone in awake animals and man is extremely low but can be very vigorously activated by even a minimal decrease in blood pressure. This enormous reserve of activity is a reflection of the powerful ongoing inhibition of the RVLM that originates from the arterial baroreceptors, is transmitted via the CVLM and is modulated there. Even a modest decrease in baroreceptor-mediated activation of CVLM neurons by elements of the central respiratory pattern generator could increase resting sympathetic tone enormously. This increase would naturally occur in bursts synchronized with respiration, exactly as observed. The likely antagonism between baroreceptor activation and respiratory inhibition of CVLM neurons provides a simple and compelling explanation of the waxing and waning of the sympathetic outflow with respiration and of the variation in the strength of the sympathetic baroreflex with the phase of the central respiratory cycle. Finally, the multiplicity of respiratory patterns found in sympathetic efferents may also have its origin in the differential control of subgroups of CVLM neurons by the respiratory pattern generator.

## References


1. Aicher, S. A., Saravay, R. H., Cravo, S., Jeske, I., Morrison, S. F., Reis, D. J., and Milner, T. A. (1996). Monosynaptic projections from the nucleus tractus solitarii to C1 adrenergic neurons in the rostral ventrolateral medulla: Comparison with input from the caudal ventrolateral medulla. *Journal of Comparative Neurology* 373, 62–75.
2. Bachoo, M., and Polosa, C. (1986). The pattern of sympathetic neurone activity during expiration in the cat. *Journal of Physiology* 378, 375–390.
3. Bailey, T. W., Hermes, S. M., Andresen, M. C., and Aicher, S. A. (2006). Cranial visceral afferent pathways through the nucleus of the solitary tract to caudal ventrolateral medulla or paraventricular hypothalamus: Target-specific synaptic reliability and convergence patterns. *Journal of Neuroscience* 26, 11893–11902.
4. Barman, S. M., and Gebber, G. L. (1997). Subgroups of rostral ventrolateral medullary and caudal medullary raphe neurons based on patterns of relationship to sympathetic nerve discharge and axonal projections. *Journal of Neurophysiology* 77, 65–75.
5. Blain, G. M., Smith, C. A., Henderson, K. S., and Dempsey, J. A. (2010). Peripheral chemoreceptors determine the respiratory sensitivity of central chemoreceptors to CO(2). *Journal of Physiology* 588, 2455–2471.
6. Blessing, W. W. (1997). *The Lower Brainstem and Homeostasis*. New York: Oxford University Press.
7. Card, J. P., Sved, J. C., Craig, B., Raizada, M., Vazquez, J., and Sved, A. F. (2006). Efferent projections of rat rostroventrolateral medulla C1 catecholamine neurons: Implications for the central control of cardiovascular regulation. *Journal of Comparative Neurology* 499, 840–859.
8. Coleridge, H. M., and Coleridge, J. C. (2001). Afferent innervation of lungs, airways, and pulmonary artery. In I. H. Zucker and J. P. Gilmore (Eds.), *Reflex Control of the Circulation*, pp. 579–607. Boca Raton: CRC Press.
9. Coleridge, H. M., and Coleridge, J. C. (1994). Pulmonary reflexes: Neural mechanisms of pulmonary defense. *Annual Review of Physiology* 56, 69–91.
10. Curran, A. K., Rodman, J. R., Eastwood, P. R., Henderson, K. S., Dempsey, J. A., and Smith, C. A. (2000). Ventilatory responses to specific CNS hypoxia in sleeping dogs. *Journal of Applied Physiology* 88, 1840–1852.
11. Cushing, H. (1901). Concerning a definitive regulatory mechanism of the vaso-motor centre which controls blood pressure during cerebral compression. *Bulletin of the Johns Hopkins Hospital* 12, 290–292.
12. Daly, M. D. (1986). Interactions between respiration and circulation. In N. S. Cherniack and J. G. Widdicombe (Eds.), *Section 3: The Respiratory System*, pp. 529–594. Bethesda, MD: American Physiological Society.
13. Daly, M. d. B., Ward, J., and Wood, L. M. (1986). Modification by lung inflation of the vascular responses from the carotid body chemoreceptors and other receptors in dogs. *Journal of Physiology* 378, 13–30.
14. Dempsey, J. A., Sheel, A. W., St. Croix, C. M., and Morgan, B. J. (2002). Respiratory influences on sympathetic vasomotor outflow in humans. *Respiratory Physiology & Neurobiology* 130, 3–20.
15. Deuchars, J., Li, Y. W., Kasparov, S., and Paton, J. F. R. (2000). Morphological and electrophysiological properties of neurones in the dorsal vagal complex of the rat activated by arterial baroreceptors. *Journal of Comparative Neurology* 417, 233–249.
16. Dimicco, J. A., Samuels, B. C., Zaretskaia, M. V., and Zaretsky, D. V. (2002). The dorsomedial hypothalamus and the response to stress: Part renaissance, part revolution. *Pharmacology, Biochemistry and Behavior* 71, 469–480.
17. Dutschmann, M., and Herbert, H. (1998). The medial nucleus of the solitary tract mediates the

trigeminally evoked pressor response. *NeuroReport* 9, 1053–1057.

18. Dutschmann, M., and Herbert, H. (1998). NMDA and GABAA receptors in the rat Kolliker-Fuse area control cardiorespiratory responses evoked by trigeminal ethmoidal nerve stimulation. *Journal of Physiology* 510 (Pt 3), 793–804.
19. Dutschmann, M., and Paton, J. F. (2002). Influence of nasotrigeminal afferents on medullary respiratory neurones and upper airway patency in the rat. *Pflugers Archiv European Journal of Physiology* 444, 227–235.
20. Eckberg, D. L. (2003). The human respiratory gate. *Journal of Physiology* 548, 339–352.
21. Eldridge, F. L., Millhorn, D. E., Kiley, J. P., and Waldrop, T. G. (1985). Stimulation by central command of locomotion, respiration and circulation during exercise. *Respiratory Physiology* 59, 313–337.
22. Eldridge, F. L., Millhorn, D. E., and Waldrop, T. G. (1981). Exercise hyperpnea and locomotion: Parallel activation from the hypothalamus. *Science* 211, 844–846.
23. Feldman, J. L., and Del Negro, C. A. (2006). Looking for inspiration: New perspectives on respiratory rhythm. *Nature Reviews in Neuroscience* 7, 232–242.
24. Feldman, J. L., and McCrimmon, D. R. (1999). Neural control of breathing. In M. J. Zigmond, F. E. Bloom, S. C. Landis, J. L. Roberts, and L. R. Squire (Eds.), *Fundamental Neuroscience*, pp. 1063–1090. San Diego, CA: Academic Press.
25. Feldman, J. L., Mitchell, G. S., and Nattie, E. E. (2003). Breathing: Rhythmicity, plasticity, chemosensitivity. *Annual Review of Neuroscience* 26, 239–266.
26. Gallagher, K. M., Fadel, P. J., Smith, S. A., Stromstad, M., Ide, K., Secher, N. H., and Raven, P. B. (2006). The interaction of central command and the exercise pressor reflex in mediating baroreflex resetting during exercise in humans. *Experimental Physiology* 91, 79–87.
27. Gebber, G. L., Das, M., and Barman, S. M. (2005). Dynamic changes in baroreceptor-sympathetic coupling during the respiratory cycle. *Brain Research* 1046, 216–223.
28. Gilbey, M. P., Jordan, D., Richter, D. W., and Spyer, K. M. (1984). Synaptic mechanisms involved in the inspiratory modulation of vagal cardio-inhibitory neurones in the cat. *Journal of Physiology* 356, 65–78.
29. Gourine, A. V., Kasymov, V., Marina, N., Tang, F., Figueiredo, M. F., Lane, S., Teschemacher, A. G., Spyer, K. M., Deisseroth, K., and Kasparov, S. (2010). Astrocytes control breathing through pH-dependent release of ATP. *Science* 329, 571–575.
30. Gourine, A. V., Llaudet, E., Dale, N., and Spyer, K. M. (2005). Release of ATP in the ventral medulla during hypoxia in rats: Role in hypoxic ventilatory response. *Journal of Neuroscience* 25, 1211–1218.
31. Guyenet, P. G. (2006). The sympathetic control of blood pressure. *Nature Reviews in Neuroscience* 7, 335–346.
32. Guyenet, P. G. (2000). Neural structures that mediate sympathoexcitation during hypoxia. *Respiratory Physiology* 121, 147–162.
33. Guyenet, P. G., Darnall, R. A., and Riley, T. A. (1990). Rostral ventrolateral medulla and sympathorespiratory integration in rats. *American Journal of Physiology: Regulatory, Integrative and Comparative Physiology* 259, R1063–R1074.
34. Guyenet, P. G., Koshiya, N., Huangfu, D., Verberne, A. J. M., and Riley, T. A. (1993). Central respiratory control of A5 and A6 pontine noradrenergic neurons. *American Journal of Physiology: Regulatory, Integrative and Comparative Physiology* 264, R1035–R1044.
35. Guyenet, P. G., Stornetta, R. L., and Bayliss, D. A. (2010). Central respiratory chemoreception. *Journal of Comparative Neurology* 518, 3883–3906.
36. Hanna, B. D., Lioy, F., and Polosa, C. (1981). Role of carotid and central chemoreceptors in the $CO_2$ response of sympathetic preganglionic neurons. *Journal of the Autonomic Nervous System* 3, 421–435.
37. Haouzi, P. (2006). Theories on the nature of the coupling between ventilation and gas exchange during exercise. *Respiratory Physiology & Neurobiology* 151, 267–279.
38. Haselton, J. R., and Guyenet, P. G. (1989). Central respiratory modulation of medullary sympathoexcitatory neurons in rat. *American Journal of Physiology: Regulatory, Integrative and Comparative Physiology* 256, R739–R750.
39. Hilaire, G., Viemari, J. C., Coulon, P., Simonneau, M., and Bevengut, M. (2004). Modulation of the respiratory rhythm generator by the pontine noradrenergic A5 and A6 groups in rodents. *Respiratory Physiology & Neurobiology* 143, 187–197.
40. Huangfu, D., Hwang, L. J., Riley, T. A., and Guyenet, P. G. (1992). Splanchnic nerve response to A5-area stimulation in rats. *American Journal of Physiology: Regulatory, Integrative and Comparative Physiology* 263, R437–R446.
41. Huckstepp, R. T., Id, B. R., Eason, R., Spyer, K. M., Dicke, N., Willecke, K., Marina, N., Gourine, A. V., and Dale, N. (2010). Connexin hemichannel-mediated $CO_2$-dependent release of ATP in the medulla oblongata contributes to central respiratory chemosensitivity. *Journal of Physiology* 588, 3901–3920.

42. Janig, W., and Habler, H. J. (2003). Neurophysiological analysis of target-related sympathetic pathways—from animal to human: Similarities and differences. *Acta Physiologica Scandinavica* 177, 255–274.
43. Jansen, A. S. P., Wessendorf, M. W., and Loewy, A. D. (1995). Transneuronal labeling of CNS neuropeptide and monoamine neurons after pseudorabies virus injections into the stellate ganglion. *Brain Research* 683, 1–24.
44. Jiang, C., and Lipski, J. (1990). Extensive monosynaptic inhibition of ventral respiratory group neurons by augmenting neurons in the Botzinger complex in the cat. *Experimental Brain Research* 81(3), 639–648.
45. Kaufman, M. P., and Hayes, S. G. (2002). The exercise pressor reflex. *Clinical Autonomic Research* 12, 429–439.
46. Kawahara, K., Kumagai, S., Nakazono, Y., and Miyamoto, Y. (1989). Coupling between respiratory and stepping rhythms during locomotion in decerebrate cats. *Journal of Applied Physiology* 67, 110–115.
47. Kawai, A., Ballantyne, D., Muckenhoff, K., and Scheid, P. (1996). Chemosensitive medullary neurones in the brainstem—spinal cord preparation of the neonatal rat. *Journal of Physiology* 492, 277–292.
48. Keay, K. A., and Bandler, R. (2001). Parallel circuits mediating distinct emotional coping reactions to different types of stress. *Neuroscience and Biobehavioral Reviews* 25, 669–678.
49. Kerman, I. A., Akil, H., and Watson, S. J. (2006). Rostral elements of sympatho-motor circuitry: A virally mediated transsynaptic tracing study. *Journal of Neuroscience* 26, 3423–3433.
50. Kerman, I. A., Enquist, L. W., Watson, S. J., and Yates, B. J. (2003). Brainstem substrates of sympatho-motor circuitry identified using transsynaptic tracing with pseudorabies virus recombinants. *Journal of Neuroscience* 23, 4657–4666.
51. Koshiya, N., and Guyenet, P. G. (1996). NTS neurons with carotid chemoreceptor inputs arborize in the rostral ventrolateral medulla. *American Journal of Physiology: Regulatory, Integrative and Comparative Physiology* 270, R1273–R1278.
52. Koshiya, N., and Guyenet, P. G. (1994). Role of the pons in the carotid sympathetic chemoreflex. *American Journal of Physiology: Regulatory, Integrative and Comparative Physiology* 267, R508–R518.
53. Kubin, L., Alheid, G. F., Zuperku, E. J., and McCrimmon, D. R. (2006). Central pathways of pulmonary and lower airway vagal afferents. *Journal of Applied Physiology* 101, 618–627.
54. Lazarenko, R. M., Milner, T. A., Depuy, S. D., Stornetta, R. L., West, G. H., Kievits, J. A., Bayliss, D. A., and Guyenet, P. G. (2009). Acid sensitivity and ultrastructure of the retrotrapezoid nucleus in Phox2b-EGFP transgenic mice. *Journal of Comparative Neurology* 517, 69–86.
55. Levy, E. I., Scarrow, A. M., and Jannetta, P. J. (2001). Microvascular decompression in the treatment of hypertension: Review and update. *Surgical Neurology* 55, 2–10.
56. Lindsey, B. G., Arata, A., Morris, K. F., Hernandez, Y. M., and Shannon, R. (1998). Medullary raphe neurones and baroreceptor modulation of the respiratory motor pattern in the cat. *Journal of Physiology* 512 (Pt 3), 863–882.
57. Lioy, F., Hanna, B. D., and Polosa, C. (1981). Cardiovascular control by medullary surface chemoreceptors. *Journal of the Autonomic Nervous System* 3, 9–24.
58. Loeschcke, H. H. (1982). Central chemosensitivity and the reaction theory. *Journal of Physiology* 332, 1–24.
59. Macefield, V. G., and Wallin, B. G. (1995). Modulation of muscle sympathetic activity during spontaneous and artificial ventilation and apnoea in humans. *Journal of the Autonomic Nervous System* 53, 137–147.
60. Macefield, V. G., Wallin, B. G., and Vallbo, Å. B. (1994). The discharge behaviour of single vasoconstrictor motoneurones in human muscle nerves. *Journal of Physiology* 481, 799–809.
61. Malpas, S. C. (1998). The rhythmicity of sympathetic nerve activity. *Progress in Neurobiology* 56, 65–96.
62. Mandel, D. A., and Schreihofer, A. M. (2006). Central respiratory modulation of barosensitive neurones in rat caudal ventrolateral medulla. *Journal of Physiology* 572, 881–896.
63. Mazza, E., Thakkar-Varia, S., Tozzi, C. A., and Neubauer, J. A. (2001). Expression of heme oxygenase in the oxygen-sensing regions of the rostral ventrolateral medulla. *Journal of Applied Physiology* 91, 379–385.
64. McCulloch, P. F., Panneton, W. M., and Guyenet, P. G. (1999). The rostral ventrolateral medulla mediates the sympathoactivation produced by chemical stimulation of the rat nasal mucosa. *Journal of Physiology* 516, 471–484.
65. McDowall, L. M., Horiuchi, J., and Dampney, R. A. (2007). Effects of disinhibition of neurons in the dorsomedial hypothalamus on central respiratory drive. *American Journal of Physiology: Regulatory, Integrative and Comparative Physiology* 293, R1728–R1735.

66. McDowall, L. M., Horiuchi, J., Killinger, S., and Dampney, R. A. (2006). Modulation of the baroreceptor reflex by the dorsomedial hypothalamic nucleus and perifornical area. *American Journal of Physiology: Regulatory, Integrative and Comparative Physiology* 290, R1020–R1026.
67. McIlveen, S. A., Hayes, S. G., and Kaufman, M. P. (2001). Both central command and exercise pressor reflex reset carotid sinus baroreflex. *American Journal of Physiology: Heart and Circulatory Physiology* 280, H1454–H1463.
68. Mifflin, S. W., Spyer, K. M., and Withington-Wray, D. J. (1988). Baroreceptor inputs to the nucleus tractus solitarius in the cat: Modulation by the hypothalamus. *Journal of Physiology* 399, 369–387.
69. Millhorn, D. E. (1986). Neural respiratory and circulatory interaction during chemoreceptor stimulation and cooling of ventral medulla in cats. *Journal of Physiology* 370, 217–231.
70. Miyawaki, T., Goodchild, A. K., and Pilowsky, P. M. (2002). Evidence for a tonic GABA-ergic inhibition of excitatory respiratory-related afferents to presympathetic neurons in the rostral ventrolateral medulla. *Brain Research* 924, 56–62.
71. Miyawaki, T., Minson, J., Arnolda, L., Chalmers, J., Llewellyn-Smith, I., and Pilowsky, P. (1996). Role of excitatory amino acid receptors in cardiorespiratory coupling in ventrolateral medulla. *American Journal of Physiology: Regulatory, Integrative and Comparative Physiology* 271, R1221–R1230.
72. Miyawaki, T., Pilowsky, P., Sun, Q. J., Minson, J., Suzuki, S., Arnolda, L., Llewellyn-Smith, I., and Chalmers, J. (1995). Central inspiration increases barosensitivity of neurons in rat rostral ventrolateral medulla. *American Journal of Physiology: Regulatory, Integrative and Comparative Physiology* 268, R909–R918.
73. Moreira, T. S., Takakura, A. C., Colombari, E., and Guyenet, P. G. (2006). Central chemoreceptors and sympathetic vasomotor outflow. *Journal of Physiology* 577, 369–386.
74. Morgado-Valle, C., Baca, S. M., and Feldman, J. L. (2010). Glycinergic pacemaker neurons in pre-Botzinger complex of neonatal mouse. *Journal of Neuroscience* 30, 3634–3639.
75. Morrison, S. F. (2001). Differential regulation of brown adipose and splanchnic sympathetic outflows in rat: Roles of raphe and rostral ventrolateral medulla neurons. *Clinical and Experimental Pharmacology and Physiology* 28, 138–143.
76. Mulkey, D. K., Stornetta, R. L., Weston, M. C., Simmons, J. R., Parker, A., Bayliss, D. A., and Guyenet, P. G. (2004). Respiratory control by ventral surface chemoreceptor neurons in rats. *Nature Neuroscience* 7, 1360–1369.
77. Nattie, E. (2006). Why do we have both peripheral and central chemoreceptors? *Journal of Applied Physiology* 100, 9–10.
78. Nattie, E. E. (2001). Central chemosensitivity, sleep, and wakefulness. *Respiratory Physiology* 129, 257–268.
79. Nattie, E. E. (2007). Chemoreceptors, breathing, and pH. In R. J. Alpern and S. C. Hebert (Eds.), *Seldin and Giebisch's The Kidney, vols. 1–2*, pp. 1587–1600. New York: Elsevier.
80. Neff, R. A., Wang, J., Baxi, S., Evans, C., and Mendelowitz, D. (2003). Respiratory sinus arrhythmia: Endogenous activation of nicotinic receptors mediates respiratory modulation of brainstem cardioinhibitory parasympathetic neurons. *Circulation Research* 93, 565–572.
81. Osborn, J. W., Jacob, F., and Guzman, P. (2005). A neural set point for the long-term control of arterial pressure: Beyond the arterial baroreceptor reflex. *American Journal of Physiology: Regulatory, Integrative and Comparative Physiology* 288, R846–R855.
82. Panneton, W. M., McCulloch, P. F., and Sun, W. (2000). Trigemino-autonomic connections in the muskrat: The neural substrate for the diving response. *Brain Research* 874, 48–65.
83. Pascual, O., Denavit-Saubie, M., Dumas, S., Kietzmann, T., Ghilini, G., Mallet, J., and Pequignot, J. M. (2001). Selective cardiorespiratory and catecholaminergic areas express the hypoxia-inducible factor-1alpha (HIF-1alpha) under in vivo hypoxia in rat brainstem. *European Journal of Neuroscience* 14, 1981–1991.
84. Paton, J. F., Abdala, A. P., Koizumi, H., Smith, J. C., and St-John, W. M. (2006). Respiratory rhythm generation during gasping depends on persistent sodium current. *Nature Neuroscience* 9, 311–313.
85. Paton, J. F., Boscan, P., Pickering, A. E., and Nalivaiko, E. (2005). The yin and yang of cardiac autonomic control: vago-sympathetic interactions revisited. *Brain Research Brain Research Reviews* 49, 555–565.
86. Paton, J. F., Deuchars, J., Li, Y. W., and Kasparov, S. (2001). Properties of solitary tract neurones responding to peripheral arterial chemoreceptors. *Neuroscience* 105, 231–248.
87. Paton, J. F. R. (1998). Pattern of cardiorespiratory afferent convergence to solitary tract neurons driven by pulmonary vagal C-fiber stimulation in the mouse. *Journal of Neurophysiology* 79, 2365–2373.
88. Paton, J. F. R. (1999). Nucleus tractus solitarii: Integrating structures. *Experimental Physiology* 84, 815–833.

89. Paton, J. F. R., Li, Y. W., Deuchars, J., and Kasparov, S. (2000). Properties of solitary tract neurons receiving inputs from the sub-diaphragmatic vagus nerve. *Neuroscience* 95, 141–153.
90. Pickering, A. E., Boscan, P., and Paton, J. F. (2003). Nociception attenuates parasympathetic but not sympathetic baroreflex via NK1 receptors in the rat nucleus tractus solitarii. *Journal of Physiology* 551, 589–599.
91. Pickering, A. E., and Paton, J. F. (2006). A decerebrate, artificially perfused in situ preparation of rat: Utility for the study of autonomic and nociceptive processing. *Journal of Neuroscience Methods* 155, 260–271.
92. Pilowsky, P. M., Miyawaki, T., Minson, J. B., Sun, Q. J., Arnolda, L. F., Llewellyn-Smith, I. J., and Chalmers, J. P. (1995). Bulbospinal sympatho-excitatory neurons in the rat caudal raphe. *Journal of Hypertension* 13, 1618–1623.
93. Potts, J. T., Paton, J. F., Mitchell, J. H., Garry, M. G., Kline, G., Anguelov, P. T., and Lee, S. M. (2003). Contraction-sensitive skeletal muscle afferents inhibit arterial baroreceptor signalling in the nucleus of the solitary tract: Role of intrinsic GABA interneurons. *Neuroscience* 119, 201–214.
94. Putnam, R. W., Filosa, J. A., and Ritucci, N. A. (2004). Cellular mechanisms involved in CO(2) and acid signaling in chemosensitive neurons. *American Journal of Physiology: Cell Physiology* 287, C1493–C1526.
95. Reis, D. J., Golanov, E. V., Galea, E., and Feinstein, D. L. (1997). Central neurogenic neuroprotection: Central neural systems that protect the brain from hypoxia and ischemia. *Annals of the New York Academy of Sciences* 835, 168–186.
96. Richerson, G. B. (2004). Serotonergic neurons as carbon dioxide sensors that maintain pH homeostasis. *Nature Reviews in Neuroscience* 5, 449–461.
97. Richter, D. W., and Spyer, K. M. (1990). Cardiorespiratory control. In A. D. Loewy and K. M. Spyer (Eds.), *Central Regulation of Autonomic Functions*, pp. 189–207. New York: Oxford University Press.
98. Roux, J. C., Pequignot, J. M., Dumas, S., Pascual, O., Ghilini, G., Pequignot, J., Mallet, J., and Denavit-Saubié M. (2000). $O_2$–sensing after carotid chemodenervation: Hypoxic ventilatory responsiveness and upregulation of tyrosine hydroxylase mRNA in brainstem catecholaminergic cells. *European Journal of Neuroscience* 12, 3181–3190.
99. Ruggiero, D. A., Giuliano, R., Anwar, M., Stornetta, R., and Reis, D. J. (1990). Anatomical substrates of cholinergic-autonomic regulation in the rat. *Journal of Comparative Neurology* 292, 1–53.
100. Rybak, I. A., Shevtsova, N. A., Paton, J. F., Dick, T. E., St-John, W. M., Morschel, M., and Dutschmann, M. (2004). Modeling the pontomedullary respiratory network. *Respiratory Physiology & Neurobiology* 143, 307–319.
101. Sapru, H. N., Gonzalez, E., and Krieger, A. J. (1981). Aortic nerve stimulation in the rat: Cardiovascular and respiratory responses. *Brain Research Bulletin* 6, 393–398.
102. Sawchenko, P. E., Li, H. Y., and Ericsson, A. (2000). Circuits and mechanisms governing hypothalamic responses to stress: A tale of two paradigms. *Progress in Brain Research* 122, 61–78.
103. Scheid, P.: guest editors: Putnam, R. W., Dean, J. B., and Ballantyne, D. (2001). Special issue: Central chemosensitivity. *Respiratory Physiology & Neurobiology* 129, 1–278.
104. Schmidt, C. F. (1932). Carotid sinus reflexes to the respiratory center: I. *Identification. American Journal of Physiology* 102, 94–118.
105. Schreihofer, A. M., and Guyenet, P. G. (2003). Baroactivated neurons with pulse-modulated activity in the rat caudal ventrolateral medulla express GAD67 mRNA. *Journal of Neurophysiology* 89, 1265–1277.
106. Schreihofer, A. M., Stornetta, R. L., and Guyenet, P. G. (1999). Evidence for glycinergic respiratory neurons: Bötzinger neurons express mRNA for glycinergic transporter 2. *Journal of Comparative Neurology* 407, 583–597.
107. Seals, D. R., Suwarno, N. O., Joyner, M. J., Iber, C., Copeland, J. G., and Dempsey, J. A. (1993). Respiratory modulation of muscle sympathetic nerve activity in intact and lung denervated humans. *Circulation Research* 72, 440–454.
108. Shao, X. M., and Feldman, J. L. (2000). Acetylcholine modulates respiratory pattern: Effects mediated by M3-like receptors in pre-Botzinger complex inspiratory neurons. *Journal of Neurophysiology* 83, 1243–1252.
109. Simms, A. E., Paton, J. F., and Pickering, A. E. (2006). Disinhibition of the cardiac limb of the arterial baroreflex in rat: A role for metabotropic glutamate receptors in the nucleus tractus solitarii. *Journal of Physiology* 575, 727–738.
110. Smith, C. A., Rodman, J. R., Chenuel, B. J., Henderson, K. S., and Dempsey, J. A. (2006). Response time and sensitivity of the ventilatory response to CO2 in unanesthetized intact dogs: Central vs. peripheral chemoreceptors. *Journal of Applied Physiology* 100, 13–19.
111. Spyer, K. M. (1994). Annual review prize lecture—Central nervous mechanisms contributing to cardiovascular control. *Journal of Physiology* 474, 1–20.

112. Spyer, K. M. (1990). The central nervous organization of reflex circulatory control. In A. D. Loewy and K. M. Spyer (Eds.), *Central Regulation of Autonomic Functions*, pp. 168–188. New York: Oxford University Press.
113. Stephenson, R. (2005). A theoretical analysis of diving performance in the Weddell seal (*Leptonychotes weddelli*). *Physiology Biochemistry Zoology* 78, 782–800.
114. Sun, M. K., and Reis, D. J. (1994). Central neural mechanisms mediating excitation of sympathetic neurons by hypoxia. *Progress in Neurobiology* 44, 197–219.
115. Sun, M. K., and Reis, D. J. (1994). Hypoxia-activated Ca2+ currents in pacemaker neurones of rat rostral ventrolateral medulla in vitro. *Journal of Physiology* 476, 101–116.
116. Sun, Q. J., Minson, J., Llewellyn-Smith, I. J., Arnolda, L., Chalmers, J., and Pilowsky, P. (1997). Bötzinger neurons project towards bulbospinal neurons in the rostral ventrolateral medulla of the rat. *Journal of Comparative Neurology* 388, 23–31.
117. Takakura, A. C., Moreira, T. S., Colombari, E., West, G. H., Stornetta, R. L., and Guyenet, P. G. (2006). Peripheral chemoreceptor inputs to retrotrapezoid nucleus (RTN) CO2–sensitive neurons in rats. *Journal of Physiology* 572, 503–523.
118. Tanaka, M., Owens, N. C., Nagashima, K., Kanosue, K., and McAllen, R. M. (2006). Reflex activation of rat fusimotor neurons by body surface cooling, and its dependence on the medullary raphe. *Journal of Physiology* 572, 569–583.
119. Thornton, J. M., Guz, A., Murphy, K., Griffith, A. R., Pedersen, D. L., Kardos, A., Leff, A., Adams, L., Casadei, B., and Paterson, D. J. (2001). Identification of higher brain centres that may encode the cardiorespiratory response to exercise in humans. *Journal of Physiology* 533, 823–836.
120. Vatner, S. F., and Uemura, N. (2001). Integrative cardiovascular control by pulmonary inflation reflexes. In I. H. Zucker and J. P. Gilmore (Eds.), *Reflex Control of the Circulation*, pp. 609–626. Boca Raton, FL: CRC Press.
121. Verberne, A. J., Saita, M., and Sartor, D. M. (2003). Chemical stimulation of vagal afferent neurons and sympathetic vasomotor tone. *Brain Research Reviews* 41, 288–305.
122. Waldrop, T. G., Iwamoto, G. A., and Haouzi, P. (2006). Point : Counterpoint: Supraspinal locomotor centers do/do not contribute significantly to the hyperpnea of dynamic exercise. *Journal of Applied Physiology* 100, 1077–1083.
123. Westerhaus, M. J., and Loewy, A. D. (2001). Central representation of the sympathetic nervous system in the cerebral cortex. *Brain Research* 903, 117–127.
124. Yasui, Y., Breder, C. D., Saper, C. B., and Cechetto, D. F. (1991). Autonomic responses and efferent pathways from the insular cortex in the rat. *Journal of Comparative Neurology* 303, 355–374.
125. Yasui, Y., Cechetto, D. F., and Saper, C. B. (1990). Evidence for a cholinergic projection from the pedunculopontine tegmental nucleus to the rostral ventrolateral medulla in the rat. *Brain Research* 517, 19–24.
126. Zanella, S., Roux, J. C., Viemari, J. C., and Hilaire, G. (2006). Possible modulation of the mouse respiratory rhythm generator by A1/C1 neurones. *Respiratory Physiology & Neurobiology* 153, 126–138.
127. Zucker, I. H., and Gilmore, J. P. (1991). *Reflex Control of the Circulation*. Boston: CRC Press.

# 11

# Modulation of Autonomic Function by the Cerebral Cortex

ANTHONY J. M. VERBERNE

Modulation of autonomic function by the cerebral cortex has been recognized for many decades, although the place of the cerebral cortex in the hierarchy of central autonomic regulatory circuits has only been identified relatively recently (for reviews, see sources [28,121,148]). Thoughts or imagined situations can obviously evoke visceromotor responses, even when these responses seem to serve no obvious purpose[123]. Similarly, strong emotional stimuli, such as the sight of blood, can trigger fainting (syncope) associated with a profound decrease in heart rate mediated by the vagus nerve[84]. This chapter will describe several regions of the cortex that are likely to participate in the autonomic responses associated with emotional stimuli and specific behavioral states, with an emphasis on the roles of these regions in circulatory control.

Connections between the cortex and brain regions involved in central autonomic control were first identified using conventional neuroanatomical tracers. Building on these investigations, trans-synaptic viral tracing studies have identified several cortical areas that project polysynaptically to a range of central and peripheral targets, suggesting that specific regions of the cerebral cortex have the potential to modulate blood flow, motility, and secretion in a wide range of organ systems[150].

Central autonomic control involves all levels of the neuraxis, including selected regions of the cerebral cortex[120]. This conclusion is supported by a variety of experimental and clinical observations, including studies on the responses to stimulation of cortical structures in anesthetized animals, neuroanatomical investigations using trans-synaptic viral tracers, brain imaging in awake human subjects, deficits caused by lesions to cortical structures, or autonomic manifestations of epileptic seizures. The areas that have received the closest attention with respect to central autonomic control are the medial prefrontal cortex and the insular cortex (Figure 11–1). Emerging evidence from brain imaging studies suggests that these cortical regions modulate various aspects of autonomic function, such as circulatory control, micturition, gastrointestinal function, and the neuroendocrine components of the stress response[36,37,40,137] (see also Chapter 19).

## CORTICAL CONNECTIONS WITH CENTRAL AUTONOMIC PATHWAYS

Labeling after injection of neurotropic viruses into peripheral targets is frequently observed in two major cortical regions, the medial prefrontal cortex and the insular cortex[19,56,113,134]. While the medial prefrontal cortex is a recognized visceromotor region, the insular cortex is generally regarded as a viscerosensory region because it processes gustatory, gastrointestinal, and cardiopulmonary afferent information. However, visceromotor responses have also been elicited from the insular cortex[117,154], so these distinctions are somewhat arbitrary.

### Medial Prefrontal Cortex

The projections of the medial prefrontal cortex have been studied in considerable detail and in several

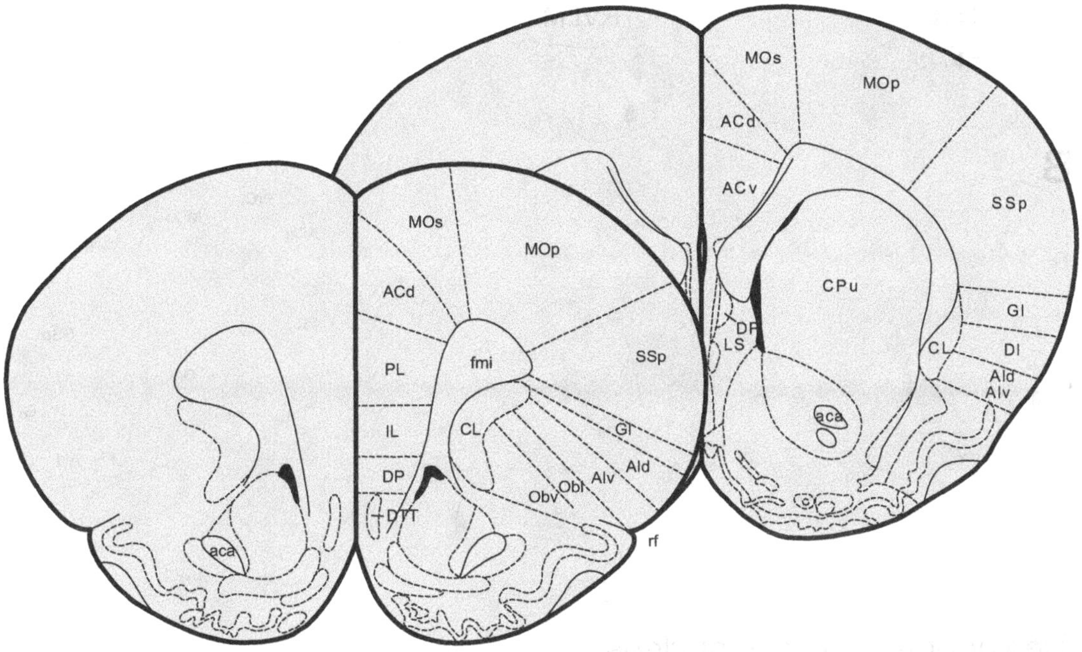


Figure 11–1 Cortical regions involved in central autonomic control. The principal cortical loci that are involved in central autonomic networks are in the medial prefrontal cortex and the insular cortex. *A:* Diagram showing the regions of the medial prefrontal cortex, which comprises the dorsal and ventral anterior cingulate cortex (ACd and ACv), the prelimbic area (PL) and the infralimbic area (IL). *B:* Diagram showing the insular cortex, which is subdivided into several sub-regions (AId, dorsal agranular insular cortex; AIv, ventral agranular insular cortex; GI, granular insular cortex). aca, anterior part of the anterior commissure; Cl, claustrum; CPu, caudate putamen; DI, dysgranular insular cortex; DP, dorsal peduncular cortex; DTT, dorsal tenia tecta; fmi, forceps minor; LS, lateral septum; MOp, primary motor cortex; MOs, secondary motor cortex; Obl, lateral orbital cortex; Obv, ventral orbital cortex; rf, rhinal fissure; SSp, primary somatosensory cortex.

species (for review, see [148]). Because the medial prefrontal cortex projects to medullary targets, including the solitary tract nucleus (NTS) and the rostral ventrolateral medulla(RVLM), this cortical region has been described as the "visceromotor cortex"[135,136,142,143]. An alternative, and perhaps more appropriate, term is "emotional motor cortex"[121]. Several of the brainstem projections of the medial prefrontal cortex have been documented in reasonable detail[53,141,149] (Figure 11–2). While the infralimbic area, prelimbic area, and anterior cingulate cortex all project to the lateral hypothalamus, the infralimbic area is the main source of afferents to the NTS. Most of the afferents from the medial prefrontal cortex to the RVLM come from the infralimbic and prelimbic areas, whereas the corticospinal projection from the medial prefrontal cortex arises predominantly from the prelimbic area and the anterior cingulate cortex. These observations suggest that the entire medial prefrontal cortex may be involved in modulation of autonomic function.

More detailed studies of projections from the prelimbic and infralimbic regions have shown that neurons in the infralimbic area primarily target other brain areas that are involved in central autonomic regulatory circuits. In contrast, prelimbic neurons have projection patterns consistent with a strong involvement in cognitive function[53,149]. Indeed, it has been suggested that there is a dorsoventral transition in function in the medial prefrontal cortex from a "cognitive" role to a "visceromotor" role[65]. Anatomical experiments that have identified the innervation targets of subregions of the medial prefrontal cortex have supported this contention[68,149].

Both the medial and lateral regions of the prefrontal cortex (anterior insular cortex) project to the NTS and RVLM[53], and activation of these cortical regions inhibits the discharge of presympathetic vasomotor RVLM neurons[130,145]. The medial prefrontal projection to medullary structures has been demonstrated in the rat, rabbit, and cat, but not in the macaque[51,148].

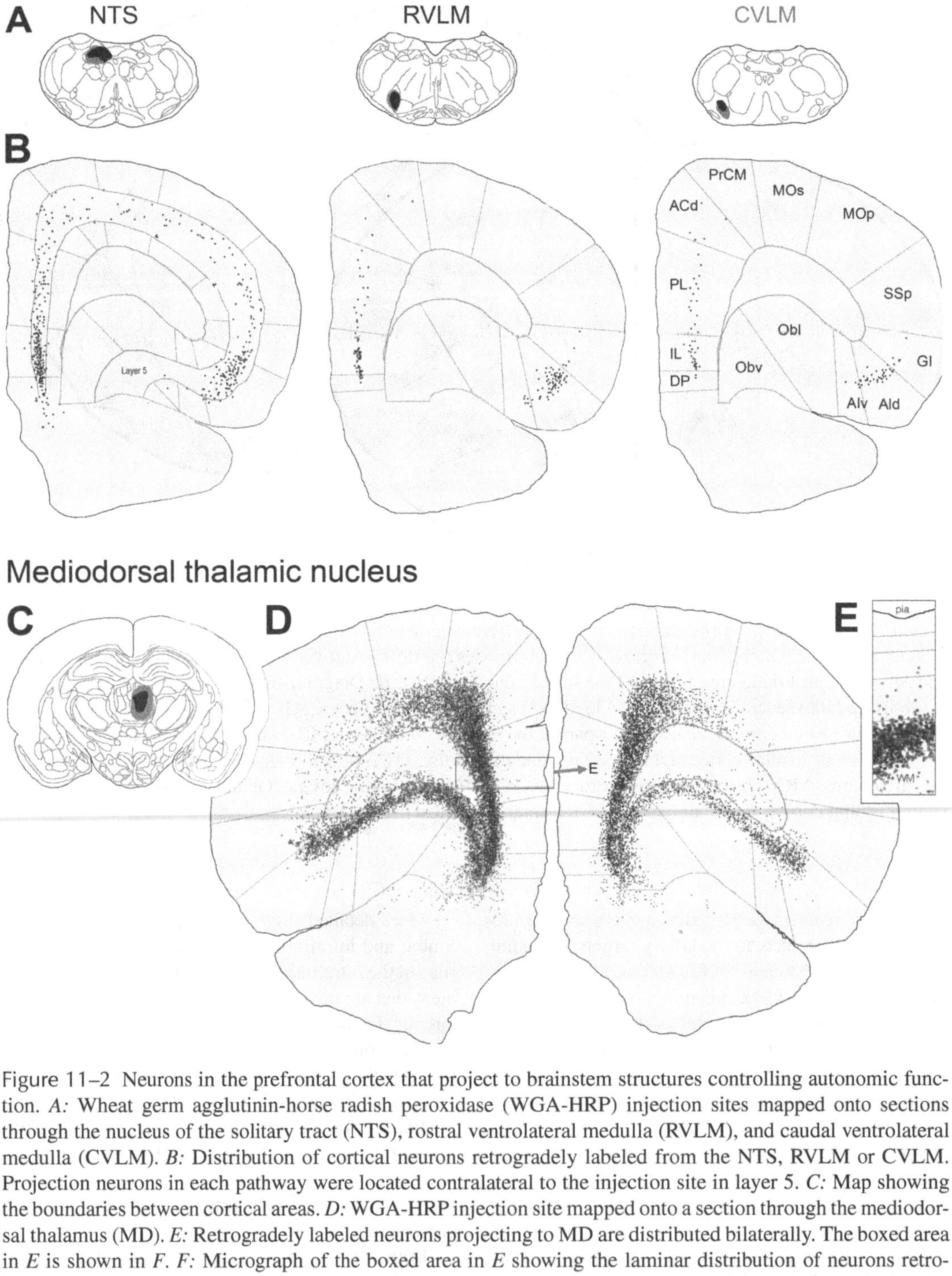


Figure 11–2 Neurons in the prefrontal cortex that project to brainstem structures controlling autonomic function. *A:* Wheat germ agglutinin-horse radish peroxidase (WGA-HRP) injection sites mapped onto sections through the nucleus of the solitary tract (NTS), rostral ventrolateral medulla (RVLM), and caudal ventrolateral medulla (CVLM). *B:* Distribution of cortical neurons retrogradely labeled from the NTS, RVLM or CVLM. Projection neurons in each pathway were located contralateral to the injection site in layer 5. *C:* Map showing the boundaries between cortical areas. *D:* WGA-HRP injection site mapped onto a section through the mediodorsal thalamus (MD). *E:* Retrogradely labeled neurons projecting to MD are distributed bilaterally. The boxed area in *E* is shown in *F*. *F:* Micrograph of the boxed area in *E* showing the laminar distribution of neurons retrogradely labeled from the ipsilateral MD. ACd, dorsal anterior cingulate cortex; AId, dorsal agranular insular cortex; AIv, ventral agranular insular cortex; DP, dorsal peduncular cortex; GI, granular insular cortex; IL, infralimbic area; MOp, primary motor cortex; MOs, secondary motor cortex; NTS, nucleus of the solitary tract; Obl, lateral orbital cortex; Obv, ventral orbital cortex; PL, prelimbic area; PrCM, precentral motor cortex; SSp, primary somatosensory cortex; VP, ventral peduncular cortex. Reproduced from Gabbott et al. (2005)[53], with permission.

### *Corticospinal Neurons of the Medial Prefrontal Cortex*

Corticospinal neurons are located in layer 5 of the medial prefrontal cortex[53,88]. However, the majority of corticospinal neurons found at this level of the neuraxis are located in the motor cortex (Figure 11–3). Prelimbic and infralimbic neurons project to the intermediolateral cell column and the central autonomic area of the thoracic spinal cord which are known to contain sympathetic interneurons[7,70,144]. This corticospinal pathway could be an additional route through which the medial prefrontal cortex influences autonomic outflow, but there is little direct evidence for this role at present.

### *Prefrontal projections to the medulla oblongata*

NTS neurons receive afferent input, not only from peripheral visceral sources, but also from supramedullary structures, including the medial prefrontal cortex[18,70,92,100,118,132,143,152]. This observation led to speculation that the cardiovascular and/or gastrointestinal motility responses evoked from prefrontal cortical areas may be mediated by NTS neurons. The termination sites of both cortical and cardiopulmonary visceral afferents overlap considerably within the NTS[117,142], suggesting that cortical neurons that project to the NTS may modulate visceral reflex function. Ultrastructural studies have now established that the projection from the infralimbic area to the contralateral commissural NTS is glutamatergic[139], and a proportion of this input appears to target catecholaminergic NTS neurons[54]. This pathway could be the reason that stimulation of the infralimbic depressor area induces Fos expression in the NTS[99], perhaps through activation of baroreceptor-related NTS neurons. Stimulation of the infralimbic depressor area also increases Fos-immunoreactivity in the caudal ventrolateral medulla (CVLM), an observation that is consistent with cortical activation of the baroreflex pathway[148].

The infralimbic area projects sparsely to the RVLM[70,136,141], and a small proportion of this input is onto

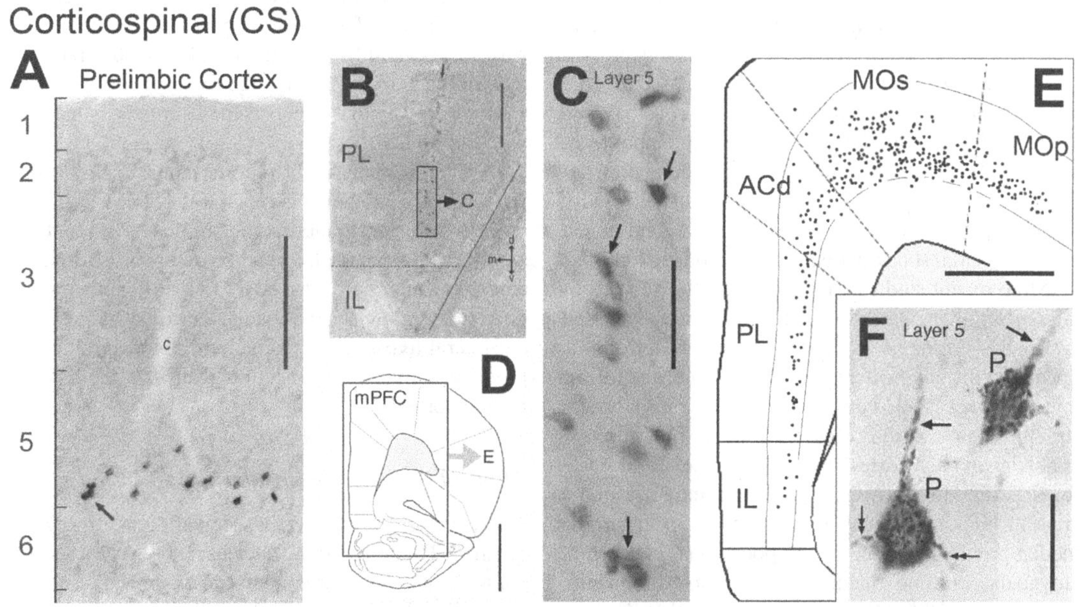


Figure 11–3 Spinally projecting neurons of the prefrontal cortex. *A:* Injection of WGA-HRP into the thoracic spinal cord (SC) retrogradely labeled corticospinal neurons (*arrow*) in layer 5 of the prelimbic (PL) area of the medial prefrontal cortex (mPFC). *B:* Corticospinal neurons (*arrow*) in layer 5 of ventral PL and infralimbic (IL) cortices. *C:* Micrograph of the boxed area in *B* showing corticospinal neurons in layer 5 (*arrows*). *D:* Coronal section expanded in *E. E:* Distribution of corticospinal neurons. *F:* Corticospinal PL pyramidal cells (P) retrogradely labeled with WGA-HRP. Apical (*single-headed arrows*) and basal dendritic processes (*double-headed arrows*) are indicated. ACd, dorsal anterior cingulate cortex; c, capillary; IL, infralimbic area; MOp, primary motor cortex; MOs, secondary motor cortex. Reproduced from Gabbott et al. (2005)[53], with permission.

C1 (adrenergic) RVLM neurons[54]. Similar to the infralimbic input to the NTS, boutons in the RVLM anterogradely labeled after injections of biotin-dextran amine into the infralimbic cortex make asymmetrical synapses and so are presumed to excite their target neurons[54].

### Afferent Input to the Medial Prefrontal Cortex

The prelimbic area of the medial prefrontal cortex receives afferent input from a number of limbic regions. In contrast, the infralimbic area receives input from structures associated with visceral sensory and motor function and from the prelimbic area. The afferent inputs to the medial prefrontal cortex have been described in detail previously (for review, see [148]). A sparse projection to the medial prefrontal cortex arises from the ventral medulla oblongata[87,142,156]. C1 cells of the RVLM send ascending collaterals to the lateral hypothalamus[63], but whether these ascend as far as the cortex is uncertain.

The medial prefrontal cortex is defined anatomically by its afferent input from the mediodorsal thalamic nucleus[81,114], and these areas are reciprocally connected[53] (Figure 11–2D). The prelimbic area receives afferents predominantly from the medial and lateral mediodorsal thalamic nucleus[31], but these projections do not appear to target the infralimbic area[81]. Stimulation of the medial prefrontal cortex in awake rabbits produced depressor and bradycardic responses and an increased uptake of $^{3}$H-2-deoxyglucose in the mediodorsal thalamic nucleus[16,17]. Although the precise role of the input from the mediodorsal thalamic nucleus to the medial prefrontal cortex is unknown, it may be important in bradycardic responses in rabbits that have been conditioned by a paraorbital shock paired with an acoustic tone[107].

More recent studies have identified the sources of afferent input to various subdivisions of the medial prefrontal cortex[68]. Microinjections of retrograde tracer into the anterior cingulate, prelimbic, and infralimbic cortices labeled unique sets of neurons. Cortical structures such as the orbitomedial prefrontal cortex, agranular insular cortex, perirhinal cortex, and entorhinal cortex. innervated the prelimbic and infralimbic areas, which also received afferent input from the medial basal forebrain, the hippocampus, claustrum, amygdala, midline thalamic nuclei, and brainstem. These anatomical data support the view that the prelimbic area has an important role in cognitive functions. In contrast, the infralimbic area appears to represent a visceromotor center[68].

## Insular Cortex

The insular cortex (Figure 11–1) consists of the dorsal section of the rhinal sulcus and is bounded dorsally by somatosensory areas I and II. It extends rostrally to the level of the olfactory bulb and caudally to the level of the amygdala.

#### Insular cortical projections to the medulla oblongata

In mouse, rat, rabbit, and cat, the posterior insular cortex projects to the caudal NTS[76,92,117,119,126,142,154,155]. The rostral dysgranular region of the insular cortex (gustatory cortex) also projects to the gustatory area of the rostral NTS[119,151]. Insular cortex neurons that innervate the NTS lie in layer 5[76], and ultrastructural studies suggest that the projection is glutamatergic[138]. Insular cortex neurons are labeled after injection of transsynaptic viral tracers into the rabbit vagus or aortic depressor nerve[10,56], suggesting that the insular cortex may modulate the activity of NTS neurons that receive input from aortic baroreceptors and other viscerosensory. afferents. Nevertheless, a direct cortico-solitary pathway is unlikely to mediate the cardiovascular responses elicited by insular cortex stimulation. Ibotenic acid lesions of the lateral hypothalamus reduce the depressor responses evoked by insular cortex stimulation[62], and the sympathoexcitatory response elicited by stimulation of the rostral posterior insular cortex was not blocked by interruption of synaptic transmission in the NTS[25]. Presumably, the insular cortex activates a pathway that connects the lateral hypothalamus with the RVLM[131].

Although many early reports failed to find a projection from the insular cortex to the RVLM[117,119,141,154], more recent retrograde tracing studies have identified a projection from the lateral prefrontal cortex or dorsal anterior insular cortex to the RVLM[6,53]. The rostral and posterior regions of the insular cortex also innervate the lateral hypothalamic area but this pathway is less prominent than the projection from the medial prefrontal cortex[60,82,154].

### Afferent Input to the Insular Cortex

The insular cortex receives visceral afferent information via the NTS, parabrachial nucleus, and visceral sensory thalamic nuclei[24]. These inputs are organized viscerotopically[27]. Other inputs arise from the mediodorsal thalamic nucleus[81,119], the ventroposterolateral parvicellular thalamic nucleus[4], and the lateral hypothalamic area[4,119]. Since stimulation of the vagus nerve evokes potentials in the insular cortex, these pathways probably convey viscerosensory and nociceptive information to the insular cortex[72–74]. Interestingly, in some patients with intractable epilepsy, vagus nerve stimulation also activates the insular cortex[90].

## CORTICAL MODULATION OF SYMPATHETIC VASOMOTOR FUNCTION

Modulation of arterial blood pressure and sympathetic vasomotor function by the cortex was first demonstrated in the early twentieth century (see [28]) and has been the subject of two reviews[109,148]. More recent discoveries are highlighted below.

### Medial Prefrontal Cortex, Arterial Blood Pressure and Sympathetic Vasomotor Function

A significant body of evidence suggests that neurons in the medial prefrontal cortex influence sympathetic vasomotor and parasympathetic cardiomotor outflow[148]. Cardiovascular responses have been elicited from both the prelimbic and infralimbic areas of the medial prefrontal cortex. However, the mechanisms that underpin these responses are likely to be different, because the projection patterns of the prelimbic and infralimbic areas are dissimilar[149] (Figure 11–4). Nevertheless, the depressor responses evoked by stimulation of either the infralimbic and prelimbic areas are accompanied by hindquarter vasodilatation[34,102].

Inhibition of NTS neurons led to simultaneous blockade of the baroreceptor reflex and attenuation of the cardiovascular responses[99] evoked from medial prefrontal cortex. Furthermore, interruption of either excitatory neurotransmission in the caudal ventrolateral medulla or GABAergic transmission in the RVLM also attenuated these responses[101]. These findings suggest that the medial prefrontal cortex–NTS circuit may contribute, at least in part, to sympathetic vasomotor inhibition evoked from the medial prefrontal cortex.

An alternative mechanism for the medial prefrontal cortex–evoked depressor response may be associated with a direct projection to the RVLM[70,136,141]. Although this projection appears sparse, sympathoexcitatory RVLM neurons are inhibited by stimulation of the medial prefrontal cortex[145]. Whether or not sympathoinhibition mediated by the medial prefrontal cortex proceeds through a relay in the NTS, stimulation of the medial prefrontal cortex has been shown to inhibit the activity of sympathoexcitatory RVLM neurons and sympathetic nerve discharge[145], and this probably represents the final output pathway mediating the hypotension and sympathoinhibition evoked by stimulation of the medial prefrontal cortex.

An additional mechanism for these inhibitory responses may involve the connections of the medial prefrontal cortex with the lateral hypothalamic area[69,70,82,124]. Excitotoxic lesions of the lateral hypothalamus reduced the depressor responses induced by microinjection of acetylcholine into the medial prefrontal cortex[103].

Taken together, the data above indicate that potential pathways that could account for the cardiovascular responses elicited from the medial prefrontal cortex include a hypothalamic relay, a direct projection to the NTS, a direct projection to the RVLM, or a direct projection to the spinal cord.

Anesthesia may influence the direction of changes in blood pressure or heart rate that occur after chemical or electrical stimulation of the medial prefrontal cortex[21,48]. Stimulation of medial prefrontal glutamate receptors resulted in pressor and tachycardic responses that were not associated with gross behavioral changes[108]. In awake rats, microinjection of noradrenaline into the prelimbic area produced a pressor response associated with an increase in plasma vasopressin that was blocked by inhibition of neurons in the paraventricular nucleus of the hypothalamus[48,49]. A cholinergic link in the lateral septal area has also been implicated in this response[50]. The vasopressin response to activation of the prelimbic area is markedly reduced by general anesthesia. An interpretation of these findings is that there are multiple pathways arising from the medial prefrontal cortex that influence cardiovascular function by modulation of vasopressin release or sympathetic vasomotor outflow. Neurons associated with these pathways in the medial prefrontal cortex may be intermingled and so are activated simultaneously when stimulated chemically or electrically.

Microinjection of the excitatory amino acid, glutamate, into the infralimbic area in awake spontaneously hypertensive rats produced hypotension and bradycardia, in stark contrast to the hypertension and tachycardia observed in normotensive rats[112]. Pharmacological analysis of the cardiovascular response in the hypertensive rats suggested that excitation of neurons in the infralimbic area is associated with sympathetic vasomotor withdrawal and cardiovagal activation. Thus, inhibitory drive from the infralimbic area to neurons that control sympathetic vasomotor output may be less in hypertensive than in normotensive rats. Alternatively, the higher resting sympathetic vasomotor drive in the spontaneously hypertensive rat could magnify the depressor response to infralimbic stimulation[75].

### Medial Prefrontal Cortex and the Baroreceptor Reflex

The medial prefrontal cortex facilitates the baroreceptor heart rate reflex[148]. Excitotoxic destruction of the medial prefrontal cortex reduces the gain of the baroreceptor heart rate reflex[91,147], but the effect on the sympathetic vasomotor baroreflex has not yet been examined in awake animals. In both awake and anesthetized animals, activation of the medial prefrontal cortex mainly facilitates the parasympathetic

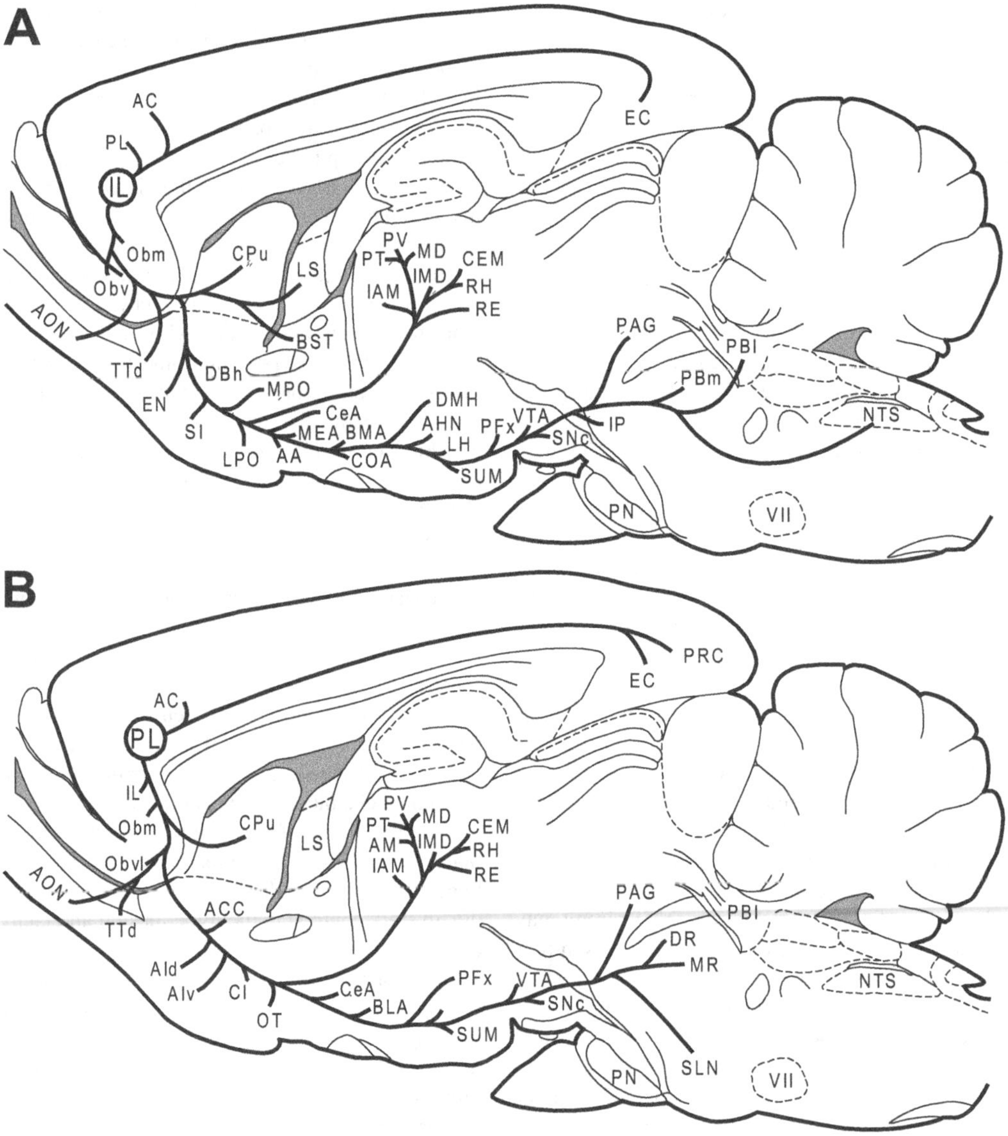


Figure 11–4 Innervation targets of the infralimbic and prelimbic areas of the medial prefrontal cortex. *A:* Brain regions innervated by the infralimbic area (IL) of the medial prefrontal cortex mapped onto a sagittal section of the rat brain. *B:* Brain regions innervated by the prelimbic area (PL) of the medial prefrontal cortex mapped onto a sagittal section of the rat brain. AA, anterior area of amygdala; AC, anterior cingulate cortex; ACC, nucleus accumbens; AHN, anterior hypothalamic nucleus; AId, dorsal agranular insular cortex; AIv, ventral agranular insular cortex; AM anteromedial nucleus of thalamus; AON, anterior olfactory nucleus; BLA, basolateral nucleus of the amygdala; BMA, basomedial nucleus of the amygdala; BST, bed nucleus of the stria terminalis; CeA, central nucleus of the amygdala; CEM, central medial nucleus of the thalamus; Cl, claustrum; COA, cortical nucleus of the amygdala; CPu, caudate putamen; DBh, diagonal band of Broca, horizontal limb; DMH, dorsomedial hypothalamic nucleus; DR, dorsal raphé nucleus; EC, entorhinal cortex; EN, endopiriform nucleus; IAM, interanteromedial nucleus of the thalamus; IC, inferior colliculus; IL, infralimbic area; IMD, intermediodorsal nucleus of the thalamus; IP, interpeduncular nucleus; LHy, lateral hypothalamic area; LPO, lateral preoptic area; LS, lateral septum; MD, mediodorsal thalamic nucleus; MEA medial nucleus of amygdala; MPO, medial preoptic area; NTS, nucleus of the solitary tract; Obm, medial orbital cortex; Obv, ventral orbital cortex; Obvl, ventral lateral orbital cortex; OT, olfactory tubercle; PAG, periaqueductal gray area; PBl, lateral parabrachial

Figure 11–4 *(Continued)*
nucleus; PBm, medial parabrachial nucleus; PFx, perifornical region of hypothalamus; PL, prelimbic area; PN, nucleus of the pons; PRC, perirhinal cortex; PT, paratenial nucleus of the thalamus; PV, paraventricular nucleus of the thalamus; RE, reunions nucleus; RH, rhomboid nucleus; SI, substantia innominata; SLN, supralemniscal nucleus; SNc, substantia nigra compacta; SUM, supramammillary nucleus; TTd, dorsal taenia tecta; VTA, ventral tegmental area; VII, facial nucleus. Reproduced from Vertes (2004)[149], with permission.

component of the baroreflex[110,111,125]. The primary locus for this response may reside in the infralimbic area, since its activation facilitates bradycardia induced by aortic nerve stimulation via a mechanism dependent on 5-$HT_{2A}$ receptors in the NTS[125]. Inhibition of NTS neurons blocked both the sympathoinhibitory response to medial prefrontal cortex stimulation and baroreflex-induced sympathoinhibition[99]. Hence, activation of the infralimbic input to the NTS may activate the baroreflex pathway[148].

Lesions of the medial prefrontal cortex in spontaneously hypertensive rats do not produce impairment of the baroreceptor heart rate reflex[109,146], probably because the vagal component of the reflex is already impaired in this rat strain[64]. This defect may arise from an age-related loss in cardiovagal motor neurons in spontaneously hypertensive rats[32]. Nevertheless, a vagally mediated bradycardic response has been reported after glutamate stimulation of the infralimbic area in this rat strain[112].

It has been suggested that cortical modulation of the baroreflex may participate in the recovery from a stressful event[93]. Baroreceptor unloading produced by lower body negative pressure in healthy volunteers was associated with reduced activity of neurons in the right anterior cingulate cortex and the orbitofrontal cortex[79], indicating that cortical modulation of baroreflex function may also occur in man.

### Dopamine Release in the Medial Prefrontal Cortex: Stress and Fear Conditioning

Dopamine neurons of the ventral tegmental area project to the medial prefrontal cortex[94]. A broad range of stressors, including hypotension, activate the mesocortical dopaminergic input to the medial prefrontal cortex[78,106]. Increased neuronal expression of Fos indicates that a wide variety of stressors also activate neurons in the medial prefrontal cortex[33,47,86,128]. Dopamine release in the medial prefrontal cortex also accompanies fear conditioning produced by footshock in rats[45], which evokes a behavioral response (freezing, ultrasonic vocalization) and autonomic responses (blood pressure elevation and tachycardia)[23] (see Chapter 12). In addition, blockade of NMDA receptors in the prelimbic and infralimbic cortices did not prevent extinction of the classical fear conditioning response but impaired its subsequent recall[20].

Inhibition of medial prefrontal cortex neurons by bilateral microinjection of the -$\gamma$-aminobutyric acid (GABA) agonist, muscimol, did not alter the pressor and tachycardic responses to restraint stress. However, inhibition of neurons in the dorsomedial hypothalamus did block these effects. Inhibition of the medial prefrontal cortex led to increased expression of Fos in response to restraint in the dorsomedial hypothalamic nucleus, medial amygdala, and medial NTS[86]. These data suggest that dopaminergic transmission in the infralimbic area mainly modulates conditioned fear extinction. In contrast, the prelimbic area is required for expression of the conditioned fear response, perhaps due to its involvement in the process of perception of the fearful situation or retrieval of its memory[106].

### Summary

The medial prefrontal cortex is a complex brain region that participates in a number of cognitive, emotional, and autonomic control processes. Although it remains uncertain how these different functions are related, the medial prefrontal cortex may be a site at which circuits controlling these functions converge, allowing emotionally significant situations to evoke changes in autonomic function.

## INSULAR CORTEX, ARTERIAL BLOOD PRESSURE, AND SYMPATHETIC VASOMOTOR FUNCTION

Predominantly depressor responses occur upon stimulation of the rostral insular area (or lateral prefrontal cortex)[61,62,130]. The effects of the rostral insular cortex on regional sympathetic nerve discharge are not known, but the depressor responses are mediated by inhibition of sympathoexcitatory RVLM neurons via a GABAergic mechanism[130]. While only depressor responses were reported upon stimulation of the rostral insular cortex[130], a small number of sympathoexcitatory RVLM neurons were activated. These findings suggest that regions within, or close to, the rostral insular cortex are involved in sympathoexcitation, and these may include the sympathoexcitatory areas of the posterior insular cortex described by others[3,22,117,154]. Stimulation of the posterior insular cortex elicits pressor responses associated with tachycardia or depressor responses associated with bradycardia, depending on the precise location of the stimulation[25,117,154]. Pressor and tachycardic responses associated with renal sympathoexcitation are elicited from rostral sites within the posterior insular cortex, while depressor and bradycardic sites are encountered in the caudal section of the posterior insular cortex[26]. Electrical stimulation of the posterior insular cortex that is synchronized with the electrocardiogram (2-7 Hz) elicits only changes in heart rate[95].

The cardiovascular responses to chemical stimulation of the posterior insular cortex have been examined in several rat strains in the awake and anesthetized states[22,117]. The cardiovascular responses elicited from the posterior insular cortex are mediated by a relay in the lateral hypothalamus[25,62,98]. Cobalt microinjection into the ventrolateral medulla attenuated both the pressor and sympathoexcitatory responses[26]. However, the most effective microinjection sites did not appear to coincide with the area that had the highest density of presympathetic neurons; i.e., the RVLM. Instead, the most effective site was in the CVLM. Taken together, these findings support the view that the cardiovascular responses elicited from both the rostral and posterior divisions of the insular cortex are mediated by a synaptic relay in the lateral hypothalamus, which then modulates the activity of presympathetic RVLM neurons, perhaps via the CVLM.

## CORTICAL MODULATION OF GASTROINTESTINAL FUNCTION

Neurons in the agranular and dysgranular insular cortex project to an area of the dorsal vagal complex that also receives input from gastric afferents[2]. Electrical stimulation of this area evokes excitatory and inhibitory effects on gastric motor function but no change in blood pressure or respiratory rate[2,8]. There is some evidence for a viscerotopic organization of circuits that control gastric, cardiovascular, and respiratory function within the insular cortex[1,8], with electrical stimulation of more caudal regions evoking respiratory responses. However, the relationships between the cardiovascular, gastrointestinal, and respiratory responses to stimulation of the insular cortex are unknown and may occur because functionally distinct populations of neurons coexist in close proximity in the insular cortex.

Trans-synaptic labeling occur in the medial prefrontal cortex and insular cortex after injection of viral tracers into the ventral stomach wall, probably because both cortical areas project to the dorsal vagal complex[113]. Hurley-Gius and Neafsey demonstrated a vagally mediated, inhibitory influence of the medial prefrontal cortex on gastric tone[71]. The infralimbic area is the most important region of the medial prefrontal cortex for this effect, and peripheral muscarinic receptor blockade reduced and vagotomy abolished the gastric relaxation induced by infralimbic stimulation[104]. Stimulation of the medial prefrontal cortex inhibits vagal sensory transmission by modulating the activity of NTS neurons[9].

## CORTICAL MODULATION OF UROGENITAL FUNCTION

Although the storage and release of urine are simple, the central processes that modulate micturition are intricate and involve sensation of bladder fullness and voluntary control related to the social appropriateness of micturition[13] (see Chapter 19). In addition to selected motor cortical regions, electrical stimulation of specific sub-areas of the anterior cingulate cortex in anesthetized cats produced both excitatory and inhibitory effects on micturition[57,58]. The central circuitry controlling micturition is complex and incompletely understood[11]. The micturition reflex is largely controlled by premotor neurons in Barrington's nucleus of the dorsal pons. These neurons project to the sacral spinal cord to innervate parasympathetic preganglionic neurons that control the bladder[46,122] (see Chapter 19). In addition, neurons in the dorsolateral pons project to neurons in Onuf's nucleus in the sacral spinal cord. The neurons in Onuf's nucleus control the tone of the pelvic floor and the urethral and anal sphincters[13].

Injection of trans-synaptic viral tracers into the urinary bladder labels neurons in several regions of the cerebral cortex, including the insular cortex, primary motor cortex, and anterior cingulate cortex[105,129,158]. While primary motor cortical areas are likely to control voluntary micturition, prefrontal cortical areas are probably involved in the decision to initiate micturition[11]. Excitotoxic lesions of the anterior cingulate cortex result in a prolongation of the interval between volume-evoked bladder contractions[85]. Prefrontal and insular cortical neurons also connect with neurons that innervate the bulbospongiosus muscles that are involved in penile erection and ejaculation[133].

Neurons in layers 5 and 6 of the prelimbic and infralimbic areas project to the laterodorsal tegmental nucleus and Barrington's nucleus[124,140,149,157], suggesting that both the prelimbic area and the infralimbic areas may modulate micturition. There is also evidence that the mediodorsal thalamus and other groups of thalamic neurons relay osmotic and thirst-related information to the anterior cingulate and insular cortex[67].

Functional magnetic resonance imaging in humans has identified several cortical areas whose activity is modulated by bladder filling[13,14,77]. These include the insular cortex, anterior cingulate gyrus, and regions of the prefrontal cortex. The insular cortex is probably involved in integration of visceral signals arising from bladder afferents, while the anterior cingulate cortex may be involved in the perception of a full bladder. It has been suggested that the prefrontal cortex is involved in deciding whether or not micturition should occur[77]. Thus, the prefrontal cortex may be important for the development of urinary control as a child matures. The right dorsolateral prefrontal cortex is active when micturition takes place and also when micturition is allowed but does not occur[12].

### Summary

Central autonomic control pathways involve all levels of the neuraxis, including selected regions of the cerebral cortex. At present, little is known about the properties of individual neurons in insular and medial prefrontal cortex that participate in central autonomic control. The precise conditions under which these cortical areas are recruited are also poorly understood. Defining these parameters for autonomic neurons in the cerebral cortex should be a fertile field for future research.

## CEREBRAL CORTICAL MODULATION OF AUTONOMIC FUNCTION IN HUMANS

Information regarding how the cerebral cortex modulates autonomic function in humans has been derived from patients with trauma to specific cortical areas or from autonomic symptoms of epileptic seizures with foci in specific cortical loci[28]. In addition, neuronal stimulation in humans has shown that insular cortex stimulation is associated with a variety of cardiovascular responses[96].

Transcranial magnetic stimulation and other techniques have indicated that the cerebral cortex influences human autonomic function. Sweating responses to transcranial magnetic stimulation are readily demonstrated and are independent of sensory nerves[115,116,127]. Transcranial magnetic stimuli applied over the vertex in humans elicits reductions in muscle sympathetic activity when the stimuli are applied within 200 ms–400 ms after the electrocardiographic R-wave[83]. This observation suggests that in humans, the cerebral cortex is also capable of reducing sympathetic vasomotor outflow to the skeletal muscle vasculature.

Since the first edition of this book, a range of brain-imaging techniques, particularly blood-oxygen–level dependent functional magnetic resonance imaging, have provided more specific answers about cortical involvement in central autonomic processes in humans (see [36] for an overview). These new findings have largely confirmed the primary roles of the medial prefrontal and insular cortices in central autonomic control.

### Medial Prefrontal Control of Autonomic Function in Humans

In 1848, a tamping rod propelled by exploding blasting powder went through the skull of a railway worker, Phineas Gage, obliterating his left prefrontal cortex. As a consequence of his injury, Gage changed from a reliable worker with a position of responsibility to a profane, irresponsible, capricious, and irreverent man[44]. In 1994, Damasio analyzed Gage's behavioral changes and became the first to pinpoint the importance of the prefrontal cortex in human behavior. This study led to new approaches for understanding the role of the prefrontal cortex in processing emotion. However, links between the human prefrontal cortex and autonomic control have only emerged relatively recently.

Humans with lesions to the ventromedial prefrontal cortex show no major changes in cardiovascular function at rest or during presentation of non-emotional stimulation[66]. However, patients with right-sided, but not left-sided, ventromedial prefrontal cortex lesions displayed increases in heart rate and blood pressure upon emotional stimulation. These observations suggests that, similar to the insular cortex (see below), lateralization of function may also occur in the medial prefrontal cortex.

Handgrip exercise in normal humans elicits increases in heart rate and blood pressure but not muscle sympathetic nerve activity. The tachycardic response is not sensitive to β-adrenoceptor blockade and is largely mediated by withdrawal of cardiovagal tone. These physiological changes occur in conjunction with reduced activity of the ventral medial prefrontal cortex[153] assessed by functional magnetic resonance imaging, suggesting that reduced activity of the ventromedial prefrontal cortex is associated with reduced cardiac parasympathetic outflow.

In human studies, several indices of autonomic function have been used to identify cortical modulation of central autonomic function. The skin conductance response is a readily measurable index of sympathetic outflow to sweat glands. This response is represented in, and probably generated within, the medial prefrontal cortex[38]. Activation of the cerebral cortex in man probably inhibits sympathetic vasomotor outflow to muscle, since transcranial magnetic stimulation of the cortex underlying the vertex elicits inhibition of muscle sympathetic nerve activity[83].

Hypoglycemia, a stimulus that originates from within the body (interoceptive stimulus), causes bilateral activation of the medial prefrontal cortex as well as activating sympathetic and parasympathetic outflow[35,137]. The prefrontal cortex may be associated with the development of hypoglycemia-associated autonomic failure, a condition in which autonomic responses to hypoglycemia are shifted to a lower glycemic threshold as a result of antecedent hypoglycemia[43]. In the heartbeat detection task, which involves another interoceptive stimulus, increased activity occurs in the insular and anterior cingulate cortices. The right anterior insular cortex also appears to be involved in interoceptive awareness[42].

Mental stress induced by performance of a mathematical task in patients with cardiac dysfunction evoked increases in skin conductance, heart rate, and blood pressure. In addition, a heartbeat-evoked cerebral cortical potential correlated with the stress-induced changes in cardiac output[59]. Baroreceptor unloading caused by lower body negative pressure increases muscle sympathetic nerve activity, induces tachycardia, and reduces stroke volume to a greater degree in men than women. This maneuver also increases neuronal activity in the dorsal and ventral cingulate cortex and the right amygdala based on blood-oxygen level–dependent functional magnetic resonance. The degree of neuronal activation matched the changes in cardiovascular parameters[80].

Engagement in difficult cognitive tasks increases heart rate and decreases variability in high-frequency heart period, a measure of cardiac parasympathetic activity. Regional cerebral blood flow measurement with $H_2{}^{15}O$ positron emission tomography indicates that these responses are associated with reduced activity in the ventromedial prefrontal cortex and insular cortex, and there is also increased activity in the anterior cingulate cortex[55]. The latter finding is consistent with the observation that patients with lesions in the anterior cingulate cortex display blunted pressor responses to mental stress[40].

In general, the human medial prefrontal cortex seems to be associated with parasympathetic activation and sympathetic vasomotor inhibition, as occurs in anesthetized animals.

### Insular Cortical Control of Autonomic Function in Humans

Lesions of the left insular cortex in humans may increase cardiac sympathetic tone[97]. Furthermore, there may be a link between sudden death as a result of cardiac arrhythmia and altered activity of the right insular cortex[29]. Stroke patients with involvement of the right insular cortex had a higher incidence of complex cardiac arrhythmias and showed reduced heart rate variability. These findings suggest that damage to the insular cortex alters cardiac sympathetic/parasympathetic balance[30].

A wide range of cardiovascular symptoms has been observed during epileptic seizures and includes changes in heart rhythm, blood pressure, and the electrocardiogram[52]. Patients with seizures involving the temporal lobes are more likely to show reduced heart rates during seizures, but this response is not associated with a particular cerebral hemisphere[15].

Presentation of images depicting facial expressions with differing emotional impact result in changes in heart rate that correlate with the type of facial expression. Activity in the insular cortex, anterior cingulate cortex, and amygdala increased when subjects were shown angry or sad faces, leading to increases in heart rate[41]. The James-Lange interpretation of this data is that we feel an emotional response to the sad or angry faces *because* of the visceral autonomic response (e.g., the increase in heart rate)[89]. This interpretation has been criticized largely because feedback from visceral reactions is unlikely to be specific enough to give rise to the full range of human emotions. Alternatively, visceral responses might occur only after cognitive appraisal of a situation leads to the emotional feelings. In support of this idea, individuals with pure autonomic failure still experienced feelings of emotion, albeit of a reduced intensity, despite the absence of the visceral responses[39]. Importantly, arousal but not conscious awareness of the stimulus modulated the activation of the amygdala, whereas activity in the right insular cortex was dependent on both arousal and conscious awareness. Hence, the insular cortex may be important in the process that leads to generation of emotional feelings, especially pain[5]. This notion is consistent with the view that the insular cortex is a "viscerosensory" brain region.

Mental stress and physical exercise not only cause sympathetic activation but also activation of the right anterior cingulate cortex and the right insular cortex[37]. In contrast, cardiovascular activation was associated with reduced activity in the right ventromedial prefrontal cortex. Earlier studies, including ones in which stimulation of the right insular cortex resulted in tachycardia and hypertension, had already pointed to this lateralization of function[96].

## GENERAL SUMMARY

Over the last two decades, our understanding of how the cerebral cortex influences the autonomic control of diverse physiological systems has steadily advanced.

Research has identified the major pathways and connections of the medial prefrontal cortex and insular cortices, but the relative importance of these pathways in mediating changes in autonomic function is still emerging.

Cortical modulation of autonomic function in humans appears to follow the principles that have emerged from studies performed in laboratory animals. Although novel observations about cortical influences on autonomic processing are coming from modern imaging techniques, their relatively low spatial resolution limits the ability of researchers to identify the cortical neurons that influence central autonomic control in humans.

It remains to be determined how other functions of the prefrontal and the insular cortex relate to their influence on autonomic function. Alterations in autonomic function may be triggered by recollection of events with significant emotional relevance. In this context, it is interesting to note that brainstem-projecting neurons in the medial prefrontal cortex receive input from the ventral hippocampus[118].

Research over the past 20 years has answered some of the questions posed by Cechetto and Saper[28] in the first edition of this book, but new questions have also emerged. The cerebral cortex is now known to influence gastrointestinal function, regional hemodynamics, and sympathetic vasomotor outflow. The neural pathways that mediate cortically evoked changes in autonomic function are better understood than 20 years ago, but much remains to be learned. In particular, the precise relationships between behavior and the influence of the cortex on autonomic function should be a major focus of future investigation.

ACKNOWLEDGEMENTS The author thanks Dr. Neil Owens and Dr. Daniela Sartor for their important contributions to studies of the medial prefrontal cortex and circulatory control. The critical comments and permission to reproduce figures provided by Drs. Paul Gabbott and Robert Vertes is also sincerely appreciated. These studies were supported by the National Health and Medical Research Council of Australia, the Heart Foundation of Australia, and the Austin Hospital Medical Research Foundation.

## References

1. Aleksandrov, V. G., Aleksandrova, N. P., and Bagaev, V. A. (2000). Identification of a respiratory related area in the rat insular cortex. *Canadian Journal of Physiology and Pharmacology* 78, 582–586.
2. Aleksandrov, V. G., Bagaev, V. A., Nozdrachev, A. D., and Panteleev, S. S. (1996). Identification of gastric related neurones in the rat insular cortex. *Neuroscience Letters* 216, 5–8.
3. Allen, G. V., and Cechetto, D. F. (1995). Neurotensin in the lateral hypothalamic area: Origin and function. *Neuroscience* 69, 533–544.
4. Allen, G. V., Saper, C. B., Hurley, K. M., and Cechetto, D. F. (1991). Organization of visceral and limbic connections in the insular cortex of the rat. *Journal of Comparative Neurology* 311, 1–16.
5. Aziz, Q., Schnitzler, A., and Enck, P. (2000). Functional neuroimaging of visceral sensation. *Journal of Clinical Neurophysiology* 17, 604–612.
6. Ba M'hamed, S., Sequeira, H., Poulain, P., Bennis, M., and Roy, J. C. (1993). Sensorimotor cortex projections to the ventrolateral and dorsomedial medulla oblongata in the rat. *Neuroscience Letters* 164, 195–198.
7. Bacon, S. J., and Smith, A. D. (1993). A monosynaptic pathway from an identified vasomotor centre in the medial prefrontal cortex to an autonomic area in the thoracic spinal cord. *Neuroscience* 54, 719–728.
8. Bagaev, V., and Aleksandrov, V. (2006). Visceral-related area in the rat insular cortex. *Autonomic Neuroscience* 125, 16–21.
9. Bagaev, V. A., and Panteleev, S. S. (1994). Limbic cortical influences to the vagal input neurones of the solitary tract nucleus. *Neuroreport* 5, 1705–1708.
10. Blessing, W. W., Li, Y. W., and Wesselingh, S. L. (1991). Transneuronal transport of herpes simplex virus from the cervical vagus to brain neurons with axonal inputs to central vagal sensory nuclei in the rat. *Neuroscience* 42, 261–274.
11. Blok, B. F. (2002). Central pathways controlling micturition and urinary continence. *Urology* 59, 13–17.
12. Blok, B. F., and Holstege, G. (1999). The central control of micturition and continence: Implications for urology. *British Journal of Urology International* 83, 1–6.
13. Blok, B. F., Sturms, L. M., and Holstege, G. (1998). Brain activation during micturition in women. *Brain* 121, 2033–2042.
14. Blok, B. F., Willemsen, A. T., and Holstege, G. (1997). A PET study on brain control of micturition in humans. *Brain* 120, 111–121.
15. Britton, J. W., Ghearing, G. R., Benarroch, E. E., and Cascino, G. D. (2006). The ictal bradycardia syndrome: Localization and lateralization. *Epilepsia* 47, 737–744.
16. Buchanan, S. L., and Powell, D. A. (1987). 3H-2-deoxyglucose uptake after electrical stimulation of cardioactive sites in insular cortex and mediodorsal nucleus of the thalamus in rabbits. *Brain Research Bulletin* 19, 439–452.
17. Buchanan, S. L., Powell, D. A., and Buggy, J. (1984). 3H-2-deoxyglucose uptake after electrical stimulation of cardioactive sites in anterior medial

cortex in rabbits. *Brain Research Bulletin* 13, 371–382.

18. Buchanan, S. L., Thompson, R. H., Maxwell, B. L., and Powell, D. A. (1994). Efferent connections of the medial prefrontal cortex in the rabbit. *Experimental Brain Research* 100, 469–483.
19. Buijs, R. M., Chun, S. J., Niijima, A., Romijn, H. J., and Nagai, K. (2001). Parasympathetic and sympathetic control of the pancreas: A role for the suprachiasmatic nucleus and other hypothalamic centers that are involved in the regulation of food intake. *Journal of Comparative Neurology* 431, 405–423.
20. Burgos-Robles, A., Vidal-Gonzalez, I., Santini, E., and Quirk, G. J. (2007). Consolidation of fear extinction requires NMDA receptor-dependent bursting in the ventromedial prefrontal cortex. *Neuron* 53, 871–880.
21. Burns, S. M., and Wyss, J. M. (1985). The involvement of the anterior cingulate cortex in blood pressure control. *Brain Research* 340, 71–77.
22. Butcher, K. S., and Cechetto, D. F. (1995). Autonomic responses of the insular cortex in hypertensive and normotensive rats. *American Journal of Physiology* 268, R214–R222.
23. Carrive, P. (2000). Conditioned fear to environmental context: Cardiovascular and behavioral components in the rat. *Brain Research* 858, 440–445.
24. Cechetto, D. F. (1987). Central representation of visceral function. *Federation Proceedings* 46, 17–23.
25. Cechetto, D. F., and Chen, S. J. (1990). Subcortical sites mediating sympathetic responses from insular cortex in rats. *American Journal of Physiology* 258, R245–R255.
26. Cechetto, D. F., and Chen, S. J. (1992). Hypothalamic and cortical sympathetic responses relay in the medulla of the rat. *American Journal of Physiology* 263, R544–R552.
27. Cechetto, D. F., and Saper, C. B. (1987). Evidence for a viscerotopic sensory representation in the cortex and thalamus in the rat. *Journal of Comparative Neurology* 262, 27–45.
28. Cechetto, D. F., and Saper, C. B. (1990). Role of the cerebral cortex in autonomic function. In A. D. Loewy and K. M. Spyer (Eds.), *Central Regulation of Autonomic Functions*, pp. 208–223. New York: Oxford University Press.
29. Cheung, R. T., and Hachinski, V. (2000). The insula and cerebrogenic sudden death. *Archives of Neurology* 57, 1685–1688.
30. Colivicchi, F., Bassi, A., Santini, M., and Caltagirone, C. (2004). Cardiac autonomic derangement and arrhythmias in right-sided stroke with insular involvement. *Stroke* 35, 2094–2098.
31. Conde, F., Audinat, E., Maire-Lepoivre, E., and Crepel, F. (1990). Afferent connections of the medial frontal cortex of the rat. A study using retrograde transport of fluorescent dyes. I. Thalamic afferents. *Brain Research Bulletin* 24, 341–354.
32. Corbett, E. K., Mary, D. A., McWilliam, P. N., and Batten, T. F. (2007). Age-related loss of cardiac vagal preganglionic neurones in spontaneously hypertensive rats. *Experimental Physiology* 92, 1005–1013.
33. Crane, J. W., Ebner, K., and Day, T. A. (2003). Medial prefrontal cortex suppression of the hypothalamic-pituitary-adrenal axis response to a physical stressor, systemic delivery of interleukin-1β. *European Journal of Neuroscience* 17, 1473–1481.
34. Crippa, G. E., Lewis, S. J., Johnson, A. K., and Correa, F. M. (2000). Medial prefrontal cortex acetylcholine injection-induced hypotension: The role of hindlimb vasodilation. *Journal of the Autonomic Nervous System* 79, 1–7.
35. Critchley, H. D. (2004). The human cortex responds to an interoceptive challenge. *Proceedings of the National Academy of Sciences, USA* 101, 6333–6334.
36. Critchley, H. D. (2005). Neural mechanisms of autonomic, affective, and cognitive integration. *Journal of Comparative Neurology* 493, 154–166.
37. Critchley, H. D., Corfield, D. R., Chandler, M. P., Mathias, C. J., and Dolan, R. J. (2000). Cerebral correlates of autonomic cardiovascular arousal: A functional neuroimaging investigation in humans. *Journal of Physiology* 523, 259–270.
38. Critchley, H. D., Elliott, R., Mathias, C. J., and Dolan, R. J. (2000). Neural activity relating to generation and representation of galvanic skin conductance responses: A functional magnetic resonance imaging study. *Journal of Neuroscience* 20, 3033–3040.
39. Critchley, H. D., Mathias, C. J., and Dolan, R. J. (2002). Fear conditioning in humans: The influence of awareness and autonomic arousal on functional neuroanatomy. *Neuron* 33, 653–663.
40. Critchley, H. D., Mathias, C. J., Josephs, O., O'Doherty, J., Zanini, S., Dewar, B.-K., Cipolotti, L., Shallice, T., and Dolan, R. J. (2003). Human cingulate cortex and autonomic control: Converging neuroimaging and clinical evidence. *Brain* 126, 2139–2152.
41. Critchley, H. D., Rotshtein, P., Nagai, Y., O'Doherty, J., Mathias, C. J., and Dolan, R. J. (2005). Activity in the human brain predicting differential heart rate responses to emotional facial expressions. *Neuroimage* 24, 751–762.
42. Critchley, H. D., Wiens, S., Rotshtein, P., Ohman, A., and Dolan, R. J. (2004). Neural systems supporting interoceptive awareness. *Nature Neuroscience* 7, 189–195.

43. Cryer, P. E. (2005). Mechanisms of hypoglycemia-associated autonomic failure and its component syndromes in diabetes. *Diabetes* 54, 3592–3601.
44. Damasio, H., Grabowski, T., Frank, R., Galaburda, A. M., and Damasio, A. R. (1994). The return of Phineas Gage: Clues about the brain from the skull of a famous patient. *Science* 264, 1102–1105.
45. Davis, M., Hitchcock, J. M., Bowers, M. B., Berridge, C. W., Melia, K. R., and Roth, R. H. (1994). Stress-induced activation of prefrontal cortex dopamine turnover: Blockade by lesions of the amygdala. *Brain Research* 664, 207–210.
46. De Groat, W. C., and Steers, W. D. (1990). Autonomic regulation of the urinary bladder and sexual organs. In A. D. Loewy and K. M. Spyer (Eds.), *Central Regulation of Autonomic Functions*, pp.310-333. New York: Oxford University Press.
47. Deutch, A. Y., Lee, M. C., Gillham, M. H., Cameron, D. A., Goldstein, M., and Iadarola, M. J. (1991). Stress selectively increases Fos protein in dopamine neurons innervating the prefrontal cortex. *Cerebral Cortex* 1, 273–292.
48. Fernandes, K. B., Crippa, G. E., Tavares, R. F., Antunes-Rodrigues, J., and Correa, F. M. (2003). Mechanisms involved in the pressor response to noradrenaline injection into the cingulate cortex of unanesthetized rats. *Neuropharmacology* 44, 757–763.
49. Fernandes, K. B., Tavares, R. F., Pelosi, G. G., and Correa, F. M. (2007). The paraventricular nucleus of hypothalamus mediates the pressor response to noradrenergic stimulation of the medial prefrontal cortex in unanesthetized rats. *Neuroscience Letters* 426, 101–105.
50. Fernandes, K. B. P., Tavares, R. F., and Correa, F. M. A. (2005). The lateral septal area is involved in the pressor pathway activated by microinjection of norepinephrine into the rat brain cingulate cortex. *Neuropharmacology* 49, 564–571.
51. Freedman, L. J., Insel, T. R., and Smith, Y. (2000). Subcortical projections of area 25 (subgenual cortex) of the macaque monkey. *Journal of Comparative Neurology* 421, 172–188.
52. Freeman, R. (2006). Cardiovascular manifestations of autonomic epilepsy. *Clinical Autonomic Research* 16, 12–17.
53. Gabbott, P. L., Warner, T. A., Jays, P. R., Salway, P., and Busby, S. J. (2005). Prefrontal cortex in the rat: Projections to subcortical autonomic, motor, and limbic centers. *Journal of Comparative Neurology* 492, 145–177.
54. Gabbott, P. L. A., Warner, T., and Busby, S. J. (2007). Catecholaminergic neurons in medullary nuclei are among the post-synaptic targets of descending projections from infralimbic area 25 of the rat medial prefrontal cortex. *Neuroscience* 144, 623–635.
55. Gianaros, P. J., Van Der Veen, F. M., and Jennings, J. R. (2004). Regional cerebral blood flow correlates with heart period and high-frequency heart period variability during working-memory tasks: Implications for the cortical and subcortical regulation of cardiac autonomic activity. *Psychophysiology* 41, 521–530.
56. Gieroba, Z. J., Li, Y. W., Wesselingh, S. L., and Blessing, W. W. (1991). Transneuronal labeling of neurons in rabbit brain after injection of herpes simplex virus type 1 into the aortic depressor nerve. *Brain Research* 558, 264–272.
57. Gjone, R. (1966). Excitatory and inhibitory bladder responses to stimulation of "limbic," diencephalic and mesencephalic structures in the cat. *Acta Physiologica Scandinavica* 66, 91–102.
58. Gjone, R., and Setekleiv, J. (1963). Excitatory and inhibitory bladder responses to stimulation of the cerebral cortex in the cat. *Acta Physiologica Scandinavica* 59, 337–348.
59. Gray, M. A., Taggart, P., Sutton, P. M., Groves, D., Holdright, D. R., Bradbury, D., Brull, D., and Critchley, H. D. (2007). A cortical potential reflecting cardiac function. *Proceedings of the National Academy of Sciences, U S A* 104, 6818–6823.
60. Hardy, S. G. P. (1994). Anatomical data supporting the concept of prefrontal influences upon hypothalamo-medullary relays in the rat. *Neuroscience Letters* 169, 17–20.
61. Hardy, S. G. P., and Holmes, D. E. (1988). Prefrontal stimulus-produced hypotension in rat. *Experimental Brain Research* 73, 249–255.
62. Hardy, S. G. P., and Mack, S. M. (1990). Brainstem mediation of prefrontal stimulus-produced hypotension. *Experimental Brain Research* 79, 393–399.
63. Haselton, J. R., and Guyenet, P. G. (1990). Ascending collaterals of medullary barosensitive neurons and C1 cells in rats. *American Journal of Physiology* 258, R1051–R1063.
64. Head, G. A. (1994). Cardiac baroreflexes and hypertension. *Clinical and Experimental Pharmacology and Physiology* 21, 791–802.
65. Heidbreder, C. A., and Groenewegen, H. J. (2003). The medial prefrontal cortex in the rat: Evidence for a dorso-ventral distinction based upon functional and anatomical characteristics. *Neuroscience and Biobehavioral Reviews* 27, 555–579.
66. Hilz, M. J., Devinsky, O., Szczepanska, H., Borod, J. C., Marthol, H., and Tutaj, M. (2006). Right ventromedial prefrontal lesions result in paradoxical cardiovascular activation with emotional stimuli. *Brain* 129, 3343–3355.

67. Hollis, J. H., McKinley, M. J., D'Souza, M., Kampe, J., and Oldfield, B. J. (2008). The trajectory of sensory pathways from the lamina terminalis to the insular and cingulate cortex; A neuroanatomical framework for the generation of thirst. *American Journal of Physiology. Regulatory, Integrative and Comparative Physiology* 294, R1390–R1401.
68. Hoover, W. B., and Vertes, R. P. (2007). Anatomical analysis of afferent projections to the medial prefrontal cortex in the rat. *Brain Structure and Function* 212, 149–179.
69. Hosoya, Y., and Matsushita, M. (1980). Cells of origin of the descending afferents to the lateral hypothalamic area in the rat, studied with the horseradish peroxidase method. *Neuroscience Letters* 18, 231–236.
70. Hurley, K. M., Herbert, H., Moga, M. M., and Saper, C. B. (1991). Efferent projections of the infralimbic cortex of the rat. *Journal of Comparative Neurology* 308, 249–276.
71. Hurley-Gius, K. M., and Neafsey, E. J. (1986). The medial frontal cortex and gastric motility: Microstimulation results and their possible significance for the overall pattern of organization of rat frontal and parietal cortex. *Brain Research* 365, 241–248.
72. Ito, S. (1992). Multiple projection of vagal non-myelinated afferents to the anterior insular cortex in rats. *Neuroscience Letters* 148, 151–154.
73. Ito, S. (1994). Electrophysiological evidence for projections of myelinated and non-myelinated primary vagal afferents to the rat insular cortex. *Neuroscience Letters* 179, 29–32.
74. Ito, S. I. (1998). Possible representation of somatic pain in the rat insular visceral sensory cortex: A field potential study. *Neuroscience Letters* 241, 171–174.
75. Judy, W. V., Watanabe, A. M., Henry, D. P., Besch, H., Jr., Murphy, W. R., and Hockel, G. M. (1976). Sympathetic nerve activity: Role in regulation of blood pressure in the spontaneously hypertensive rat. *Circulation Research* 38, 21–29.
76. Kapp, B. S., Schwaber, J. S., and Driscoll, P. A. (1985). The organization of insular cortex projections to the amygdaloid central nucleus and autonomic regulatory nuclei of the dorsal medulla. *Brain Research* 360, 355–360.
77. Kavia, R. B., Dasgupta, R., and Fowler, C. J. (2005). Functional imaging and the central control of the bladder. *Journal of Comparative Neurology* 493, 27–32.
78. Kawahara, Y., Kawahara, H., and Westerink, B. H. (2002). Hypotension-induced dopamine release in prefrontal cortex is mediated by local glutamatergic projections at the level of nerve terminals. *Journal of Neurochemistry* 81, 285–291.
79. Kimmerly, D. S., O'Leary, D. D., Menon, R. S., Gati, J. S., and Shoemaker, J. K. (2005). Cortical regions associated with autonomic cardiovascular regulation during lower body negative pressure in humans. *Journal of Physiology* 569, 331–345.
80. Kimmerly, D. S., Wong, S., Menon, R., and Shoemaker, J. K. (2007). Forebrain neural patterns associated with sex differences in autonomic and cardiovascular function during baroreceptor unloading. *American Journal of Physiology. Regulatory, Integrative and Comparative Physiology* 292, R715–R722.
81. Krettek, J. E., and Price, J. L. (1977). The cortical projections of the mediodorsal nucleus and adjacent thalamic nuclei in the rat. *Journal of Comparative Neurology* 171, 157–192.
82. Luiten, P. G., Ter Horst, G. J., and Steffens, A. B. (1987). The hypothalamus, intrinsic connections and outflow pathways to the endocrine system in relation to the control of feeding and metabolism. *Progress in Neurobiology* 28, 1–54.
83. Macefield, V. G., Taylor, J. L., and Wallin, B. G. (1998). Inhibition of muscle sympathetic outflow following transcranial cortical stimulation. *Journal of the Autonomic Nervous System* 68, 49–57.
84. Marks, I. (1988). Blood-injury phobia: A review. *American Journal of Psychiatry* 145, 1207–1213.
85. Matsumoto, S., Hanai, T., Yoshioka, N., Shimizu, N., Sugiyama, T., and Uemura, H. (2006). Medial prefrontal cortex lesions inhibit reflex micturition in anesthetized rats. *Neuroscience Research* 54, 66–70.
86. McDougall, S. J., Widdop, R. E., and Lawrence, A. J. (2004). Medial prefrontal cortical integration of psychological stress in rats. *European Journal of Neuroscience* 20, 2430–2440.
87. Meyer, G., Galindo-Mireles, D., Gonzalez-Hernandez, T., Castaneyra-Perdomo, A., and Ferres-Torres, R. (1986). Direct projections from the reticular formation of the medulla oblongata to the anterior cingulate cortex in the mouse and the rat. *Brain Research* 398, 207–211.
88. Miller, M. W. (1987). The origin of corticospinal projection neurons in rat. *Experimental Brain Research* 67, 339–351.
89. Morris, J. S. (2002). How do you feel? *Trends in Cognitive Sciences* 6, 317–319.
90. Narayanan, J. T., Watts, R., Haddad, N., Labar, D. R., Li, P. M., and Filippi, C. G. (2002). Cerebral activation during vagus nerve stimulation: A functional MR study. *Epilepsia* 43, 1509–1514.
91. Neafsey, E. J. (1990). Prefrontal cortical control of the autonomic nervous system: Anatomical and

physiological observations. *Progress in Brain Research* 85, 147–165.

92. Neafsey, E. J., Hurley-Gius, K. M., and Arvanitis, D. (1986). The topographical organization of neurons in the rat medial frontal, insular and olfactory cortex projecting to the solitary nucleus, olfactory bulb, periaqueductal gray and superior colliculus. *Brain Research* 377, 561–570.
93. Nosaka, S. (1996). Modifications of arterial baroreflexes: Obligatory roles in cardiovascular regulation in stress and post-stress recovery. *Japanese Journal of Physiology* 46, 271–288.
94. Ongur, D., and Price, J. L. (2000). The organization of networks within the orbital and medial prefrontal cortex of rats, monkeys and humans. *Cerebral Cortex* 10, 206–219.
95. Oppenheimer, S. M., and Cechetto, D. F. (1990). Cardiac chronotropic organization of the rat insular cortex. *Brain Research* 533, 66–72.
96. Oppenheimer, S. M., Gelb, A., Girvin, J. P., and Hachinski, V. C. (1992). Cardiovascular effects of human insular cortex stimulation. *Neurology* 42, 1727–1732.
97. Oppenheimer, S. M., Kedem, G., and Martin, W. M. (1996). Left-insular cortex lesions perturb cardiac autonomic tone in humans. *Clinical Autonomic Research* 6, 131–140.
98. Oppenheimer, S. M., Saleh, T., and Cechetto, D. F. (1992). Lateral hypothalamic area neurotransmission and neuromodulation of the specific cardiac effects of insular cortex stimulation. *Brain Research* 581, 133–142.
99. Owens, N. C., Sartor, D. M., and Verberne, A. J. M. (1999). Medial prefrontal cortex depressor response: Role of the solitary tract nucleus in the rat. *Neuroscience* 89, 1331–1346.
100. Owens, N. C., and Verberne, A. J. M. (1996). An electrophysiological study of the medial prefrontal cortical projection to the nucleus of the solitary tract in rat. *Experimental Brain Research* 110, 55–61.
101. Owens, N. C., and Verberne, A. J. M. (2000). Medial prefrontal depressor response: Involvement of the rostral and caudal ventrolateral medulla in the rat. *Journal of the Autonomic Nervous System* 78, 86–93.
102. Owens, N. C., and Verberne, A. J. M. (2001). Regional haemodynamic responses to activation of the medial prefrontal cortex depressor region. *Brain Research* 919, 221–231.
103. Pajolla, G. P., Crippa, G. E., Correa, S. A., Moreira, K. B., Tavares, R. F., and Correa, F. M. (2001). The lateral hypothalamus is involved in the pathway mediating the hypotensive response to cingulate cortex-cholinergic stimulation. *Cellular and Molecular Neurobiology* 21, 341–356.
104. Panteleev, S., and Grundy, D. (2000). Descending influences from the infralimbic cortex on vago-vagal reflex control of gastric motor activity in the rat. *Autonomic Neuroscience* 86, 78–83.
105. Park, M., Kim, J., Bae, Y., Son, B., Park, Y., Lee, B., Cho, K., Kim, D., Sung, E., and Yoon, Y. W. (1997). CNS innervation of the urinary bladder demonstrated by immunohistochemical study for c-Fos and pseudorabies virus. *Journal of Korean Medical Science* 12, 340–352.
106. Pezze, M. A., and Feldon, J. (2004). Mesolimbic dopaminergic pathways in fear conditioning. *Progress in Neurobiology* 74, 301–320.
107. Powell, D. A., Buchanan, S. L., and Gibbs, C. M. (1990). Role of the prefrontal-thalamic axis in classical conditioning. *Progress in Brain Research* 85, 433–465.
108. Resstel, L. B., and Correa, F. M. (2006). Injection of l-glutamate into medial prefrontal cortex induces cardiovascular responses through NMDA receptor–nitric oxide in rat. *Neuropharmacology* 51, 160–167.
109. Resstel, L. B., and Correa, F. M. (2006). Involvement of the medial prefrontal cortex in central cardiovascular modulation in the rat. *Autonomic Neuroscience* 126–127, 130–138.
110. Resstel, L. B., and Correa, F. M. (2006). Medial prefrontal cortex NMDA receptors and nitric oxide modulate the parasympathetic component of the baroreflex. *European Journal of Neuroscience* 23, 481–488.
111. Resstel, L. B., Fernandes, K. B., and Correa, F. M. (2004). Medial prefrontal cortex modulation of the baroreflex parasympathetic component in the rat. *Brain Research* 1015, 136–144.
112. Resstel, L. B. M., and Correa, F. M. A. (2008). Cardiovascular effects of l-glutamate injected in the medial prefrontal cortex of spontaneously hypertensive rats. *European Journal of Pharmacology* 580, 372–379.
113. Rinaman, L., Levitt, P., and Card, J. P. (2000). Progressive postnatal assembly of limbic-autonomic circuits revealed by central transneuronal transport of pseudorabies virus. *Journal of Neuroscience* 20, 2731–2741.
114. Rose, J. E., and Woolsey, C. N. (1948). Structure and relations of limbic cortex and anterior thalamic nucleus in rabbit and cat. *Journal of Comparative Neurology* 89, 279–347.
115. Rossini, P. M., Massa, R., Sancesario, G., and Boccasena, P. (1993). Sudomotor skin responses to brain stimulation do not depend on nerve sensory fiber functionality. *Electroencephalography and Clinical Neurophysiology* 89, 447–451.

116. Rossini, P. M., Opsomer, R. J., and Boccasena, P. (1993). Sudomotor skin responses following nerve and brain stimulation. *Electroencephalography and Clinical Neurophysiology* 89, 442–446.
117. Ruggiero, D. A., Mraovitch, S., Granata, A. R., Anwar, M., and Reis, D. J. (1987). A role of insular cortex in cardiovascular function. *Journal of Comparative Neurology* 257, 189–207.
118. Ruit, K. G., and Neafsey, E. J. (1990). Hippocampal input to a "visceral motor" corticobulbar pathway: An anatomical and electrophysiological study in the rat. *Experimental Brain Research* 82, 606–616.
119. Saper, C. B. (1982). Convergence of autonomic and limbic connections in the insular cortex of the rat. *Journal of Comparative Neurology* 210, 163–173.
120. Saper, C. B. (1995). Central autonomic system. In G. Paxinos (ed.), *The Rat Nervous System*, pp. 107–135. San Diego, CA: Academic Press.
121. Saper, C. B. (2002). The central autonomic nervous system: Conscious visceral perception and autonomic pattern generation. *Annual Review of Neuroscience* 25, 433–469.
122. Satoh, K., Shimizu, N., Tohyama, M., and Maeda, T. (1978). Localization of the micturition reflex center at the dorsolateral pontine tegmentum of the rat. *Neuroscience Letters* 8, 27–33.
123. Schwartz, G. E., Weinberger, D. A., and Singer, J. A. (1981). Cardiovascular differentiation of happiness, sadness, anger, and fear following imagery and exercise. *Psychosomatic Medicine* 43, 343–364.
124. Sesack, S. R., Deutch, A. T., Roth, R. H., and Bunney, B. S. (1989). Topographical organization of the efferent projections of the medial prefrontal cortex in the rat: An anterograde tract-tracing study with *Phaseolus vulgaris* Leucoagglutinin. *Journal of Comparative Neurology* 290, 213–242.
125. Sevoz-Couche, C., Comet, M. A., Bernard, J. F., Hamon, M., and Laguzzi, R. (2006). Cardiac baroreflex facilitation evoked by hypothalamus and prefrontal cortex stimulation: Role of the nucleus tractus solitarius (NTS) 5-$HT2_A$ receptors. *American Journal of Physiology. Regulatory, Integrative and Comparative Physiology* 291, R1007–R1015.
126. Shipley, M. T. (1982). Insular cortex projection to the nucleus of the solitary tract and brainstem visceromotor regions in the mouse. *Brain Research Bulletin* 8, 139–148.
127. Silber, D. H., Sinoway, L. I., Leuenberger, U. A., and Amassian, V. E. (2000). Magnetic stimulation of the human motor cortex evokes skin sympathetic nerve activity. *Journal of Applied Physiology* 88, 126–134.
128. Spencer, S. J., Ebner, K., and Day, T. A. (2004). Differential involvement of rat medial prefrontal cortex dopamine receptors in modulation of hypothalamic-pituitary-adrenal axis responses to different stressors. *European Journal of Neuroscience* 20, 1008–1016.
129. Sugaya, K., Roppolo, J. R., Yoshimura, N., Card, J. P., and De Groat, W. C. (1997). The central neural pathways involved in micturition in the neonatal rat as revealed by the injection of pseudorabies virus into the urinary bladder. *Neuroscience Letters* 223, 197–200.
130. Sun, M. K. (1992). Medullospinal vasomotor neurones mediate hypotension from stimulation of prefrontal cortex. *Journal of the Autonomic Nervous System* 38, 209–218.
131. Sun, M. K., and Guyenet, P. G. (1986). Hypothalamic glutamatergic input to medullary sympathoexcitatory neurons in rats. *American Journal of Physiology* 251, R798–R810.
132. Takagishi, M., and Chiba, T. (1991). Efferent projections of the infralimbic (area 25) region of the medial prefrontal cortex in the rat: An anterograde tracer PHA-L study. *Brain Research* 566, 26–39.
133. Tang, Y., Rampin, O., Giuliano, F., and Ugolini, G. (1999). Spinal and brain circuits to motoneurons of the bulbospongiosus muscle: Retrograde transneuronal tracing with rabies virus. *Journal of Comparative Neurology* 414, 167–192.
134. Ter Horst, G. J., and Postema, F. (1997). Forebrain parasympathetic control of heart activity: Retrograde transneuronal viral labeling in rats—Rapid communication. *American Journal of Physiology* 42, H2926–H2930.
135. Terreberry, R. R., and Neafsey, E. J. (1983). Rat medial frontal cortex: A visceral motor region with a direct projection to the solitary nucleus. *Brain Research* 278, 245–249.
136. Terreberry, R. R., and Neafsey, E. J. (1987). The rat medial frontal cortex projects directly to autonomic regions of the brainstem. *Brain Research Bulletin* 19, 639–649.
137. Teves, D., Videen, T. O., Cryer, P. E., and Powers, W. J. (2004). Activation of human medial prefrontal cortex during autonomic responses to hypoglycemia. *Proceedings of the National Academy of Sciences, USA* 101, 6217–6221.
138. Torrealba, F., and Muller, C. (1996). Glutamate immunoreactivity of insular cortex afferents to the nucleus tractus solitarius in the rat—A quantitative electron microscopic study. *Neuroscience* 71, 77–87.

139. Torrealba, F., and Muller, C. (1999). Ultrastructure of glutamate and GABA immunoreactive axon terminals of the rat nucleus tractus solitarius, with a note on infralimbic cortex afferents. *Brain Research* 820, 20–30.
140. Valentino, R. J., Page, M. E., Luppi, P. H., Zhu, Y., Van Bockstaele, E., and Aston-Jones, G. (1994). Evidence for widespread afferents to Barrington's nucleus, a brainstem region rich in corticotropin-releasing hormone neurons. *Neuroscience* 62, 125–143.
141. Van Bockstaele, E. J., Pieribone, V. A., and Aston-Jones, G. (1989). Diverse afferents converge on the nucleus paragigantocellularis in the rat ventrolateral medulla: Retrograde and anterograde tracing studies. *Journal of Comparative Neurology* 290, 561–584.
142. Van Der Kooy, D., Koda, L. Y., McGinty, J. F., Gerfen, C. R., and Bloom, F. E. (1984). The organization of projections from the cortex, amygdala, and hypothalamus to the nucleus of the solitary tract in rat. *Journal of Comparative Neurology* 224, 1–24.
143. Van Der Kooy, D., McGinty, J. F., Koda, L. Y., Gerfen, C. R., and Bloom, F. E. (1982). Visceral cortex: A direct connection from prefrontal cortex to the solitary nucleus in rat. *Neuroscience Letters* 33, 123–127.
144. Van Eden, C. G., and Buijs, R. M. (2000). Functional neuroanatomy of the prefrontal cortex: Autonomic interactions. *Progress in Brain Research* 126, 49–62.
145. Verberne, A. J. M. (1996). Medullary sympathoexcitatory neurons are inhibited by activation of the medial prefrontal cortex in the rat. *American Journal of Physiology* 270, R713–R719.
146. Verberne, A. J. M., Lewis, S. J., Jarrott, B., and Louis, W. J. (1988). Medial prefrontal cortical lesions and baroreceptor heart rate reflex sensitivity in the spontaneously hypertensive rat. *Journal of Hypertension* 6, 123–127.
147. Verberne, A. J. M., Lewis, S. J., Worland, P. J., Beart, P. M., Jarrott, B., Christie, M. J., and Louis, W. J. (1987). Medial prefrontal cortical lesions modulate baroreflex sensitivity in the rat. *Brain Research* 426, 243–249.
148. Verberne, A. J. M., and Owens, N. C. (1998). Cortical modulation of the cardiovascular system. *Progress in Neurobiology* 54, 149–168.
149. Vertes, R. P. (2004). Differential projections of the infralimbic and prelimbic cortex in the rat. *Synapse* 51, 32–58.
150. Westerhaus, M. J., and Loewy, A. D. (2001). Central representation of the sympathetic nervous system in the cerebral cortex. *Brain Research* 903, 117–127.
151. Whitehead, M. C., Bergula, A., and Holliday, K. (2000). Forebrain projections to the rostral nucleus of the solitary tract in the hamster. *Journal of Comparative Neurology* 422, 429–447.
152. Willett, C. J., Gwyn, D. G., Rutherford, J. G., and Leslie, R. A. (1986). Cortical projections to the nucleus of the tractus solitarius: An HRP study in the cat. *Brain Research Bulletin* 16, 497–505.
153. Wong, S. W., Masse, N., Kimmerly, D. S., Menon, R. S., and Shoemaker, J. K. (2007). Ventral medial prefrontal cortex and cardiovagal control in conscious humans. *Neuroimage* 35, 698–708.
154. Yasui, Y., Breder, C. D., Saper, C. B., and Cechetto, D. F. (1991). Autonomic responses and efferent pathways from the insular cortex in the rat. *Journal of Comparative Neurology* 303, 355–374.
155. Yasui, Y., Itoh, K., Shigemoto, R., and Mizuno, N. (1991). Topographical projections from the cerebral cortex to the nucleus of the solitary tract in the cat. *Experimental Brain Research* 85, 75–84.
156. Zagon, A., Totterdell, S., and Jones, R. S. (1994). Direct projections from the ventrolateral medulla oblongata to the limbic forebrain: Anterograde and retrograde tract-tracing studies in the rat. *Journal of Comparative Neurology* 340, 445–468.
157. Zeng, D., and Stuesse, S. L. (1993). Topographic organization of efferent projections of medial frontal cortex. *Brain Research Bulletin* 32, 195–200.
158. Zermann, D. H., Ishigooka, M., Doggweiler, R., and Schmidt, R. A. (1998). Central autonomic innervation of the lower urinary tract—A neuroanatomy study. *World Journal of Urology* 16, 417–422.

12

# Central Circulatory Control: Psychological Stress and the Defense Reaction

PASCAL CARRIVE

This chapter will review the history and our current understanding of the central pathways mediating cardiovascular responses to psychological stress. Physical stressors, such as pain, cold and hemorrhage, have well-defined physical properties and are relatively easy to recognize, either because they are directly harmful to the body or because they challenge homeostatic regulation. Psychological stressors, on the other hand, are subtler. In this case, the stimuli that trigger psychological stress are not directly harmful to the body but are perceived by the individual as potentially harmful. The underlying cause may be an association with unpleasant memories, a conflict with learned rules, or a chronic pathological state (e.g., paranoia). Like physical stress, however, psychological stress can be associated with marked autonomic and cardiovascular changes. Presumably, these changes prepare the organism for an active response in case it is needed to face or escape from the expected challenge (i.e., fight or flight). They appear preprogrammed and can sometimes be difficult to consciously prevent from happening.

Obviously, psychological stress can only be studied in conscious animals. This constraint makes the recording of cardiovascular variables difficult, which is probably why progress in this field has been slow. However, an important finding in the 1940s provided an early start and a way to bypass this methodological problem. This was the discovery by Hess and Brugger[54] that electrical stimulation of the hypothalamus in the cat could evoke integrated emotional responses that appeared identical to the natural defensive reactions of this animal. Hess and Brugger gave it a name: *affektiven abwehrreaktion,* or defense reaction. This simple way of activating the circuitry of defensive reactions provided a convenient means to study emotional stress responses. Most important, because the same stimulation could be done under anesthesia, it also made investigation of their cardiovascular components possible. This approach was very successful and led to major discoveries. It will certainly continue to do so; however, it is important to recognize its limitations. Intracerebral stimulation may activate a network, but activation of that network by a natural stressor may be very different in space and time. Cardiovascular regulation may still occur under anesthesia, but anesthetics almost certainly modify the way that neuronal networks operate. Thus, experiments in anesthetized animals cannot replace experiments in conscious animals, which are the critical ones.

The chapter is divided into two parts. The first part deals with the circuitry of central circulatory control as revealed by direct activation of the neural substrate mediating the defense reaction, mostly in anesthetized preparations. The second part deals with the same circuitry as revealed by the effect of lesions on naturally evoked psychological stress responses in the awake animal. Since the focus of this chapter is primarily on central control, there will be no review of the different patterns of cardiovascular response to the various forms of stress in humans and animals. These have been reviewed elsewhere[53,64,79].

## THE DEFENSE REACTION AND ITS NEURAL SUBSTRATE: A HISTORICAL PERSPECTIVE

### Electrical Stimulation and the Defense Reaction in the Cat

The term "defense reaction" (*Abwehrreaktion*) was first introduced by Hess and Brugger[54] to describe the effect of electrical stimulation in the hypothalamus of conscious cats. The responses they observed were well coordinated, had a clear emotional component, and looked similar to the characteristic patterns of defensive behavior seen in normal cats[86,98]. A typical response would begin with an increased level of alertness, followed by growling and hissing, and, when the intensity of the stimulation was increased, would culminate in flight or fight. The most responsive area of the hypothalamus was in the dorsal part of the tuberal hypothalamus, medial, around and lateral to the fornix. Following in the footsteps of Hess, Hunsperger[60] showed that the region from which the defense reaction could be evoked extended caudally into the periaqueductal gray and rostrally into the amygdala and bed nucleus of the stria terminalis[46] (Figure 12–1). Further investigations[47] led to the conclusion that the defense reaction was integrated along a system descending from the amygdala to the midbrain via the hypothalamus.

Although Hess and Brugger were the first to comprehensively describe the effect of hypothalamic stimulation in the conscious cat, they were not the first to stimulate this brain region. Cardiovascular physiologists had been exploring this area in the anesthetized animal since the 1920s. By the end of the 1940s, Ranson, Magoun, and Kabat[65,87] had generated accurate maps of the hypothalamus and midbrain showing an extensive pressor zone extending from the tuberal hypothalamus to the midbrain periaqueductal gray and dorsal tegmentum. The next milestone was the discovery that the pressor response evoked from these areas was associated with a characteristic pattern of blood flow redistribution that consisted of a marked sympathetic vasodilatation in skeletal muscles associated with sympathetic vasoconstriction in the intestines and skin[44,69,70]. The muscle vasodilatation, which was mediated by cholinergic sympathetic fibers in the cat, would later become the hallmark of the defense reaction[2]. These investigators also traced the descending pathway mediating this pattern and showed that it traveled in the ventrolateral tegmentum of the midbrain, pons, and medulla[69]. Most important, the pattern they had revealed was consistent with the one originally proposed by Cannon[16] for what he called "emergency reactions," i.e., reactions necessary for vigorous responses, such as fight and flight.

Finally, Abrahams et al.[1] put the behavioral and cardiovascular studies together by demonstrating that the same sites that produced the defense reaction in the conscious cat also produced the redistribution of blood flow described previously in the anesthetized animal. Abrahams et al.[1] mapped these sites in the hypothalamus and rostral midbrain and showed that the most effective region extended from the dorsomedial/perifornical/lateral hypothalamus to the dorsal periaqueductal gray and adjacent tegmentum (Figure 12–2). They also showed that the pathway mediating the cholinergic vasodilatation, and to a large extent the rest of the cardiovascular response, descended through the ventrolateral midbrain tegmentum. Using the same conscious/anesthetized approach, subsequent workers[58,111] extended the findings of Abrahams et al.[1] to the medial amygdala and showed that it is connected to the hypothalamus and midbrain via the ventral amygdalofugal pathway (Figure 12–2).

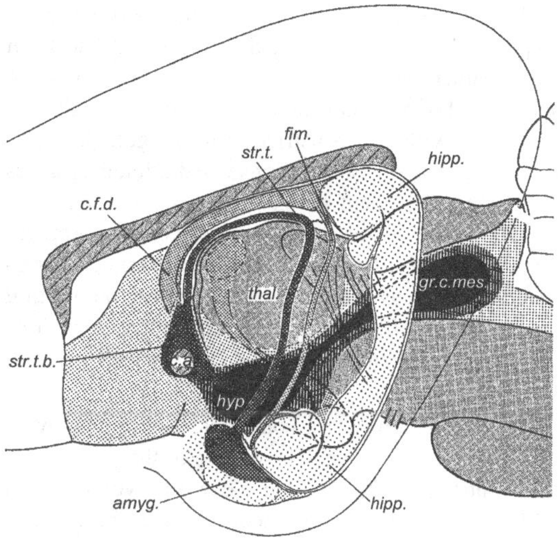


Figure 12–1 Brain regions involved in the defense reaction in the conscious cat. Schematic diagram of a sagittal view through the forebrain and midbrain showing areas from which electrical stimulation evokes the defense reaction in the cat. Cross-hatched areas correspond to the medial part of the amygdala, stria terminalis, and bed nucleus of the stria terminalis. Black areas correspond to the tuberal hypothalamus, periventricular gray, and periaqueductal gray. amyg., amygdala; c.a., anterior commissure; c.f.d., descending column of the fornix; gr.c.mes., central gray matter of the mesencephalon (periaqueductal gray); fim, fimbria; hipp., hippocampus; hyp., hypothalamus; str.t., stria terminalis; str.t.b., bed nucleus of the stria terminalis; thal., thalamus. Reproduced from Fernandez De Molina and Hunsperger (1959)[46], with permission.

By the end of the 1960s, the cardiovascular response of the defense reaction in the cat had been well characterized. The reaction's hallmark was the active cholinergic muscle vasodilatation, which was associated with vasoconstriction in the gut, skin, and kidney, and a pressor response. Additional features were tachycardia and an increase in cardiac output[88]. These cardiovascular changes were seen as a preparatory response for fight and flight, which could be triggered as early as the commencement of the alerting stage of the defense reaction[2]. This set of reactions would later become known as the *visceral alerting response*[55].

Attention then focused on the descending pathway of the defense reaction. The course of the pathway in the ventrolateral pons and near the ventrolateral surface of the rostral medulla had been well characterized[69,70,94]. However, it was not clear if the projection was direct to the thoracic spinal cord or if a relay in the lower brainstem was involved. The discovery by Feldberg and Guertzenstein[45] of a vasomotor area near the ventrolateral surface of the rostral medulla (i.e., the rostral ventrolateral medulla [RVLM]) raised the possibility of a relay in this region. Indeed, this relay was confirmed when it was shown that glycine application in the RVLM almost abolished all components of the visceral alerting response, including the muscle vasodilatation[56]. Kainic acid lesions[82] and kynurenic acid inhibition[109] of the RVLM proved its involvement in the vasoconstrictor and pressor components of the reaction. The tachycardic component, however, could not be abolished by drug application in the RVLM[82,109].

Thus, within 40 years of the discovery of the hypothalamic defense reaction by Hess and Brugger[54], a descending pathway connecting the amygdala with the thoracic cord had been delineated for the expression of emotionally coupled cardiovascular responses. However, controversies about the significance of the alerting visceral response remained. For Hilton and coworkers, the response was a set pattern that was activated from the alerting stages to the full expression of the defense response[55]. Mancia and Zanchetti[77-79], on the other hand, maintained that the muscle vasodilatation was only evoked with movement of the limbs; i.e., during fight or flight. Immobile confrontation with an angry cat, for example, did not evoke muscle vasoconstriction but muscle vasoconstriction. Hilton's concept was simple and attractive; but it was based on studies conducted in anesthetized animals using electrical stimulation, a rather crude method to produce defensive responses. Mancia and Zanchetti worked in the conscious animal and made their observations during natural defensive responses. As shown in the next section, Mancia and Zanchetti's suggestion that there maybe more than one pattern of response was actually correct.

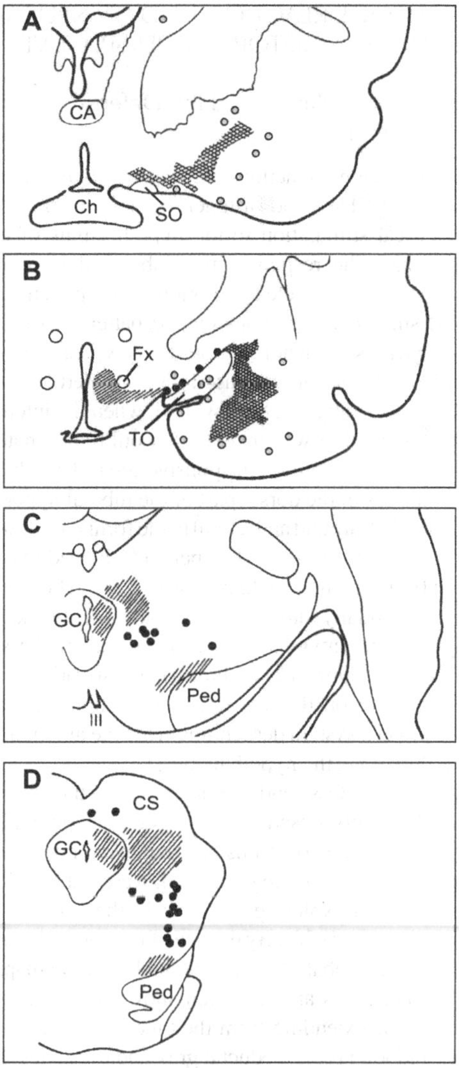


Figure 12–2 Forebrain and midbrain sites from which the defense reaction can be evoked in the anesthetized cat. Transverse sections through the forebrain and midbrain of the cat showing areas where the defense reaction and its cardiovascular component can be evoked by electrical stimulation in the cat. III, oculomotor nerve; CA, anterior commissure; Ch, optic chiasm; CS, superior colliculus; Fx, fornix; GC, central gray (periaqueductal gray); Ped, cerebral peduncle; SO, supraoptic nucleus; TO, optic tract. Reproduced from Abrahams et al. (1960)[1] and Hilton and Zbrozyna (1963)[58], with permission.

## Excitatory Amino Acid Activation and Shift to the Periaqueductal Gray

To circumvent the problem of electrical stimulation, which activates both cell bodies and fibers of passage, Goodchild, Dampney and Bandler[52] introduced the method of injecting excitatory amino acids (e.g., glutamate) to try identify the exact location of the neuronal cell groups in the hypothalamus and periaqueductal gray (PAG) that mediated the defense reaction. This study led to the surprising finding that injection of excitatory amino acids into the hypothalamus of the cat did not evoke defensive responses[7]. In contrast, excitatory amino acids injection in the PAG evoked a strong facio-vocal response similar to the one caused by electrical stimulation[9,12]. In the rat, excitatory amino acids in the PAG also produced the same flight response as electrical stimulation[57]. Furthermore, the full visceral alerting response could not be evoked by injection of an excitatory amino acid into the hypothalamus of an anesthetized cat[7]. Although iliac vasodilatation occurred, it was not accompanied by its pressor and vasoconstrictor components. The same observation was made after excitatory amino acid injections into the amygdala. Injection into the amygdala of anesthetized rats also failed to evoke the pressor component of the reaction[4] and evoked depressor responses instead[50,61]. In contrast, excitatory amino acid injections in the PAG of anesthetized rats, at sites that evoked defensive behavior, was associated with the full pattern of the visceral alerting response[57]. The simplest interpretation of these findings was that the defense reaction evoked by electrical stimulation in the hypothalamus or amygdala was due to activation of fibers of passage rather than cell bodies[8,50,57]. Although this interpretation was not correct (see following section), it dealt a serious blow to the hypothalamus as the seat of the defense reaction; and, as a result, attention shifted to the PAG.

Dampney, Bandler, and Carrive used unanesthetized, unparalyzed precollicular decerebrate cats to understand how the PAG could integrate both somatic and cardiovascular components of the defense reaction[10,13,21,31]. This powerful approach allowed simultaneous recording of cardiovascular and behavioral changes and led to major discoveries (Figure 12–3A). The most important was that different types of basic defensive behavior were topographically represented along a longitudinal column of neurons extending along the lateral PAG (Figure 12–3B). Thus, activation of the middle third of this lateral PAG column with an excitatory amino acid evoked a strong facio-vocal response characterized by hissing, intense vocalizations, and tonic extension of the limbs, but without stepping movement. This behavioral response is typically seen in defending cats and is known as "threat display." The associated cardiovascular changes consisted of a rise in blood pressure and heart rate, moderate renal vasoconstriction, carotid vasodilatation, and hindlimb vasoconstriction[20,25,29] (Figure 12–3C, D). This was exactly the pattern observed by Mancia and Zanchetti during immobile confrontation with an angry cat[77,78]. In contrast, excitatory amino acid activation of the caudal third of the lateral PAG column evoked few vocalizations and no hissing but vigorous movements of the limbs as in a flight response (Figure 12–3B). The cardiovascular changes associated with this response consisted of a rise in blood pressure and heart rate, a strong renal and carotid vasoconstriction, and a marked atropine-sensitive iliac vasodilatation[25,27] (Figure 12–3C, D); i.e., the visceral alerting response that had been described previously. Further experiments in the intact, freely moving animal showed that this latter response was indeed a flight response[115]. Thus, contrary to Hilton's hypothesis of one defense reaction associated with a unique visceral alerting response, there are at least two different defensive responses associated with perfectly adapted visceral changes (vasodilatation in active vascular beds coupled with vasoconstriction in inactive vascular beds).

Anatomical experiments have confirmed the topographical representation of these two responses in the lateral PAG. First, the topographic representation of the two responses is perfectly aligned with the terminal fields of ascending sensory projections originating from the trigeminal nucleus (to the middle third of the PAG, where threat display is represented) and lumbar dorsal horn (to the caudal third of the PAG, where flight is represented)[13,21]. Second, the iliac and renal vasoconstrictor regions of the lateral PAG (middle and caudal third, respectively) project directly to the iliac and renal vasoconstrictor regions of the RVLM[26,28,72,81]. This latter finding also indicates that the lateral PAG is viscerotopically organized and has a relay in the RVLM.

Because activation of the lateral PAG column always evoked pressor responses, it was referred to as "the pressor column"[20] to distinguish it from a "depressor column" that was later discovered in the caudal half of the ventrolateral PAG[26] (Figure 12–3C). Activation of this second column with an excitatory amino acid evokes depressor and bradycardic responses associated with cessation of spontaneous activity and a quiescent response[115]. It has the same viscerotopic organization as the lateral column and also projects to the RVLM[26]. Although all this work was carried out in the cat, there is good evidence that a similar topographic organization exists in the rat, although it may not be as clear-cut. On the behavioral side, this was elegantly demonstrated by Depaulis, Keay, and Bandler using excitatory amino acid injections made in rats tested in the resident-intruder paradigm[11,39,40]. On the cardiovascular side, Lovick demonstrated the pressor and depressor columns in anesthetized rats using excitatory amino acid injection and also showed that activation of the pressor and depressor columns produced activation and inhibition, respectively, of bulbospinal neurons in the RVLM[73–75].

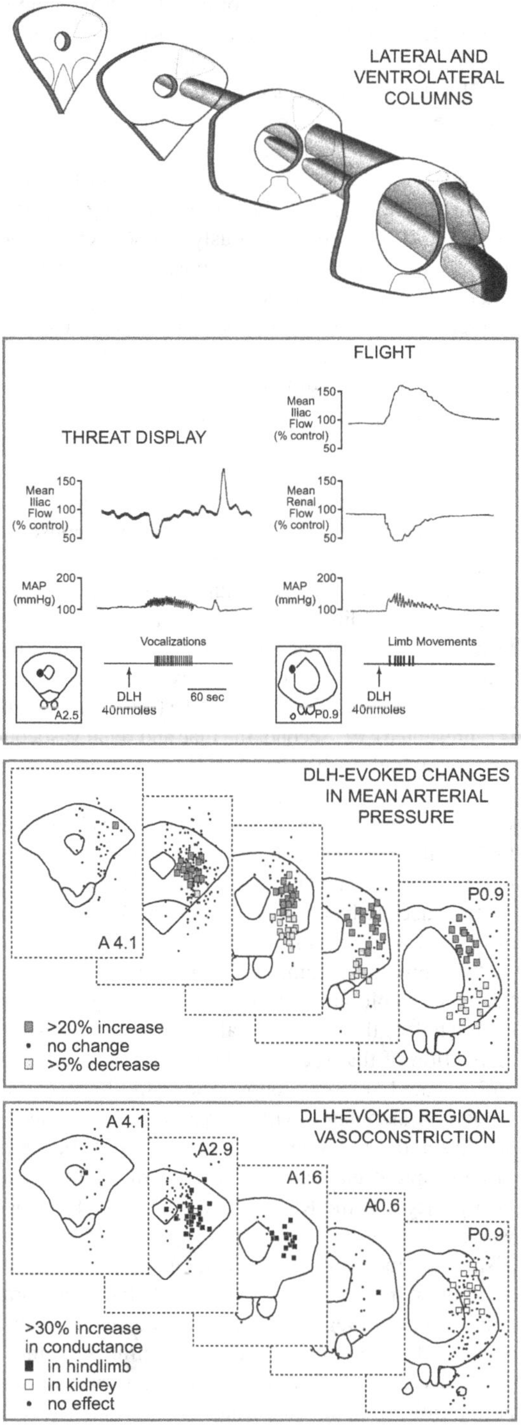


Figure 12–3 The periaqueductal gray and its involvement in the defense reaction in the unparalyzed, decerebrate cat. Representation of defensive behavior and its cardiovascular components in the periaqueductal gray. *Top panel,* Schematic representation of the lateral and ventrolateral columns of the periaqueductal gray. *Second panel,* Somatic and cardiovascular responses evoked by microinjections of D,L-homocysteic acid (DLH) in the rostral (*left*) and caudal (*right*) parts of the lateral column in the unparalyzed, precollicular decerebrate cat. *Insets,* sites at which DLH was injected. *Third panel,* Functional map showing sites at which DLH evoked increases (*dark gray squares*) or decreases (*pale gray squares*) in mean arterial pressure or had no effect (*small black circles*) when microinjected in the precollicular decerebrate cat. Pressor and depressor responses were evoked from the lateral and ventrolateral columns, respectively. *Bottom panel,* Functional map showing sites at which DLH evoked vasoconstriction in the hindlimb (*black squares*) or kidney (*white squares*) or had no effect (*small black circles*) when microinjected in the precollicular decerebrate cat. Vasoconstriction in the hindlimb and kidney were evoked from the rostral and caudal parts of the lateral column, respectively. The antero-posterior coordinates of the PAG sections are indicated in millimeters anterior (A) or posterior (P) to the interaural line. Adapted from Carrive (1991, 1993)[20,21], with permission.

Thus, within 10 years of the introduction of the excitatory amino acid microinjection technique, a column of neurons had been identified in the PAG that could mediate not one but at least two different patterns of coordinated defensive behavior. Furthermore, this column had both a somatotopic and a viscerotopic organization. Evidence for the role of PAG neurons in the control of defensive behavior appeared to be overwhelming. In contrast, excitatory amino acid injections had failed to reveal neurons integrating defensive responses in the hypothalamus. These observations suggested that the final integrating center for defensive behavior, and possibly other forms of emotional behavior, was the PAG. However, this inference would turn out to be wrong. The excitatory amino acid injection technique also had limitations and the lack of effect in the hypothalamus was wrongly interpreted.

## GABA Disinhibition and the Renaissance of The Hypothalamus

One reason for rejecting the hypothalamus as a defense integrating center was that microinjections of excitatory amino acid in anesthetized animals evoked depressor rather than pressor effects from this area[57,51,106,107], even though other work had shown that higher doses of excitatory amino acids injected into the perifornical area could produce moderate rises in blood pressure[5,109]. One problem may have been anesthesia. When injections were made in conscious rats, clear pressor and marked tachycardic effects could be evoked from the dorsomedial hypothalamus[38,104,105]. This cardiovascular response was also associated with running and rearing[105] (Carrive, personal observation). Thus, anesthesia is an important limiting factor in pressor responses evoked by excitatory amino acid in the hypothalamus. Another limiting factor may be the low density of pressor neurons. Excitatory amino acids may be less effective in areas where output neurons are scattered, especially if they are mixed with inhibitory neurons, because co-activation of inhibitory interneurons by excitatory amino acids would result in no net effect or even an inhibition of pressor neurons[37].

A more effective way to activate hypothalamic neurons is by disinhibition with microinjection of $GABA_A$ receptor antagonists, such as bicuculline. Early work by DiMicco had revealed the presence of a tonic GABAergic inhibition in the posterior hypothalamus. Blocking this tonic inhibition could produce marked tachycardia and clear pressor responses in anesthetized rats[3,43] and even greater effects in conscious rats[38]. Bicuculline microinjection in the dorsal tuberal hypothalamus of conscious rats could evoke fast running and rearing, and injection in the dorsomedial hypothalamus evoked jumping[15,42,93,96]. These behaviors correspond to a flight response, which appears more coordinated and less explosive than that evoked from the PAG[42]. As a result, bicuculline microinjection has now become the best method to activate hypothalamic sympathoexcitatory neurons in anesthetized animals; and numerous reports have confirmed its pressor and tachycardic effects when injected in the dorsomedial, perifornical, and lateral hypothalamic regions[17,32,38,48,59,84,90]. In addition to its pressor and tachycardic components, the response is also associated with an increase in renal nerve activity, which indicates that vasoconstriction occurs in this territory[17,48,59,84]. Thus, the hypothalamic defense area contains neurons that can mediate flight responses associated with the appropriate cardiovascular changes, and these neurons are under tonic GABAergic inhibition. For reasons that are still not entirely clear, removal of this inhibition is more effective than direct activation by excitatory amino acids.

Current work is now focusing on the output relays of the dorsomedial hypothalamus and, in particular, on the role of the RVLM. Recent studies have shown that the RVLM is a necessary relay for the renal nerve response because it is blocked by bilateral inhibition of the RVLM with muscimol[17,48,59]. The results are less clear for the pressor response. Fontes et al.[48] have shown that bilateral muscimol abolishes it, but Cao et al.[17] did not find any significant reduction. What is clear, however, is that the tachycardic response is not reduced[17,48], which confirms earlier observations[56,82]. The tachycardia may, in part, be mediated by the raphé pallidus because muscimol inhibition of this region reduces it by half[59,89]. Inhibition of raphé pallidus also reduces the pressor response by half or more, but the fact that RVLM inhibition blocks the pressor effect evoked by direct disinhibition of the raphé pallidus[18] suggests that this reduction is mediated by an additional relay in the RVLM. Interestingly, injections of kynurenic acid in the raphé pallidus do not reduce the pressor and tachycardic response evoked from the dorsomedial hypothalamus, suggesting that the transmission is not glutamatergic[19]. Thus, there is good evidence now that the RVLM and raphé pallidus mediate at least a large part of the vasopressor and tachycardic responses to disinhibition of the dorsomedial hypothalamus. However, it is not known if this link is direct or not. The existence of direct projections from the dorsomedial hypothalamus to the RVLM and raphé pallidus[37,89] suggests that this connection could be direct. On the other hand, recent work by Fontes and collaborators in the conscious rat[35,36] shows that the pressor and tachycardic responses evoked by disinhibition of the dorsomedial hypothalamus are practically abolished by muscimol or NMDA-antagonist injections into the ipsilateral lateral PAG but not the ventrolateral PAG. If correct, this suggests an intermediate relay in the lateral PAG, at least for the tachycardic and vasopressor components of the response.

Finally, disinhibition of GABAergic transmission with bicuculline was also found to be effective in the amygdala, where it could evoke clear pressor and tachycardic responses when injected in the basolateral nucleus but not the central nucleus of conscious rats[91,103,104]. However, bicuculline had no effect when the injections were repeated in the anesthetized animal[91]. Nevertheless, the bicuculline-evoked cardiovascular response obtained from the basolateral nucleus in the conscious animal is abolished by microinjections of excitatory amino acid antagonists in the dorsomedial hypothalamus. This finding suggests that the dorsomedial hypothalamus is an important relay of the amygdala, confirming the original observations of Hilton and Zbrozyna[58] with electrical stimulation.

Thus, the last 15 years have seen a recognition of the role of hypothalamic neurons in the defense reaction. So far, chemical stimulation experiments have confirmed the general organization of the neural substrate for the defense reaction that was originally defined by electrical stimulation. There is now a better understanding of the location, organization, and functions of the neurons that form this network, from the amygdala to the hypothalamus, PAG, and rostral ventral medulla.

### Overview of the Defense Reaction and its Neural Substrate

The defense reaction evoked by stimulation of the hypothalamus has taught us a great deal about the central control of cardiovascular responses associated with emotional behavior. It has revealed the existence of a periventricular network whose neurons are organized in such a way that they can coordinate the autonomic and behavioral components of different patterns of defensive responses. It has also revealed links with premotor sympathetic centers in the lower brainstem for the expression of the cardiovascular components of these responses. However, as pointed out in the introduction to this chapter, these studies have two major limitations. One is the artificial means of evoking the emotional behavior. The other is the use of anesthetics to study the cardiovascular changes. The risk with this approach is that it may be too reductionist and reveal details of organization that are not relevant to the expression of stress responses in the conscious, freely behaving animal. Therefore, it is important to consider other approaches that do not have these limitations.

## NATURALLY EVOKED PSYCHOLOGICAL STRESS AND ITS NEURAL SUBSTRATE

In the other experimental approach that has been used to study the neural substrate of psychological stress, the stress response is evoked by environmental stimuli in the conscious animal rather than by intracerebral stimulation in an anesthetized or decerebrate preparation. This approach focuses on a given stress response and tries to identify the neural structures mediating its components. Interventions used in these studies include chemical lesions or temporary chemical blockade of neurotransmission in target areas that have often been identified previously by functional anatomical mapping using the expression of immediate early genes, such as *c-fos*. A major advantage of this combined functional and anatomical approach is that a brain structure or pathway can be directly linked to an integrated response known to be part of the behavioral repertoire of the animal. However, working in the conscious animal imposes serious technical and ethical challenges for the physiologist, so that there are only a few studies of this kind. Nevertheless, those few studies have led to important findings that partly confirm and partly challenge those revealed by studies of the defense reaction in anesthetized or decerebrate preparations.

Different models have been developed to induce psychological stress in the animal. Any form of stress may have a psychological component if it is tested in the conscious animal. However, there are forms of stress that we instantly recognize as more psychological than others, such as those that are triggered by innocuous but cognitively salient stimuli. For example, fear evoked by the reactivation of an unpleasant memory (i.e., conditioned fear) may be considered the purest form of psychological stress. Psychosocial stress may also be considered a pure form of psychological stress, because it depends on learned rules of dominance and submission. On the other hand, air-jet stress and restraint stress are not pure because the stimuli or conditions that trigger them have a strong physical component and are immediate rather than anticipatory. Because these stimuli are neither noxious nor resistant to anesthesia, they cannot be considered physical stressors and therefore fall into a lower category of psychological stress. As will be discussed, these different forms of stress may also differ in terms of the organization of their neural substrate.

### Conditioned Fear

Smith et al.[102] developed a fear-conditioning paradigm in baboons that consisted of pairing a one-minute sound with an electric shock delivered to the abdomen. After conditioning, the cardiovascular response to presentation of the sound consisted of a rapid increase in mean arterial pressure (+15 mmHg) and heart rate (+35 beats per minute: bpm) associated with a marked renal vasoconstriction and hindlimb vasodilatation; i.e., the classic visceral alerting response. Subsequent work showed that electrolytic and excitotoxic lesions of a hypothalamic area that included the perifornical and medial part of lateral hypothalamus—i.e., the central and lateral parts of the hypothalamic defense region—completely abolished the cardiovascular response of conditioned fear without affecting other cardiovascular responses, such as those associated with exercise[99,101]. Similar lesions of the paraventricular nucleus of the hypothalamus had no effect. Retrograde tracing studies from this hypothalamic area revealed afferents from medial preoptic and supraoptic regions, nucleus of the diagonal band of Broca, lateral septum, and medial, cortical, and basal subnuclei of the amygdala[41]. Anterograde tracing revealed direct projections from the same hypothalamic area to the PAG, parabrachial area, rostral ventromedial medulla, RVLM, and the intermediolateral column of the thoracic cord[100].

In the rat, Iwata, LeDoux, and colleagues confirmed and extended the work of Smith and coworkers with a conditioned-fear paradigm that paired a one-second sound with a 10-second electric shock to the footpad as the conditioned stimulus. The cardiovascular response to this stimulus consisted of a 15 mmHg increase in mean arterial pressure and was associated with a characteristic behavioral response known as "freezing immobility"[63]. Both components of the response were completely abolished by large excitotoxic lesions of the amygdala that included the central and medial nuclei[62]. Bilateral excitotoxic lesions of the lateral hypothalamic area, which included lateral parts of the perifornical hypothalamus, abolished the conditioned component of the pressor response but did not reduce the freezing response[63,67] (Figure 12–4). Neither component was affected by bilateral excitotoxic lesions of the medial hypothalamus that included the dorsomedial hypothalamus[63]. Electrolytic lesions of

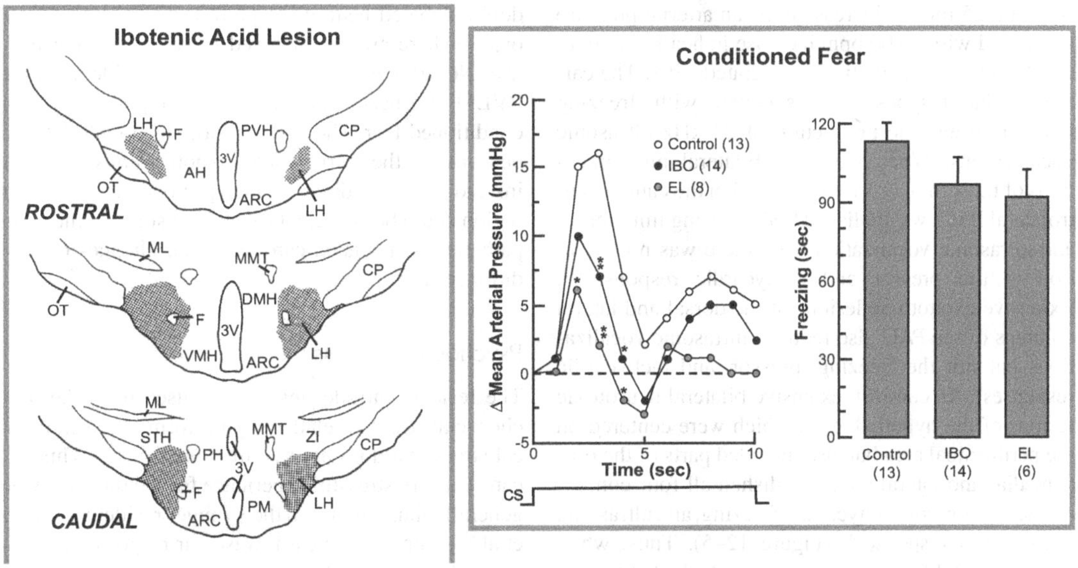


Figure 12–4 Effects of hypothalamic lesions on the response to conditioned fear in the conscious rat. Effects of bilateral lateral hypothalamus lesions on the arterial pressure and freezing responses of conditioned fear to a tone in the rat. *Left,* example of a bilateral lesion with ibotenic acid. *Right,* changes in mean arterial pressure and freezing in unlesioned (Control), ibotenic acid lesioned (IBO) and electrolytically lesioned (EL) rats. Note the reduction in the pressor but not the freezing responses after lesions. 3V, third ventricle; AH, anterior hypothalamus; ARC, arcuate nucleus; CS, conditioned stimulus (tone); CP, cerebral peduncle; DMH, dorsomedial hypothalamic nucleus; *F:* fornix; LH, lateral hypothalamus; ML, medial lemniscus; MMT, mammillothalamic tract; PVH, paraventricular hypothalamic nucleus; OT, optic tract; PH, posterior hypothalamic nucleus; PM, posteromedial hypothalamic nucleus; STH, subthalamic nucleus; VMH, ventromedial hypothalamic nucleus; ZI, zona incerta. *, $P<0.05$; **, $P<0.01$. Modified from LeDoux et al. (1988)[67], with permission.

the rostral and caudal PAG did not affect the pressor response but abolished the freezing response; and excitotoxic lesions of the caudal PAG, but not the rostral PAG, abolished the freezing response[67]. Hence, the amygdala controls both pressor and behavioral components; the lateral hypothalamus, only the pressor component; the caudal PAG, only the behavioral component. In addition, the descending projections mediating the pressor response from the lateral hypothalamus do not traverse the PAG; and the dorsomedial hypothalamus is not involved in the response. This pathway also appears specific to the conditioned response because the pressor response to the unconditioned response (i.e., to the shock itself, a physical stressor) was unaffected by amygdala or lateral hypothalamus lesion[62,67].

Fear conditioning to sound, as in the studies described above, only produces conditioned responses of short duration. However, longer responses can be evoked with conditioned fear to context. In this paradigm, the conditioned stimulus is the environment or context—e.g., the shock chamber itself—and the response can last for 30 to 40 minutes. In the model of contextual fear that we have developed, the cardiovascular response is recorded by radiotelemetry and consists of a 25 mmHg increase in mean arterial pressure associated with a 100 bpm increase in heart rate, both of which are sympathetically mediated[22–24,33]. The cardiovascular response is associated with freezing immobility and the production of 22 kHz ultrasonic vocalizations. When we made bilateral microinjections of muscimol or kynurenic acid in the caudal ventrolateral PAG, we abolished both freezing immobility and ultrasonic vocalizations; but there was no reduction in the pressor and tachycardic responses[113]. Extensive excitotoxic lesions of the dorsal and lateral columns of the PAG also reduced ultrasonic vocalizations but not the freezing, pressor, and tachycardic responses[68]. In contrast, extensive bilateral neurotoxic lesions of the hypothalamus, which were centered on the perifornical area but also included parts of the dorsomedial and lateral areas, abolished all four components; i.e., pressor, tachycardic, freezing, and ultrasonic vocalization responses[49] (Figure 12–5). Thus, while there may be differences with respect to the behavioral component of the response, as far as the cardiovascular component is concerned, our findings support those of Smith, Iwata, and LeDoux. Our data also strongly suggest that the hypothalamic defense area is necessary for mediating the cardiovascular response of conditioned fear, whereas the PAG is not.

An important question is what is the output pathway mediating the pressor response from the hypothalamus. Although anatomical tracing studies had raised the possibility that the pressor effect might be mediated by direct projections to the cord, experiments in anaesthetized animals suggested that the pressor response evoked from the hypothalamic defense area relays in the RVLM (see above). To answer this question, we used a functional anatomical approach combining Fos immunohistochemistry with retrograde tracing from the thoracic cord[30]. When we processed the brains of rats injected in the upper, middle, or lower thoracic cord and tested for contextual conditioned fear, we found that four main groups of neurons were double-labeled for Fos and the retrograde tracer (Figure 12–6). The largest group, which accounted for 21% of all the double-labeled neurons, was in the perifornical hypothalamus. The other groups were the PVN, the pontine A5 noradrenergic group, and the rostral ventromedial medulla (15%, 16%, and 10%, respectively). The caudal raphé nuclei, including the raphé pallidus, accounted for 4%; and the RVLM, for only 1% of all the double-labeled neurons, with less than 2% of all spinally projecting RVLM neurons being double-labeled for Fos.

This result must be interpreted with caution, because we do not know what activation of 2% of RVLM bulbospinal neurons represents in terms of cardiovascular changes. It may also be that the other double-labeled neurons in perifornical hypothalamus or elsewhere are not involved in cardiovascular control. Nevertheless, it casts doubts on the idea that the RVLM is a necessary relay of the hypothalamus for conditioned fear. The large number of double-labeled neurons in the perifornical hypothalamus suggests instead that the direct spinal projections from this region could be sufficient to mediate some of the sympathetically mediated cardiovascular changes of conditioned fear.

## Psychosocial Stress

The resident-intruder test can be used to evoke psychosocial stress, a relatively pure form of psychological stress that does not require conditioning. This test can be a very stressful experience for the intruder, who generally must submit to the stronger resident. Kayaba et al.[66] compared the cardiovascular response of wild-type mice to orexin knock-out mice in this stress paradigm. This study is particularly relevant because it directly addresses the role of a subgroup of cells found exclusively in the perifornical hypothalamus. Orexin (also known as hypocretin) is a neuropeptide produced by a restricted group of neurons located in the perifornical hypothalamus. Orexin has been implicated in the control of wakefulness and of many autonomic functions, including cardiovascular control[85,92,97,110]. Orexinergic neurons project to the spinal cord, and intrathecal orexin injections evoke significant pressor

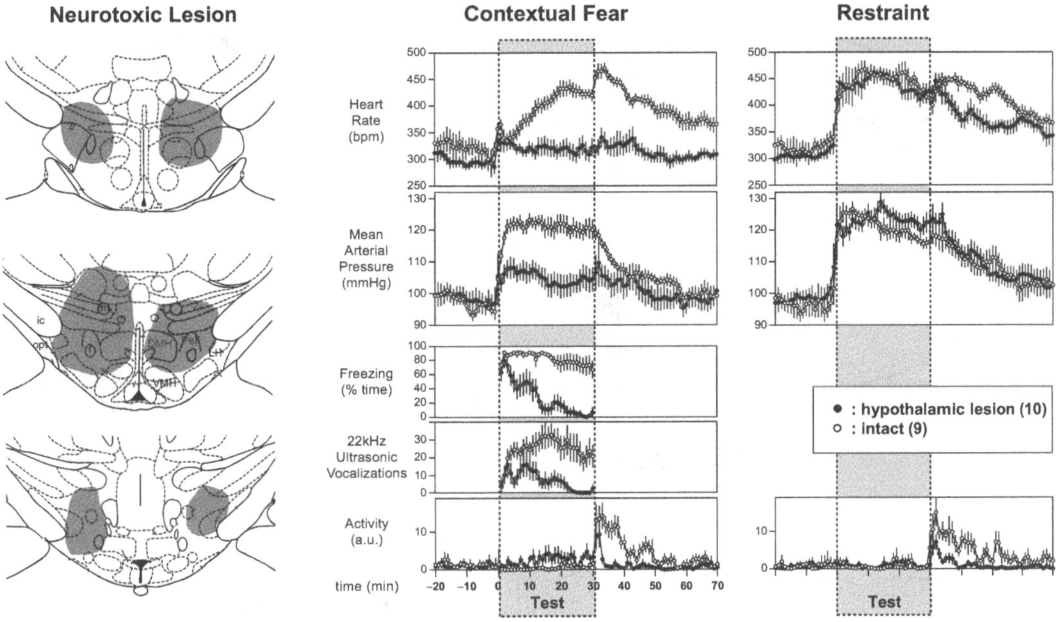


Figure 12–5 Effects of hypothalamic lesions on the response to conditioned fear in the conscious rat. Effects of bilateral neurotoxic lesions of the perifornical hypothalamus on the heart rate, arterial pressure, freezing, ultrasonic vocalizations, and activity responses of conditioned fear to context and restraint in rats. *Left,* Example of a bilateral neurotoxic lesion. The neurotoxin was hypocretin2/orexinB-saporin, which was supposed to destroy only cells with hypocretin receptors. However, the toxin was found to be non-specific and destroyed all neurons within the injected area. *Right,* Average effect (mean ± SEM) of lesions similar to that in the *left panel* on the two stress responses tested in the same group of rats. Note that the lesions markedly reduced all components of the fear response by approximately 70% but had no effect on the cardiovascular response to restraint. DMH, dorsomedial hypothalamic nucleus; f, fornix; ic, internal capsule; LH, lateral hypothalamus; mt, mammillothalamic tract; opt, optic tract; PeF, perifornical hypothalamic area; VMH, ventromedial hypothalamic nucleus; ZI, zona incerta. Modified from Furlong and Carrive (2007)[49], with permission.

and tachycardic effects[6,71,112]. Orexinergic neurons also project to the RVLM and medullary raphé nuclei, and orexin injections into these regions also produce tachycardic and pressor effects[14,34,76]. Orexin knock-out mice lack these neurons. The study by Kayaba et al.[66] showed that the pressor and tachycardic responses of the intruder (+15 mmHg, +100 bpm) were practically abolished in orexin knock-out mice (Figure 12–7). The pressor and tachycardic responses evoked by disinhibition of the perifornical hypothalamus under anesthesia were also markedly reduced in the knock-out mice. However, the pressor and tachycardic response (+15 mmHg, +40 bpm) to a physical stressor, in this case a noxious pinch of the tail, remained unaffected. This study confirms the role of the perifornical hypothalamus in the cardiovascular response to psychological stress but not physical stress and implicates the orexin neurons in the response to psychological stress. It also supports the idea that the response could be mediated (at least in part) by direct spinal projections since orexin terminals are found in the thoracic cord, and orexin administered intrathecally has pressor and tachycardic effects.

## Air-Jet Stress

As mentioned earlier, air-jet stress is another form of psychological stress, although it may not be as pure as conditioned fear or psychosocial stress. In the rat model of air-jet stress, the cardiovascular response consists of a rise in mean arterial pressure (+25 mmHg) and heart rate (+150 bpm) lasting for 10 to 30 minutes. In this model, temporary bilateral blockade of the dorsomedial hypothalamus with muscimol or kynurenic acid markedly reduces the cardiovascular response, whereas injections of muscimol in the PVN

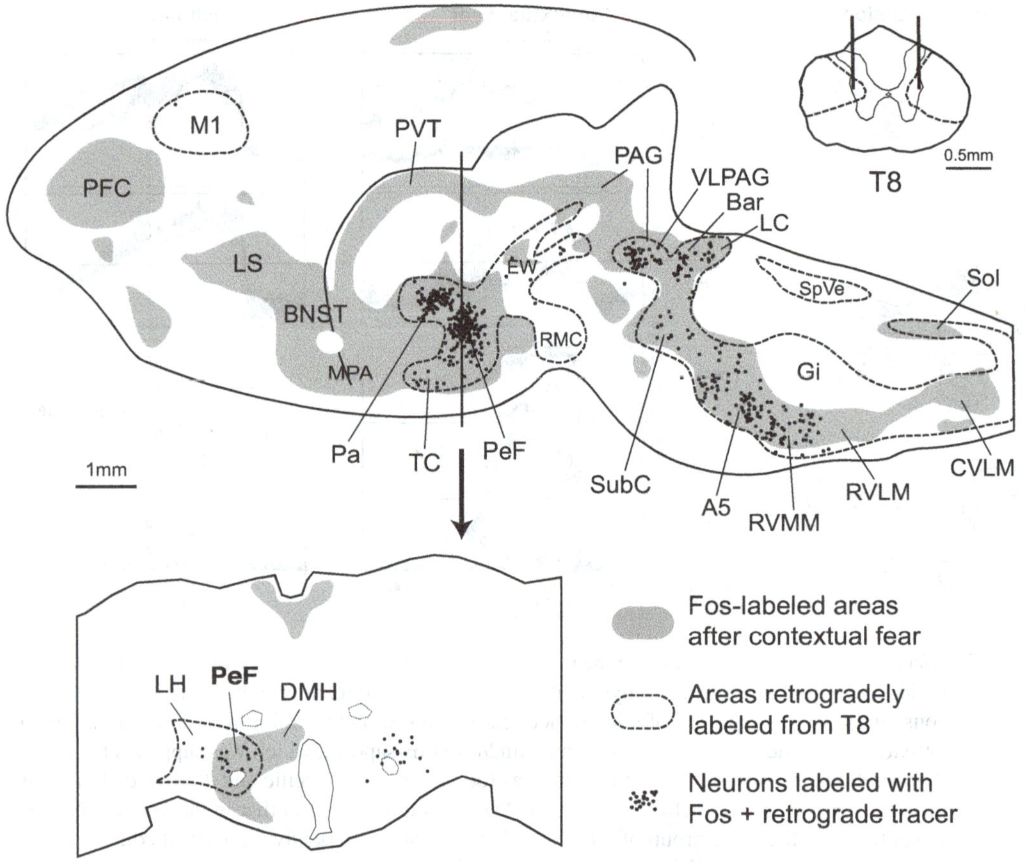


Figure 12–6 Central autonomic neurons that mediate the response to conditioned fear to context in the rat. Diagram showing the location of putative premotor sympathetic neurons that mediate responses to conditioned fear to context in the rat. The neurons were revealed by double immunolabeling for Fos (evoked by contextual fear) and a retrograde tracer (cholera toxin B subunit) injected bilaterally into the thoracic cord. Injections centered on the intermediolateral column. *Top,* Sagittal projection of one brain showing the distribution of the double-labeled neurons, overlaid on the areas single labeled for Fos (marked with *gray shading*) or the retrograde tracer (demarcated by the *dashed line*). In this rat, the injection site for the retrograde tracer was in T8 and is shown in the inset. *Bottom,* A single transverse section through the tuberal hypothalamus from the same brain as in the top panel. Note the high density of double-labeled cells in the perifornical area (PeF). In this particular case, the PeF contained 25% of all the double-labeled neurons and was the group with the most extensive double labeling. In contrast, no double labeling was found in the RVLM. A5, A5 noradrenergic group; Bar, Barrington's nucleus; BNST, bed nucleus of the stria terminalis; CVLM, caudal ventrolateral medulla; DMH, dorsomedial hypothalamic nucleus; EW, Edinger-Westphal nucleus; Gi, gigantocellular reticular nucleus; LC, locus coeruleus; LH, lateral hypothalamic area; LS, lateral septum; M1, primary motor cortex; MPA, medial preoptic area; Pa, paraventricular hypothalamic nucleus; PAG, periaqueductal gray; PeF, perifornical hypothalamic area; PFC, prefrontal cortex; PVT, paraventricular thalamic nucleus; RMC, red nucleus magnocellular part; RVLM, rostral ventrolateral medulla, RVMM, rostral ventromedial medulla; Sol, nucleus of the solitary tract; SpVe, spinal vestibular nucleus; SubC, subcoeruleus nucleus; TC, tuber cinereum hypothalamic area; VLPAG, ventrolateral periaqueductal gray. Modified from Carrive and Gorissen (2008)[30], with permission.

have no effect[105,108]. These observations implicate the dorsomedial hypothalamus in the response to air-jet stress, which is interesting because medial hypothalamic lesions did not affect the response to conditioned fear[63]. This issue needs to be further investigated, because it raises the possibility that stressors that are

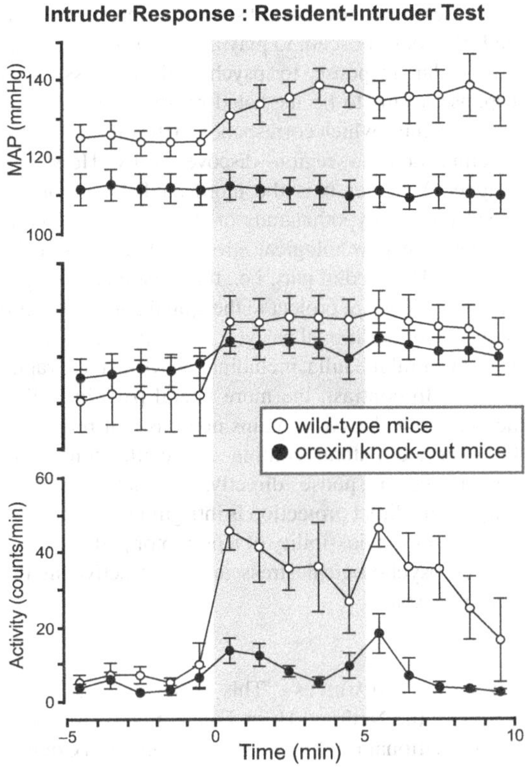


Figure 12–7 Cardiovascular and behavioral responses to the resident intruder test in orexin knock-out and wild-type mice. Changes in mean arterial pressure (MAP), heart rate and activity evoked by the resident-intruder test in orexin/hypocretin knock-out mice and wild-type mice. The responses of the intruder are shown. The gray area indicates the time during which the intruder mouse was present in the resident mouse's cage. Note the marked reduction of all parameters in the knock-out mice. Reproduced from Kayaba et al. (2003)[66], with permission.

primarily psychological relay in more lateral regions of the hypothalamus. The involvement of the perifornical hypothalamus and lateral hypothalamus in responses to air-jet stress should also be explored.

In a more recent study on conscious rats, muscimol injections into the raphé pallidus were found to abolish the tachycardic response but they did not significantly reduce the pressor response to air-jet stress[114]. The role of the RVLM has not been investigated in the rat; but in the conscious rabbit, blockade of the RVLM with kynurenic acid reduces the increase in renal sympathetic nerve activity evoked by air-jet stress[80], consistent with results obtained in anesthetized animals[59,89,90]. These studies are also the first demonstrations that medullary structures can relay the cardiovascular components of a form of psychological stress.

## Restraint

Restraint or immobilization is a commonly used stressor, often classified as a psychological stressor. However, restraint should be considered a mixed form of physical and psychological stress because the squeeze and struggle in the restrainer is itself a strong physical stimulus in this test. The cardiovascular response to restraint is of similar magnitude to the one evoked by air-jet stress (+28 mmHg and +130 bpm); and, as with air-jet stress, it is reduced by muscimol inhibition of the dorsomedial hypothalamus[83]. However, we have reported that large neurotoxic lesions of the hypothalamus that included the dorsomedial hypothalamus—i.e., the same lesions that abolished the cardiovascular response to conditioned fear (see above)—had no effect on the pressor and tachycardic responses to restraint (Figure 12–5)[49]. This intriguing finding suggests that the dorsomedial hypothalamus can contribute to but is not necessary for the cardiovascular response to restraint, unlike conditioned fear and psychosocial stress. Other centers, presumably located at lower levels of the neuraxis, may be sufficient to mediate the cardiovascular response to restraint if dorsomedial hypothalamic neurons have been permanently lesioned. It would be interesting to know if this is also true for air-jet stress, which, like restraint, is not a pure form of psychological stress. Taken together, these data indicate that the dorsal tuberal hypothalamus may be necessary for the purer forms of psychological stress but not for those that are associated with a strong physical stimulus. This suggestion is consistent with the lack of effect of hypothalamic lesions (selective or not) on the cardiovascular response to physical stressors, such as electric footshocks or noxious tail pinch[63,66,67].

Interestingly, a study combining immunohistochemistry for Fos and retrograde tracing from the middle thoracic cord revealed only two main groups of possible sympathetic premotor neurons for the response to restraint, the A5 catecholaminergic group and the raphé pallidus[95], with practically no double labeling occurring in the hypothalamus. This finding is in sharp contrast to the predominantly hypothalamic location of the premotor sympathetic neurons involved in the response to conditioned fear[30] (see above). Thus, functional anatomical evidence supports the idea that mixed forms of psychological stress (e.g., restraint) do not activate premotor sympathetic neurons in the hypothalamus, whereas the purer forms of stress (e.g., conditioned fear) do.

### Overview of Naturally Evoked Psychological Stress Responses and their Neural Substrate

The studies carried out in conscious baboons, rats, and mice show that neurons located in the hypothalamic defense region play an important role in mediating the expression of the cardiovascular response to psychological stress. More specifically, these neurons appear to be necessary for the responses to the purest forms of psychological stress but are not so important for response to stressors that have a significant physical component or are purely physical. Neurons in the PAG, on the other hand, do not appear to play a critical role in these cardiovascular responses, and neither does the PVN, at least for the sympathetic component of the response. What is less clear, however, is how the hypothalamus transmits its effects to sympathetic preganglionic neurons in the thoracic spinal cord. There may be relays in the lower brainstem, especially in the RVLM and raphé pallidus. There may also be direct projections from the perifornical area to the spinal cord that could be sufficient to mediate the cardiovascular effects, at least for the purest forms of psychological stress. These direct and indirect projections could be in part orexinergic.

One could speculate that the direct projection from the hypothalamus to the cord plays a greater role during psychological stress than during physical stress. This direct pathway could bypass the basic homeostatic regulation performed by centers in the lower brainstem, an idea that is consistent with autonomic responses to psychological stress being emergency responses. Finally, the direct pathway may be more sensitive to anesthetics than the indirect pathway, since anesthetics are very effective at blocking responses to psychological stress. This differential sensitivity to anesthetics and the fact that most of the work has been done under anesthesia could explain why more is known about the indirect pathways than the direct one.

## SUMMARY

Periventricular structures in the forebrain and midbrain play an important role in the integration of the somatic and autonomic components of complex behaviors, including emotional responses. We are just starting to understand how this network is organized and how it integrates the different forms of emotional responses with their cardiovascular components. In the PAG, there is a functional organization based on topographical representation of the body and internal organs. The circuitry in the PAG may be involved in integrating basic forms of defensive behavior, probably in response to intense external or visceral sensory stimuli. However, the PAG does not seem to play a major role in the cardiovascular response to psychological stress. This response seems to be mediated by the dorsal tuberal hypothalamus, which corresponds to the original hypothalamic defense region discovered by Hess and Brugger. Whether it is the more medial part of the dorsal tuberal hypothalamus or its more lateral parts that mediate psychological stress still remains to be clarified. The medial part, i.e., the dorsomedial hypothalamus, does not project to the spinal cord, implying the need for additional relay(s), most probably in the rostral ventral medulla, including the RVLM and raphé pallidus. In contrast, the more lateral part, including the perifornical area, contains neurons that project to the intermediolateral column and could potentially mediate the response directly, without additional relays. This direct projection is intriguing, and its existence raises the possibility of a premotor pathway specific to psychological stress and only active in the conscious state.

ACKNOWLEDGEMENTS This research was supported by the National Heart Foundation of Australia and the National Health and Medical Research Council of Australia.

### References

1. Abrahams, V. C., Hilton, S. M., and Zbrozyna, A. (1960). Active muscle vasodilation produced by stimulation of the brainstem: Its significance in the defence reaction. *Journal of Physiology* 154, 491–513.
2. Abrahams, V. C., Hilton, S. M., and Zbrozyna, A. W. (1964). The role of active muscle vasodilatation in the early stage of the defence reaction. *Journal of Physiology* 171, 189–202.
3. Abshire, V. M., Hankins, K. D., Roehr, K. E., and Dimicco, J. A. (1988). Injection of L-allylglycine into the posterior hypothalamus in rats causes decreases in local GABA which correlate with increases in heart rate. *Neuropharmacology* 27, 1171–1177.
4. Al Maskati, H. A., and Zbrozyna, A. W. (1989). Cardiovascular and motor components of the defense reaction elicited in rats by electrical and chemical stimulation in amygdala. *Journal of the Autonomic Nervous System* 28, 127–131.
5. Allen, G. V., and Cechetto, D. F. (1992). Functional and anatomical organization of cardiovascular pressor and depressor sites in the lateral hypothalamic area: I. Descending projections. *Journal of Comparative Neurology* 315, 313–332.

6. Antunes, V. R., Brailoiu, G. C., Kwok, E. H., Scruggs, P., and Dun, N. J. (2001). Orexins/hypocretins excite rat sympathetic preganglionic neurons in vivo and in vitro. *American Journal of Physiology. Regulatory, Integrative and Comparative Physiology* 281, R1801–R1807.
7. Bandler, R. (1982). Induction of 'rage' following microinjections of glutamate into midbrain but not hypothalamus of cats. *Neuroscience Letters* 30, 183–188.
8. Bandler, R. (1988). Brain mechanisms of aggression as revealed by electrical and chemical stimulation: Suggestion of a central role for the midbrain periaqueductal gray region. In A. Epstein and A. Morrison (Eds.), *Progress in Psychobiology and Physiological Psychology, vol. 13*, pp. 67–153. New York: Academic Press.
9. Bandler, R., and Carrive, P. (1988). Integrated defence reaction elicited by excitatory amino acid microinjection in the midbrain periaqueductal grey region of the unrestrained cat. *Brain Research* 439, 95–106.
10. Bandler, R., Carrive, P., and Depaulis, A. (1991). Emerging principles of organization of the midbrain periaqueductal gray matter. In A. Depaulis and R. Bandler (Eds.), *The Midbrain Periaqueductal Gray Matter: Functional, Anatomical and Immunohistochemical Organization*, pp. 1–8. London: Plenum.
11. Bandler, R., and Depaulis, A. (1991). Midbrain periaqueductal gray control of defensive behavior in the cat and rat. In A. Depaulis and R. Bandler (Eds.), *The Midbrain Periaqueductal Gray Matter: Functional, Anatomical and Immunohistochemical Organization*, pp. 175–198. London: Plenum.
12. Bandler, R., Prineas, S., and McCulloch, T. (1985). Further localization of midbrain neurones mediating the defence reaction in the cat by microinjections of excitatory amino acids. *Neuroscience Letters* 56, 311–316.
13. Bandler, R., and Shipley, M. T. (1994). Columnar organization in the midbrain periaqueductal gray: Modules for emotional expression? *Trends in Neuroscience* 17, 379–389.
14. Berthoud, H. R., Patterson, L. M., Sutton, G. M., Morrison, C., and Zheng, H. (2005). Orexin inputs to caudal raphé neurons involved in thermal, cardiovascular, and gastrointestinal regulation. *Histochemistry and Cell Biology* 123, 147–156.
15. Brandao, M. L., Di Scala, G., Bouchet, M. J., and Schmitt, P. (1986). Escape behavior produced by the blockade of glutamic acid decarboxylase (GAD) in mesencephalic central gray or medial hypothalamus. *Pharmacology, Biochemistry and Behavior* 24, 497–501.
16. Cannon, W. C. (1929). *Bodily Changes in Pain, Hunger, Fear and Rage, 2nd ed.* New York: D. Appleton & Co.
17. Cao, W. H., Fan, W., and Morrison, S. F. (2004). Medullary pathways mediating specific sympathetic responses to activation of dorsomedial hypothalamus. *Neuroscience* 126, 229–240.
18. Cao, W. H., and Morrison, S. F. (2003). Disinhibition of rostral raphé pallidus neurons increases cardiac sympathetic nerve activity and heart rate. *Brain Research* 980, 1–10.
19. Cao, W. H., and Morrison, S. F. (2006). Glutamate receptors in the raphé pallidus mediate brown adipose tissue thermogenesis evoked by activation of dorsomedial hypothalamic neurons. *Neuropharmacology* 51, 426–437.
20. Carrive, P. (1991). Functional organization of midbrain periaqueductal grey neurons controlling regional vascular beds. In A. Depaulis and R. Bandler (Eds.), *The Midbrain Periaqueductal Gray Matter: Functional, Anatomical and Immunohistochemical Organization*, pp. 67–100. London: Plenum.
21. Carrive, P. (1993). The periaqueductal gray and defensive behavior: Functional representation and neuronal organization. *Behavioral Brain Research* 58, 27–47.
22. Carrive, P. (2000). Conditioned fear to environmental context: Cardiovascular and behavioral components in the rat. *Brain Research* 858, 440–445.
23. Carrive, P. (2002). Cardiovascular and behavioural components of conditioned fear to context after ganglionic and alpha-adrenergic blockade. *Autonomic Neuroscience* 98, 90–93.
24. Carrive, P. (2006). Dual activation of cardiac sympathetic and parasympathetic components during conditioned fear to context in the rat. *Clinical and Experimental Pharmacology and Physiology* 33, 1260–1263.
25. Carrive, P., and Bandler, R. (1991). Control of extracranial and hindlimb blood flow by the midbrain periaqueductal grey of the cat. *Experimental Brain Research* 84, 599–606.
26. Carrive, P., and Bandler, R. (1991). Viscerotopic organization of neurons subserving hypotensive reactions within the midbrain periaqueductal grey: A correlative functional and anatomical study. *Brain Research* 541, 206–215.
27. Carrive, P., Bandler, R., and Dampney, R. A. (1989). Somatic and autonomic integration in the midbrain of the unanesthetized decerebrate cat: A distinctive pattern evoked by excitation of neurones in the subtentorial portion of the midbrain periaqueductal grey. *Brain Research* 483, 251–258.

28. Carrive, P., Bandler, R., and Dampney, R. A. (1989). Viscerotopic control of regional vascular beds by discrete groups of neurons within the midbrain periaqueductal gray. *Brain Research* 493, 385–390.
29. Carrive, P., Dampney, R. A., and Bandler, R. (1987). Excitation of neurones in a restricted portion of the midbrain periaqueductal grey elicits both behavioural and cardiovascular components of the defence reaction in the unanaesthetised decerebrate cat. *Neuroscience Letters* 81, 273–278.
30. Carrive, P., and Gorissen, M. (2008). Premotor sympathetic neurons of conditioned fear in the rat. *European Journal of Neuroscience* 28, 428–446.
31. Carrive, P., and Morgan, M. M. (2003). The periaqueductal gray. In G. Paxinos (Ed.), *The Human Nervous System, 2nd ed.*, pp. 393–423. San Diego, CA: Academic Press.
32. Cerri, M., and Morrison, S. F. (2005). Activation of lateral hypothalamic neurons stimulates brown adipose tissue thermogenesis. *Neuroscience* 135, 627–638.
33. Choi, E. A., Leman, S., Vianna, D. M., Waite, P. M., and Carrive, P. (2005). Expression of cardiovascular and behavioural components of conditioned fear to context in T4 spinally transected rats. *Autonomic Neuroscience* 120, 26–34.
34. Ciriello, J., Li, Z., and De Oliveira, C. V. (2003). Cardioacceleratory responses to hypocretin-1 injections into rostral ventromedial medulla. *Brain Research* 991, 84–95.
35. Da Silva, L. G., De Menezes, R. C., Dos Santos, R. A., Campagnole-Santos, M. J., and Fontes, M. A. (2003). Role of periaqueductal gray on the cardiovascular response evoked by disinhibition of the dorsomedial hypothalamus. *Brain Research* 984, 206–214.
36. Da Silva, L. G., Jr., Menezes, R. C., Villela, D. C., and Fontes, M. A. (2006). Excitatory amino acid receptors in the periaqueductal gray mediate the cardiovascular response evoked by activation of dorsomedial hypothalamic neurons. *Neuroscience* 139, 1129–1139.
37. Dampney, R. A. (1994). Functional organization of central pathways regulating the cardiovascular system. *Physiological Reviews* 74, 323–364.
38. De Novellis, V., Stotz-Potter, E. H., Morin, S. M., Rossi, F., and Dimicco, J. A. (1995). Hypothalamic sites mediating cardiovascular effects of microinjected bicuculline and EAAs in rats. *American Journal of Physiology* 269, R131–R140.
39. Depaulis, A., Keay, K. A., and Bandler, R. (1992). Longitudinal neuronal organization of defensive reactions in the midbrain periaqueductal gray region of the rat. *Experimental Brain Research* 90, 307–318.
40. Depaulis, A., Keay, K. A., and Bandler, R. (1994). Quiescence and hyporeactivity evoked by activation of cell bodies in the ventrolateral midbrain periaqueductal gray of the rat. *Experimental Brain Research* 99, 75–83.
41. Devito, J. L., and Smith, O. A. (1982). Afferent projections to the hypothalamic area controlling emotional responses (HACER). *Brain Research* 252, 213–226.
42. Di Scala, G., Schmitt, P., and Karli, P. (1984). Flight induced by infusion of bicuculline methiodide into periventricular structures. *Brain Research* 309, 199–208.
43. Dimicco, J. A., and Abshire, V. M. (1987). Evidence for GABAergic inhibition of a hypothalamic sympathoexcitatory mechanism in anesthetized rats. *Brain Research* 402, 1–10.
44. Eliasson, S., Folkow, B., Lindgren, P., and Uvnäs, B. (1951). Activation of sympathetic vasodilator nerves to skeletal muscles in the cat by hypothalamic stimulation. *Acta Physiologica Scandinavica* 23, 333–351.
45. Feldberg, W., and Guertzenstein, P. G. (1972). A vasodepressor effect of pentobarbitone sodium. *Journal of Physiology* 224, 83–103.
46. Fernandez De Molina, A., and Hunsperger, R. W. (1959). Central representation of affective reactions in forebrain and brainstem. Electrical stimulation of amygdala, stria terminalis and adjacent structures. *Journal of Physiology* 153, 251–265.
47. Fernandez De Molina, A., and Hunsperger, R. W. (1962). Organization of the subcortical system governing defence and flight reactions in the cat. *Journal of Physiology* 160, 200–213.
48. Fontes, M. A., Tagawa, T., Polson, J. W., Cavanagh, S. J., and Dampney, R. A. (2001). Descending pathways mediating cardiovascular response from dorsomedial hypothalamic nucleus. *American Journal of Physiology. Heart and Circulatory Physiology* 280, H2891–H2901.
49. Furlong, T., and Carrive, P. (2007). Effects of neurotoxic lesions centered on the perifornical hypothalamus on the cardiovascular and behavioural responses to contextual fear and restraint. *Brain Research* 1128, 107–109.
50. Gelsema, A. J., McKitrick, D. J., and Calaresu, F. R. (1987). Cardiovascular responses to chemical and electrical stimulation of amygdala in rats. *American Journal of Physiology* 253, R712–R718.
51. Gelsema, A. J., Roe, M. J., and Calaresu, F. R. (1989). Neurally mediated cardiovascular responses to stimulation of cell bodies in the hypothalamus of the rat. *Brain Research* 482, 67–77.

52. Goodchild, A. K., Dampney, R. A., and Bandler, R. (1982). A method for evoking physiological responses by stimulation of cell bodies, but not axons of passage, within localized regions of the central nervous system. *Journal of Neuroscience Methods* 6, 351–363.
53. Herd, J. A. (1991). Cardiovascular response to stress. *Physiological Reviews* 71, 305–330.
54. Hess, W. R., and Brugger, M. (1943). Das Subkorticale Zentrum der affektiven Abwehrreaktion. *Helvetical Physiologica Pharmacologica Acta* 1, 33–52. Translated in: K. Akert (Ed.), *Biological Order and Brain Organization. Selected Works of W. R. Hess*, pp. 182–202. New York: Springer-Verlag.
55. Hilton, S. M. (1982). The defence-arousal system and its relevance for circulatory and respiratory control. *Journal of Experimental Biology* 100, 159–174.
56. Hilton, S. M., Marshall, J. M., and Timms, R. J. (1983). Ventral medullary relay neurones in the pathway from the defence areas of the cat and their effect on blood pressure. *Journal of Physiology* 345, 149–166.
57. Hilton, S. M., and Redfern, W. S. (1986). A search for brain stem cell groups integrating the defence reaction in the rat. *Journal of Physiology* 378, 213–228.
58. Hilton, S. M., and Zbrozyna, A. W. (1963). Amygdaloid region of the defence reaction and its efferent pathway to the brainstem. *Journal of Physiology* 165, 160–173.
59. Horiuchi, J., McAllen, R. M., Allen, A. M., Killinger, S., Fontes, M. A., and Dampney, R. A. (2004). Descending vasomotor pathways from the dorsomedial hypothalamic nucleus: Role of medullary raphé and RVLM. *American Journal of Physiology. Regulatory, Integrative and Comparative Physiology* 287, R824–R832.
60. Hunsperger, R. W. (1956). Affektreaktionen auf electrische reizung im Hirnstamm der katze. (Defense reaction evoked by electrical stimulation of the cat brainstem) *Helvetica Physiologica et Pharmacologica Acta* 14, 70–92.
61. Iwata, J., Chida, K., and Ledoux, J. E. (1987). Cardiovascular responses elicited by stimulation of neurons in the central amygdaloid nucleus in awake but not anesthetized rats resemble conditioned emotional responses. *Brain Research* 418, 183–188.
62. Iwata, J., Ledoux, J. E., Meeley, M. P., Arneric, S., and Reis, D. J. (1986). Intrinsic neurons in the amygdaloid field projected to by the medial geniculate body mediate emotional responses conditioned to acoustic stimuli. *Brain Research* 383, 195–214.
63. Iwata, J., Ledoux, J. E., and Reis, D. J. (1986). Destruction of intrinsic neurons in the lateral hypothalamus disrupts the classical conditioning of autonomic but not behavioral emotional responses in the rat. *Brain Research* 368, 161–166.
64. Jordan, D. (1990). Autonomic changes in affective behavior. In: A. D. Loewy and K. M. Spyer (Eds.), *Central Regulation of Autonomic Function*, pp. 349–366. New York: Oxford University Press.
65. Kabat, H., Magoun, H. W., and Ranson, J. W. (1935). Electrical stimulation of points in the forebrain and midbrain. *Archives of Neurology* 34, 931–955.
66. Kayaba, Y., Nakamura, A., Kasuya, Y., Ohuchi, T., Yanagisawa, M., Komuro, I., Fukuda, Y., and Kuwaki, T. (2003). Attenuated defense response and low basal blood pressure in orexin knockout mice. *American Journal of Physiology. Regulatory, Integrative and Comparative Physiology* 285, R581–R593.
67. Ledoux, J. E., Iwata, J., Cicchetti, P., and Reis, D. J. (1988). Different projections of the central amygdaloid nucleus mediate autonomic and behavioral correlates of conditioned fear. *Journal of Neuroscience* 8, 2517–2529.
68. Leman, S., Dielenberg, R. A., and Carrive, P. (2003). Effect of dorsal periaqueductal gray lesion on cardiovascular and behavioural responses to contextual conditioned fear in rats. *Behavioural Brain Research* 143, 169–176.
69. Lindgren, P., Rosen, A., Stranberg, P., and Uvnäs, B. (1956). The sympathetic vasodilator outflow. *Journal of Comparative Neurology* 105, 95–109.
70. Lindgren, P., and Uvnäs, B. (1953). Activation of sympathetic vasodilator and vasoconstrictor neurons by electrical stimulation in the medulla of the dog and cat. *Circulation Research* 1, 479–485.
71. Llewellyn-Smith, I. J., Martin, C. L., Marcus, J. N., Yanagisawa, M., Minson, J. B., and Scammell, T. E. (2003). Orexin-immunoreactive inputs to rat sympathetic preganglionic neurons. *Neuroscience Letters* 351, 115–119.
72. Lovick, T. A. (1987). Differential control of cardiac and vasomotor activity by neurones in nucleus paragigantocellularis lateralis in the cat. *Journal of Physiology* 389, 23–35.
73. Lovick, T. A. (1992). Inhibitory modulation of the cardiovascular defence response by the ventrolateral periaqueductal grey matter in rats. *Experimental Brain Research* 89, 133–139.
74. Lovick, T. A. (1992). Midbrain influences on ventrolateral medullo-spinal neurones in the rat. *Experimental Brain Research* 90, 147–152.
75. Lovick, T. A. (1993). The periaqueductal gray-rostral medulla connection in the defence reaction: Efferent pathways and descending control mechanisms. *Behavioural Brain Research* 58, 19–25.

76. Machado, B. H., Bonagamba, L. G., Dun, S. L., Kwok, E. H., and Dun, N. J. (2002). Pressor response to microinjection of orexin/hypocretin into rostral ventrolateral medulla of awake rats. *Regulatory Peptides* 104, 75–81.
77. Mancia, G., Baccelli, G., and Zanchetti, A. (1972). Hemodynamic responses to different emotional stimuli in the cat: Patterns and mechanisms. *American Journal of Physiology* 223, 925–933.
78. Mancia, G., Baccelli, G., and Zanchetti, A. (1974). Regulation of renal circulation during behavioral changes in the cat. *American Journal of Physiology* 227, 536–542.
79. Mancia, G., and Zanchetti, A. (1981). Hypothalamic control of autonomic functions. In P. J. Morgane and J. Panksepp (Eds.), *Handbook of the Hypothalamus*, pp. 147–201. New York: Decker.
80. Mayorov, D. N., and Head, G. A. (2002). Ionotropic glutamate receptors in the rostral ventrolateral medulla mediate sympathetic responses to acute stress in conscious rabbits. *Autonomic Neuroscience* 98, 20–23.
81. McAllen, R. M., and Dampney, R. A. (1990). Vasomotor neurons in the rostral ventrolateral medulla are organized topographically with respect to type of vascular bed but not body region. *Neuroscience Letters* 110, 91–96.
82. McAllen, R. M., Neil, J. J., and Loewy, A. D. (1982). Effects of kainic acid applied to the ventral surface of the medulla oblongata on vasomotor tone, the baroreceptor reflex and hypothalamic autonomic responses. *Brain Research* 238, 65–76.
83. McDougall, S. J., Widdop, R. E., and Lawrence, A. J. (2004). Medial prefrontal cortical integration of psychological stress in rats. *European Journal of Neuroscience* 20, 2430–2440.
84. McDowall, L. M., Horiuchi, J., Killinger, S., and Dampney, R. (2006). Modulation of the baroreceptor reflex by the dorsomedial hypothalamic nucleus and perifornical area. *American Journal of Physiology. Regulatory, Integrative and Comparative Physiology* 290, R1020–R1026.
85. Mochizuki, T., and Scammell, T. E. (2003). Orexin/Hypocretin: Wired for wakefulness. *Current Biology* 13, R563–564.
86. Nakao, H. (1958). Emotional behaviour produced by hypothalamic stimulation. *American Journal of Physiology* 194, 411–418.
87. Ranson, S. W., and Magoun, H. W. (1939). The hypothalamus. *Ergebnisse der Physiologie, biologischen Chemie und experimentellen Pharmakologie* 41, 56–163.
88. Rosen, A. (1961). Augmented cardiac contraction, heart acceleration and skeletal muscle vasodilatation produced by hypothalamic stimulation in cats. *Acta Physiologica Scandinavica* 52, 291–300.
89. Samuels, B. C., Zaretsky, D. V., and Dimicco, J. A. (2002). Tachycardia evoked by disinhibition of the dorsomedial hypothalamus in rats is mediated through medullary raphé. *Journal of Physiology* 538, 941–946.
90. Samuels, B. C., Zaretsky, D. V., and Dimicco, J. A. (2004). Dorsomedial hypothalamic sites where disinhibition evokes tachycardia correlate with location of raphé-projecting neurons. *American Journal of Physiology. Regulatory, Integrative and Comparative Physiology* 287, R472–R478.
91. Sanders, S. K., and Shekhar, A. (1991). Blockade of GABAA receptors in the region of the anterior basolateral amygdala of rats elicits increases in heart rate and blood pressure. *Brain Research* 567, 101–110.
92. Saper, C. B., Chou, T. C., and Scammell, T. E. (2001). The sleep switch: Hypothalamic control of sleep and wakefulness. *Trends in Neurosciences* 24, 726–731.
93. Schmitt, P., Carrive, P., Di Scala, G., Jenck, F., Brandao, M., Bagri, A., Moreau, J. L., and Sandner, G. (1986). A neuropharmacological study of the periventricular neural substrate involved in flight. *Behavioral Brain Research* 22, 181–190.
94. Schramm, L. P., and Bignall, K. E. (1971). Central neural pathways mediating active sympathetic muscle vasodilation in cats. *American Journal of Physiology* 221, 754–767.
95. Senba, E., Matsunaga, K., Tohyama, M., and Noguchi, K. (1993). Stress-induced c-fos expression in the rat brain: Activation mechanism of sympathetic pathway. *Brain Research Bulletin* 31, 329–344.
96. Shekhar, A., and Dimicco, J. A. (1987). Defense reaction elicited by injection of GABA antagonists and synthesis inhibitors into the posterior hypothalamus in rats. *Neuropharmacology* 26, 407–417.
97. Shirasaka, T., Nakazato, M., Matsukura, S., Takasaki, M., and Kannan, H. (1999). Sympathetic and cardiovascular actions of orexins in conscious rats. *American Journal of Physiology* 277, R1780–R1785.
98. Skultety, F. M. (1963). Stimulation of periaqueductal gray and hypothalamus. *Archives of Neurology* 8, 608–620.
99. Smith, O. A., Astley, C. A., Devito, J. L., Stein, J. M., and Walsh, K. E. (1980). Functional analysis of hypothalamic control of the cardiovascular responses accompanying emotional behavior. *Federation Proceedings* 39, 2487–2494.

100. Smith, O. A., and Devito, J. L. (1984). Central neural integration for the control of autonomic responses associated with emotion. *Annual Review of Neuroscience* 7, 43–65.
101. Smith, O. A., Devito, J. L., and Astley, C. A. (1990). Neurons controlling cardiovascular responses to emotion are located in lateral hypothalamus-perifornical region. *American Journal of Physiology* 259, R943–R954.
102. Smith, O. A., Hohimer, A. R., Astley, C. A., and Taylor, D. J. (1979). Renal and hindlimb vascular control during acute emotion in the baboon. *American Journal of Physiology* 236, R198–R205.
103. Soltis, R. P., Cook, J. C., Gregg, A. E., and Sanders, B. J. (1997). Interaction of GABA and excitatory amino acids in the basolateral amygdala: Role in cardiovascular regulation. *Journal of Neuroscience* 17, 9367–9374.
104. Soltis, R. P., Cook, J. C., Gregg, A. E., Stratton, J. M., and Flickinger, K. A. (1998). EAA receptors in the dorsomedial hypothalamic area mediate the cardiovascular response to activation of the amygdala. *American Journal of Physiology.* 275, R624–R631.
105. Soltis, R. P., and Dimicco, J. A. (1992). Hypothalamic excitatory amino acid receptors mediate stress-induced tachycardia in rats. *American Journal of Physiology.* 262, R689–R697.
106. Spencer, S. E., Sawyer, W. B., and Loewy, A. D. (1989). Cardiovascular effects produced by L-glutamate stimulation of the lateral hypothalamic area. *American Journal of Physiology* 257, H540–H552.
107. Spencer, S. E., Sawyer, W. B., and Loewy, A. D. (1990). L-glutamate mapping of cardioreactive areas in the rat posterior hypothalamus. *Brain Research* 511, 149–157.
108. Stotz-Potter, E. H., Willis, L. R., and Dimicco, J. A. (1996). Muscimol acts in dorsomedial but not paraventricular hypothalamic nucleus to suppress cardiovascular effects of stress. *Journal of Neuroscience* 16, 1173–1179.
109. Sun, M. K., and Guyenet, P. G. (1986). Hypothalamic glutamatergic input to medullary sympathoexcitatory neurons in rats. *American Journal of Physiology* 251, R798–810.
110. Sutcliffe, J. G., and De Lecea, L. (2002). The hypocretins: Setting the arousal threshold. *Nature Reviews Neuroscience* 3, 339–349.
111. Timms, R. J. (1981). A study of the amygdaloid defence reaction showing the value of Althesin anaesthesia in studies of the functions of the fore-brain in cats. *Pflugers Archives* 391, 49–56.
112. Van Den Pol, A. N. (1999). Hypothalamic hypocretin (orexin): Robust innervation of the spinal cord. *Journal of Neuroscience* 19, 3171–3182.
113. Walker, P., and Carrive, P. (2003). Role of ventrolateral periaqueductal gray neurons in the behavioral and cardiovascular responses to contextual conditioned fear and poststress recovery. *Neuroscience* 116, 897–912.
114. Zaretsky, D. V., Zaretskaia, M. V., Samuels, B. C., Cluxton, L. K., and Dimicco, J. A. (2003). Microinjection of muscimol into raphé pallidus suppresses tachycardia associated with air stress in conscious rats. *Journal of Physiology* 546, 243–250.
115. Zhang, S. P., Bandler, R., and Carrive, P. (1990). Flight and immobility evoked by excitatory amino acid microinjection within distinct parts of the subtentorial midbrain periaqueductal gray of the cat. *Brain Research* 520, 73–82.

# 13

# Central Autonomic Regulation of the Airways

BRENDAN J. CANNING

The airways serve as a conduit to and from the gas-exchanging regions of the lungs. Airway smooth muscle controls the diameter and length of the airways, while mucus glands and the vasculature of the bronchial mucosa regulate the composition, depth, volume, and/or clearance of luminal and interstitial fluid contents. Defensive reflexes, including cough and mucus secretion, facilitate clearance and inactivation of accumulated secretions, irritants, and pathogens, and so serve the essential role of maintaining airway patency and preserving lung capacity for gas exchange. During cough, airway smooth muscle may modify airflow by altering airway diameter, thus maximizing clearance. Smooth muscle tone also regulates dead space and resistance to airflow, matching the demands for respiration by optimizing the work of breathing.

The autonomic nervous system plays an essential role in regulating the tone of airway and bronchial vascular smooth muscle, and mucus secretion[15,25,94,155]. Autonomic nerves also regulate pulmonary vascular tone, matching ventilation with perfusion in response to the ever-changing physiological demands for gas exchange[8]. Dysfunction of the autonomic nervous system accounts, in part, for the symptoms of pulmonary disorders, including asthma, chronic obstructive pulmonary disease, pulmonary hypertension, pulmonary embolism, neurogenic pulmonary edema, and possibly sleep-disordered breathing[8,15,26,57,138,142]. In all species, autonomic tone in the airways and lungs is necessarily dependent upon sympathetic and parasympathetic preganglionic input arising from the central nervous system (reviewed by [15]).

Methods for studying airway autonomic nerves and reflexes have been reviewed elsewhere[16]. The efferent innervation of the airways and the properties of the various subtypes of afferent nerves regulating airway autonomic tone have also been extensively reviewed[8,15,17,55,94]. This chapter focuses on the control of airway autonomic nerves by the CNS. By necessity, a brief overview of the efferent and afferent innervation of the airways precedes discussions of their control by the CNS. The primary objective of the chapter is to summarize what is known about the anatomy, physiology, and pharmacology of control of the airways by the CNS. The chapter also highlights the many gaps in our understanding of airway neural regulation. These uncertainties preclude development of a working model of function of nerves that control the airways in health and disease.

## AUTONOMIC REGULATION OF AIRWAY FUNCTION

Post-ganglionic sympathetic nerves arising from paravertebral and superior cervical ganglia innervate the airways and lungs of all species. Stimulation of sympathetic nerves can evoke contractions of the pulmonary and bronchial vasculature and relaxations of airway smooth muscle through the release of noradrenaline, which acts on $\alpha$- and $\beta$-adrenoceptors, respectively[8,14,15,25,30,63,90,94,113,131]. Smooth muscle of the bronchial and pulmonary vasculature may also contract in response to stimulation of sympathetic nerves due to the actions of neuropeptide Y, which is co-released with noradrenaline from post-ganglionic sympathetic nerves[39,90]. Sympathetic innervation of mucus glands in the airways has been described anatomically, but its physiological function is unclear[155].

Post-ganglionic parasympathetic neurons also innervate the airways and lungs, regulating mucus secretion and dilatation of bronchial and pulmonary blood vessels, as well as contractions and relaxations of airway smooth muscle (Figure 13–1). These effects have been attributed primarily to acetylcholine acting at muscarinic type 3 receptors but also to peptide transmitters, such as vasoactive intestinal peptide, pituitary adenylate cyclase activating polypeptide, peptide histidine isoleucine or peptide histidine methionine, and/or the gaseous transmitter nitric oxide[8,14,15,19,25,30,83,94,152,155].

The distribution and function of the parasympathetic-cholinergic innervation of the airways is well conserved amongst species, as is the sympathetic innervation of the pulmonary and bronchial vasculature. In contrast, the distribution and function of the sympathetic and non-cholinergic parasympathetic innervation of airway smooth muscle varies considerably between species. In humans and non-human primates, airway smooth muscle is largely devoid of noradrenergic sympathetic innervation[15,104]. Non-adrenergic, non-cholinergic neurotransmitters, which are probably derived from parasympathetic nerves, mediate nerve-dependent relaxations of human airway smooth muscle. In some species (dogs, rabbits, rats, mice) but not in others (humans, guinea pigs), stimulation of sympathetic nerves following blockade of β-adrenoceptors evokes contractions of airway smooth muscle through the effects of noradrenaline acting on α-adrenoceptors[15]. In dogs, only the noradrenergic innervation of airway smooth muscle induces relaxation[14,131]. Airway smooth muscle in rats and mice

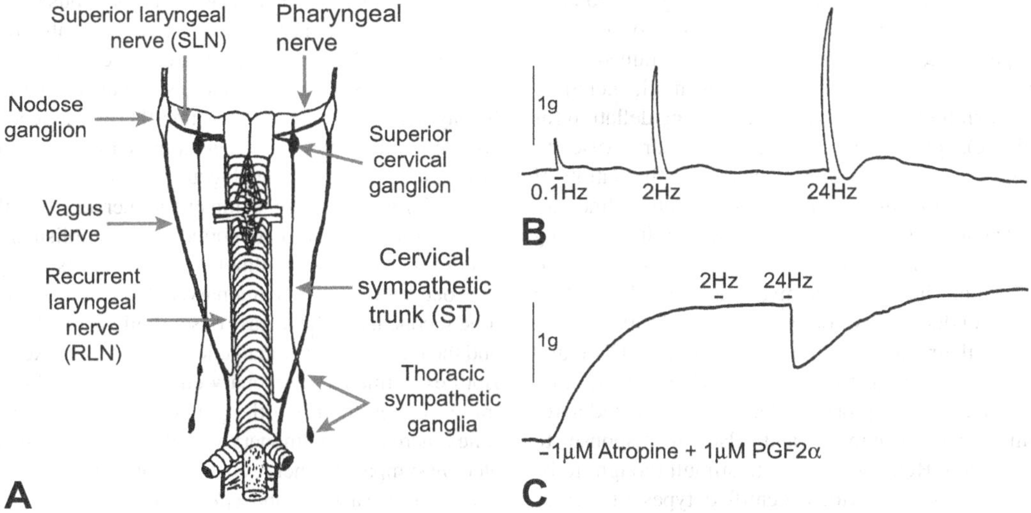


Figure 13–1 Extrinsic innervation of the guinea pig airways and the effects of cholinergic and non-adrenergic, non-cholinergic nerves on trachealis activity. *A:* Diagram showing the extrinsic innervation of the airways in an isolated, innervated preparation of the guinea pig trachea. The airways receive innervation from vagal sensory neurons and sympathetic and parasympathetic post-ganglionic neurons. The preparation illustrated here allows the autonomic innervation of the trachealis to be studied in vitro by monitoring changes in isometric tension in an open segment of the trachea evoked by electrically stimulating the extrinsic nerves. *B:* Cholinergic contractions of the trachealis evoked by bilateral stimulation (10-second trains) of the vagus nerve at optimal stimulation intensities using suction electrodes. *C:* Non-adrenergic, non-cholinergic relaxations of the trachealis evoked by bilateral stimulation of the vagus nerve following atropine pretreatment and pre-contraction of the trachealis with prostaglandin $F_{2\alpha}$ ($PGF_{2\alpha}$). Note that only relaxations occurred in the precontracted preparations pre-treated with atropine. These relaxations were abolished by the ganglionic blockers/ nicotinic receptor antagonists hexamethonium, trimethaphan, and mecamylamine, but were unaffected by the β-adrenoceptor antagonist, propranolol (*not shown*). Also note that higher stimulation frequencies were required to evoke the non-cholinergic relaxations of the trachealis. Reproduced from Canning and Undem (1993)[19,20], with permission.

appears to be devoid of a direct, functional relaxant innervation (reviewed in[15]).

Studies in cats and guinea pigs have shown that non-cholinergic transmitters released from parasympathetic post-ganglionic axons do not come from the same population of nerves that release acetylcholine. Rather, an anatomically and functionally distinct parasympathetic pathway regulates non-adrenergic, non-cholinergic responses in the airways[15,19,38,91]. Reflexes differentially regulate these cholinergic and non-cholinergic parasympathetic pathways[65,96]. Circumstantial evidence suggests that the parasympathetic innervation of human airways is similar to that of cats and guinea pigs[15,152].

## SENSORY AFFERENT NEURONS THAT INNERVATE THE AIRWAYS AND LUNGS

Bronchopulmonary afferent nerves can be subdivided into mechanoreceptors and chemosensitive, nociceptor-like afferent nerves[15,17,147]. Mechanoreceptors are identified by their responsiveness to lung inflation and can be subdivided into rapidly and slowly adapting receptors, based on their responses to sustained, static lung inflations. Other mechanical stimuli, including airway smooth muscle contractions, lung deflation (or collapse), pulmonary edema, pulmonary vascular congestion, and punctate mechanical stimulation of the airway mucosa, also activate bronchopulmonary mechanoreceptors, particularly the rapidly adapting receptors. Additional characteristics of airway mechanoreceptors include their myelination (and therefore their conduction velocity), their activity during eupnea, their sites of termination within the CNS, and their relative insensitivity to direct chemical stimulation. Mechanoreceptors regulate respiration and autonomic tone at eupnea and also in response to stimulation. Reflex responses to stimuli thought to be selective for the various identified types of airway mechanoreceptors help differentiate the known subtypes (Figure 13–2).

The physiological properties of airway mechanoreceptors contrast with those of the chemically sensitive, nociceptor-like vagal afferent nerves that innervate the airways and lungs[15,25,147]. Nociceptors are relatively insensitive to mechanical stimuli and so are mostly inactive during eupnea (Figure 13–2). Noxious chemical (e.g., capsaicin, acid, hypertonic saline, bradykinin, serotonin, adenosine) and mechanical (e.g., lung hyperinflation) stimuli do, however, activate bronchopulmonary nociceptors. Not surprisingly, their activation is associated with airway defensive reflexes, including cough, reflex bronchospasm, mucus secretion, and inhibition of sympathetic vasomotor outflow. The majority of the bronchopulmonary nociceptor-like afferent neurons are of the unmyelinated C-fiber type; but small, myelinated afferent neurons displaying nociceptive properties have also been described[15].

Sensory neurons with cell bodies in the thoracic dorsal root ganglia also innervate the airways and lungs[86,90,113,151]. The functions of these primary afferent neurons, particularly in relation to neural control of the airways, remain poorly defined. Both mechanoreceptors and chemically sensitive nociceptors have been identified amongst the afferent nerves innervating the airways. Spinal terminations of afferent nerves innervating the airways and lungs have not been studied.

## CNS REGULATION OF AIRWAY SYMPATHETIC NEURONS

Reflex-induced alterations in pulmonary and bronchial sympathetic vasomotor tone in response to several stimuli have been studied to some extent[3,8,9,25,63,94,125]. Recordings from pre- and post-ganglionic sympathetic nerves that may regulate airway smooth muscle and bronchial or pulmonary vascular tone have also been reported[5,43,66,136,153]. However, there are essentially no studies of CNS control of airway sympathetic outflow. It may seem reasonable to assume that the ascending and descending pathways regulating sympathetic outflow to other organs are analogous to those that regulate the activity of airway sympathetic nerves, but this assumption is not well supported by the published literature. For example, pulmonary embolism is thought to evoke alterations in pulmonary and systemic vascular tone secondary to the release of serotonin from platelets and the initiation of sympathetic vasomotor reflexes[15,46]. Both experimental pulmonary embolism and administration of serotonin via the pulmonary artery evoke a reflex increase in pulmonary vascular tone that is mediated by sympathetic nerves but a *decrease* in renal sympathetic nerve activity and a *decrease* in systemic blood pressure[125,148,151]. Clearly, control of airway sympathetic outflow by the CNS is a grossly under-studied field of investigation, despite its probable importance in life-threatening acute conditions, such as pulmonary embolism, neurogenic pulmonary edema, and altitude sickness, as well as its involvement in chronic diseases, such as pulmonary hypertension, and chronic obstructive lung disease[8,15,26,126,138,142].

Several novel aspects of CNS control of airway sympathetic nerves have been described. Stimulation of the posterior hypothalamus evoked a sympathetic nerve-dependent decrease in tracheal smooth muscle tone with a concomitant increase in blood pressure and heart rate[66]. These responses were attributed to the activation of histaminergic neurons in the hypothalamus,

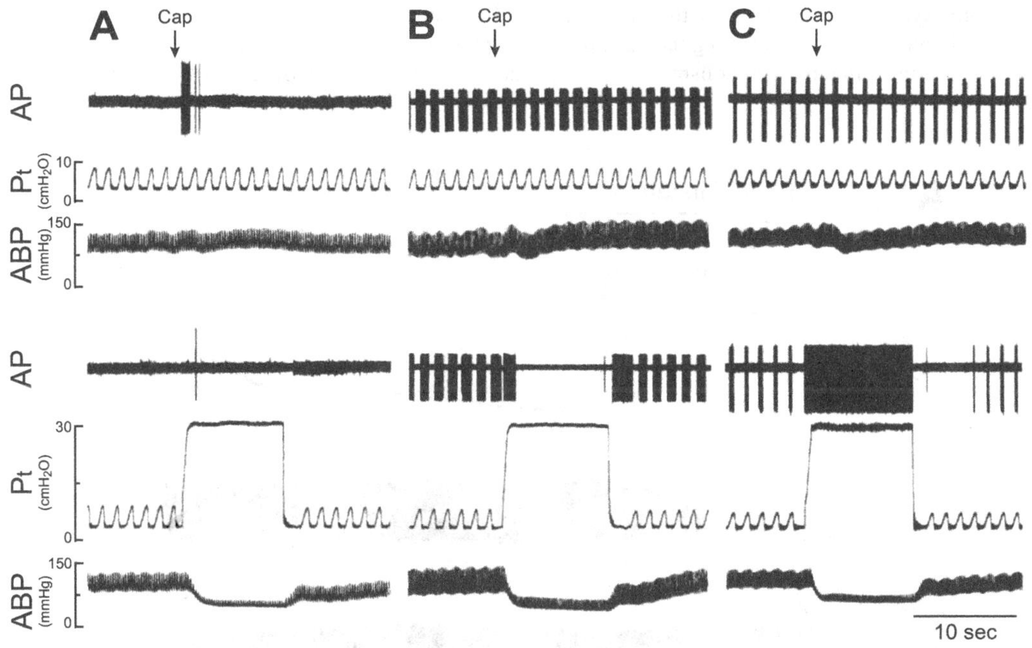


Figure 13–2 Responses to chemical and mechanical stimulation in different subtypes of vagal afferent nerves that innervate the airways and lungs. *A:* Chemical stimuli, such as capsaicin (CAP) vigorously activate C-fiber afferents with unmyelinated axons (*top 3 traces*); but these afferent are relatively insensitive to changes in airway intraluminal pressures (*bottom 3 traces*). *B:* Rapidly adapting receptors (RARs) are insensitive to CAP (*top 3 traces*) but are activated by changes in airway luminal pressure (*bottom 3 traces*). Note that these afferents quickly adapt and cease firing with sustained lung hyperinflation. *C:* Slowly adapting receptors (SARs) are insensitive to CAP (*top 3 traces*) but are vigorously activated in a non-adapting manner by lung inflation and positive luminal airway pressure (*bottom 3 traces*). Also note that RARs and SARs are tonically active at eupnea and thus regulate baseline autonomic outflow to multiple organs, including the airways. These representative traces are from experiments performed on more than 10 anesthetized, paralyzed rats with open chests. ABP, blood pressure; AP, action potentials; PT, tracheal pressure. Reproduced from Ho et al. (2001)[65], with permission.

since the responses were abolished by administering a histamine $H_1$ receptor antagonist into the fourth ventricle. In a subsequent study in anesthetized, paralyzed, and artificially ventilated rabbits, hyperthermia replicated the effects of hypothalamic stimulation[74]. Microdialysis experiments confirmed that histamine was released in the nucleus of the solitary tract (NTS), raphé magnus, and the rostral ventrolateral medulla (RVLM) during hyperthermia. Microinjection of a histamine $H_1$ receptor antagonist into the RVLM almost abolished the effects of hyperthermia on tracheal and vascular tone.

The reflex described above suggests that sympathetic nerves supplying the airways and sympathetic nerves supplying the extrapulmonary vasculature are activated in a similar fashion in response to posterior hypothalamic stimulation or hyperthermia, but this may not always be the case[113]. Following vagotomy and pre-contraction of the trachealis with histamine, aerosol administration of capsaicin into the lower airways evoked a pronounced fall in tracheal smooth muscle tone (Figure 13–3). This relaxation was abolished by pretreatment with propranolol, hexamethonium, tetrodotoxin applied topically to the tracheal mucosa, extrinsic (efferent) denervation of the trachea, or sectioning the dorsal roots of thoracic spinal segments 1 through 4. The pronounced fall in tracheal tone occurred independently of any changes in heart rate or blood pressure. The dissociation of the effects on airway and systemic vasculature was not due to a subtlety of the cardiovascular response, because asphyxia, which produced a comparable propranolol-sensitive fall in tracheal tone, evoked a profound increase in heart rate and blood pressure. Hence, activation of capsaicin-sensitive sensory nerves innervating the airways and lungs can selectively increase non-vasomotor sympathetic outflow to the airways. These same afferent nerves may also regulate sympathetic reflexes during pulmonary embolism.

Interestingly, systemically administered tachykinin receptor antagonists also abolished the airway sympathetic reflex evoked by aerosol administration of

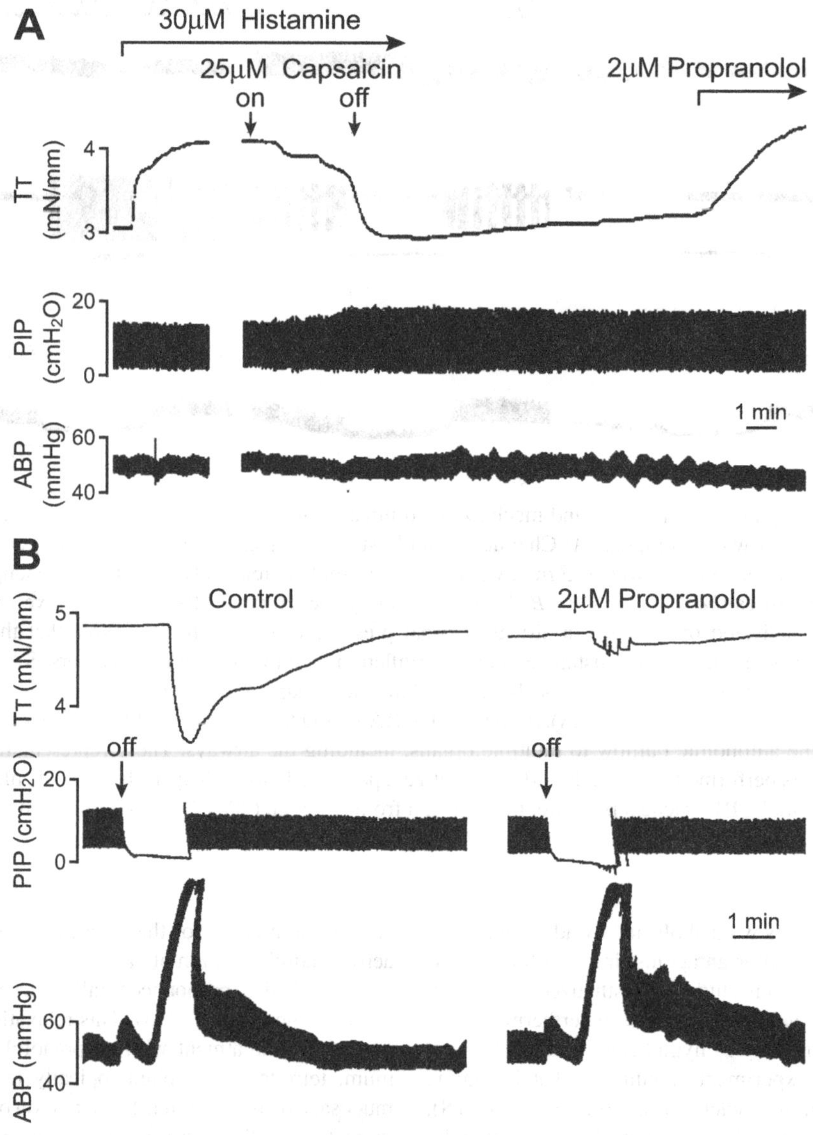


Figure 13–3 Responses of the guinea-pig trachealis to reflexes mediated by sympathetic nerves Isometric tracheal tension (TT) in a segment of the in situ extrathoracic trachea of an anesthetized, paralyzed, vagotomized, mechanically ventilated guinea-pig. *A:* Capsaicin inhalation for four minutes evoked a nearly complete reversal of a histamine-induced contraction of the in situ trachealis. This relaxation was completely reversed by the β-adrenoceptor antagonist propranolol and was prevented by ganglionic blockade or extrinsic denervation of the trachealis (*not shown*). Note that the capsaicin aerosol had no effect on arterial blood pressure (ABP). *B:* Hypoxia/hypercapnea evoked by shutting the ventilator off for 90 seconds produced a profound reversal of the histamine-evoked contraction, accompanied by a sharp increase in both ABP and heart rate (*not shown*). Pretreatment with propranolol abolished the effect on the histamine-evoked contraction but did not affect the cardiovascular response. PIP, pulmonary inflation pressure. Reproduced from Oh et al. (2006)[116], with permission.

capsaicin[113]. Parallel retrograde tracing and electrophysiological and immunohistochemical analyses showed that the majority of sensory nerves supplying the airways and lungs of guinea pigs were capsaicin-sensitive and immunoreactive for substance P. Perhaps tachykinins augment synaptic transmission in the spinal cord and thus augment basal sympathetic outflow to the airways. This may account for the selective effects of inhaled capsaicin on airway sympathetic nerves.

Vagal afferents also regulate the activity of sympathetic vasomotor nerves[5,7,43,64,76,77,134,149]. Electrical stimulation of the central cut end of the vagus nerve following bilateral vagotomy has been shown to evoke a pronounced propranolol-sensitive relaxation of the pre-contracted trachealis *in situ*, which commenced only after the stimulation had ceased[113]. These relaxations were accompanied by a characteristic fall in blood pressure followed by a rebound increase in blood pressure that coincided with relaxation of the tracheal smooth muscle. The vagal pathways that regulate alterations in airway sympathetic outflow have not been characterized.

## TERMINATION SITES OF AIRWAY VAGAL AFFERENT NEURONS IN THE BRAINSTEM

Neuroanatomical tract tracing studies indicate that the majority of vagal afferent neurons innervating the airways and lungs terminate in the NTS[44,54,69,70,88]. Other brainstem locations directly innervated by vagal afferent nerves, including the area postrema and the dorsal motor nucleus of the vagus (dorsal vagal nucleus [DVN]), receive far less direct synaptic input from sensory neurons. Terminations are primarily ipsilateral in the rostral portions of the NTS, whereas contralateral terminations are more common in the commissural subnucleus of the NTS and in NTS subnuclei at the level of the obex; i.e., the caudal-most point of the fourth ventricle. The terminations of airway and non-airway vagal afferent nerves overlap extensively in NTS (see also Chapter. 2), and there is direct evidence for convergent afferent input to second-order NTS neurons, particularly in the commissural subnucleus[97,99,105,117,118,137,143]. Not surprisingly, then, reflex bronchospasm and/or mucus secretion is evoked, not only by activation of bronchopulmonary C-fibers and rapidly adapting receptors, but also by vagal afferent nerves innervating the esophagus, heart, and stomach[15,18,41,96,97]. Similarly, activation of vagal afferents innervating the airways initiates changes in heart rate and basal sympathetic nerve activity[2,24,76,77]. There is also ample divergence of CNS termination sites to account for the distinct reflexes reliably evoked in response to stimuli selective for the various subtypes of afferent nerves[88].

Patterns of termination for the various subtypes of bronchopulmonary vagal afferents have been described. C-fibers, which represent the majority of vagal afferents that innervate the airways and lungs, terminate extensively and often bilaterally in the NTS, particularly in the commissural and medial subnuclei[12,88,89,97]. Rapidly adapting receptors also terminate in caudal locations in the NTS, including the commissural and medial subnuclei[27,72,73,88]. Slowly adapting receptors terminate primarily ipsilateral to their vagal side of origin, rostral to obex in the lateral and interstitial subnuclei of the NTS[13,28,37,71,88].

## BRAINSTEM ORIGIN OF AIRWAY PARASYMPATHETIC PREGANGLIONIC NERVES

Since reflexes differentially regulate the parasympathetic post-ganglionic cholinergic and non-cholinergic nerves that control airway smooth muscle tone[65,96], it follows that distinct populations of preganglionic neurons almost certainly control these opposing effects at the end organs[19,91]. Functional and tract tracing studies have identified parasympathetic preganglionic neurons with cell bodies in the nucleus ambiguus that regulate cholinergic contractions of airway smooth muscle in dogs and guinea pigs (Figure 13–4)[21,44,45,47,51,55,79,95,111]. The preganglionic nerves that innervate airway non-cholinergic parasympathetic post-ganglionic neurons may be unmyelinated and originate from a distinct location in the nucleus ambiguus or may be derived from the DVN[19,91]. Subtypes of parasympathetic preganglionic neurons in the nucleus ambiguus have not been identified[54,55,100]. Neurons in the DVN have been retrogradely labeled from the airways and from the neuronal plexuses containing the cholinergic and non-cholinergic parasympathetic post-ganglionic neurons. However, airway DVN neurons are far outnumbered by the neurons in the nucleus ambiguus that project to the airways[44,54,70,121]. To date, no function has been ascribed to the preganglionic neurons with cell bodies in the DVN[55,81]. A relaxant innervation of the airways from the DVN would parallel a relaxant innervation of the stomach and esophagus from the DVN[87,130]. In the guinea pig at least, the non-cholinergic parasympathetic post-ganglionic nerves regulating non-adrenergic relaxations of airway smooth muscle emanate from the adjacent esophagus[19,38].

There is circumstantial evidence both for and against the hypotheses that parasympathetic reflexes differentially regulate different airway segments and that the right and left vagus nerves differentially

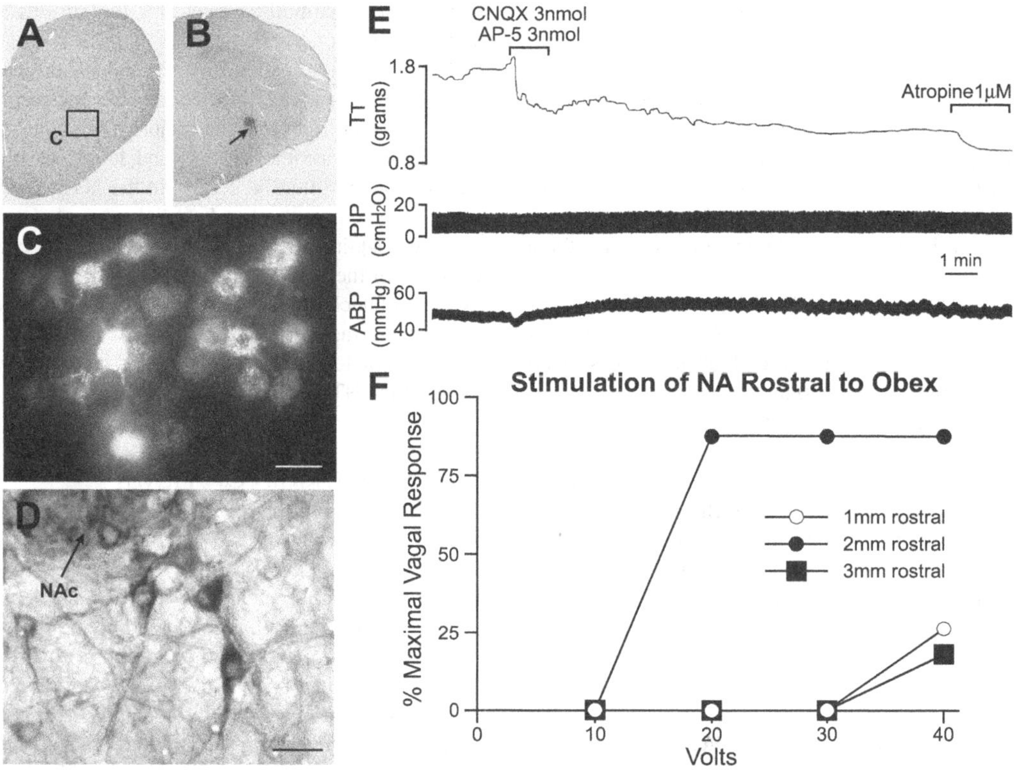


Figure 13–4 Cholinergic contractions of the guinea pig trachea regulated by parasympathetic preganglionic neurons in the nucleus ambiguus. *A:* Section of the guinea-pig brainstem, approximately 2 mm rostral to obex (the caudal-most point of the fourth ventricle). The boxed area shows the location of nucleus ambiguus and the location of preganglionic parasympathetic nerves projecting to the trachea. *B:* Section of the rat brainstem approximately 2 mm rostral to obex stained to show immunoreactivity for choline acetyltransferase, which is present in all parasympathetic preganglionic neurons. Nucleus ambiguus neurons are located bilaterally in the ventrolateral medulla and are stained black. The boxed area is shown at higher magnification in *D*. Bar, 0.5 mm. *C:* Neurons in the NA are retrogradely labeled after injection of the tracer, DiI, into the guinea-pig trachealis. Scale bar, 40 μm. *D:* Parasympathetic preganglionic neurons in NA showing immunoreactivity for choline acetyltransferase. Three neurons lie ventral to the nucleus ambiguus pars compacta (NAc), where neurons are packed so tightly that it is impossible to appreciate the structure of their dendrites. Bar, 50 μm. *E:* Bilateral microinjection of an NMDA receptor antagonist (AP-5) plus a non-NMDA receptor antagonist (CNQX) into the NA at about 2 mm rostral to the obex substantially reduces cholinergic tone in the guinea-pig trachea in situ. ABP, arterial blood pressure; PIP, pulmonary inflation pressure; TT, tracheal tension. *F:* Cholinergic contractions of the guinea-pig trachealis measured in an isolated innervated trachea/ brainstem preparation with extrinsic innervation of the trachea intact and attached to the brainstem. A concentric bipolar electrode was placed stereotaxically into various locations within the NA and electrical stimulation of increasing voltage was applied. Cholinergic contractions evoked by NA stimulation were compared with the response obtained from stimulating the vagus nerve. The contractions were most reliably evoked from areas identified by tracing and microinjection studies to be the likely origin of the parasympathetic preganglionic-neurons regulating cholinergic contractions of the trachealis; i.e., approximately 2 mm rostral to obex. *E* reproduced from Mazzone and Canning (2002)[97], with permission.

regulate the airways[19,44,54,85,95,96,111]. It is unclear what possible physiological role these differences would play in adult vertebrates, which have roughly symmetrical lungs that move air by creating pressure gradients in the airways secondary to changes in thoracic volume and not by peristaltic contractions of smooth muscle (as in amphibians). In general, for mammals, reflexes that alter tracheal/extrathoracic smooth muscle tone also alter bronchial/intrathoracic airway caliber. Gap junctions between neurons in the nucleus ambiguus that project to the airways may be one way in which airway tone is coordinated throughout the airways[139].

It is not known whether distinct subpopulations of parasympathetic preganglionic neurons regulate airway smooth muscle, smooth muscle of the bronchial and pulmonary vasculature, and mucus glands. For the most part, the effects of parasympathetic reflexes occur simultaneously in all of these end-organ targets in the airway wall[18,25,29,31,47,48,53,58,96,97,122,123,124,133,146,156]. The lack of effect on airway caliber of DVN lesions led to the speculation that the DVN may specifically regulate mucus secretion in the airways[81]. However, this now seems unlikely[47].

## BRAINSTEM PATHWAYS THAT REGULATE AIRWAY AUTONOMIC TONE

The brainstem networks that control airway autonomic tone are largely unknown and unstudied. Nearly all of the literature on this topic relates only to cholinergic parasympathetic nerves supplying the airways. No aspect of CNS regulation of the activity of noncholinergic parasympathetic nerves supplying the airways has been studied, and only one study indirectly related to airway sympathetic nerve activity has been published. Even the CNS pathways that regulate cholinergic parasympathetic nerves innervating the airways are poorly described. For example, unlike for cardiac, esophageal, laryngeal, and gastric parasympathetic pathways[1,40,61,62], no studies have directly demonstrated that NTS relay neurons receiving afferent input from the airways project directly to the parasympathetic preganglionic neurons that regulate airway function. Monosynaptic reflexes, such as those that have been described for the gastrointestinal tract[128], have also not been described or even studied for the airways.

The limited information that is available on the brainstem regulation of airway autonomic tone suggests a complex and interconnected system with multiple parallel, and either opposing, additive, or synergistic pathways that increase or decrease autonomic outflow to the airways (Figure 13–5)[55]. Tracing studies using pseudorabies virus have confirmed the extensive network of airway vagal afferent endings in the NTS and a preponderance of projections of airway parasympathetic preganglionic neurons projecting from the nucleus ambiguus[44,54]. Second-order transneuronal viral labeling was found in the hypothalamus, midbrain, pons, and brainstem nuclei, including ventral medullary raphé nuclei, the A5 noradrenergic cell group, the locus coeruleus, and the Kölliker-Fuse nucleus. Anatomical and electrophysiological studies of second-order NTS neurons that receive slowly and rapidly adapting receptor input from the airways have confirmed projections to nucleus ambiguus and to adjacent ipsilateral and contralateral NTS subnuclei[37,88,114,115]. Anatomical studies of second-order NTS neurons that receive input from bronchopulmonary C-fibers have not been conducted.

Functional studies confirm the complexity and interconnectivity of the groups of CNS neurons that regulate the tone of airway smooth muscle implied from the anatomical analyses described above. Neurons in the paraventricular nucleus of the hypothalamus project directly to the nucleus ambiguus and elsewhere in the brainstem[78]. Hypothalamic stimulation evokes either an increase or a decrease in the activity of airway parasympathetic nerves, depending on the specific stimulation site[10,66,144]. Neurons in the periaqueductal gray that release $\gamma$-aminobutyric acid (GABA) also project to the nucleus ambiguus, and their activation initiates withdrawal of airway parasympathetic tone[60]. Serotonergic neurons from the medullary raphé nuclei and noradrenergic neurons in the locus coeruleus may also innervate airway parasympathetic preganglionic neurons in the nucleus ambiguus[50]. Thus, stimulation of medullary raphé produces withdrawal of cholinergic tone that is prevented by microinjection of a serotonin receptor antagonist into the nucleus ambiguus, while locus coeruleus stimulation produces an $\alpha_2$-adrenoceptor-dependent withdrawal of airway cholinergic tone that is accompanied by noradrenaline release in the nucleus ambiguus[56].

Interactions within and between NTS subnuclei also regulate airway autonomic function. Neurons that receive input from slowly adapting receptors project to the parabrachial nucleus[33,37]. The airway dilatation associated with the Hering-Breuer reflex, which depends on slowly adapting receptors and occurs through a withdrawal of cholinergic nerve activity, is inhibited by glutamate receptor antagonists microinjected into the parabrachial nucleus[110]. Pump cells, another subpopulation of neurons that receive input from slowly adapting receptors, project to subnuclei in the caudal NTS. These projections from pump cells overlap with the terminals of rapidly adapting receptors and bronchopulmonary C-fibers[37]. Electrophysiological studies show that activation of pump cells inhibits synaptic transmission at second-order NTS neurons with rapidly adapting receptor

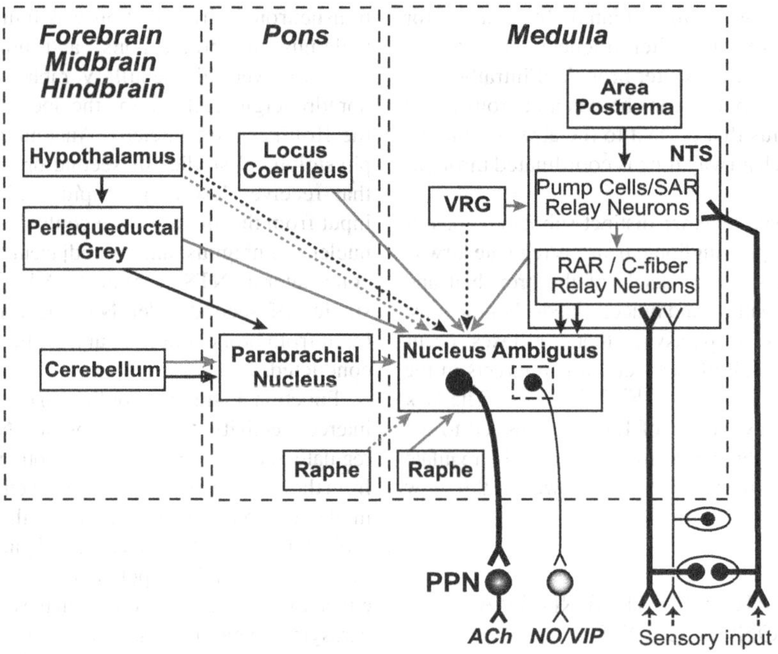


Figure 13–5 Central neural circuitry regulating the parasympathetic innervation of the airways. The *black lines* indicate excitatory pathways while the *gray lines* are inhibitory pathways. Pathways with direct evidence for a role in regulating the activity of airway parasympathetic nerves are indicated by *solid lines*. Pathways with only circumstantial evidence for a role in regulating airway parasympathetic nerves are indicated by dotted *lines*. The precise location of the cell bodies for the parasympathetic preganglionic neurons that regulate non-cholinergic relaxations has not been firmly established. Functional studies in cats and guinea pigs suggest, that, in contrast to the parasympathetic preganglionic nerves mediating contractions of airway smooth muscle, the parasympathetic preganglionic nerves mediating relaxations are unmyelinated. See text for further details. ACh, acetylcholine; NO, nitric oxide; NTS, nucleus of the solitary tract; PPN, parasympathetic preganglionic neuron; RAR, rapidly adapting receptor; SAR, slowly adapting receptors; VIP, vasoactive intestinal peptide; VRG, ventral respiratory group.

input through the release of GABA and possibly glycine[35]. Conversely, pump cells are innervated by neurons of the ventral respiratory group, which regulates generation of central respiratory rhythm and apparently also pump cell activity[107].

Although there is no direct evidence for an effect on airway function, neurons in the nucleus ambiguus may reciprocally regulate neurons in the rostral and caudal ventrolateral medulla that, in turn, regulate both sympathetic and parasympathetic nerve function[102,103]. Other likely projections and nuclei that regulate the activity of airway autonomic nerves include the area postrema, the spinal trigeminal nuclei, the cerebellum, ascending spinal tracts, and several forebrain and midbrain nuclei[11,15,35,45,52,55,57,93,101,109,116,119,132,135]. Although not yet directly studied, cortical structures almost certainly regulate airway autonomic tone and function.

## AUTONOMIC REGULATION OF THE AIRWAYS AT REST

Cholinergic and non-cholinergic parasympathetic nerves and noradrenergic sympathetic nerves are tonically active at eupnea[8,15,47,63,67,82,83,84,106,111,113,146,153]. This explains the marked dilatation of the airways evoked by anti-cholinergic drugs and the constrictions and contractions evoked when β-adrenoceptors are blocked or nitric oxide synthase is inhibited[15,82,83,96,97,106,113]. Basal cholinergic tone is readily demonstrable in all species, while basal noradrenergic and non-noradrenergic relaxant tone is highly variable even within species. Ganglionic blockade (all preganglionic neurons that regulate the airways are cholinergic [Figure 13–4][19,55,80,113]), preganglionic nerve transection, or vagal cooling effectively abolish all baseline cholinergic tone in airway smooth muscle, indicating that basal activity in these nerves requires ongoing preganglionic input arising from the CNS[15,59,82,83,84,95,96,146].

The mechanisms that regulate basal autonomic tone in the airways are not fully understood. The few published studies addressing this issue have primarily focused on cholinergic innervation of the airways. From these studies, it seems clear that vagal afferent nerves play an essential role in regulating basal cholinergic tone[59,67,82,83]. CNS pathways also regulate autonomic outflow to the airways both at rest and upon reflex activation[15,52,55,84], and central regulation of airway autonomic tone may be closely coupled to central respiratory rhythm generation. For example, Mitchell and colleagues[106] (Figure 13–6), studied baseline cholinergic tone in the airways of anesthetized and paralyzed cats and noted an inspiratory rhythm in smooth muscle tone, which increased or decreased as integrated phrenic nerve activity increased or decreased in response to various interventions (e.g., sodium cyanide, positive end-expiratory pressure, hyperventilation, inhalation of $CO_2$). These data led to the conclusion that basal cholinergic tone was coupled to central respiratory drive[106]. Consistent with this notion, Roberts et al.[129] found evidence for a basal level of tone in the trachea of dogs that was insensitive to cooling of vagal afferent nerves. However, some studies show independent regulation of breathing and baseline cholinergic tone in the airways[6,31,49,140].

Basal activity in the multiple autonomic pathways innervating the airways, and their dependence on ongoing activity in sensory afferent nerves innervating the airways, has several functional consequences. Thus, contractions and relaxations can be mediated reflexively either by augmenting or by withdrawing activity in one of these opposing afferent and efferent neuronal pathways[18,82,96,106,127,129,141,144]. In addition, reflex effects initiated by activation of afferent nerves or by CNS pathways regulating autonomic outflow must integrate into a tonically active system. This can have a profound influence over the resulting effects measured in the airways and lungs[31,49,97,140,141].

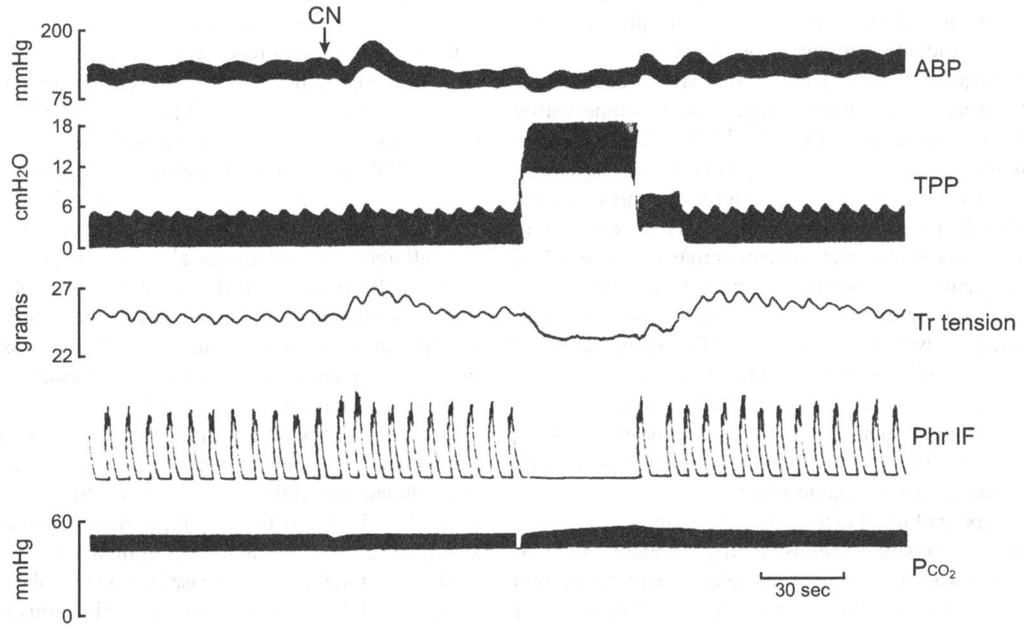


Figure 13–6 Inspiratory rhythm of airway cholinergic tone in the cat. Blood pressure (ABP; *top trace*), transpulmonary pressure (TPP; *second trace* from the top), isometric tracheal tension (Tr tension; *third trace* from the top), phrenic nerve activity (Phr IF; *fourth trace* from the top); and expiratory $CO_2$ ($P_{CO2}$; *bottom trace*) were monitored in an anesthetized, paralyzed cat ventilated by forced oscillation. Changes in central respiratory drive were evoked by intravenous administration of sodium cyanide (CN) and by the Hering-Breuer reflex, induced by increasing end expiratory pressure. Note that TPP and tracheal tension increased during peak phrenic nerve activity and fell during a central apnea induced by positive end expiratory pressure. Reproduced from Michell et al. (1985)[109], with permission.

Attributing reflex effects to activation of any single type of afferent nerve should be done cautiously, given the many converging and parallel inputs that regulate basal and evoked alterations in the tone of airway smooth muscle. The highly predictable presence and level of basal tone in the airways of all species studied to date also suggest the existence of a "set point" for smooth muscle contraction, perhaps optimized such that a withdrawal or augmentation of tone can be rapidly achieved in response to physiological and pathophysiological stimuli. In this way, alterations in afferent or efferent nerve function may contribute to airways' hyper-responsiveness and airways' obstruction in diseases such as asthma and chronic obstructive pulmonary disease[15].

## BRAINSTEM SYNAPTIC MECHANISMS THAT REGULATE AIRWAY PARASYMPATHETIC NEURONS

Neurotransmission at the synapses between identified vagal sensory neurons innervating the airways and the second-order NTS neurons that receive their input has been studied using physiological and electrophysiological methods. Electrophysiological analyses identify glutamate acting at both *N*-methyl-D-aspartate (NMDA) and non-NMDA receptors as the primary transmitter of vagal afferents innervating the airways (Figure 13–7)[4,11,23,36,59,75,154]. The actions of glutamate are mediated primarily through non-NMDA receptors at vagal afferent synapses in the NTS. Nitric oxide released in the NTS secondary to activation of glutamate receptors may enhance, while presynaptic metabotropic glutamate receptors may attenuate or modulate, the actions of glutamate during airway reflexes[20,22,42,92]. Glutamate acting at NMDA and non-NMDA receptors has also been implicated at synapses in the nucleus ambiguus, the parabrachial nucleus, and the hypothalamus in studies on the role of these brain structures in regulating airway parasympathetic tone[47,51,79,95,111]. Other transmitters, including tachykinins, serotonin, noradrenaline, adenosine, adenosine triphosphate, GABA, angiotensin, calcitonin gene-related peptide, carbon monoxide, and ligands for the transient receptor potential vanilloid type 1 receptor, may also regulate synaptic transmission in the NTS and consequently airway autonomic reflexes[32,42,50,55,56,68,69,74,98,120,145,150].

As mentioned above, the tachykinins substance P and neurokinin A acting at neurokinin-1, neurokinin-2 and neurokinin-3 receptors may play a role in modulating or mediating synaptic transmission at synapses made by bronchopulmonary C-fibers in the NTS[18,90,97,98,99,113]. The many tachykinin-containing afferent neurons that innervate the airways of several species and convey information to the brain through the vagus or via spinal pathways may not co-release glutamate, so their primary transmitters may indeed be tachykinins[90,97,108,113,147]. Surprisingly, a role for endogenous tachykinins in mediating or even modulating synaptic transmission at NTS neurons that receive input from the airways has not been evident in most electrophysiological studies[23,59,154]. It is unclear why such disparate effects of the tachykinin receptor antagonists are seen in these functional and electrophysiological studies. Perhaps tachykinins are co-released with glutamate and simply facilitate synaptic transmission and thus amplify reflex effects[15,58,99,112]. This amplification may not be evident when a single synapse is studied over short stimulation periods or when the solitary tract is stimulated with single pulses. Alternatively, the time-course and intensity of stimulation required for reflexes evoked through vagal afferent pathways may not be reliably mimicked when studies are performed in slices using patch-clamp recordings and electrical stimulation of the solitary tract, or when intracellular or extracellular recordings are made *in vivo* or *in vitro* during transient afferent nerve stimulation.

There is evidence that airway afferent sensory neurons as well as baroreceptors and perhaps afferent nerves supplying the pharynx and esophagus provide convergentsynapticinputstoNTSneurons[15,97,105,117,137,143]. Functional studies are consistent with the hypothesis that multiple populations of vagal afferents converge in the NTS to regulate airway parasympathetic reflexes. For example, stimulation of both gastric and esophageal afferent nerves initiates airway parasympathetic reflexes. Both anatomical and electrophysiological data are consistent with the hypothesis that gastric and esophageal afferents terminate in NTS locations that overlap with and/or are adjacent to regions where airway afferent nerves terminate[15,41,96].

Different types of sensory nerves innervating the airways may also converge centrally to regulate airway parasympathetic reflexes (Figure 13–8). Capsaicin applied topically to the laryngeal mucosa evoked a slowly developing but long-lasting increase in airway cholinergic tone[97]. This increase in tone was abolished by laryngeal denervation or topical application of capsazepine, an antagonist at transient receptor potential vanilloid type 1 receptors, and mimicked by the C-fiber stimulants, bradykinin, and 15-hydroxyeicosatetraenoic acid, which also work entirely or partly through activation of the transient receptor potential vanilloid type 1 receptor. Antagonists at the neurokinin-1, -2, or -3 receptor applied topically to the tracheal and laryngeal mucosa did not affect this reflex, whereas atropine completely reversed the reflex and also abolished

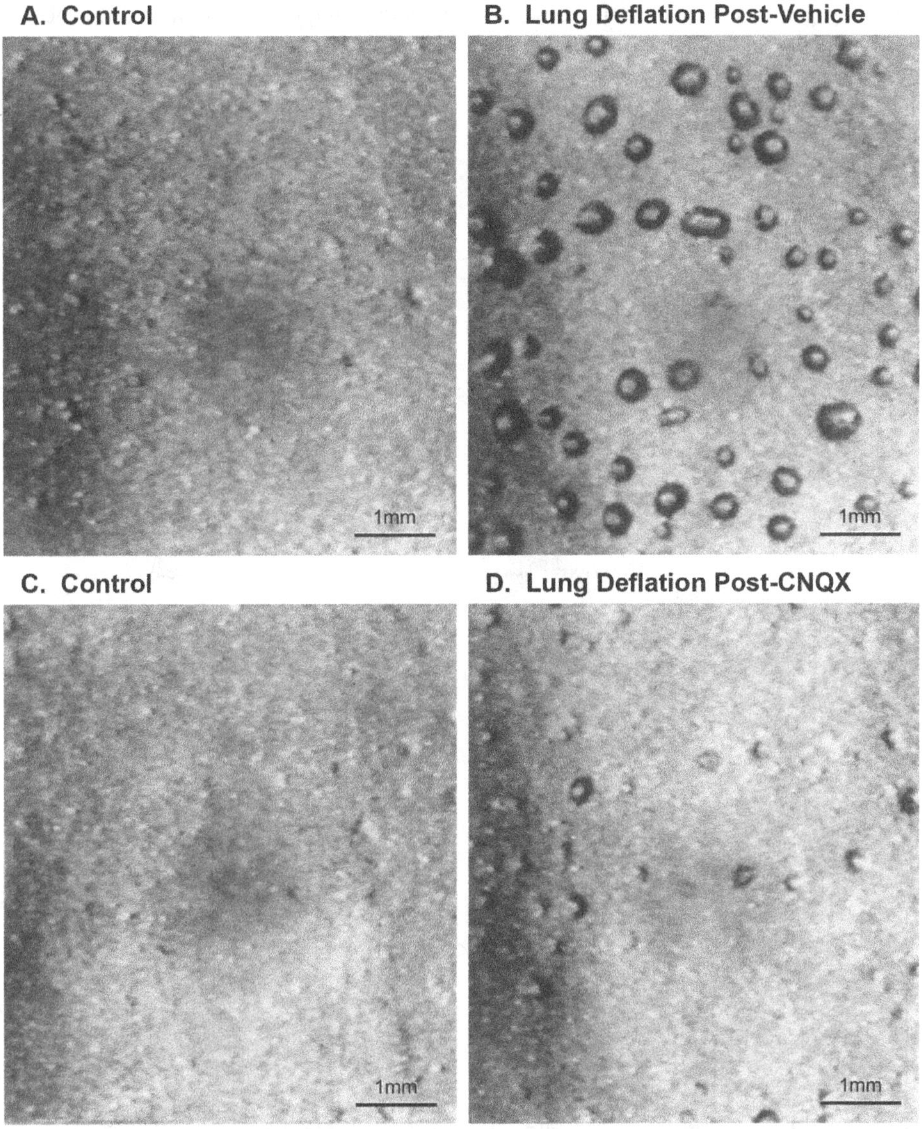


Figure 13–7 Reflex mucus secretion mediated by parasympathetic nerves in the dog trachea Photomicrographs were taken before. (*A*) and after (*B*) activation of rapidly adapting receptors induced by lung deflation. Mucus hillocks on the tracheal mucosa were produced in situ and then photographed one minute after visualization with tantalum. *C* and *D:* similarly prepared mucosa from dogs treated with the non-NMDA receptor antagonist CNQX into the fourth ventricle before lung deflation. Reproduced from Haxhiu at al. (2000)[48], with permission.

basal cholinergic tone in the trachea. Because basal cholinergic tone in the airways is absolutely dependent upon ongoing activity in vagal afferents innervating the intrapulmonary airways and lungs[82], it is possible that challenge with laryngeal capsaicin reflexly increases airway parasympathetic tone by amplifying the synaptic transmission that regulates baseline cholinergic tone. Consistent with this hypothesis, selective denervation of the intrapulmonary airways, which leaves intact the afferent and efferent innervation of the trachea and larynx, completely abolishes the increases in tracheal cholinergic tone evoked by laryngeal application of capsaicin. Pharmacological studies implicated tachykinins in this capsaicin-evoked reflex because intracerebroventricular administration of tachykinin receptor antagonists had no effect on baseline cholinergic tone but prevented or reversed the reflex effects initiated by laryngeal capsaicin challenge.

Results from studies on the synergistic interactions between bradykinin, which stimulates C-fiber afferents, and histamine, which stimulates rapidly adapting receptors, on airway cholinergic tone are consistent with the interpretation of the reflex evoked by laryngeal capsaicin described above[97]. Central administration of substance P mimicked the effects of laryngeal capsaicin on cholinergic tone. As with the reflex response to laryngeal capsaicin, centrally administered neurokinin receptor antagonists prevented the enhancement of cholinergic tone evoked by histamine. A conventional dual tracing study from the airways and brainstem identified discrete locations in the commissural subnucleus of the NTS as potential sites of airway C-fiber and rapidly adapting receptor

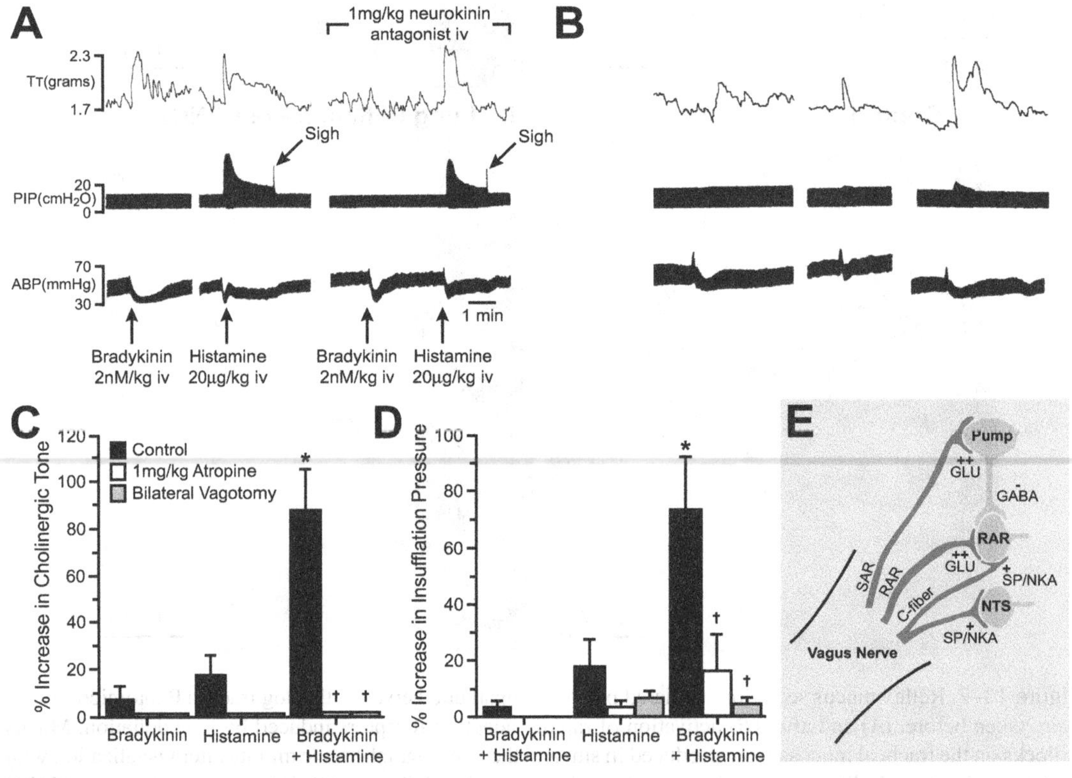


Figure 13–8 Parasympathetic cholinergic reflexes evoked by histamine and bradykinin in anesthetized guinea-pigs. *A:* Reflex tracheal contractions evoked by intravenously administered histamine and bradykinin in the absence and presence of neurokinin receptor antagonists in anesthetized, paralyzed, mechanically ventilated guinea pigs. Bradykinin evokes parasympathetic reflexes secondary to activation of tachykinin-containing bronchopulmonary C-fibers. Histamine evokes parasympathetic reflexes indirectly by inducing contractions of the tracheal smooth muscle that activate rapidly adapting receptors. *B:* Synergistic effect of histamine and bradykinin on tracheal cholinergic tone and pulmonary inflation pressure. *C* and *D:* bar histograms summarizing the effects of histamine, bradykinin and histamine+bradykinin on tracheal cholinergic tone and pulmonary inflation pressure, respectively, after various interventions. Data are presented as mean±s.e.m. The results suggest a synergistic interaction between these two autacoids, which activate different types of vagal afferent nerves. *E:* Hypothetical interactions between bronchopulmonary vagal afferent nerve subtypes in NTS. Reproduced from Canning et al. (2001)[18] and Mazzone and Canning (2002)[98,100], with permission

termination and perhaps convergence. More recent studies of cough support a role for synergistic interactions and convergence of airway afferents in the regulation of airway defensive reflexes[99].

The data above suggest that bronchopulmonary C-fibers and rapidly adapting receptors converge centrally in the NTS and synergistically increase cholinergic parasympathetic tone in the airways[15,97,99]. In contrast, slowly adapting receptors may inhibit increases in parasympathetic nerve activity that depend on rapidly adapting receptors. Ezure and colleagues reported that sustained lung inflation, which tonically activates slowly adapting receptors and induces a withdrawal of cholinergic tone[82,106,110,127,129], reduces synaptic transmission in NTS neurons receiving input from rapidly adapting receptors[34]. Subsequent studies showed that pump cells driven by slowly adapting receptors project caudally in the NTS to regions containing second-order neurons with rapidly adapting receptor input[37]. GABA and glycine mediate the pump cell–dependent inhibition of synaptic transmission at the rapidly adapting receptor second-order neurons[35].

## FUTURE DIRECTIONS

Multiple parasympathetic and sympathetic efferent pathways control airway function. Reflexes differentially regulate the activity in these efferent pathways, either increasing or decreasing autonomic drive in response to homeostatic demands or in response to noxious stimulation. Multiple subtypes of sensory afferent neurons regulate airway autonomic reflexes. These afferent and efferent pathways interact centrally through an interconnected neural network involving multiple brainstem, midbrain, and forebrain structures.

Future studies are needed to unravel some of the complexities of airway autonomic control. For example, in essentially every mammalian species, there are opposing excitatory and inhibitory autonomic nerves. Nevertheless, the central preganglionic origins of the excitatory and inhibitory innervation have not been identified for any target tissue in the airways. Interactions between airway sympathetic and parasympathetic pathways have also gone unstudied. What role in airway function, if any, is played by preganglionic neurons in the DVN should also be addressed. Finally, the importance of the autonomic nervous system in diseases of the airways and lung, such as asthma, chronic obstructive pulmonary disease, pulmonary hypertension, neurogenic pulmonary edema, and pulmonary thromboembolism, is obvious. Therefore, understanding how central autonomic control of airway function affects disease outcomes and changes with chronic illness will probably yield insights into novel therapeutic approaches that prevent or limit illness.

ACKNOWLEDGMENTS Dr. Canning's research is supported by a grant from the National Institutes of Health (HL083192).

## References

1. Agassandian, K., Fazan, V. P., Adanina, V., and Talman, W. T. (2002). Direct projections from the cardiovascular nucleus tractus solitarii to pontine preganglionic parasympathetic neurons: A link to cerebrovascular regulation. *Journal of Comparative Neurology* 452, 242–254.
2. Allen, D. A., Schertel, E. R., and Bailey, J. E. (1993). Reflex cardiovascular effects of continuous prostacyclin administration into an isolated in situ lung in the dog. *Journal of Applied Physiology* 74, 2928–2934.
3. Aviado, D. M., Jr., Ling, J. S., and Schmidt, C. F. (1957). Effects of anoxia on pulmonary circulation: Reflex pulmonary vasoconstriction. *American Journal of Physiology* 189, 253–262.
4. Aylwin, M. L., Horowitz, J. M., and Bonham, A. C. (1997). NMDA receptors contribute to primary visceral afferent transmission in the nucleus of the solitary tract. *Journal of Neurophysiology* 77, 2539–2548.
5. Bachoo, M., and Polosa, C. (1987). Properties of the inspiration-related activity of sympathetic preganglionic neurones of the cervical trunk in the cat. *Journal of Physiology* 385, 545–564.
6. Baker, D. G., and Don, H. (1988). Reversal of the relation between respiratory drive and airway tone in cats. *Respiration Physiology* 73, 21–30.
7. Barman, S. M., and Gebber, G. L. (1976). Basis for synchronization of sympathetic and phrenic nerve discharges. *American Journal of Physiology* 231, 1601–1607.
8. Barnes, P. J., and Liu, S. F. (1995). Regulation of pulmonary vascular tone. *Pharmacological Reviews* 47, 87–131.
9. Barthelemy, P., Sabeur, G., and Jammes, Y. (1996). Assessment of an airway-to-pulmonary circulation reflex in cats. *Neuroscience Letters* 211, 89–92.
10. Beyaert, C. A., Hill, J. M., Lewis, B. K., and Kaufman, M. P. (1998). Effect on airway caliber of stimulation of the hypothalamic locomotor region. *Journal of Applied Physiology* 84, 1388–1394.
11. Bonham, A. C., and Hasser, E. M. (1993). Area postrema and aortic or vagal afferents converge to excite cells in nucleus tractus solitarius. *American Journal of Physiology* 264, H1674–H1685.

12. Bonham, A. C., and Joad, J. P. (1991). Neurones in commissural nucleus tractus solitarii required for full expression of the pulmonary C fibre reflex in rat. *Journal of Physiology* 441, 95–112.
13. Bonham, A. C., and McCrimmon, D. R. (1990). Neurones in a discrete region of the nucleus tractus solitarius are required for the Breuer-Hering reflex in rat. *Journal of Physiology* 427, 261–280.
14. Cabezas, G. A., Graf, P. D., and Nadel, J. A. (1971). Sympathetic versus parasympathetic nervous regulation of airways in dogs. *Journal of Applied Physiology* 31, 651–655.
15. Canning, B. J. (2006). Reflex regulation of airway smooth muscle tone. *Journal of Applied Physiology* 101, 971–985.
16. Canning, B. J., and Mazzone, S. B. (2005). Reflexes initiated by activation of the vagal afferent nerves innervating the airways and lungs. In B. J. Undem and D. Weinreich (Eds), *Advances in Vagal Afferent Neurobiology*, pp. 403-430. Boca Raton, Florida: CRC Taylor and Francis.
17. Canning, B. J., Mori, N., and Mazzone, S. B. (2006). Vagal afferent nerves regulating the cough reflex. *Respiratory Physiology and Neurobiology* 152, 223–242.
18. Canning, B. J., Reynolds, S. M., and Mazzone, S. B. (2001). Multiple mechanisms of reflex bronchospasm in guinea pigs. *Journal of Applied Physiology* 91, 2642–2653.
19. Canning, B. J., and Undem, B. J. (1993). Evidence that distinct neural pathways mediate parasympathetic contractions and relaxations of guinea-pig trachealis. *Journal of Physiology* 471, 25–40.
20. Canning, B. J., and Undem, B. J. (1993). Relaxant innervation of the guinea-pig trachealis: Demonstration of capsaicin-sensitive and -insensitive vagal pathways. *Journal of Physiology* 460, 719–739.
21. Chen, C. Y., Ling Eh, E. H., Horowitz, J. M., and Bonham, A. C. (2002). Synaptic transmission in nucleus tractus solitarius is depressed by Group II and III but not Group I presynaptic metabotropic glutamate receptors in rats. *Journal of Physiology* 538, 773–786.
22. Chen, Y., Li, M., Liu, H., and Wang, J. (2007). The airway-related parasympathetic motoneurones in the ventrolateral medulla of newborn rats were dissociated anatomically and in functional control. *Experimental Physiology* 92, 99–108.
23. Chianca, D. A., Jr., Lin, L. H., Dragon, D. N., and Talman, W. T. (2004). NMDA receptors in nucleus tractus solitarii are linked to soluble guanylate cyclase. *American Journal of Physiology. Heart and Circulatory Physiology* 286, H1521–H1527.
24. Chianca, D. A., Jr. and Machado, B. H. (1996). Microinjection of NMDA antagonist into the NTS of conscious rats blocks the Bezold-Jarisch reflex. *Brain Research* 718, 185–188.
25. Clozel, J. P., Roberts, A. M., Hoffman, J. I., Coleridge, H. M., and Coleridge, J. C. (1985). Vagal chemoreflex coronary vasodilation evoked by stimulating pulmonary C-fibers in dogs. *Circulation Research* 57, 450–460.
26. Coleridge, H. M., and Coleridge, J. C. (1994). Neural regulation of bronchial blood flow. *Respiration Physiology* 98, 1–13.
27. Colice, G. L. (1985). Neurogenic pulmonary edema. *Clinics in Chest Medicine* 6, 473–489.
28. Davies, R. O., and Kubin, L. (1986). Projection of pulmonary rapidly adapting receptors to the medulla of the cat: An antidromic mapping study. *Journal of Physiology* 373, 63–86.
29. Davies, R. O., Kubin, L., and Pack, A. I. (1987). Pulmonary stretch receptor relay neurones of the cat: Location and contralateral medullary projections. *Journal of Physiology* 383, 571–585.
30. Davis, B., Chinn, R., Gold, J., Popovac, D., Widdicombe, J. G., and Nadel, J. A. (1982). Hypoxemia reflexly increases secretion from tracheal submucosal glands in dogs. *Journal of Applied Physiology* 52, 1416–1419.
31. Diamond, L., and O'Donnell, M. (1980). A nonadrenergic vagal inhibitory pathway to feline airways. *Science* 208, 185–188.
32. Dickstein, J., Greenberg, A., Kruger, J., Robicsek, A., Silverman, J. A., Sommer, L. Z., Sommer, D. D., Volgyesi, G. A., Iscoe, S., and Fisher, J. A. (1996). PCO2 affects tracheal tone during apnea in anesthetized dogs. *Journal of Applied Physiology* 81, 1184–1189.
33. Doyle, M. W., Bailey, T. W., Jin, Y. H., and Andresen, M. C. (2002). Vanilloid receptors presynaptically modulate cranial visceral afferent synaptic transmission in nucleus tractus solitarius. *Journal of Neuroscience* 22, 8222–8229.
34. Ezure, K. (2004). Respiration-related afferents to parabrachial pontine regions. *Respiratory Physiology and Neurobiology* 143, 167–175.
35. Ezure, K., and Tanaka, I. (2000). Lung inflation inhibits rapidly adapting receptor relay neurons in the rat. *Neuroreport* 11, 1709–1712.
36. Ezure, K., and Tanaka, I. (2004). GABA, in some cases together with glycine, is used as the inhibitory transmitter by pump cells in the Hering-Breuer reflex pathway of the rat. *Neuroscience* 127, 409–417.
37. Ezure, K., Tanaka, I., and Miyazaki, M. (1999). Electrophysiological and pharmacological analysis of synaptic inputs to pulmonary rapidly adapting receptor relay neurons in the rat. *Experimental Brain Research* 128, 471–480.

38. Ezure, K., Tanaka, I., Saito, Y., and Otake, K. (2002). Axonal projections of pulmonary slowly adapting receptor relay neurons in the rat. *Journal of Comparative Neurology* 446, 81–94.
39. Fischer, A., Canning, B. J., Undem, B. J., and Kummer, W. (1998). Evidence for an esophageal origin of VIP-IR and NO synthase-IR nerves innervating the guinea pig trachealis: A retrograde neuronal tracing and immunohistochemical analysis. *Journal of Comparative Neurology* 394, 326–334.
40. Franco-Cereceda, A., Matran, R., Alving, K., and Lundberg, J. M. (1995). Sympathetic vascular control of the laryngeo-tracheal, bronchial and pulmonary circulation in the pig: Evidence for non-adrenergic mechanisms involving neuropeptide Y. *Acta Physiologica Scandinavica* 155, 193–204.
41. Gai, W. P., Messenger, J. P., Yu, Y. H., Gieroba, Z. J., and Blessing, W. W. (1995). Nitric oxide-synthesising neurons in the central subnucleus of the nucleus tractus solitarius provide a major innervation of the rostral nucleus ambiguus in the rabbit. *Journal of Comparative Neurology* 357, 348–361.
42. German, V. F., Corrales, R., Ueki, I. F., and Nadel, J. A. (1982). Reflex stimulation of tracheal mucus gland secretion by gastric irritation in cats. *Journal of Applied Physiology* 52, 1153–1155.
43. Glaum, S. R., and Miller, R. J. (1993). Zinc protoporphyrin-IX blocks the effects of metabotropic glutamate receptor activation in the rat nucleus tractus solitarii. *Molecular Pharmacology* 43, 965–969.
44. Habler, H. J., Janig, W., and Michaelis, M. (1994). Respiratory modulation in the activity of sympathetic neurones. *Progress in Neurobiology* 43, 567–606.
45. Hadziefendic, S., and Haxhiu, M. A. (1999). CNS innervation of vagal preganglionic neurons controlling peripheral airways: A transneuronal labeling study using pseudorabies virus. *Journal of the Autonomic Nervous System* 76, 135–145.
46. Haselton, J. R., Solomon, I. C., Motekaitis, A. M., and Kaufman, M. P. (1992). Bronchomotor vagal preganglionic cell bodies in the dog: An anatomic and functional study. *Journal of Applied Physiology* 73, 1122–1129.
47. Hatridge, J., Haji, A., Perez-Padilla, J. R., and Remmers, J. E. (1989). Rapid shallow breathing caused by pulmonary vascular congestion in cats. *Journal of Applied Physiology* 67, 2257–2264.
48. Haxhiu, M. A., Chavez, J. C., Pichiule, P., Erokwu, B., and Dreshaj, I. A. (2000). The excitatory amino acid glutamate mediates reflexly increased tracheal blood flow and airway submucosal gland secretion. *Brain Research* 883, 77–86.
49. Haxhiu, M. A., Cherniack, N. S., and Strohl, K. P. (1991). Reflex responses of laryngeal and pharyngeal submucosal glands in dogs. *Journal of Applied Physiology* 71, 1669–1673.
50. Haxhiu, M. A., Deal, E. C., and Cherniack, N. S. (1989). Influence of respiratory drive on airway responses to excitation of lung C-fibers. *Journal of Applied Physiology* 67, 203–209.
51. Haxhiu, M. A., Erokwu, B., Bhardwaj, V., and Dreshaj, I. A. (1998). The role of the medullary raphé nuclei in regulation of cholinergic outflow to the airways. *Journal of the Autonomic Nervous System* 69, 64–71.
52. Haxhiu, M. A., Erokwu, B., and Dreshaj, I. A. (1997). The role of excitatory amino acids in airway reflex responses in anesthetized dogs. *Journal of the Autonomic Nervous System* 67, 192–199.
53. Haxhiu, M. A., Erokwu, B. O., and Cherniack, N. S. (1996). The brainstem network involved in coordination of inspiratory activity and cholinergic outflow to the airways. *Journal of the Autonomic Nervous System* 61, 155–161.
54. Haxhiu, M. A., Haxhiu-Poskurica, B., Moracic, V., Carlo, W. A., and Martin, R. J. (1990). Reflex and chemical responses of tracheal submucosal glands in piglets. *Respiration Physiology* 82, 267–277.
55. Haxhiu, M. A., Jansen, A. S., Cherniack, N. S., and Loewy, A. D. (1993). CNS innervation of airway-related parasympathetic preganglionic neurons: A transneuronal labeling study using pseudorabies virus. *Brain Research* 618, 115–134.
56. Haxhiu, M. A., Kc, P., Moore, C. T., Acquah, S. S., Wilson, C. G., Zaidi, S. I., Massari, V. J., and Ferguson, D. G. (2005). Brain stem excitatory and inhibitory signaling pathways regulating bronchoconstrictive responses. *Journal of Applied Physiology* 98, 1961–1982.
57. Haxhiu, M. A., Kc, P., Neziri, B., Yamamoto, B. K., Ferguson, D. G., and Massari, V. J. (2003). Catecholaminergic microcircuitry controlling the output of airway-related vagal preganglionic neurons. *Journal of Applied Physiology* 94, 1999–2009.
58. Haxhiu, M. A., Rust, C. F., Brooks, C., and Kc, P. (2006). CNS determinants of sleep-related worsening of airway functions: Implications for nocturnal asthma. *Respiratory Physiology and Neurobiology* 151, 1–30.
59. Haxhiu, M. A., Van, L. E., and Cherniack, N. S. (1991). Central effects of tachykinin peptide on tracheal secretion. *Respiration Physiology* 86, 405–414.
60. Haxhiu, M. A., Yamamoto, B., Dreshaj, I. A., Bedol, D., and Ferguson, D. G. (2000). Involvement

of glutamate in transmission of afferent constrictive inputs from the airways to the nucleus tractus solitarius in ferrets. *Journal of the Autonomic Nervous System* 80, 22–30.

61. Haxhiu, M. A., Yamamoto, B. K., Dreshaj, I. A., and Ferguson, D. G. (2002). Activation of the midbrain periaqueductal gray induces airway smooth muscle relaxation. *Journal of Applied Physiology* 93, 440–449.
62. Hayakawa, T., Takanaga, A., Maeda, S., Ito, H., and Seki, M. (2000). Monosynaptic inputs from the nucleus tractus solitarii to the laryngeal motoneurons in the nucleus ambiguus of the rat. *Anatomy and Embryology* 202, 411–420.
63. Hayakawa, T., Zheng, J. Q., and Yajima, Y. (1997). Direct synaptic projections to esophageal motoneurons in the nucleus ambiguus from the nucleus of the solitary tract of the rat. *Journal of Comparative Neurology* 381, 18–30.
64. Hennessy, E., White, S., van der Touw, T., Quail, A., Porges, W., and Glenfield, P. (1993). Control of resting bronchial hemodynamics in the awake dog. *American Journal of Physiology* 265, H649–H660.
65. Ho, C. Y., Gu, Q., Lin, Y. S., and Lee, L. Y. (2001). Sensitivity of vagal afferent endings to chemical irritants in the rat lung. *Respiration Physiology* 127, 113–124.
66. Huangfu, D. H., and Guyenet, P. G. (1991). Sympatholytic response to stimulation of superior laryngeal nerve in rats. *American Journal of Physiology* 260, R290–R297.
67. Inoue, H., Ichinose, M., Miura, M., Katsumata, U., and Takishima, T. (1989). Sensory receptors and reflex pathways of nonadrenergic inhibitory nervous system in feline airways. *American Review of Respiratory Disease* 139, 1175–1178.
68. Iwase, M., Kanamaru, M., Kanamaru, A., and Homma, I. (1998). Central histaminergic neurons regulate rabbit tracheal tension through the cervical sympathetic nerve. *Journal of the Autonomic Nervous System* 74, 23–32.
69. Jammes, Y., and Mei, N. (1979). Assessment of the pulmonary origin of bronchoconstrictor vagal tone. *Journal of Physiology* 291, 305–316.
70. Jeggo, R. D., Kellett, D. O., Wang, Y., Ramage, A. G., and Jordan, D. (2005). The role of central 5-HT3 receptors in vagal reflex inputs to neurones in the nucleus tractus solitarius of anaesthetized rats. *Journal of Physiology* 566, 939–953.
71. Kalia, M., Fuxe, K., Hokfelt, T., Johansson, O., Lang, R., Ganten, D., Cuello, C., and Terenius, L. (1984). Distribution of neuropeptide immunoreactive nerve terminals within the subnuclei of the nucleus of the tractus solitarius of the rat. *Journal of Comparative Neurology* 222, 409–444.
72. Kalia, M., and Mesulam, M. M. (1980). Brain stem projections of sensory and motor components of the vagus complex in the cat: II. Laryngeal, tracheobronchial, pulmonary, cardiac, and gastrointestinal branches. *Journal of Comparative Neurology* 193, 467–508.
73. Kalia, M., and Richter, D. (1985). Morphology of physiologically identified slowly adapting lung stretch receptor afferents stained with intra-axonal horseradish peroxidase in the nucleus of the tractus solitarius of the cat. I. A light microscopic analysis. *Journal of Comparative Neurology* 241, 503–520.
74. Kalia, M., and Richter, D. (1988). Rapidly adapting pulmonary receptor afferents: I. Arborization in the nucleus of the tractus solitarius. *Journal of Comparative Neurology* 274, 560–573.
75. Kalia, M., and Richter, D. (1988). Rapidly adapting pulmonary receptor afferents: II. Fine structure and synaptic organization of central terminal processes in the nucleus of the tractus solitarius. *Journal of Comparative Neurology* 274, 574–594.
76. Kanamaru, M., Iwase, M., and Homma, I. (2001). Neuronal histamine release elicited by hyperthermia mediates tracheal dilation and pressor response. *American Journal of Physiology. Regulatory, Integrative and Comparative Physiology* 280, R1748 R1754.
77. Karius, D. R., Ling, L., and Speck, D. F. (1994). Nucleus tractus solitarius and excitatory amino acids in afferent-evoked inspiratory termination. *Journal of Applied Physiology* 76, 1293–1301.
78. Kato, H., Menon, A. S., Chen, F. J., and Slutsky, A. S. (1988). Contribution of pulmonary receptors to the heart rate response to acute hypoxemia in rabbits. *Circulation* 78, 1260–1266.
79. Kaufman, M. P., Iwamoto, G. A., Ashton, J. H., and Cassidy, S. S. (1982). Responses to inflation of vagal afferents with endings in the lung of dogs. *Circulation Research* 51, 525–531.
80. Kc, P., Karibi-Ikiriko, A., Rust, C. F., Jayam-Trouth, A., and Haxhiu, M. A. (2006). Phenotypic traits of the hypothalamic PVN cells innervating airway-related vagal preganglionic neurons. *Respiratory Physiology and Neurobiology* 154, 319–330.
81. Kc, P., and Martin, R. J. (2010). Role of central neurotransmission and chemoreception on airway control. *Respiratory Physiology and Neurobiology*, in press.
82. Kc, P., Mayer, C. A., and Haxhiu, M. A. (2004). Chemical profile of vagal preganglionic motor cells innervating the airways in ferrets: The absence

of noncholinergic neurons. *Journal of Applied Physiology* 97, 1508–1517.
83. Kerr, F. W. (1969). Preserved vagal visceromotor function following destruction of the dorsal motor nucleus. *Journal of Physiology* 202, 755–769.
84. Kesler, B. S., and Canning, B. J. (1999). Regulation of baseline cholinergic tone in guinea-pig airway smooth muscle. *Journal of Physiology* 518 (Pt 3), 843–855.
85. Kesler, B. S., Mazzone, S. B., and Canning, B. J. (2002). Nitric oxide-dependent modulation of smooth-muscle tone by airway parasympathetic nerves. *American Journal of Respiratory and Critical Care Medicine* 165, 481–488.
86. Kondo, T., Kobayashi, I., Hayama, N., Tazaki, G., and Ohta, Y. (2000). Respiratory-related bronchial rhythmic constrictions in the dog with extracorporeal circulation. *Journal of Applied Physiology* 88, 2031–2036.
87. Kondo, T., Kobayashi, I., Hirokawa, Y., Suda, S., Ohta, Y., and Arita, H. (1995). Differences in motor control in the bronchus and extrathoracic trachea. *Journal of the Autonomic Nervous System* 55, 1–8.
88. Kostreva, D. R., Zuperku, E. J., Hess, G. L., Coon, R. L., and Kampine, J. P. (1975). Pulmonary afferent activity recorded from sympathetic nerves. *Journal of Applied Physiology* 39, 37–40.
89. Krowicki, Z. K., and Hornby, P. J. (2000). Substance P in the dorsal motor nucleus of the vagus evokes gastric motor inhibition via neurokinin 1 receptor in rat. *Journal of Pharmacology and Experimental Therapeutics* 293, 214–221.
90. Kubin, L., Alheid, G. F., Zuperku, E. J., and McCrimmon, D. R. (2006). Central pathways of pulmonary and lower airway vagal afferents. *Journal of Applied Physiology* 101, 618–627.
91. Kubin, L., Kimura, H., and Davies, R. O. (1991). The medullary projections of afferent bronchopulmonary C fibres in the cat as shown by antidromic mapping. *Journal of Physiology* 435, 207–228.
92. Kummer, W., Fischer, A., Kurkowski, R., and Heym, C. (1992). The sensory and sympathetic innervation of guinea-pig lung and trachea as studied by retrograde neuronal tracing and double-labellingimmunohistochemistry. *Neuroscience* 49, 715–737.
93. Lama, A., Delpierre, S., and Jammes, Y. (1988). The effects of electrical stimulation of myelinated and non-myelinated vagal motor fibres on airway tone in the rabbit and the cat. *Respiration Physiology* 74, 265–274.
94. Lawrence, A. J., Castillo-Melendez, M., McLean, K. J., and Jarrott, B. (1998). The distribution of nitric oxide synthase-, adenosine deaminase- and neuropeptide Y-immunoreactivity through the entire rat nucleus tractus solitarius: Effect of unilateral nodose ganglionectomy. *Journal of Chemical Neuroanatomy* 15, 27–40.
95. Loewy, A. D. (1991). Forebrain nuclei involved in autonomic control. *Progress in Brain Research* 87, 253–268.
96. Matran, R. (1991). Neural control of lower airway vasculature. Involvement of classical transmitters and neuropeptides. *Acta Physiologica Scandinavica* 601, S1–S54.
97. Mazzone, S. B., and Canning, B. J. (2002). An in vivo guinea pig preparation for studying the autonomic regulation of airway smooth muscle tone. *Autonomic Neuroscience* 99, 91–101.
98. Mazzone, S. B., and Canning, B. J. (2002). Central nervous system control of the airways: Pharmacological implications. *Current Opinion in Pharmacology* 2, 220–228.
99. Mazzone, S. B., and Canning, B. J. (2002). Evidence for differential reflex regulation of cholinergic and noncholinergic parasympathetic nerves innervating the airways. *American Journal of Respiratory and Critical Care Medicine* 165, 1076–1083.
100. Mazzone, S. B., and Canning, B. J. (2002). Synergistic interactions between airway afferent nerve subtypes mediating reflex bronchospasm in guinea pigs. *American Journal of Physiology. Regulatory, Integrative and Comparative Physiology* 283, R86–R98.
101. Mazzone, S. B., and Geraghty, D. P. (1999). Respiratory action of capsaicin microinjected into the nucleus of the solitary tract: Involvement of vanilloid and tachykinin receptors. *British Journal of Pharmacology* 127, 473–481.
102. Mazzone, S. B., Mori, N., and Canning, B. J. (2005). Synergistic interactions between airway afferent nerve subtypes regulating the cough reflex in guinea-pigs. *Journal of Physiology* 569, 559–573.
103. McAllen, R. M., and Spyer, K. M. (1978). Two types of vagal preganglionic motoneurones projecting to the heart and lungs. *Journal of Physiology* 282, 353–364.
104. McCallister, L. W., McCoy, K. W., Connelly, J. C., and Kaufman, M. P. (1986). Stimulation of groups III and IV phrenic afferents reflexly decreases total lung resistance in dogs. *Journal of Applied Physiology* 61, 1346–1351.
105. McKitrick, D. J., and Calaresu, F. R. (1996). Nucleus ambiguus inhibits activity of cardiovascular units in RVLM. *Brain Research* 742, 203–210.
106. McKitrick, D. J., and Calaresu, F. R. (1997). Reciprocal connection between nucleus

ambiguus and caudal ventrolateral medulla. *Brain Research* 770, 213–220.
107. Middendorf, W. F., and Russell, J. A. (1980). Innervation of airway smooth muscle in the baboon: Evidence for a nonadrenergic inhibitory system. *Journal of Applied Physiology* 48, 947–956.
108. Mifflin, S. W. (1996). Convergent carotid sinus nerve and superior laryngeal nerve afferent inputs to neurons in the NTS. *American Journal of Physiology* 271, R870–R880.
109. Mitchell, R. A., Herbert, D. A., and Baker, D. G. (1985). Inspiratory rhythm in airway smooth muscle tone. *Journal of Applied Physiology* 58, 911–920.
110. Miyazaki, M., Arata, A., Tanaka, I., and Ezure, K. (1998). Activity of rat pump neurons is modulated with central respiratory rhythm. *Neuroscience Letters* 249, 61–64.
111. Morris, J. L., Konig, P., Shimizu, T., Jobling, P., and Gibbins, I. L. (2005). Most peptide-containing sensory neurons lack proteins for exocytotic release and vesicular transport of glutamate. *Journal of Comparative Neurology* 483, 1–16.
112. Motekaitis, A. M., and Kaufman, M. P. (1996). Stimulation of the mesencephalic locomotor region constricts the airways of cats. *Respiration Physiology* 106, 263–271.
113. Motekaitis, A. M., Solomon, I. C., and Kaufman, M. P. (1995). Role of the parabrachial nuclei in the airway dilation evoked by the Hering-Breuer reflex. *Brain Research* 671, 314–316.
114. Mueller, P. J., Buckwalter, J. B., and Clifford, P. S. (2004). Tracheal tone and the role of ionotropic glutamate receptors in the nucleus ambiguus. *Brain Research* 1021, 54–62.
115. Mutoh, T., Bonham, A. C., and Joad, J. P. (2000). Substance P in the nucleus of the solitary tract augments bronchopulmonary C fiber reflex output. *American Journal of Physiology. Regulatory, Integrative and Comparative Physiology* 279, R1215–R1223.
116. Oh, E. J., Mazzone, S. B., Canning, B. J., and Weinreich, D. (2006). Reflex regulation of airway sympathetic nerves in guinea-pigs. *Journal of Physiology* 573, 549–564.
117. Otake, K., Ezure, K., Lipski, J., and Wong She, R. B. (1992). Projections from the commissural subnucleus of the nucleus of the solitary tract: An anterograde tracing study in the cat. *Journal of Comparative Neurology* 324, 365–378.
118. Otake, K., Nakamura, Y., Tanaka, I., and Ezure, K. (2001). Morphology of pulmonary rapidly adapting receptor relay neurons in the rat. *Journal of Comparative Neurology* 430, 458–470.
119. Padrid, P. A., Haselton, J. R., and Kaufman, M. P. (1991). Role of caudal ventrolateral medulla in reflex and central control of airway caliber. *Journal of Applied Physiology* 71, 2274–2282.
120. Paton, J. F. (1998). Pattern of cardiorespiratory afferent convergence to solitary tract neurons driven by pulmonary vagal C-fiber stimulation in the mouse. *Journal of Neurophysiology* 79, 2365–2373.
121. Paton, J. F., Li, Y. W., Deuchars, J., and Kasparov, S. (2000). Properties of solitary tract neurons receiving inputs from the sub-diaphragmatic vagus nerve. *Neuroscience* 95, 141–153.
122. Paton, J. F., and Spyer, K. M. (1990). Brain stem regions mediating the cardiovascular responses elicited from the posterior cerebellar cortex in the rabbit. *Journal of Physiology* 427, 533–552.
123. Paton, J. F., Waki, H., Abdala, A. P., Dickinson, J., and Kasparov, S. (2007). Vascular-brain signaling in hypertension: Role of angiotensin II and nitric oxide. *Current Hypertension Reports* 9, 242–247.
124. Perez Fontan, J. J., and Velloff, C. R. (2001). Labeling of vagal motoneurons and central afferents after injection of cholera toxin B into the airway lumen. *American Journal of Physiology. Lung, Cellular and Molecular Physiology* 280, L152–L164.
125. Phipps, R. J., and Richardson, P. S. (1976). The effects of irritation at various levels of the airway upon tracheal mucus secretion in the cat. *Journal of Physiology* 261, 563–581.
126. Pisarri, T. E., Coleridge, J. C., and Coleridge, H. M. (1993). Capsaicin-induced bronchial vasodilation in dogs: Central and peripheral neural mechanisms. *Journal of Applied Physiology* 74, 259–266.
127. Pisarri, T. E., and Giesbrecht, G. G. (1997). Reflex tracheal smooth muscle contraction and bronchial vasodilation evoked by airway cooling in dogs. *Journal of Applied Physiology* 82, 1566–1572.
128. Rapaport, E., Rolston, W. A., and Stern, S. (1977). The role of adrenergic receptor blockade in serotonin-induced changes in the pulmonary circulation. *Journal of Physiology* 273, 83–107.
129. Raupach, T., Bahr, F., Herrmann, P., Luethje, L., Heusser, K., Hasenfuss, G., Bernardi, L., and Andreas, S. (2008). Slow breathing reduces sympathoexcitation in COPD. *European Respiratory Journal* 32, 387–392.
130. Richardson, C. A., Herbert, D. A., and Mitchell, R. A. (1984). Modulation of pulmonary stretch receptors and airway resistance by parasympathetic

efferents. *Journal of Applied Physiology* 57, 1842–1849.
131. Rinaman, L., Card, J. P., Schwaber, J. S., and Miselis, R. R. (1989). Ultrastructural demonstration of a gastric monosynaptic vagal circuit in the nucleus of the solitary tract in rat. *Journal of Neuroscience* 9, 1985–1996.
132. Roberts, A. M., Coleridge, H. M., and Coleridge, J. C. (1988). Reciprocal action of pulmonary vagal afferents on tracheal smooth muscle tension in dogs. *Respiration Physiology* 72, 35–46.
133. Rossiter, C. D., Norman, W. P., Jain, M., Hornby, P. J., Benjamin, S., and Gillis, R. A. (1990). Control of lower esophageal sphincter pressure by two sites in dorsal motor nucleus of the vagus. *American Journal of Physiology* 259, G899–G906.
134. Russell, J. A. (1980). Noradrenergic inhibitory innervation of canine airways. *Journal of Applied Physiology* 48, 16–22.
135. Rybicki, K. J., Longhurst, J. C., and Kaufman, M. P. (1983). Stimulation of splanchnic afferents reflexly relaxes tracheal smooth muscle in dogs. *Journal of Applied Physiology* 55, 427–432.
136. Schultz, H. D., Roberts, A. M., Bratcher, C., Coleridge, H. M., Coleridge, J. C., and Davis, B. (1985). Pulmonary C-fibers reflexly increase secretion by tracheal submucosal glands in dogs. *Journal of Applied Physiology* 58, 907–910.
137. Seals, D. R., Suwarno, N. O., Joyner, M. J., Iber, C., Copeland, J. G., and Dempsey, J. A. (1993). Respiratory modulation of muscle sympathetic nerve activity in intact and lung denervated humans. *Circulation Research* 72, 440–454.
138. Shapiro, R. E., and Miselis, R. R. (1985). The central neural connections of the area postrema of the rat. *Journal of Comparative Neurology* 234, 344–364.
139. Shirai, M., Matsukawa, K., Nishiura, N., and Ninomiya, I. (1995). Effects of baroreceptor reflex on efferent pulmonary sympathetic nerve activity in anesthetized cat. *American Journal of Physiology* 268, R1078–R1083.
140. Silva-Carvalho, L., Paton, J. F., Rocha, I., Goldsmith, G. E., and Spyer, K. M. (1998). Convergence properties of solitary tract neurons responsive to cardiac receptor stimulation in the anesthetized cat. *Journal of Neurophysiology* 79, 2374–2382.
141. Smulders, Y. M. (2000). Pathophysiology and treatment of haemodynamic instability in acute pulmonary embolism: The pivotal role of pulmonary vasoconstriction. *Cardiovascular Research* 48, 23–33.
142. Solomon, I. C., and Dean, J. B. (2002). Gap junctions in $CO_{(2)}$-chemoreception and respiratory control. *Respiratory Physiology and Neurobiology* 131, 155–173.
143. Sorkness, R. L., and Vidruk, E. H. (1986). Ventilatory responses to hypoxia nullify hypoxic tracheal constriction in awake dogs. *Respiration Physiology* 66, 41–52.
144. Stein, J. F., and Widdicombe, J. G. (1975). The interaction of chemo- and mechanoreceptor signals in the control of airway calibre. *Respiration Physiology* 25, 363–376.
145. Stratmann, G., and Gregory, G. A. (2003). Neurogenic and humoral vasoconstriction in acute pulmonary thromboembolism. *Anesthesia and Analgesia* 97, 341–354.
146. Takagi, S., Umezaki, T., and Shin, T. (1995). Convergence of laryngeal afferents with different natures upon cat NTS neurons. *Brain Research Bulletin* 38, 261–268.
147. Tatsuta, H., and Arita, H. (1996). Nonadrenergic relaxation of the cat cervical trachea evoked by stimulation in the lateral hypothalamic area. *Neuroscience Research* 26, 315–322.
148. Torrealba, F. (1992). Calcitonin gene-related peptide immunoreactivity in the nucleus of the tractus solitarius and the carotid receptors of the cat originates from peripheral afferents. *Neuroscience* 47, 165–173.
149. Ueki, I., German, V. F., and Nadel, J. A. (1980). Micropipette measurement of airway submucosal gland secretion. Autonomic effects. *American Review of Respiratory Disease* 121, 351–357.
150. Undem, B. J., Chuaychoo, B., Lee, M. G., Weinreich, D., Myers, A. C., and Kollarik, M. (2004). Subtypes of vagal afferent C-fibres in guinea-pig lungs. *Journal of Physiology* 556, 905–917.
151. Veelken, R., Leonard, M., Stetter, A., Hilgers, K. F., Mann, J. F., Reeh, P. W., Geiger, H., and Luft, F. C. (1997). Pulmonary serotonin 5-HT3-sensitive afferent fibers modulate renal sympathetic nerve activity in rats. *American Journal of Physiology* 272, H979–H986.
152. Verberne, A. J., and Guyenet, P. G. (1992). Medullary pathway of the Bezold-Jarisch reflex in the rat. *American Journal of Physiology* 263, R1195–R1202.
153. Wang, Y., and Ramage, A. G. (2001). The role of central 5-HT(1A) receptors in the control of B-fibre cardiac and bronchoconstrictor vagal preganglionic neurones in anaesthetized cats. *Journal of Physiology* 536, 753–767.
154. Wang, Y., Soukhova, G., Proctor, M., Walker, J., and Yu, J. (2003). Bradykinin causes hypotension by activating pulmonary sympathetic

afferents in the rabbit. *Journal of Applied Physiology* 95, 233–240.

155. Ward, J. K., Barnes, P. J., Springall, D. R., Abelli, L., Tadjkarimi, S., Yacoub, M. H., Polak, J. M., and Belvisi, M. G. (1995). Distribution of human i-NANC bronchodilator and nitric oxide-immunoreactive nerves. *American Journal of Respiratory Cell and Molecular Biology* 13, 175–184.
156. Widdicombe, J. G. (1966). Action potentials in parasympathetic and sympathetic efferent fibres to the trachea and lungs of dogs and cats. *Journal of Physiology* 186, 56–88.
157. Wilson, C. G., Zhang, Z., and Bonham, A. C. (1996). Non-NMDA receptors transmit cardiopulmonary C fibre input in nucleus tractus solitarii in rats. *Journal of Physiology* 496, 773–785.
158. Wine, J. J. (2007). Parasympathetic control of airway submucosal glands: Central reflexes and the airway intrinsic nervous system. *Autonomic Neuroscience* 133, 35–54.
159. Zimmerman, M. P., and Pisarri, T. E. (2000). Bronchial vasodilation evoked by increased lower airway osmolarity in dogs. *Journal of Applied Physiology* 88, 425–432.

14

# Central Control of Gastrointestinal Function

PAMELA J. HORNBY AND PAUL R. WADE

Neurons controlling the gastrointestinal tract integrate digestion and absorption of nutrients, secretion, passage of digesta and defecation, tissue defense, and vascular perfusion. This chapter will focus on the normal control of passage of digesta through the gastrointestinal tract and how alterations in normal control can lead to pathophysiology.

The study of the neural control of the gut has a long history. By the start of the twentieth century, Ivan Pavlov had determined that the vagus nerve was responsible for the conditioned secretion and motor functions of the gut; Canon[22] had demonstrated the presence of neural reflexes that coordinated swallowing with gastric relaxation, and Langley had recognized the "enteric nervous system" within the gut, as a separate part of the autonomic nervous system[59].

## The Gut is Controlled by Intrinsic and Extrinsic Nerves

The ganglia of the enteric nervous system are collections of sensory neurons, motor neurons, and interneurons that lie within the wall of the gastrointestinal tract[37]. These interconnected ganglia occur in two principal networks, the myenteric and submucosal plexuses, which primarily control contraction and relaxation of the gastrointestinal smooth muscle and absorption and secretion, through the mucosal epithelium, respectively. The enteric nervous system is a large division of the autonomic nervous system, containing as many neurons as in the spinal cord. The enteric nervous system has all the features of the central nervous system (CNS) in terms of diversity of neurotransmitters and neuromodulators, ion channels, receptors, and transporters.

The extrinsic parasympathetic innervation of the gut arises from the dorsal motor nucleus of the vagus (dorsal vagal nucleus [DVN]), which innervates gastrointestinal smooth muscle from the distal esophagus to mid/distal colon, and from the sacral spinal cord, which innervates the most distal segments of the gastrointestinal tract[98]. Initially, Langley[60] and later Wood[120] hypothesized that each vagal preganglionic axon contacts "command" enteric ganglia, which then convey information throughout the gut via enteric networks. However, individual vagal fibers form varicose endings around almost all neurons of the myenteric plexus and could coordinate activities of potentially disparate regions of the gut[79]. Thus, the "command ganglia" hypothesis has been challenged, and it is now largely accepted that governance of the gut by extrinsic control (i.e., the CNS) can override the enteric nervous system in certain situations. However, oversight by the CNS is permissive of the independent decision-making activity of the enteric nervous system for moment-to-moment regulation of gastrointestinal function.

Sympathetic innervation of the upper gastrointestinal tract is via the splanchnic nerves. These nerves contain the axons of sympathetic preganglionic neurons in the intermediolateral cell column of the fifth through ninth thoracic spinal segments and enter the celiac ganglion. Sympathetic post-ganglionic neurons supplying the upper gastrointestinal tract are found close to the enteric ganglia and blood vessels[42] and presynaptically inhibit cholinergic excitatory drive from extrinsic and intrinsic neurons.

## VAGAL INNERVATION OF THE GASTROINTESTINAL TRACT

### Organization of Afferent Innervation from the Gut

The afferent innervation of the gastrointestinal tract involves the vagus and splanchnic nerves and utilizes several different types of specialized transducers of mechanical or chemical stimuli. Overall, spinal afferents, including the afferents that travel in the splanchnic nerve, carry either low- or high-threshold mechano- or chemo-receptor signals and are nociceptive[96]. In contrast, afferents that travel in the vagus convey low threshold mechano- and chemoreceptor signals conveying information on the movement and digestion of nutrients[80]. (A recent review describes the three types of vagal mechanoreceptors in more detail[80].) Two types of mechanosensitive afferent detect tension and distention in the gut. One is the intraganglionic laminar ending that receives sensory information from overlapping receptive fields in the wall of the gut. The second is the intramuscular array that contacts smooth muscle cells and specialized pacemaker cells called *interstitial cells of Cajal*[78]. The interstitial cells of Cajal help coordinate gut motility by interfacing with enteric nerves and smooth muscle[117]. A third type of receptor is a mucosal vagal afferent receptor[26], which is thought to respond to light stroking of the gastrointestinal mucosa[76]. The cell bodies of these vagal afferents reside in the nodose ganglion, where there is a limited viscerotopic gastrointestinal organization and some processing between gastrointestinal and non-gastrointestinal visceral information[19].

### Organization of Efferent Projections to the Gut

Parasympathetic preganglionic neurons innervating different regions of the gastrointestinal tract are organized in columns within the DVN; populations of neurons from medial to lateral innervate the upper stomach, antrum, intestine and colon (Figure 14–1)[75,98]. Vagal efferents mediate an increase in the force and amplitude of gut contraction via activation of nicotinic acetylcholine receptors on cholinergic post-ganglionic/enteric neurons, which in turn release acetylcholine to stimulate muscarinic acetylcholine receptors on smooth muscle. Vagal efferents can also inhibit gut contractility and tone via non-adrenergic, non-cholinergic (NANC) post-ganglionic/enteric neurons that release transmitters, such as nitric oxide and vasoactive intestinal polypeptide[41]. The preganglionic neurons in the DVN are functionally organized with excitatory pathways predominantly in the rostral DVN and inhibitory responses in the caudal DVN (Figure 14–1)[2].

### Vago-Vagal Reflexes

Vago-vagal reflex pathways are composed of vagal afferents that synapse with interneurons in the nucleus of the solitary tract (NTS) which, in turn, contact DVN neurons to convey motor information to the gut[87]. Low-pressure distention of the gut initiates vago-vagal reflexes. For example, esophageal distention evokes a receptive relaxation of the stomach that prepares the stomach to accommodate a bolus arriving from the esophagus. Duodenal[8] and colonic distention[15] also evoke gastric relaxation, thus preventing too-rapid emptying of the stomach while the intestines are distended.

Typically in vago-vagal reflexes, distention results in release of an excitatory transmitter (glutamate) from vagal primary afferents in the NTS; then second-order interneurons communicate to DVN motor neurons via inhibitory synapses that release GABA and catecholamines. Evidence for this reflex pathway is as follows: (a) stimulation of the gut results in excitation of NTS neurons and inhibition of DVN neurons[123]; (b) NTS stimulation evokes gastric relaxation[83]; and (c) gastric motor activity is increased *in vivo* when bicuculline, a $GABA_A$ receptor antagonist, is microinjected into the DVN[101]. Vago-vagal reflexes in the dorsal vagal complex are amenable to modulation by opioids and their signaling pathways[20] and provide a high degree of integration at the level of the brainstem. For example, distention of the small bowel in humans results in reflex gastric relaxation whether or not there is conscious perception of the distention[8].

There is also integration of vago-vagal and cardiorespiratory reflexes at the medullary reticular level; for example, in the case of retching and expulsion of stomach contents during emesis (vomiting)[49]. Output neurons in the dorsomedial medulla, ventrolateral medulla, nucleus ambiguus, and retrofacial nucleus control muscles involved in emesis (inspiratory, diaphragm, tongue, larynx, pharynx, heart, blood vessels, lower esophageal sphincter, and gastric fundus). Since these neurons are scattered throughout the medulla and must be activated in sequence to coordinate the behavior, they are referred to as the *medullary central pattern generator*[69]. The area postrema detects humoral factors that initiate nausea, and this information is integrated with sensory information from the abdominal vagal afferents in the NTS. Anti-emetics work by inhibiting activation of abdominal vagal afferents (for example, serotonin [$5\text{-}HT_3$] receptor antagonists[47]) or act centrally by inhibiting the dorsal vagal complex (for example, cannabinoid 1 receptor agonists[111]).

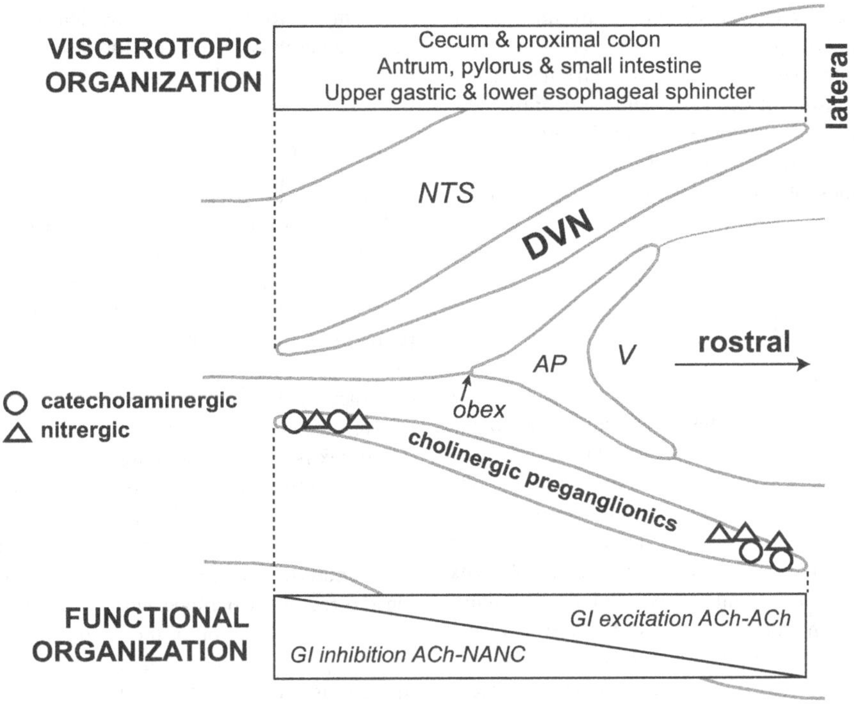


Figure 14–1 The viscerotopic, functional and neurochemical organization of the dorsal motor nucleus of the vagus (DVN). These viscerotopic aspects of DVN organization are superimposed on one side of a diagram showing the dorsal surface of the medulla and the functional and neurochemical aspects on the other. The *top* of the diagram shows that the neurons innervating the gastrointestinal tract are loosely organized in overlapping longitudinal columns. These columns innervate from medial to lateral: lower esophageal sphincter, gastric fundus, and cardia antrum pylorus with the small intestine interspersed, then cecum and proximal colon. The *bottom* shows that the functional organization of the upper GI tract is predominantly inhibitory in the caudal DVN, and predominantly excitatory motor in the rostral DVN. Cecal inhibitory responses, which are evoked in the rostral DVN, are not shown. All of the motor neurons in the DVN are cholinergic. However, neurons that use nitric oxide or catecholamines as neurotransmitters occur at both rostral and caudal poles of the DVN. AP, area postrema; NTS, nucleus of the solitary tract; *V:* fourth ventricle.

## The Vagus and Inflammation

Early evidence for an important anti-inflammatory role of the vagus was the demonstration that vagal de-afferentation exacerbated colonic inflammation[65]. More recently, electrical stimulation of the vagus has been shown to inhibit cytokine release from macrophages[16,109] and the release of the cytokine tumor necrosis factor in models of surgery-induced inflammation of the gut[31]. A mechanism involving nicotinic acetylcholine receptors on immune cells has been postulated, in part because the effect is attenuated in mice deficient in alpha7 nicotinic acetylcholine receptors[115], and because macrophages are a primary target for this neuroimmune axis[38]. Selective lesioning of the celiac branch of the vagus nerve prevented the vagal anti-inflammatory reflex, suggesting that the spleen is a pivotal site in this response[51].

Mast cells increase in number and are found in close anatomical association with vagal afferents in an inflamed gut; conversely, vagotomy reduces mast cell density[103]. Cytokines, such as tumor necrosis factor, can also activate cachexia-related behavior (i.e., behavior that leads to weight loss) by a direct action in the brain. Suppression of gastric motor function is associated with cachexia/emesis, so it is interesting that gastric motility is suppressed by microinjection of tumor necrosis factor into the dorsal vagal complex[35]. Systemic lipopolysaccharide administration also suppressed contractile activity of the stomach, and this effect was prevented by immunoneutralization of tumor necrosis factor in the region of the dorsal vagal complex[45].

The clinical relevance of this neuroimmune-gut axis is still emerging, but there seems to be a two-way communication. Neuronal activity contributes to the level of expression of cytokines and other inflammatory mediators in inflammatory bowel diseases[28,38]. Conversely, colonic inflammation can alter the vagovagal functions of the gut[70] that may contribute to symptoms associated with colitis.

## THE OROPHARYNX AND PHARYNX

### Neuroanatomical Pathways

Cranial motor neurons in the trigeminal, facial, vagal, and hypoglossal nerves are those most directly involved in the control of swallowing. Afferents from the body of the tongue and the hard palate end in the rostral portion of the lateral subnucleus of the NTS, while those from the root of the tongue and soft palate and pharynx terminate in the dorsal half of the medial NTS, intermediate NTS, and interstitial NTS[30,44]. Afferents from the esophageal body terminate entirely within the central subnucleus of the NTS[18], and esophageal distention activates neurons of the central subnucleus that contain catecholamines and nitric oxide. Gastric relaxation evoked by esophageal distention can be abolished by $\alpha$-adrenoceptor blockade in the DVN[89].

Premotor neurons in the NTS contact ipsilateral motor neurons within the nucleus ambiguus that innervate laryngeal muscles and the esophagus[30]. These premotor neurons are considered to be key coordinators of the central program generator that controls swallowing. For example, in a reduced *in vitro* neonatal rat brainstem preparation, blockade of $GABA_A$ receptors in the NTS results in oropharyngeal movements when the activity of the fourth cervical ventral nerve is inhibited[56], suggesting reciprocal coordination of swallowing and respiration.

Motor neurons within the nucleus ambiguus are viscerotopically organized. Motor neurons innervating the esophagus occur within the compact formation; those projecting to the pharynx lie within the adjacent semi-compact formation, and those innervating the intrinsic laryngeal muscles are within the loose formation[4,11]. There also appears to be a functional organization for activation of different phases of swallowing. Activation of neurons, as indicated by expression of the immediate early gene *c-fos*, occurs preferentially in motor neurons located in the dorsal portion of the nucleus ambiguus after the pharyngeal phase of swallowing. The pharyngeal and esophageal phases of swallowing are associated with activation of the caudal and rostral DVN, respectively[58]. The extensive bundling of dendrites within the semi-compact and compact formation of the nucleus ambiguus could be the anatomical substrate for motor neuronal integration controlling different aspects of swallowing[18].

### Pathophysiology

The circuits described above underlie the protective reflexes coordinating swallowing and respiration[3]. Dysphagia is a decompensation of swallowing and airway protective mechanisms, which can lead to increased incidence of aspiration. It is a significant problem in patients with gastroesophageal reflux and results in coughing and damage to the larynx[97]. Contraction of the upper esophageal sphincter is a protective mechanism preventing aspiration. This protective reflex is impaired with age, which may be due to changes in the sensory inputs to the swallowing central program generator[54], the location of which is described in the previous section. Dysphagia can result from infarctions involving the medulla, and correlating the region of damage with severity of dysphagia can reveal the location of the central program generator. In patients with Wallenberg's syndrome, the infarctions were situated in the rostral third of the medulla and affected the nucleus ambiguus, NTS, and surrounding reticular formation. These dysphagic patients have significantly worse outcomes than those with Avellis' syndrome involving infarctions of only the nucleus ambiguus and its surrounding reticular formation[81].

Afferents in the esophageal mucosa that are sensitive to distention and pH could provide the painful symptoms of gastroesophageal reflux disease[96]. Central sensitization of vagal afferents in the NTS resulting from acid and pepsin infusion into the esophagus may also contribute to this painful sensation[68]. Spinal afferents conveying painful sensations from the esophagus and the heart enter at the same level of the spinal cord, which may account for the similarity in referred pain observed in cardiac patients and in patients with non-cardiac chest pain.

## THE LOWER ESOPHAGEAL SPHINCTER AND STOMACH

### Neuroanatomical Pathways

The gastroesophageal junction forms a zone of high intraluminal pressure that prevents reflux of the gastric contents into the esophagus. Relaxation of the lower esophageal sphincter occurs transiently during swallowing and belching when gas may be vented from the stomach, and is sustained prior to, and during, emesis. About half of the DVN neurons that innervate the lower esophageal sphincter also innervate the gastric fundus[52]. These neurons coordinate the activity of both regions, and co-morbidities of the lower esophageal sphincter and stomach are frequent. For example, in 50% of patients with an inability to completely relax the lower esophageal sphincter (achalasia), there is also impaired gastric adaptive relaxation[67]. In addition, local enteric inhibitory pathways from the esophagus to the nearby stomach can transmit inhibition of smooth muscle[121]. Preganglionic DVN neurons supplying the lower esophageal sphincter express nitric oxide synthase[52]. However, relaxation of the lower esophageal sphincter is abolished by the ganglion blocker hexamethonium (a selective antagonist of nicotinic acetylcholine receptors)[2], suggesting that preganglionic neurons containing nitric oxide are not directly responsible for this relaxation.

The gut produces a wide variety of hormones related to nutritional status that act on vagal afferents[7]. Parietal cells in the stomach produce ghrelin, an appetite-stimulating hormone[108] that also promotes motility of the upper gastrointestinal tract[107]. Ghrelin also acts in the arcuate nucleus in the hypothalamus[116] to stimulate feeding. Plasma levels of ghrelin[91] are generally low, although paradoxically in anorectic patients the fasting level of ghrelin is significantly higher[72].

Nutrients are detected by specialized enteroendocrine cells in the epithelium of the small intestine. In response, some of these enteroendocrine cells secrete peptide YY. This gut hormone was the first to be identified as participating in the so-called "ileal brake" mechanism, which inhibits feeding and transit of contents through the upper gastrointestinal tract[102]. This gut-brain reflex very effectively slows down transit through the upper gastrointestinal tract and gastric emptying and is associated with a feeling of fullness. The term *ileal brake*, when coined in 1984 by Spiller, originally referred only to the action of peptide YY[102]. However, recent research has expanded our understanding of the complex mechanisms underlying the ileal brake and has identified other hormones that are involved and their effects (see "The Small Intestine" below). Other gut hormones, such as pancreatic polypeptide[88] and insulin[57], can also act directly on the area postrema and dorsal vagal complex to alter gastric contractility and tone. In the dorsal vagal complex, peptide YY directly activates Y2 receptors to reduce gastric contractility[24]; and in the arcuate nucleus, activation of Y2 receptors inhibits feeding[12].

### Pathophysiology

Gastroesophageal reflux disease is associated with a higher than normal number of transient relaxations of the lower esophageal sphincter following a meal. Attempts to modify the triggering of these transient relaxations with the $GABA_B$ agonist baclofen has reduced esophageal exposure to low pH in humans[25,62]. Since $GABA_B$ receptors are localized on DVN neurons innervating the lower esophageal sphincter in ferrets, baclofen could directly inhibit the motor pathway for this response[66], as well as altering the firing of vagal afferent neurons[77]. Thus, modulating central pathways controlling the lower esophageal sphincter is a potential approach to treating gastroesophageal reflux disease. Spinal afferents traveling with sympathetic (splanchnic) fibers from the lower esophageal sphincter are generally considered to convey painful information[96] associated with reflux disease.

Gastric emptying is abnormally slow in patients with long-standing diabetes, and the rate of gastric emptying is related to diurnal shifts in blood glucose levels in healthy as well as diabetic patients[50]. Electrical stimulation of the stomach in obese patients has resulted in weight loss in some clinical trials[39], with improvements in glycemic control in diabetic patients secondary to weight loss.

## THE SMALL INTESTINE

### Neuroanatomical Pathways

The major role of the small intestine is digestion of protein, lipids, and complex carbohydrates, which are absorbed and, depending on their composition, enter either the hepatic portal circulation or the lymphatic system via villous capillaries and lacteals. The latter drain into the thoracic duct, which empties directly into the superior vena cava. Neural and hormonal (endocrine and paracrine) signals conveying information about luminal composition and wall distention in the small intestine help to optimize the speed of transit relative to the amount of nutrient that is absorbed. For example, if undigested fatty acids pass too rapidly into the large intestine and are made available to colonizing bacteria, then this results in fatty stools and flatulence. Detection of fatty acids in the small intestine releases ileal brake hormones that slow the rate of intestinal transit into large intestine. A specific enteroendocrine cell type that releases hormones involved in the ileal brake is the L-cell, which has a regionally discrete location in the intestine, as is the case for the other types of enteroendocrine cells. L-cells are most numerous in the ileum, at the distal end of the small intestine. Upon detection of fatty acids, these L cells release glucagon-like peptide–1, which enters the mesenteric vasculature. This peptide activates glucagon-like peptide-1 receptors located on the vagus nerve[110] in close association with the hepatic portal vein and on beta cells in the pancreas.

Both distention and acidic perfusion of the small intestine excite NTS neurons and inhibit DVN neurons, which is a vagal reflex to delay gastric emptying in response to detection of acidity or increasing volume in the duodenum[122]. The sensitivity of mesenteric afferents to distention is modulated by numerous neurotransmitters[34,46,90] and hormones released by the small intestine. These hormones include peptide YY, glucagon-like peptide-1, glucagon-like peptide-2, and cholecystokinin[17]. Each of these hormones has multiple effects and sites of action depending, in part, on the amount released, diet, and the specific stimulus. For example, the chain length of free fatty acids determines the release of gut hormones in healthy volunteers with dodecanoic (12 carbon chain) but not decanoic (10 carbon chain) fatty acids increasing glucagon-like peptide and peptide YY[36]. Rats maintained on a high-fat diet have reduced neuronal activation in response to the presence of oleic acid in the intestinal lumen[29].

Lipid absorbed in the intestine through chylomicron formation stimulates cholecystokinin release, which acts on cholecystokinin type 1 receptors on vagal afferents to stimulate NTS neurons. In the NTS, selective chemical ablation of noradrenergic neurons abolishes the satiating effects of cholecystokinin[85]. Furthermore, these noradrenergic neurons innervate and activate regions of the amygdala involved in emotional learning[71]. At higher than physiological doses, cholecystokinin activates the dorsal vagal complex through pathways other than the sub-diaphragmatic vagus nerve[94]. Other neurons activated by high doses of cholecystokinin occur in the ventrolateral medulla, paraventricular and supraoptic nuclei of the hypothalamus (including neurons immunoreactive for corticotrophin-releasing factor), central nucleus of the amygdala, and bed nucleus of the stria terminalis[14]. Many of these regions are also involved in emesis. Transection of the brainstem-hypothalamic pathway attenuates the inhibitory effect of both peptide YY and glucagon-like peptide-1 on food intake[1] by preventing activation of arcuate neurons that express receptors for glucagon-like peptide-1[99]. Gastric distention activates neurons in the caudal NTS that contain glucagon-like peptide-1[114], and administration of this peptide at higher than physiological doses stimulates emetogenic pathways[84]. Thus, cholecystokinin and glucagon-like peptides 1 and 2 have dual roles in mediating satiety and taste aversion/nausea, depending in part on the level of activation of neural pathways that use these peptides for conveying information.

### Pathophysiology

In non-obese, non-diabetic, fasted individuals, the levels of glucagon-like peptide-1 are in the range of 5–10 pmol/L and increase rapidly to 15–50 pmol/L after a meal[32]. In Type 2 diabetic patients, the meal-related increase in glucagon-like peptide-1 is significantly blunted. Advances in treatment for type 2 diabetes and obesity have been made through a new class of drugs similar to glucagon-like peptide-1, termed *incretin mimetics*. The first in this class is exenatide (Byetta® Amylin/Eli Lilly), approved by the U.S. Department of Agriculture for the treatment of type 2 diabetes in 2005. Exenatide improved both glycemic control and weight loss[95]. This drug is thought to be anorectic and alter fuel homeostasis due to multiple sites of action, in addition to improving insulin sensitivity. However, increasing satiety without causing nausea limits the use of intestinal hormones in the control of obesity because similar neural circuits are activated by satiety and nausea, especially at higher hormone doses.

## THE LARGE INTESTINE

### Neuroanatomical Pathways

The celiac and accessory celiac branches of the vagus nerve innervate most of the colon[5], but the extent to which the vagus modulates colonic motor activity is unclear. For example, disinhibition of the dorsal vagal complex inhibits colonic motility. However, the inhibition is not blocked by vagotomy[40], although transneuronal labeling in the DVN after inoculation of trans-synaptic viral tracer into the colon confirms the presence of vagal as well as spinal pathways to this region of the intestine[113]. Recently, DVN stimulation has been shown to reduce phasic activity of the cecum through vagal pathways using nitric oxide as a transmitter[23] Stress-related visceral responses involving increased colonic motility and sensitization to colonic distention are due to activation of corticotropin-releasing factor type 1 receptors in the brain[106].

In addition to the vagal parasympathetic contributions described above, sympathetic innervation of the colon arrives via the splanchnic nerves. These nerves travel from the thoracolumbar spinal cord to prevertebral ganglia, which surround the three unpaired arteries of the abdominal aorta; i.e., the celiac, superior, and inferior mesenteric arteries.

Axons of these sympathetic post-ganglionic neurons in the prevertebral ganglia project through the mesenteric nerves to innervate effectors in the wall of the colon (Figure 14–2)[105]. The prevertebral ganglia historically were considered simple relay stations where preganglionic neurons communicated with noradrenergic post-ganglionic neurons via nicotinic acetylcholine receptors. However, it is now known that sympathetic post-ganglionic neurons have a complex neurochemical coding. Furthermore, the prevertebral ganglia are centers for integration of information between the CNS and the gut and are essential components in coordinating activity of the enteric nervous system in different regions of the gut[104,105].

Afferent information from the urinary bladder and colon converges in the sacral spinal cord and is relayed to the locus coeruleus complex, including Barrington's nucleus, in the pons[113]. Small-diameter unmyelinated (C-fiber) afferents signal noxious colonic distention that, in turn, activates neurons within the NTS and in Barrington's nucleus[64]. In Barrington's nucleus, neurons that respond to bladder stimulation are also activated by colonic distention, and many are immunoreactive for corticotropin-releasing factor[92]. From Barrington's nucleus, processed information relating to painful colonic stimuli is relayed to the nucleus submedius of the medial thalamus[10], where viscerosomatic inputs from colon and skin converge[53]. Hypersensitivity to somatic, urinary, and colonic stimuli can occur together, which may be due, in part, to the convergence of these inputs in the medial thalamus.

## Pathophysiology

Irritable bowel syndrome is associated with recurring constipation and/or diarrhea and abdominal discomfort and pain. The etiology of irritable bowel syndrome is not known, although stress or post-inflammatory remodeling due to previous enteritis may predispose an individual to developing this syndrome. In patients with irritable bowel syndrome, there is evidence for hypersensitivity at the level of peripheral afferent signaling, altered central processing of painful information, and descending modulatory input in the spinal

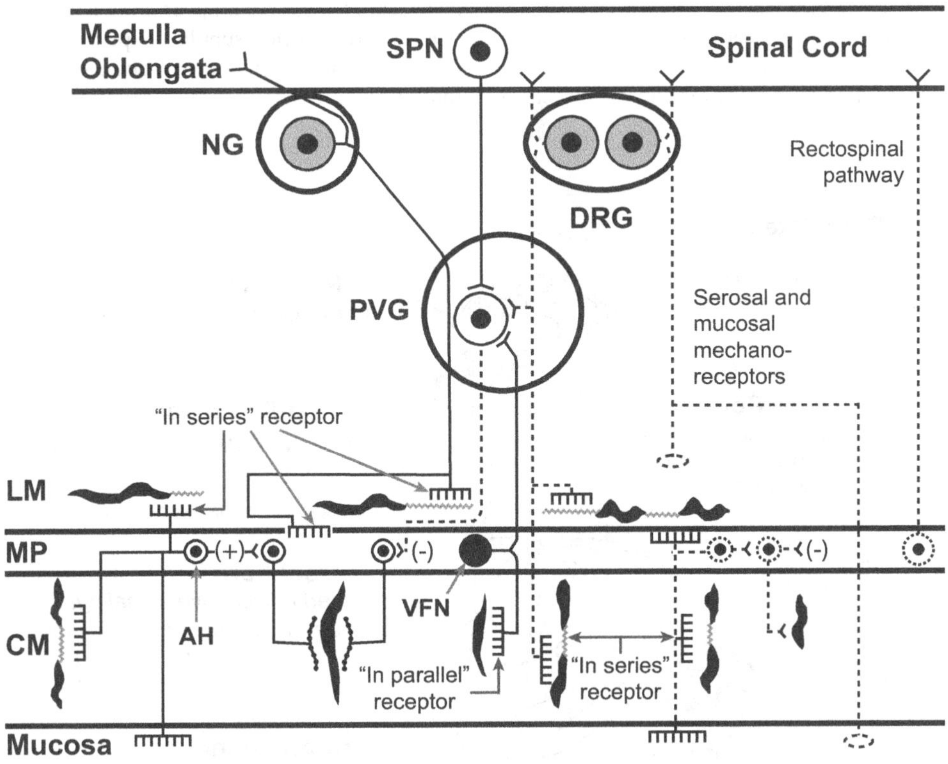


Figure 14–2 The possible arrangement of mechanosensory afferent nerves in the gut wall. Viscerofugal neurons (VFN) function as an "in parallel" arrangement to the circular muscle (CM) layer. Intrinsic sensory neurons (AH) in the longitudinal muscle (LM) layer function as an "in-series" arrangment. Receptors labeled as "in series" receptors in the longitudinal muscle and the myenteric plexus (MP) are intramuscular arrays (IMAs) and intraganglionic laminar endings (IGLEs), which function as "in series" tension receptors. IMAs occur throughout the gut; IGLEs occur only in the rectum and are not shown. The physiological significance of rectospinal neurons is not defined but they may be involved in the defecation reflex. DRG, dorsal root ganglion; NG, nodose ganglion; PVG, paravertebral ganglion; SPN, sympathetic preganglionic neuron. Modified from Szurszewski et al.[105], with permission.

cord and cortical hypervigilance[27,61,73,118]. Functional neuroimaging has identified regions of the forebrain that are activated differently in patients with irritable bowel syndrome compared to controls (Figure 14–3). These regions include the anterior insular cortex, dorsal anterior cingulate cortex, and prefrontal cortex and provide the neuroanatomical basis for what patients describe as anxiety, attention, and anticipation in response to colorectal distention. These cortical regions and the hippocampus also respond to subliminal levels of rectal distention, suggesting that there are disturbances of associative and emotional processing of visceral sensation[6,55,100].

## THE RECTOANAL REGION AND THE DEFECATION REFLEX

The rectoanal end of the gastrointestinal tract is a specialized region where autonomic and voluntary controls of a complex set of smooth and striated muscles must act in concert for proper function. Anatomically, the rectum is that part of the bowel situated between the sigmoid colon and the anal canal, from the level of the third sacral vertebra to the pelvic diaphragm. The rectum and anus function together as a unit in concert with the skeletal muscles of the pelvic floor in order to provide for fecal continence[13,82]. At rest the rectum and anus lie at an angle to each other so that the puborectalis muscle forms a sling that loops around the anorectum. Voluntary contraction of the puborectalis muscle pulls the bowel forward, creating a more acute angle to assist in maintaining continence.

The internal anal sphincter consists of a thickened layer of circular smooth muscle in the upper portions of the anal canal and provides most of the resting pressure that prevents leakage of rectal contents. Parasympathetic stimulation contracts the internal anal sphincter, whereas presacral sympathetic stimulation relaxes it. The enteric nervous system provides the circuitry for the rectoanal reflex, which produces periodic transient relaxations of the internal anal sphincter[119]. These allow the contents of the rectum to be sampled near the upper end of the anal canal, where there is a rich supply of special sensory endings near the internal anal sphincter[86]. Rectoanal inhibitory reflexes occur even if the extrinsic

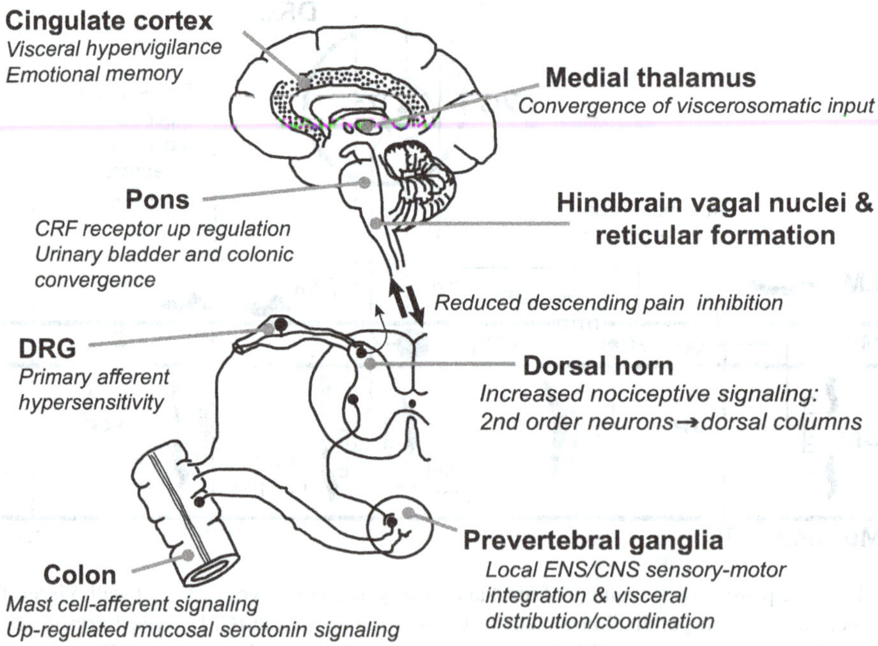


Figure 14–3 Key regions for altered colonic visceral sensation associated with irritable bowel syndrome. The diagram shows the key regions in the brain and spinal cord that are involved in irritable bowel syndrome and the roles that they may play in this condition. Several of the brain regions involved in irritable bowel syndrome are part of classic nociceptive circuitry and are sites where convergence of visceral and somatic sensory processing occurs.

hypogastric nerves are lesioned or if there is spinal cord damage. The reflex is stimulated by an increase in rectal volume so that a greater volume evokes relaxations of the internal anal sphincter that are greater in amplitude and duration. Sampling of rectal contents reaches conscious levels and allows for discrimination between gas, liquid, or solid content. Changes in rectal distention may also be sensed by sacral dorsal root ganglion neurons through specialized endings called *rectal intraganglionic laminar endings* that occur within enteric ganglia[63]. Sudden changes in rectal volume also stimulate contraction of the external anal sphincter to preserve continence. This contractile reflex is mediated by sensory input via pelvic splanchnic nerves and by motor outflow to the external anal sphincter via the pudendal nerve from a collection of sacral motor neurons known as *Onuf's nucleus*. The external anal sphincter is a band of skeletal muscle that surrounds the lower end of the anal canal and comprises a thickening of the levator ani complex, the deepest layer being continuous with the puborectalis muscle. Abrupt changes in intra-abdominal pressure, such as those brought on by a sneeze or cough, evoke a reflex contraction of puborectalis and an increase in external anal sphincter pressure.

### Pathophysiology

Clinical evidence demonstrates that the outflow from different levels of the sacral cord contributes to parasympathetic and somatic innervation to the distal colon, rectum, and anal sphincters. In patients with injuries to the cervical or upper thoracic spinal cord[112], stimulation of sacral spinal cord segment S2 evoked low-amplitude colorectal contractions. Stimulation of S3 evoked high amplitude peristaltic contractions in a frequency-dependent fashion; and S4 stimulation increased tone in the distal colon as well as the rectum. Stimulation of S2–S4 increased contractile activity of the external anal sphincter but was increasingly graded from upper to lower spinal segments[112]. Blockade of the pudendal nerve does not alter rectal sensation but interrupts the rectoanal contractile reflex because it reduces the contractions of the external anal sphincter. Resection or blockade of the pelvic splanchnic nerves abolishes rectal sensation and the defecation reflex. Blockade of the pudendal nerve blocks the function of the external anal sphincter but does not alter function of the puborectalis muscle, since these two structures have separate innervation. A concise, contemporary review of the anatomical and neural correlates of the defecation reflex and the primary functional disorder related to the rectoanal region, fecal incontinence, has recently been published[13].

## FUTURE DIRECTIONS FOR RESEARCH

Advances in the understanding of how the CNS and the gastrointestinal tract communicate are central to several areas of clinical relevance. Due to the alarming increase in prevalence of metabolic syndrome, type 2 diabetes, and obesity, a better understanding of the role of the gut-brain axis in metabolic disorders is required. For example, bariatric surgery (Roux-en-Y gastric bypass) reduces the size of the stomach and redirects the emptying of gastric contents to the terminal small intestine. In morbidly obese patients, this successfully reduces weight and, in about 75% of patients, also resolves type 2 diabetes[21]. The mechanisms underlying this improvement are being rigorously debated. On one hand, it is argued that improved glucose metabolism and insulin resistance are simply due to caloric restriction and weight loss[43]. On the other hand, gastric bypass results in considerable hormonal changes before significant weight loss occurs[93]. This highlights the need for further insight into the relationship between gut motility, gut hormones, and metabolism as a means to regulate food intake.

A second area of interest in the gut-brain axis is whether stress and traumatic events early in life predispose people to the alterations in bowel function and visceral pain associated with irritable bowel syndrome ("top down" theory), or whether bouts of pathogenic enteritis and/or alteration of colonizing bacteria leading to peripheral gut sensitization ("bottom up" 'theory) have this effect. The former theory suggests that patients would benefit from therapy that reduces cortical hypervigilance and anxiety. High-resolution functional brain imaging in patient populations with diverse diseases that may all have a component of hypervigilance, such as pelvic pain disorders and fibromyalgia, may provide insights into the neuroanatomical basis of irritable bowel syndrome[33]. Unfortunately, animal models of visceral pain with altered gastrointestinal motility do not mimic irritable bowel syndrome, because these acute models lack the hypervigilance and emotional component that cause the pain and discomfort of irritable bowel syndrome to be a "feed-forward event." If bouts of pathogenic enteritis and/or alteration of colonizing bacteria predispose patients to irritable bowel syndrome, then strategies that reduce neuroimmune dysfunction may be therapeutic. Understanding what happens at the interface of the gastrointestinal contents with the epithelium and immune cells, and how transduction by mucosal/mechanoreceptors contributes to afferent nerve signaling[48], will be invaluable to this area of research. There is excitement about the vagal anti-inflammatory reflex, in which vagally released acetylcholine inhibits inflammation by suppressing cytokine synthesis through alpha7 nicotinic acetylcholine receptors on immune cells in the spleen, liver, and gastrointestinal tract[74]. However, more research is required before determining that modulating this vagal reflex and/or selectively activating alpha7 nicotinic acetylcholine receptors could provide relief for patients with inflammatory bowel disease. In the gastrointestinal mucosa, activated mast cells in close proximity to nerves release tryptase that signals to afferent nerves by cleaving protease-activated receptors. However, the contribution of these types of neuroimmune interactions to the pathophysiology of irritable bowel syndrome[9] is yet to be established.

ACKNOWLEDGEMENTS The National Institutes of Health's National Institute of Diabetes and Digestive and Kidney Diseases 42714 (PJH) supported the studies reported here. We also appreciate the discussions with our colleagues from the Johnson & Johnson Enterology Research Team (2002–2006) and Centocor Research and Development on topics related to this chapter.

## References


1. Abbott, C. R., Monteiro, M., Small, C. J., Sajedi, A., Smith, K. L., Parkinson, J. R., Ghatei, M. A., and Bloom, S. R. (2005). The inhibitory effects of peripheral administration of peptide YY(3–36) and glucagon like peptide-1 on food intake are attenuated by ablation of the vagal-brainstem-hypothalamic pathway. *Brain Research* 1044, 127–131.
2. Abrahams, T. P., Partosoedarso, E. R., and Hornby, P. J. (2002). Lower oesophageal sphincter relaxation evoked by stimulation of the dorsal motor nucleus of the vagus in ferrets. *Neurogastroenterology and Motility* 14, 295–304.
3. Altschuler, S. M. (2001). Laryngeal and respiratory protective reflexes. *American Journal of Medicine* 111 Suppl 8A, 90S–94S.
4. Altschuler, S. M., Bao, X. M., Bieger, D., Hopkins, D. A., and Miselis, R. R. (1989). Viscerotopic representation of the upper alimentary tract in the rat: Sensory ganglia and nuclei of the solitary and spinal trigeminal tracts. *Journal of Comparative Neurology* 283, 248–268.
5. Altschuler, S. M., Escardo, J., Lynn, R. B., and Miselis, R. R. (1993). The central organization of the vagus nerve innervating the colon of the rat. *Gastroenterology* 104, 502–509.
6. Andresen, V., Bach, D. R., Poellinger, A., Tsrouya, C., Stroh, A., Foerschler, A., Georgiewa, P., Zimmer, C., and Monnikes, H. (2005). Brain activation responses to subliminal or supraliminal rectal stimuli and to auditory stimuli in irritable bowel syndrome. *Neurogastroenterology and Motility* 17, 827–837.
7. Andrews, P. L., and Sanger, G. J. (2002). Abdominal vagal afferent neurones: An important target for the treatment of gastrointestinal dysfunction. *Current Opinion in Pharmacology* 2, 650–656.
8. Azpiroz, F., and Malagelada, J. R. (1990). Perception and reflex relaxation of the stomach in response to gut distention. *Gastroenterology* 98, 1193–1198.
9. Barbara, G., Stanghellini, V., De Giorgio, R., Cremon, C., Cottrell, G. S., Santini, D., Pasquinelli, G., Morselli-Labate, A. M., Grady, E. F., Bunnett, N. W., Collins, S. M., and Corinaldesi, R. (2004). Activated mast cells in proximity to colonic nerves correlate with abdominal pain in irritable bowel syndrome. *Gastroenterology* 126, 693–702.
10. Barkova, E., Turnbull, G. K., and Downie, J. W. (2005). Colonic nociception via nucleus submedius is modulated by pontine centres in the rat. *Neuroscience Letters* 384, 193–197.
11. Barrett, R. T., Bao, X., Miselis, R. R., and Altschuler, S. M. (1994). Brain stem localization of rodent esophageal premotor neurons revealed by transneuronal passage of pseudorabies virus. *Gastroenterology* 107, 728–737.
12. Batterham, R. L., Cowley, M. A., Small, C. J., Herzog, H., Cohen, M. A., Dakin, C. L., Wren, A. M., Brynes, A. E., Low, M. J., Ghatei, M. A., Cone, R. D., and Bloom, S. R. (2002). Gut hormone PYY(3–36) physiologically inhibits food intake. *Nature* 418, 650–654.
13. Bharucha, A. E. (2006). Pelvic floor: Anatomy and function. *Neurogastroenterology and Motility* 18, 507–519.
14. Billig, I., Yates, B. J., and Rinaman, L. (2001). Plasma hormone levels and central c-Fos expression in ferrets after systemic administration of cholecystokinin. *American Journal of Physiology. Regulatory, Integrative and Comparative Physiology* 281, R1243–R1255.
15. Bojo, L., and Cassuto, J. (1992). Gastric reflex relaxation by colonic distension. *Journal of the Autonomic Nervous System* 38, 57–64.
16. Borovikova, L. V., Ivanova, S., Zhang, M., Yang, H., Botchkina, G. I., Watkins, L. R., Wang, H., Abumrad, N., Eaton, J. W., and Tracey, K. J. (2000). Vagus nerve stimulation attenuates the systemic inflammatory response to endotoxin. *Nature* 405, 458–462.
17. Bray, G. A. (2000). Afferent signals regulating food intake. *Proceedings of the Nutrition Society* 59, 373–384.
18. Broussard, D. L., and Altschuler, S. M. (2000). Brainstem viscerotopic organization of afferents

and efferents involved in the control of swallowing. *American Journal of Medicine* 108 Suppl 4a, 79S-86S.

19. Browning, K. N., and Mendelowitz, D. (2003). Musings on the wanderer: What's new in our understanding of vago-vagal reflexes?: II. Integration of afferent signaling from the viscera by the nodose ganglia. *American Journal of Physiology. Gastrointestinal and Liver Physiology* 284, G8–G14.
20. Browning, K. N., and Travagli, R. A. (2006). Short-term receptor trafficking in the dorsal vagal complex: An overview. *Autonomic Neuroscience* 126–127, 2–8.
21. Buchwald, H., Avidor, Y., Braunwald, E., Jensen, M. D., Pories, W., Fahrbach, K., and Schoelles, K. (2004). Bariatric surgery: A systematic review and meta-analysis. *Journal of the American Medical Association* 292, 1724–1737.
22. Cannon, W. B., and Leib, C. W. (1911). The receptive relaxation of the stomach. *American Journal of Physiology* 29, 267-273.
23. Cao, X., Ball, A. J., Partosoedarso, E. R., Burmeister, M. A., and Hornby, P. J. (2007). Functional effects and characteristics of cecum-projecting neurons in the dorsal motor nucleus of the vagus of rats. *Autonomic Neuroscience* 131, 1–8.
24. Chen, C. H., Stephens, R. L., Jr. and Rogers, R. C. (1997). PYY and NPY: Control of gastric motility via action on Y1 and Y2 receptors in the DVC. *Neurogastroenterology and Motility* 9, 109–116.
25. Ciccaglione, A. F., and Marzio, L. (2003). Effect of acute and chronic administration of the GABA B agonist baclofen on 24-hour pH metry and symptoms in control subjects and in patients with gastro-oesophageal reflux disease. *Gut* 52, 464–470.
26. Clerc, N., and Condamin, M. (1987). Selective labeling of vagal sensory nerve fibers in the lower esophageal sphincter with anterogradely transported WGA-HRP. *Brain Research* 424, 216–224.
27. Coffin, B., Bouhassira, D., Sabate, J. M., Barbe, L., and Jian, R. (2004). Alteration of the spinal modulation of nociceptive processing in patients with irritable bowel syndrome. *Gut* 53, 1465–1470.
28. Collins, S. M. (1996). The immunomodulation of enteric neuromuscular function: Implications for motility and inflammatory disorders. *Gastroenterology* 111, 1683–1699.
29. Covasa, M., Grahn, J., and Ritter, R. C. (2000). Reduced hindbrain and enteric neuronal response to intestinal oleate in rats maintained on high-fat diet. *Autonomic Neuroscience* 84, 8–18.
30. Cunningham, E. T., Jr., and Sawchenko, P. E. (2000). Dorsal medullary pathways subserving oromotor reflexes in the rat: Implications for the central neural control of swallowing. *Journal of Comparative Neurology* 417, 448–466.
31. De Jonge, W. J., Van Der Zanden, E. P., The, F. O., Bijlsma, M. F., Van Westerloo, D. J., Bennink, R. J., Berthoud, H. R., Uematsu, S., Akira, S., Van Den Wijngaard, R. M., and Boeckxstaens, G. E. (2005). Stimulation of the vagus nerve attenuates macrophage activation by activating the Jak2–STAT3 signaling pathway. *Nature Immunology* 6, 844–851.
32. Drucker, D. J., and Nauck, M. A. (2006). The incretin system: Glucagon-like peptide-1 receptor agonists and dipeptidyl peptidase-4 inhibitors in type 2 diabetes. *Lancet* 368, 1696–1705.
33. Dunckley, P., Aziz, Q., Wise, R. G., Brooks, J., Tracey, I., and Chang, L. (2007). Attentional modulation of visceral and somatic pain. *Neurogastroenterology and Motility* 19, 569–577.
34. Eastwood, C., and Grundy, D. (2000). Opioid-receptor-mediated excitation of rat mesenteric afferent fibres supplying the rat jejunum. *Neurogastroenterology and Motility* 12, 517–522.
35. Emch, G. S., Hermann, G. E., and Rogers, R. C. (2000). TNF-alpha activates solitary nucleus neurons responsive to gastric distension. *American Journal of Physiology. Gastrointestinal and Liver Physiology* 279, G582–G586.
36. Feltrin, K. L., Patterson, M., Ghatei, M. A., Bloom, S. R., Meyer, J. H., Horowitz, M., and Feinle-Bisset, C. (2006). Effect of fatty acid chain length on suppression of ghrelin and stimulation of PYY, GLP-2 and PP secretion in healthy men. *Peptides* 27, 1638–1643.
37. Gershon, M. D., Kirchgessner, A. L., and Wade, P. R. (1994). In L. R. Johnson (Ed.), *Physiology of the Gastrointestinal Tract, vol. 1*, pp. 381–422. New York: Raven Press.
38. Ghia, J. E., Blennerhassett, P., Kumar-Ondiveeran, H., Verdu, E. F., and Collins, S. M. (2006). The vagus nerve: A tonic inhibitory influence associated with inflammatory bowel disease in a murine model. *Gastroenterology* 131, 1122–1130.
39. Greenway, F., and Zheng, J. (2007). Electrical stimulation as a treatment for diabetes and obesity. *Journal of Diabetes Science and Technology* 2, 251–259.
40. Greenwood-Van Meerveld, B., and Barron, K. W. (1998). Tonic GABA(A) receptor-mediated neurotransmission in the dorsal vagal complex regulates intestinal motility in rats. *European Journal of Pharmacology* 346, 197–202.
41. Grundy, D., Gharib-Naseri, M. K., and Hutson, D. (1993). Role of nitric oxide and vasoactive intestinal polypeptide in vagally mediated

relaxation of the gastric corpus in the anaesthetized ferret. *Journal of the Autonomic Nervous System* 43, 241–246.

42. Grundy, D., and Schemann, M. (2002). Motor control of the stomach. In S. J. Brookes and M. Costa (Eds.), *Innervation of the Gastrointestinal Tract, vol. 14*, pp. 57–102. London: Taylor and Francis.
43. Gumbs, A. A., Modlin, I. M., and Ballantyne, G. H. (2005). Changes in insulin resistance following bariatric surgery: Role of caloric restriction and weight loss. *Obesity Surgery* 15, 462–473.
44. Hayakawa, T., Takanaga, A., Maeda, S., Seki, M., and Yajima, Y. (2001). Subnuclear distribution of afferents from the oral, pharyngeal and laryngeal regions in the nucleus tractus solitarii of the rat: A study using transganglionic transport of cholera toxin. *Neuroscience Research* 39, 221–232.
45. Hermann, G. E., Tovar, C. A., and Rogers, R. C. (2002). LPS-induced suppression of gastric motility relieved by TNFR:Fc construct in dorsal vagal complex. *American Journal of Physiology. Gastrointestinal and Liver Physiology* 283, G634–G639.
46. Hillsley, K., and Grundy, D. (1998). Sensitivity to 5-hydroxytryptamine in different afferent subpopulations within mesenteric nerves supplying the rat jejunum. *Journal of Physiology* 509, 717–727.
47. Hillsley, K., and Grundy, D. (1999). Plasticity in the mesenteric afferent response to cisplatin following vagotomy in the rat. *Journal of the Autonomic Nervous System* 76, 93–98.
48. Holzer, P. (2007). Role of visceral afferent neurons in mucosal inflammation and defense. *Current Opinion in Pharmacology* 7, 563–569.
49. Hornby, P. J. (2001). Central neurocircuitry associated with emesis. *American Journal of Medicine* 111 Suppl 8A, 106S-112S.
50. Horowitz, M., O'Donovan, D., Jones, K. L., Feinle, C., Rayner, C. K., and Samsom, M. (2002). Gastric emptying in diabetes: Clinical significance and treatment. *Diabetic Medicine* 19, 177–194.
51. Huston, J. M., Ochani, M., Rosas-Ballina, M., Liao, H., Ochani, K., Pavlov, V. A., Gallowitsch-Puerta, M., Ashok, M., Czura, C. J., Foxwell, B., Tracey, K. J., and Ulloa, L. (2006). Splenectomy inactivates the cholinergic anti-inflammatory pathway during lethal endotoxemia and polymicrobial sepsis. *Journal of Experimental Medicine* 203, 1623–1628.
52. Hyland, N. P., Abrahams, T. P., Fuchs, K., Burmeister, M. A., and Hornby, P. J. (2001). Organization and neurochemistry of vagal preganglionic neurons innervating the lower esophageal sphincter in ferrets. *Journal of Comparative Neurology* 430, 222–234.
53. Kawakita, K., Sumiya, E., Murase, K., and Okada, K. (1997). Response characteristics of nucleus submedius neurons to colo-rectal distension in the rat. *Neuroscience Research* 28, 59–66.
54. Kawamura, O., Easterling, C., Aslam, M., Rittmann, T., Hofmann, C., and Shaker, R. (2004). Laryngo-upper esophageal sphincter contractile reflex in humans deteriorates with age. *Gastroenterology* 127, 57–64.
55. Kern, M. K., and Shaker, R. (2002). Cerebral cortical registration of subliminal visceral stimulation. *Gastroenterology* 122, 290–298.
56. Kogo, M., Yamanishi, T., Koizumi, H., and Matsuya, T. (2002). Swallowing-like activity elicited in vitro in neonatal rat organ attached brainstem block preparation. *Brain Research* 955, 24–33.
57. Krowicki, Z. K., Nathan, N. A., and Hornby, P. J. (1998). Gastric motor and cardiovascular effects of insulin in dorsal vagal complex of the rat. *American Journal of Physiology* 275, G964–G972.
58. Lang, I. M., Dean, C., Medda, B. K., Aslam, M., and Shaker, R. (2004). Differential activation of medullary vagal nuclei during different phases of swallowing in the cat. *Brain Research* 1014, 145–163.
59. Langley, J. N. (1921). *The Autonomic Nervous System, Part 1*. W. Heffer, ed. Cambridge, UK.
60. Langley, J. N. (1922). Connections of the enteric nerve cells. *Journal of Physiology* 56, 39–58.
61. Lembo, T., Munakata, J., Mertz, H., Niazi, N., Kodner, A., Nikas, V., and Mayer, E. A. (1994). Evidence for the hypersensitivity of lumbar splanchnic afferents in irritable bowel syndrome. *Gastroenterology* 107, 1686–1696.
62. Lidums, I., Lehmann, A., Checklin, H., Dent, J., and Holloway, R. H. (2000). Control of transient lower esophageal sphincter relaxations and reflux by the GABA(B) agonist baclofen in normal subjects. *Gastroenterology* 118, 7–13.
63. Lynn, P. A., Olsson, C., Zagorodnyuk, V., Costa, M., and Brookes, S. J. (2003). Rectal intraganglionic laminar endings are transduction sites of extrinsic mechanoreceptors in the guinea pig rectum. *Gastroenterology* 125, 786–794.
64. Martinez, V., Wang, L., and Tache, Y. (2006). Proximal colon distension induces Fos expression in the brain and inhibits gastric emptying through capsaicin-sensitive pathways in conscious rats. *Brain Research* 1086, 168–180.
65. Mazelin, L., Theodorou, V., More, J., Fioramonti, J., and Bueno, L. (1998). Protective role of vagal afferents in experimentally induced colitis in rats. *Journal of the Autonomic Nervous System* 73, 38–45.

66. Mcdermott,C.M.,Abrahams,T.P.,Partosoedarso,E., Hyland, N., Ekstrand, J., Monroe, M., and Hornby, P. J. (2001). Site of action of GABA(B) receptor for vagal motor control of the lower esophageal sphincter in ferrets and rats. *Gastroenterology* 120, 1749–1762.
67. Mearin, F., Mourelle, M., Guarner, F., Salas, A., Riveros-Moreno, V., Moncada, S., and Malagelada, J. R. (1993). Patients with achalasia lack nitric oxide synthase in the gastro-oesophageal junction. *European Journal of Clinical Investigation* 23, 724–728.
68. Medda, B. K., Sengupta, J. N., Lang, I. M., and Shaker, R. (2005). Response properties of the brainstem neurons of the cat following intra-esophageal acid-pepsin infusion. *Neuroscience* 135, 1285–1294.
69. Miller, A. D., and Ruggiero, D. A. (1994). Emetic reflex arc revealed by expression of the immediate-early gene c-Fos in the cat. *Journal of Neuroscience* 14, 871–888.
70. Monroe, M. J., Schneider, C. R., Wallace, N. H., Hornby, P. J., and Palmer, J. L. (2004). Altered reflex control of gastric motility in mice with experimentally induced colitis. *Gastroenterology* 126 Suppl. 2, M998.
71. Myers, E. A., and Rinaman, L. (2002). Viscerosensory activation of noradrenergic inputs to the amygdala in rats. *Physiology and Behavior* 77, 723–729.
72. Nakai, Y., Hosoda, H., Nin, K., Ooya, C., Hayashi, H., Akamizu, T., and Kangawa, K. (2003). Plasma levels of active form of ghrelin during oral glucose tolerance test in patients with anorexia nervosa. *European Journal of Endocrinology* 149, R1–R3.
73. Naliboff, B. D., Munakata, J., Fullerton, S., Gracely, R. H., Kodner, A., Harraf, F., and Mayer, E. A. (1997). Evidence for two distinct perceptual alterations in irritable bowel syndrome. *Gut* 41, 505–512.
74. Oke, S. L., and Tracey, K. J. (2008). From CNI-1493 to the immunological homunculus: Physiology of the inflammatory reflex. *Journal of Leukocyte Biology* 83, 512–517.
75. Pagani, F. D., Norman, W. P., and Gillis, R. A. (1988). Medullary parasympathetic projections innervate specific sites in the feline stomach. *Gastroenterology* 95, 277–288.
76. Page, A. J., and Blackshaw, L. A. (1998). An in vitro study of the properties of vagal afferent fibres innervating the ferret oesophagus and stomach. *Journal of Physiology* 512(Pt 3), 907–916.
77. Partosoedarso, E. R., Young, R. L., and Blackshaw, L. A. (2001). GABA(B) receptors on vagal afferent pathways: Peripheral and central inhibition. *American Journal of Physiology. Gastrointestinal and Liver Physiology* 280, G658–G668.
78. Patterson, L. M., Zheng, H., Ward, S. M., and Berthoud, H. R. (2001). Immunohistochemical identification of cholecystokinin A receptors on interstitial cells of Cajal, smooth muscle, and enteric neurons in rat pylorus. *Cell and Tissue Research* 305, 11–23.
79. Powley, T. L. (2000). Vagal input to the enteric nervous system. *Gut* 47 Suppl 4, iv 30–32; discussion, iv 36.
80. Powley, T. L., and Phillips, R. J. (2002). Musings on the wanderer: What's new in our understanding of vago-vagal reflexes? I. Morphology and topography of vagal afferents innervating the GI tract. *American Journal of Physiology. Gastrointestinal and Liver Physiology* 283, G1217–G1225.
81. Prosiegel, M., Holing, R., Heintze, M., Wagner-Sonntag, E., and Wiseman, K. (2005). The localization of central pattern generators for swallowing in humans—A clinical-anatomical study on patients with unilateral paresis of the vagal nerve, Avellis' syndrome, Wallenberg's syndrome, posterior fossa tumours and cerebellar hemorrhage. *Acta Neurochirurgica* Suppl 93, 85–88.
82. Rao, S. S. (2004). Pathophysiology of adult fecal incontinence. *Gastroenterology* 126, S14–S22.
83. Raybould, H. E., Jakobsen, L. J., Novin, D., and Tache, Y. (1989). TRH stimulation and L-glutamic acid inhibition of proximal gastric motor activity in the rat dorsal vagal complex. *Brain Research* 495, 319–328.
84. Rinaman, L. (1999). A functional role for central glucagon-like peptide-1 receptors in lithium chloride-induced anorexia. *American Journal of Physiology* 277, R1537–R1540.
85. Rinaman, L. (2003). Hindbrain noradrenergic lesions attenuate anorexia and alter central c-Fos expression in rats after gastric viscerosensory stimulation. *Journal of Neuroscience* 23, 10084–10092.
86. Rogers, J. (1992). Anal and rectal sensation. In M. Henry (Ed.), *Bailliere's Clinical Gastroenterology*, pp. 179–181. London: Bailliere Tindall.
87. Rogers, R. C., Hermann, G. E., and Travagli, R. A. (2006). Brainstem control of gastric function. In L. R. Johnson (Ed.), *Physiology of the Gastrointestinal Tract, vol. 1*, pp. 851–875. London: Academic Press.
88. Rogers, R. C., McTigue, D. M., and Hermann, G. E. (1995). Vagovagal reflex control of digestion: Afferent modulation by neural and "endoneurocrine" factors. *American Journal of Physiology* 268, G1–G10.
89. Rogers, R. C., Travagli, R. A., and Hermann, G. E. (2003). Noradrenergic neurons in the rat solitary

nucleus participate in the esophageal-gastric relaxation reflex. *American Journal of Physiology. Regulatory, Integrative and Comparative Physiology* 285, R479–R489.

90. Rong, W., Hillsley, K., Davis, J. B., Hicks, G., Winchester, W. J., and Grundy, D. (2004). Jejunal afferent nerve sensitivity in wild-type and TRPV1 knockout mice. *Journal of Physiology* 560, 867–881.
91. Rose, K., Bougueleret, L., Baussant, T., Bohm, G., Botti, P., Colinge, J., Cusin, I., Gaertner, H., Gleizes, A., Heller, M., Jimenez, S., Johnson, A., Kussmann, M., Menin, L., Menzel, C., Ranno, F., Rodriguez-Tome, P., Rogers, J., Saudrais, C., Villain, M., Wetmore, D., Bairoch, A., and Hochstrasser, D. (2004). Industrial-scale proteomics: From liters of plasma to chemically synthesized proteins. *Proteomics* 4, 2125–2150.
92. Rouzade-Dominguez, M. L., Pernar, L., Beck, S., and Valentino, R. J. (2003). Convergent responses of Barrington's nucleus neurons to pelvic visceral stimuli in the rat: A juxtacellular labelling study. *European Journal of Neuroscience* 18, 3325–3334.
93. Rubino, F., Gagner, M., Gentileschi, P., Kini, S., Fukuyama, S., Feng, J., and Diamond, E. (2004). The early effect of the Roux-en-Y gastric bypass on hormones involved in body weight regulation and glucose metabolism. *Annals of Surgery* 240, 236–242.
94. Sayegh, A. I., and Ritter, R. C. (2000). Vagus nerve participates in CCK-induced Fos expression in hindbrain but not myenteric plexus. *Brain Research* 878, 155–162.
95. Schnabel, C. A., Wintle, M., and Kolterman, O. (2006). Metabolic effects of the incretin mimetic exenatide in the treatment of type 2 diabetes. *Vascular Health and Risk Management* 2, 69–77.
96. Sengupta, J. N. (2000). An overview of esophageal sensory receptors. *American Journal of Medicine* 108 Suppl 4a, 87S-89S.
97. Shaker, R. (2000). Protective mechanisms against supraesophageal GERD. *Journal of Clinical Gastroenterology* 30, S3–S8.
98. Shapiro, R. E., and Miselis, R. R. (1985). The central organization of the vagus nerve innervating the stomach of the rat. *Journal of Comparative Neurology* 238, 473–488.
99. Shughrue, P. J., Lane, M. V., and Merchenthaler, I. (1996). Glucagon-like peptide-1 receptor (GLP1–R) mRNA in the rat hypothalamus. *Endocrinology* 137, 5159–5162.
100. Sidhu, H., Kern, M., and Shaker, R. (2004). Absence of increasing cortical fMRI activity volume in response to increasing visceral stimulation in IBS patients. *American Journal of Physiology. Gastrointestinal and Liver Physiology* 287, G425–G435.
101. Sivarao, D. V., Krowicki, Z. K., and Hornby, P. J. (1998). Role of GABAA receptors in rat hindbrain nuclei controlling gastric motor function. *Neurogastroenterology and Motility* 10, 305–313.
102. Spiller, R. C., Trotman, I. F., Higgins, B. E., Ghatei, M. A., Grimble, G. K., Lee, Y. C., Bloom, S. R., Misiewicz, J. J., and Silk, D. B. (1984). The ileal brake—Inhibition of jejunal motility after ileal fat perfusion in man. *Gut* 25, 365–374.
103. Stead, R. H., Colley, E. C., Wang, B., Partosoedarso, E., Lin, J., Stanisz, A., and Hillsley, K. (2006). Vagal influences over mast cells. *Autonomic Neuroscience* 125, 53–61.
104. Szurszewski, J., and Miller, S. (1994). Physiology of Prevertebral Ganglia. In L. Johnson (Ed.), *Physiology of the Gastrointestinal Tract, vol. 1*, pp. 795–877. New York: Raven Press.
105. Szurszewski, J., and Miller, S. (2006). Physiology of prevertebral sympathetic ganglia. In L. Johnson (Ed.), *Physiology of the Gastrointestinal Tract, vol. 1*, pp. 603–627. New York: Raven Press.
106. Tache, Y., Million, M., Nelson, A. G., Lamy, C., and Wang, L. (2005). Role of corticotropin-releasing factor pathways in stress-related alterations of colonic motor function and viscerosensibility in female rodents. *Gender Medicine* 2, 146–154.
107. Tack, J., Depoortere, I., Bisschops, R., Delporte, C., Coulie, B., Meulemans, A., Janssens, J., and Peeters, T. (2006). Influence of ghrelin on interdigestive gastrointestinal motility in humans. *Gut* 55, 327–333.
108. Tanaka-Shintani, M., and Watanabe, M. (2005). Distribution of ghrelin-immunoreactive cells in human gastric mucosa: Comparison with that of parietal cells. *Journal of Gastroenterology* 40, 345–349.
109. Tracey, K. J. (2002). The inflammatory reflex. *Nature* 420, 853–859.
110. Vahl, T. P., Tauchi, M., Durler, T. S., Elfers, E. E., Fernandes, T. M., Bitner, R. D., Ellis, K. S., Woods, S. C., Seeley, R. J., Herman, J. P., and D'alessio, D. A. (2007). GLP-1 receptors expressed on nerve terminals in the portal vein mediate the effects of endogenous GLP-1 on glucose tolerance in rats. *Endocrinology* 148, 4965–4973.
111. Van Sickle, M. D., Oland, L. D., Mackie, K., Davison, J. S., and Sharkey, K. A. (2003). Delta9-tetrahydrocannabinol selectively acts on CB1 receptors in specific regions of dorsal vagal complex to inhibit emesis in ferrets. *American Journal of Physiology. Gastrointestinal and Liver Physiology* 285, G566–G576.

112. Varma, J. S., Binnie, N., Smith, A. N., Creasey, G. H., and Edmond, P. (1986). Differential effects of sacral anterior root stimulation on anal sphincter and colorectal motility in spinally injured man. *British Journal of Surgery* 73, 478–482.
113. Vizzard, M. A., Brisson, M., and De Groat, W. C. (2000). Transneuronal labeling of neurons in the adult rat central nervous system following inoculation of pseudorabies virus into the colon. *Cell and Tissue Research* 299, 9–26.
114. Vrang, N., Phifer, C. B., Corkern, M. M., and Berthoud, H. R. (2003). Gastric distension induces c-Fos in medullary GLP-1/2–containing neurons. *American Journal of Physiology. Regulatory, Integrative and Comparative Physiology* 285, R470–R478.
115. Wang, H., Yu, M., Ochani, M., Amella, C. A., Tanovic, M., Susarla, S., Li, J. H., Yang, H., Ulloa, L., Al-Abed, Y., Czura, C. J., and Tracey, K. J. (2003). Nicotinic acetylcholine receptor alpha7 subunit is an essential regulator of inflammation. *Nature* 421, 384–388.
116. Wang, L., Saint-Pierre, D. H., and Tache, Y. (2002). Peripheral ghrelin selectively increases Fos expression in neuropeptide Y-synthesizing neurons in mouse hypothalamic arcuate nucleus. *Neuroscience Letters* 325, 47–51.
117. Ward, S. M., and Sanders, K. M. (2001). Physiology and pathophysiology of the interstitial cell of Cajal: From bench to bedside. I. Functional development and plasticity of interstitial cells of Cajal networks. *American Journal of Physiology. Gastrointestinal and Liver Physiology* 281, G602–G611.
118. Wilder-Smith, C. H., Schindler, D., Lovblad, K., Redmond, S. M., and Nirkko, A. (2004). Brain functional magnetic resonance imaging of rectal pain and activation of endogenous inhibitory mechanisms in irritable bowel syndrome patient subgroups and healthy controls. *Gut* 53, 1595–1601.
119. Wood, J. (2006). Integrative functions of the enteric nervous system. In L. Johnson (Ed.), *Physiology of the Gastrointestinal Tract, vol. 1*, pp. 665–683. New York: Raven Press.
120. Wood, J. D. (1987). Physiology of the Enteric Nervous System. In L. Johnson (Ed.), *Physiology of the Gastrointestinal Tract, vol. 1*, pp. 670–709. New York: Raven Press.
121. Yuan, S., and Brookes, S. J. (1999). Neuronal control of the gastric sling muscle of the guinea pig. *Journal of Comparative Neurology* 412, 669–680.
122. Zhang, X., Renehan, W. E., and Fogel, R. (1998). Neurons in the vagal complex of the rat respond to mechanical and chemical stimulation of the GI tract. *American Journal of Physiology* 274, G331–G341.
123. Zheng, Z. L., Rogers, R. C., and Travagli, R. A. (1999). Selective gastric projections of nitric oxide synthase-containing vagal brainstem neurons. *Neuroscience* 90, 685–694.

15

# Central Autonomic Control of the Pancreas

R. ALBERTO TRAVAGLI AND KIRSTEEN N. BROWNING

The contribution of the pancreas to proper control of caloric homeostasis and nutrition is accomplished by its two major glandular functions, endocrine and exocrine. The autonomic nervous system plays a major role in controlling both of these functions, and the pancreas is abundantly innervated by parasympathetic and sympathetic as well as sensory axons.

The endocrine pancreas comprises several groups of cells organized in pancreatic islets or islets of Langerhans. The most numerous type of cell, the β-cell, secretes insulin and comprises about 70% of the cells within the islets. The remaining approximately 30% of cells comprise α-cells that secrete glucagon, δ-cells that secrete somatostatin, and cells that secrete pancreatic polypeptide. The major function of the endocrine pancreas is to maintain the concentration of glucose in the plasma within a narrow range in spite of oscillations caused by alternating periods of feeding and fasting. Glucose homeostasis is achieved through a finely tuned balance between pancreatic release of insulin (hypoglycemic) and glucagon (hyperglycemic).

The exocrine pancreas is composed of only two major types of cells, acinar cells and ductal cells. Acinar cells synthesize, store, and secrete digestive enzymes, while ductal cells secrete chloride and bicarbonate. The major function of the exocrine pancreas is to facilitate the efficient digestion of food and the absorption of micronutrients. These functions are accomplished through the release of enzymes that break down macronutrients to more elementary compounds, such as small peptides, amino acids, fatty acids, or monoglycerides, that can be more easily absorbed by the small intestine. Bicarbonate secretion from ductal cells neutralizes gastric acids and creates an intraluminal environment in which the pancreatic enzymes secreted by acinar cells can break down macromolecules.

In this chapter, we provide an overview of the central neural mechanisms controlling the pancreas. For more details, we refer the reader to specialized reviews dealing with each aspect of pancreatic function[11,39,41,75,81].

## PERIPHERAL PATHWAYS CONTROLLING THE PANCREAS AND THEIR CENTRAL NERVOUS SYSTEM (CNS) CONNECTIONS

### Parasympathetic Innervation

The parasympathetic outflow from the brainstem provides the major excitatory input to the pancreas. Cholinergic parasympathetic preganglionic neurons in the dorsal motor nucleus of the vagus (dorsal vagal nucleus [DVN]) receive a vast array of neuromodulatory inputs from brainstem reflex circuits as well as from "higher" centers in the CNS. DVN neurons then send axons through the vagus nerve to the intrinsic pancreatic ganglia, which are scattered in the exocrine parenchyma (see below). Preganglionic neurons of the DVN activate parasympathetic post-ganglionic neurons in the pancreatic ganglia principally via nicotinic acetylcholine receptors. This nicotinic transmission can be modulated within the pancreatic ganglion by several neurotransmitters and neuromodulators (reviewed recently; see [81]). Post-ganglionic neurons of the intrapancreatic ganglia then excite acinar, ductal, and islet cells either via the release of acetylcholine, acting on muscarinic receptors of the M3 and M1 subtypes, or via release of non-adrenergic non-cholinergic neurotransmitters, principally vasoactive intestinal polypeptide, gastrin-releasing peptide, pituitary adenylate cyclase-activating polypeptide, and possibly nitric oxide[39,75,81].

## Sympathetic Innervation

Sympathetic pathways to the pancreas originate from sympathetic preganglionic neurons in lower thoracic and upper lumbar segments of the spinal cord. The axons of these sympathetic preganglionic neurons exit the spinal cord through the ventral roots, either to supply the paravertebral ganglia of the sympathetic chain via (white) communicating rami of the thoracic and lumbar nerves, or to supply the celiac and mesenteric ganglia via the splanchnic nerves. The catecholaminergic neurons of the paravertebral sympathetic celiac and superior mesenteric ganglia innervate the intrapancreatic ganglia, islets, and blood vessels and, to a lesser extent, the ducts and acini. The sympathetic post-ganglionic neurotransmitters are principally noradrenaline, galanin, and neuropeptide Y, although noradrenergic axons also provide a fairly extensive innervation to the islet cells. Stimulation of the sympathetic nerves innervating the pancreas decreases insulin secretion and induces vasoconstriction of the pancreatic vasculature but appears to have little or no direct effect on ductal or acinar cells[75,81].

## Sensory Innervation

Visceral sensory information is conveyed to the CNS by vagal and spinal afferent axons that carry non-painful physiological sensations and painful stimuli, respectively[42]. Small myelinated (Aδ) and unmyelinated (C) sensory fibers from the lower thoracic and upper lumbar dorsal root ganglia project to the pancreas via the celiac and mesenteric ganglia through the splanchnic nerve. These sensory neurons use neuropeptide Y and calcitonin-gene-related peptide as neurotransmitters[113]. Pancreatic afferent fibers originating in the nodose ganglia have been detected in the vagus nerve[108] and probably use substance P as their neurotransmitter[109]. Spinal afferent fibers are mechanosensitive and associated mostly with blood vessels. These axons are also located within the pancreatic parenchyma but do not appear to innervate the ductal system[105]. Vagal afferent fibers are relatively sparse compared to spinal afferents[102,105] and are not mechanosensory[105]. The density and distribution of the pancreatic sensory innervation remains controversial. Some authors report a uniform distribution throughout the organ[108], while others indicate that the innervation decreases in density from the duodenal to the splanchnic areas[76]. Notably, the axons of sensory neurons in dorsal root ganglia have collaterals that innervate both the prevertebral and pancreatic ganglia[51], providing a possible neuronal pathway for sensory-motor axonal reflexes.

## Neurons within the Pancreas

Neurons occur within the pancreas and are organized into heterogeneous intrapancreatic ganglia that are scattered throughout the pancreatic parenchyma. The intrapancreatic neurons modulate sympathetic and parasympathetic outflow to both the exocrine and endocrine pancreas.

Two different types of ganglia are found in the pancreas. The most prevalent are large ganglia containing 10 to 50 neurons that form an interconnected network or plexus. These ganglia send axons to the surrounding acinar tissue and ducts. The second, less common, type of ganglion contains a smaller number of neurons and is associated with nerve trunks. The neurons of these small ganglia do not appear to be interconnected but rather project through, and receive inputs from, the associated nerve trunk[60].

Intrapancreatic ganglia in the cat and guinea pig contain two electrophysiological types of neurons that can be distinguished by their tonic or phasic action potential discharges in response to prolonged injections of direct depolarizing current. In contrast, only phasic firing neurons appear to exist in the rabbit[60,77,79]. The two responses to injection of depolarizing current resemble the dichotomy observed in the responses of inferior mesenteric ganglion neurons innervating the mesenteric vasculature[25]. Hence, pancreatic ganglia may be organized in a similar way to the inferior mesenteric ganglion neurons, with different subsets of neurons selectively innervating distinct pancreatic secretory elements. While pancreatic neurons have spontaneous synaptic activity, suggesting they have intrinsic circuitry capable of regulating pancreatic functions[60,79], intrapancreatic neurons also receive an extensive extrinsic innervation. As with enteric neurons[132], nicotinic, hexamethonium-sensitive fast excitatory postsynaptic potentials (EPSPs) transmit preganglionic information to intrapancreatic neurons[60,77]. However, some pancreatic neurons also display a hexamethonium-resistant component to their fast EPSPs, suggesting the presence of a neurotransmitter other than acetylcholine[77]. Indeed, rabbit pancreatic ganglion neurons receive diverse innervation from cholinergic, noradrenergic, and neuropeptide-containing axons[80].

Intrapancreatic neurons also exhibit viscerotopic diversity in their properties. For example, neurons in the head of the pancreas (i.e., close to the duodenum) respond differently from neurons in the body of the pancreas when challenged with catecholamines or with electrical stimulation of the vagus. The predominant response of neurons in the head of the pancreas is mediated by $\alpha_2$-adrenoceptors, whereas neurons in the body of the pancreas have an $\alpha_1$-adrenoceptor-mediated response[134]. Likewise, vagal stimulation activates the expression of the early gene *c-fos* in about 30% of neurons in the head of the pancreas but only 10% to 20% of neurons in the body and tail (close to the spleen)[129]. Such differential responses between the head and the body of the pancreas further suggest a differential innervation by cholinergic nerves and, possibly, a separation in the physiology of ganglionic transmission.

A differential distribution of neurochemical phenotypes within the intrapancreatic ganglia has also been reported in the guinea pig and rat. Neurons are mainly choline acetyltransferase- and/or nitric oxide synthase-immunoreactive[77,129]; but vasoactive intestinal polypeptide, calcitonin-gene-related peptide, pituitary adenylate cyclase-activating polypeptide, and neuropeptide Y-immunoreactive axons, probably of intrinsic origin, also surround the acini[80]. Intrapancreatic neurons can also have different cell shapes and sizes, with the major heterogeneity seen in neurons containing nitric oxide synthase[80].

Intrapancreatic neurons, therefore, exhibit different electrophysiological, neurochemical, and pharmacological properties, suggesting that their responses to extrinsic neural inputs may be diverse. It is probably prudent, therefore, to consider the extrinsic innervation of the pancreas as an integrative system open to extensive modulation rather than a simple neural command-follower system.

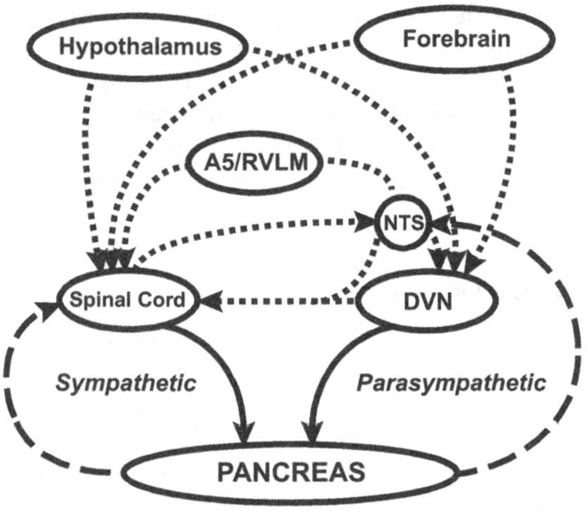


Figure 15–1 Sympathetic and parasympathetic innervation to the pancreas. Parasympathetic outflow from the brainstem provides the major excitatory input to the pancreas. Cholinergic parasympathetic preganglionic neurons of the dorsal vagal nucleus (DVN) receive neuromodulatory inputs from brainstem reflex circuits as well as from "higher" centers in the central nervous system. DVN neurons then send efferent (motor) vagal fibers to the intrinsic pancreatic ganglia that are scattered throughout the pancreatic parenchyma. Sympathetic outflow to the pancreas originates from sympathetic preganglionic neurons in the lower thoracic and upper lumbar levels of the spinal cord. Axons of these preganglionic neurons exit the ventral roots of the spinal cord to supply the paravertebral sympathetic chain (via communicating rami of the thoracic and lumbar nerves) or celiac and mesenteric ganglia (via the splanchnic nerves). Catecholaminergic neurons of celiac and superior mesenteric ganglia innervate pancreatic ganglia, islets, blood vessels, and, to a lesser extent, the pancreatic ducts and acini. Note that the same central nuclei may send information via both sympathetic and parasympathetic pathways, suggesting that an extensive degree of cross-talk exists within the central circuits that control pancreatic functions. Moreover, a large proportion of autonomic homeostatic information is received, integrated and transferred directly to the pancreas from the CNS.

## CNS PATHWAYS CONTROLLING THE PANCREAS

Trans-synaptic viral tracers, such as the Bartha strain of pseudorabies virus, have been instrumental in reconstructing the neuronal pathways in the brain that are involved in controlling the pancreas[26,78,111] (Figure 15–1).

Microinjections of attenuated virus into the pancreas of *vagotomized* rats revealed that sympathetic pathways include first-order neurons in the intermediolateral cell column (IML) of the spinal cord. Second-order neurons are scattered in the brainstem and include catecholaminergic neurons in the A5 area, the locus coeruleus, and the ventrolateral medulla, and serotonergic neurons in the caudal raphé. Second-order sympathetic neurons are also found in higher centers, such as the paraventricular nucleus (PVN) of the hypothalamus, the lateral hypothalamus, the retrochiasmatic area, and the prefrontal cortex. Third-order neurons are located in the bed nucleus of the stria terminalis, medial preoptic area, and subfornical organs; dorsomedial, ventromedial, and arcuate nuclei of the hypothalamus; as well as the central amygdala. Immunohistochemical studies of virus-labeled neurons indicate that a small percentage of these are positive for oxytocin, melanocortin-concentrating hormone, neuropeptide Y, or orexin. However, few, if any, contain choline acetyltransferase, corticotropin-releasing hormone or enkephalins.

Microinjections of attenuated viral tracer into the pancreas of *sympathectomized* rats have revealed brain parasympathetic circuitry that regulates pancreatic function. First-order neurons are scattered bilaterally throughout the rostrocaudal extent of the DVN (i.e., cholinergic parasympathetic preganglionic neurons). Two morphologically distinct cell types are labeled within the DVN; one is bipolar, while the other is multipolar with dendrites projecting toward the central canal or the area postrema[22,102,111](Figure 15–2).

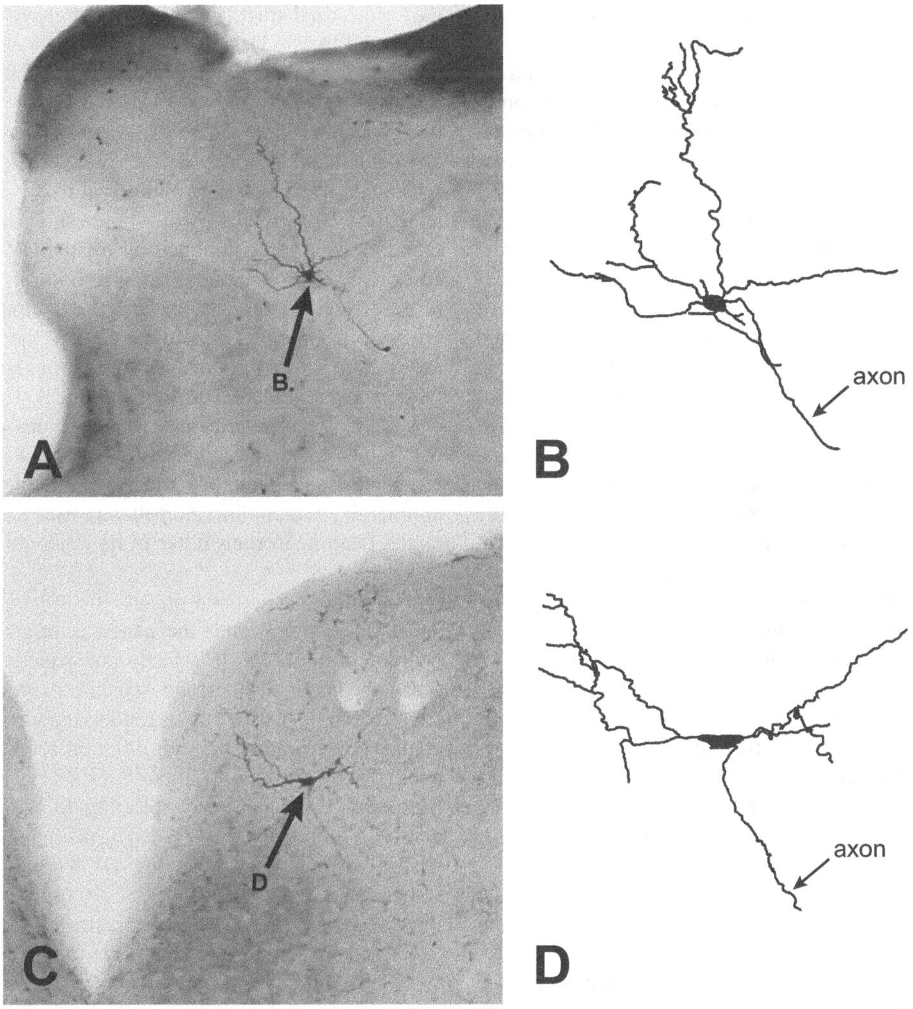


Figure 15–2 Morphology of identified pancreas-projecting DVN neurons. *A:* Low-magnification brightfield micrograph of a coronal brainstem section located approximately 1.2 mm rostral to obex. *Arrow B* indicates a filled DVN neuron that projects to the pancreas. *B:* Computer-aided reconstruction of the neuron shown in *A.* The filled neuron has a multipolar dendritic arbor. The axon could be reconstructed only as far as shown. *C:* Low-magnification brightfield micrograph of a coronal brainstem sections located approximately 1 mm rostral to obex. *Arrow D* indicates a filled DVN neuron that projects to the pancreas. *D:* Computer-aided reconstruction of the neuron shown in the micrograph above. The neuron has a bipolar dendritic arbor and some of the dendrites make contact with the ependymal layer of the fourth ventricle. The axon could be reconstructed only as far as shown. Adapted from Browning et al.[22], with permission.

Specific roles for these two types of DVN neurons in the control of pancreatic functions have not yet been established.

Parasympathetic second-order neurons are more abundant and more widely distributed than the second-order neurons of sympathetic pathways, perhaps indicating a "tighter" role for parasympathetic pathways in the control of pancreatic endocrine and exocrine secretion. Virus-labeled second-order neurons are found in the brainstem areas of the nucleus of the solitary tract (NTS), area postrema, accessory nucleus of the spinal trigeminal nerve, raphé pallidus and obscurus, substantia reticulata, ventrolateral medulla, and A5 area. Second-order neurons are also found in higher centers, such as the PVN, lateral and dorsomedial hypothalamus, arcuate nucleus, medial preoptic, retrochiasmatic, subfornical and zona incerta areas, bed nucleus of the stria terminalis, and prefrontal, piriform, and gustatory cortex. Immunohistochemical studies have revealed that the peptide content of virus-labeled neurons is similar to that of neurons participating in sympathetic circuits. However, the numbers of melanocortin concentrating hormone-, orexin- and oxytocin-containing neurons were significantly lower, while neither corticotropin-releasing hormone, neuropeptide Y, somatostatin, neurotensin, galanin, vasopressin, nor enkephalin neurons were labeled in the PVN, lateral hypothalamus, or perifornical areas.

The areas that are labeled with trans-synaptically transported viruses suggest that the same central nuclei may send information through both sympathetic and parasympathetic pathways. This anatomical arrangement also indicates that extensive cross-talk exists within the CNS. It is likely, therefore, that a large proportion of autonomic homeostatic information is received, integrated, and transferred to pancreatic secretory units directly from the CNS. In this regard, the autonomic control of the pancreas resembles that of enteric ganglia. Considerable integration probably occurs in the CNS, rather than neuronal integration being biased towards the peripheral (i.e., pancreatic or enteric ganglion) level.

## Central Parasympathetic Pathways

Visceral vagal sensory inputs are conveyed to the second-order neurons of the NTS at the level of the caudal brainstem and utilize mainly glutamate as neurotransmitter[12,54]. The rat NTS is organized such that sensory information from the gastrointestinal tract is received and processed in distinct, viscerotopically organized subnuclei (reviewed in [119]; although see Chapter 2 for more discussion about viscerotopy in the NTS). The NTS then sends projections to the efferent vagal preganglionic neurons of the DVN as well as relaying this immense volume of afferent information to higher integrative structures in the pons and the diencephalon.

The DVN also shows viscerotopic organization, but it is less rigid than that of the NTS. The DVN is organized into mediolateral columns. Neurons in the medial part of the nucleus project to the proximal gastrointestinal tract via the paired anterior and posterior gastric branches and the hepatic branch of the subdiaphragmatic vagus. DVN neurons in the lateral part of the nucleus give rise to the celiac and the accessory celiac vagal branches, which project to the more distal gastrointestinal tract, including the transverse colon (reviewed in [119]). Despite the existence of numerous, distinct neurochemical phenotypes of NTS neurons that provide inputs to the DVN, the NTS-DVN synaptic connections are mainly GABAergic, glutamatergic, or catecholaminergic (reviewed in [119]).

Vagally mediated gastrointestinal motor functions are controlled tonically by the cholinergic parasympathetic preganglionic motoneurons of the DVN. These neurons show spontaneous activity both *in vivo* and *in vitro* (reviewed in [119]). Vagal motor output is conveyed from DVN neurons in the CNS to the gastrointestinal tract via two pathways, distinguishable by their post-ganglionic neurotransmitters. An excitatory cholinergic (muscarinic) pathway provides a significant tonic input to gastrointestinal viscera and sets the contractile and secretory tone. An inhibitory non-adrenergic, non-cholinergic pathway uses nitric oxide as the main neurotransmitter to its innervation target (reviewed by [24,119]).

As with other visceral organs, the efferent (motor) vagal fibers innervating the pancreas originate from neurons in the DVN. It is likely that pancreatic functions are under distinct and separate control by the vagus nerve since exocrine and endocrine secretions are controlled separately through different types of vagal axons and neurotransmitters[3,16,18,22,23,29,52,91,92,100,126-129]. Moreover, DVN neurons projecting to the pancreas comprise subpopulations that can be distinguished from gastric- or intestinal-projecting DVN cells by their somatic and dendritic features[22,102,111], further reinforcing the possibility of selective pathways controlling exocrine versus endocrine pancreatic functions.

Many authors have demonstrated that different frequencies of vagal stimulation selectively release acetylcholine, nitric oxide, or vasoactive intestinal peptide onto the smooth muscles that control gastrointestinal motility (reviewed in [119]). Vagal activation also affects pancreatic exocrine and endocrine secretion directly[16,65,69,92,100]. As with gastrointestinal smooth muscle, the influence of the vagus on pancreatic exocrine or endocrine function appears to depend upon either the frequency of vagal stimulation or the frequency of action-potential firing that the DVN neurons are capable of sustaining. Different stimulation frequencies have divergent effects on vagally stimulated gastric acid secretion versus insulin and glucagon secretion[17]. Furthermore, electrical stimulation of gastric and hepatic branches of the vagus increase insulin secretion in a independent and additive manner[16], suggesting differences in vagal neurons that control insulin secretion or in vagal neuroeffector coupling. These observations further suggest that different vagal branches may control different populations of pancreatic islet cells.

At the level of the pancreas, vagal innervation shows a gradient. The head of the pancreas (i.e., the duodenal portion) receives a greater density of vagal axons than the tail (i.e., the splenic portion)[16,18,19,107]. The vagal influence on pancreatic function, especially endocrine secretion, also appears to depend upon the particular subdiaphragmatic vagal branch involved. Electrical stimulation of the right vagal branch, for example, induced more *c-fos* expression in the main body of the pancreas compared to stimulation of the left branch, suggesting that the vagal terminal fields do not overlap completely[16,18,19,107,129]. Despite anatomical evidence for the vagal celiac branches innervating the splenic end of the pancreas, electrical stimulation of the hepatic and gastric branches of the vagus appear solely responsible for insulin and glucagon secretion[18], suggesting that the celiac branches innervate pancreatic targets other than pancreatic $\beta$ and $\alpha$ cells. These data suggest that different regions or cell groups within the DVN regulate specific pancreatic functions, such as, for example, the release of insulin during the cephalic phase of digestion.

Several pieces of evidence highlight the importance of vagal innervation in the control of endocrine secretion:

1. An increase in plasma glucose produces an increase in vagal activity (reviewed in [90]). Since pretreatment with the non-selective muscarinic antagonist atropine attenuated and delayed the insulin response to intravenous or intragastric glucose load (reviewed in [104]), vagal pathways are involved in relaying the relevant information to the pancreatic $\beta$-cells.
2. In the basal state, plasma insulin concentration oscillates with a periodicity of approximately 14 minutes. Insulin is released in a pulsatile manner, which implies that islets secrete insulin synchronously, possibly via a coordination of the extensive inter-islet post-ganglionic pancreatic neural network[80,82]. Such pulsatile stimuli may arise from the CNS directly; or, alternatively, the vagus may play a major role in the modulation of the intrinsic pacemaker activity of the pancreas (in a similar manner to the vagal modulation of the sino-atrial node in the heart).
3. Patients with complete resection of all subdiaphragmatic vagal branches following surgical procedures have oscillations in plasma insulin with longer periodicity (33–37 minutes), and the swings are significantly larger than in normal subjects[82].
4. Finally, electrical stimulation of the DVN or NTS increases insulin secretion[52], suggesting not only that there are neurons and fibers that facilitate insulin secretion exclusively, but also that NTS activation stimulates the DVN neurons that control insulin secretion subsequently.

Together with other available information, these data provide ample evidence that the vagus is involved in the overall dynamics of insulin secretion, rather than just the cephalic phase response.

The "cephalic phase response" refers to the release of gut hormones in the initial stages of digestion when the ingested nutrients have not yet induced a systemic hormonal response. This phase appears to play an important physiological role in priming the secretory capabilities of the gut, increasing the efficiency of the subsequent gastric and intestinal phases of secretion (reviewed in [59,112]). The cephalic phase of digestion has been described in detail, both in humans and experimental animals, especially in relation to the early insulin response; i.e., the release of insulin that appears before the first noticeable increase in blood glucose. Its anatomical substrate is the inputs arising from the gustatory, piriform, and prefrontal cortices[26]. The effector portion of the cephalic phase of the insulin response is mediated by the hepatic and gastric branches of the vagus[18]; early insulin release is suppressed by subdiaphragmatic vagotomy or by prior administration of atropine[4,59,90,104,112]. The cephalic-phase response is, however, not limited to endocrine secretion but also includes exocrine secretion (also vagally mediated) that accounts for a large proportion of the total postprandial enzyme secretion[8].

As with endocrine secretion, an intact vagal innervation is necessary for the control of pancreatic exocrine secretion. A number of observations highlight the importance of vagal innervation in the control of exocrine secretion:

1. Peptides known to modulate pancreatic secretion, such as cholecystokinin, somatostatin, calcitonin gene-related peptide, and pancreatic polypeptide, or the transduction of luminal information, all exert their actions on pancreatic exocrine secretion via vagally dependent pathways[29,43,43,55,70,70,94,95,123,130,137].

2. Enzyme output cycles are significantly faster in the extrinsically denervated pancreas[138].
3. Exocrine secretion in the cephalic phase is vagally mediated and accounts for a significant portion of total postprandial enzyme secretion[8].
4. Atropine or vagotomy almost completely abolish pancreatic exocrine secretion induced by feeding or by pharmacological or electrical stimuli[31,71,72,88,89].
5. The negative feedback control of exocrine secretion exerted by circulating hormones, such as pancreatic polypeptide, is abolished by vagotomy[92].

Taken together with other information, these observations provide ample evidence that the vagus is involved in the control of pancreatic exocrine secretion.

## Sensory Innervation

Retrograde tracing studies have identified neurochemically distinct populations of sensory neurons innervating the pancreas with cell bodies located bilaterally in dorsal root ganglia of the thoracic and lumbar region (predominately thoracic spinal segments 9–12)[38,81,131]. Immunohistochemical studies in the rat identified principally calcitonin gene-related peptide and substance P-containing neurons[109,131]. However, in the mouse, most pancreas-projecting sensory neurons appear to contain transient receptor potential vanilloid 1 (TRPV1), glial derived neurotrophic factor $\alpha$, and calcitonin gene-related peptide[38]. These neurons send their axons to the pancreas via the splanchnic nerves and transmit mechanosensitive and nociceptive information to sympathetic preganglionic neurons in the IML of the spinal cord[26]. Collateral projections from these dorsal root ganglion neurons innervate prevertebral and pancreatic ganglia and may provide a mechanistic explanation for visceral reflexes[51].

The role of sensory nerves in normal physiological functions (as opposed to pathophysiological conditions; see [38,87]) is still controversial. Endocrine (insulin) secretion is certainly affected by calcitonin gene-related peptide and substance P, although species differences may exist. In the mouse and pig, for example, calcitonin gene-related peptide inhibits both basal and stimulated insulin secretion[5,99]. In the rat, calcitonin gene-related peptide stimulates basal insulin secretion but inhibits stimulated release[97,98]. In the calf, calcitonin gene-related peptide appears to have no effect upon insulin secretion[37]. Chemical ablation of pancreatic sensory nerves (via capsaicin application) has been reported to increase[56] glucose-induced insulin secretion, although other reports have noted no effect[57]. These findings suggest that these sensory nerves may exert a tonic inhibition of insulin secretion[1,99], although it is important to recognize that the indirect involvement of glucose-stimulated reflexes cannot be discounted. The effect of substance P on endocrine secretion is similarly confusing, with reports demonstrating substance P-induced stimulation[45,106] or inhibition[21] of insulin release. Glucagon secretion may also be regulated by sensory nerves. Calcitonin gene-related peptide has been reported to either stimulate[5,53] or inhibit[97] glucagon secretion; and capsaicin-induced ablation of sensory nerves has been demonstrated to either reduce[57] or have no effect upon[53] stimulated glucagon secretion. The role of sensory afferents in physiological exocrine secretion has not been established, although both calcitonin gene-related peptide and substance P have been demonstrated to inhibit exocrine secretion indirectly via actions on ganglionic transmission[63].

## Central Sympathetic Pathways

Sympathetic preganglionic (motor) neurons innervating the pancreas are located in the thoracic and lumbar segments of the spinal cord. Axons from these neurons form the thoracic and lumbar nerves that reach the paravertebral chain. Preganglionic neurons either innervate neurons within the paravertebral ganglia or pass through the splanchnic nerves to innervate the celiac and superior mesenteric ganglia. Sympathetic post-ganglionic neurons have their cell bodies in these ganglia; and an extensive and dense network of varicose catecholaminergic fibers has been observed surrounding intrapancreatic neurons, blood vessels, islets, and ducts. Interestingly, immunohistochemical evidence suggests that pancreatic acinar cells receive very little direct innervation from sympathetic axons, yet the sympathetic nervous system may exert profound effects upon exocrine secretion (see below; reviewed in [81]). The presence of adrenoceptors on acinar cells, however, suggests that catecholamines may facilitate enzyme secretion directly (reviewed in [81]). Immunohistochemical studies suggest that tyrosine-hydroxylase-immunoreactive neurons are present within pancreatic ganglia. However, these neurons do not appear to contain dopamine $\beta$-hydroxylase; hence they are probably not noradrenergic (reviewed in [81]). The precise catecholamine present within pancreatic ganglion neurons remains to be identified.

Sympathetic post-ganglionic axons innervating the pancreas release mainly noradrenaline, but prominent effects of galanin and neuropeptide Y have also been reported[2,36,81,114]. The effects of noradrenaline vary according to the pancreatic region under investigation. In the head of the pancreas, for example, noradrenaline inhibits fast excitatory synaptic transmission via actions at presynaptic $\alpha_2$-adrenoceptors. In contrast, in the body of the pancreas, noradrenaline facilitates fast (nicotinic) excitatory transmission via actions at post-synaptic $\alpha_1$-adrenoceptors (reviewed in [81]) . Large species differences may also exist in the neurochemical content of post-ganglionic sympathetic fibers. In the rabbit, for example, galanin-containing fibers are scarce, existing principally in larger nerve trunks alongside blood vessels or within intrapancreatic ganglia, suggesting expression in a distinct subpopulation of sympathetic fibers. In contrast, galanin is co-released with noradrenaline following splanchnic nerve stimulation in dogs and inhibits insulin secretion[2,36]. In the guinea pig, somatostatin-immunoreactivity is present in axons surrounding intrapancreatic ganglion neurons, yet somatostatin-positive fibers are not observed in the rabbit pancreas[62,80].

The role of the sympathetic nervous system in the neural control of pancreatic functions has been difficult to establish definitively. Stimulation of sympathetic nerves can elicit diverse effects, and there has been difficulty in separating direct actions on pancreatic exocrine and endocrine tissue from indirect effects on blood pressure, blood flow, and hormone release, as well as indirect effects to modulate ganglionic transmission. The non-selective actions of many adrenoceptor agonists and antagonists compound these difficulties, and the profound differences between *in vitro* versus *in vivo* studies and the apparently marked species differences render generalizations problematic. Nevertheless, many observations highlight the importance of the sympathetic nervous system in the neural control of the endocrine pancreas. Electrical stimulation of the splanchnic nerve lowers plasma insulin levels, possibly due to direct actions of noradrenaline on pancreatic β-cells[6,7,9,35,50]. Disruption of the splanchnic nerves increases insulin secretion, suggesting that the sympathetic nervous system exerts a tonic inhibition on endocrine secretion. Sympathetic nerve stimulation increases basal insulin secretion[1,35]. Splanchnic nerve stimulation elevates catecholamine levels, and catecholamines may inhibit insulin secretion in both *in vivo* as well as *in vitro* assays via activation of $\alpha_2$-adrenoceptors on pancreatic β-cells[35,48] (but see also [1,7]). Splanchnic nerve stimulation increases glucagon secretion, probably via activation of $\beta_2$-adrenoceptors. Similarly, adrenaline increases glucagon secretion both *in vivo* and *in vitro*[5,6,9,50]. Galanin, which is co-released with noradrenaline, decreases insulin secretion in dogs[2,36]. Consistent with the general inhibitory effect on the pancreas, adrenoceptor agonists induce vasoconstriction and decrease endocrine secretion[6,7,15]. Thus, the overall effect of sympathetic nerve stimulation on pancreatic endocrine secretion appears to be organized towards maintenance of glycemic levels during conditions of stress via inhibition of insulin secretion and stimulation of glucagon secretion.

Although the problems mentioned also apply to understanding sympathetic control of the exocrine pancreas, experimental data confirm the importance of sympathetic innervation in regulating pancreatic enzyme secretion. Electrical stimulation of the splanchnic nerves inhibited enzyme secretion. Conversely, cutting the splanchnic nerves increased enzyme secretion, suggesting that the sympathetic nervous system exerts a tonic inhibitory action on pancreatic exocrine secretion[15,49]. Denervation of the celiac ganglion in the dog reduced pancreatic secretion by approximately 70% but increased blood flow by approximately 350%, suggesting that the sympathetic nervous system exerts a tonic stimulatory effect on pancreatic secretion as well as a tonic vasoconstriction of blood vessels within the pancreas that is mediated by the rostral ventrolateral medulla[64,122]. Noradrenaline as well as selective α- and β-adrenoceptor agonists or antagonists decrease, increase, or have no effect upon exocrine secretion (reviewed in [81]). Noradrenergic vasoconstriction, however, decreases exocrine secretion[15]. In part, this may explain some of the confusion surrounding the *in vivo* results above, since it may be difficult to separate the effects of noradrenaline in decreasing secretion directly through effects on acinar tissue and indirectly via vasoconstriction. Thus, although pharmacological evidence and *in vitro* studies suggest that the sympathetic nervous system may exert profound actions to regulate pancreatic exocrine secretion, technical difficulties, allied with the apparent lack of sympathetic innervation to the acini, make interpretation of these results difficult. At the present stage, it appears more likely that the actions of the sympathetic nervous system to alter exocrine secretion occur predominantly indirectly, via alterations in pancreatic blood flow.

## NEUROTRANSMITTERS IN CENTRAL PATHWAYS REGULATING THE PANCREAS

The brainstem clearly plays a prominent role in the integration and regulation of both parasympathetic and sympathetic outflow to the pancreas. Chronic decerebration decreases basal and stimulated pancreatic secretion, but only by approximately one third, indicating that the majority of the central neural circuitry controlling the pancreas is contained entirely within the brainstem[73]. Nevertheless, the prominent reciprocal connections between the brainstem and "higher" CNS nuclei suggest the likelihood of "higher" influences on pancreatic secretion. The extensive nature of these inputs implies that many neurotransmitters and neuromodulators may influence efferent outflow to the pancreas. It is also important to recognize that the dorsal vagal complex in the brainstem is essentially a circumventricular organ with large areas being either entirely outside the blood–brain barrier (e.g., the area postrema) or having a leaky blood–brain barrier because of the presence of fenestrated capillaries (e.g., nucleus of the solitary tract and dorsal motor nucleus of the vagus)[27]. Hence, neurons within the brainstem are more accessible to circulating neuropeptides. Here we will concentrate on those peptides and transmitters that have been most extensively studied.

## GABA and Glutamate

GABA is not only the main inhibitory neurotransmitter in the CNS but also the principal brainstem neurotransmitter involved in controlling vagal outflow to the viscera. Unsurprisingly, therefore, GABA has been shown to influence pancreatic functions, particularly exocrine secretion. Microinjection of the GABA receptor antagonist bicuculline into the dorsal vagal complex increased pancreatic exocrine secretion, suggesting that vagal motor neurons innervating the pancreas are inhibited tonically by GABAergic synaptic inputs[86]. A similar inhibitory influence (tonic or stimulated) of GABAergic neurotransmission on pancreatic endocrine secretion does not appear to have been investigated. Nevertheless, inferences may be drawn from *in vitro* electrophysiological studies, which have shown that glucagon-like peptide-1 (which acts in the brainstem to modulate insulin secretion; see below) modulates GABAergic synaptic inputs onto pancreas-projecting DVN neurons[126]. Hence, GABAergic inputs onto parasympathetic preganglionic neurons may be equally important in the regulation of endocrine secretion.

The role of glutamatergic excitatory synaptic transmission in the control of brainstem vagal pathways controlling pancreatic outflow has not been elucidated fully. It is widely accepted that vagal sensory inputs into the brainstem release glutamate as their principal neurotransmitter (reviewed in [119]). The close proximity of interconnected brainstem nuclei makes it impossible to use microinjection techniques to distinguish the actions of glutamate on NTS neurons from the actions of glutamate on pancreas-projecting DVN neurons (see also Chapters 2 and 7). Nevertheless, inferences may be drawn from *in vitro* electrophysiological studies, since peptides such as glucagon-like peptide-1 and pancreatic polypeptide (which are known to act in the dorsal vagal complex to affect both endocrine and exocrine pancreatic secretion; see below) alter glutamatergic synaptic transmission to pancreas-projecting DVN neurons[23,126] (and see below). Hence, glutamatergic inputs onto parasympathetic preganglionic neurons are likely to be important not only in the regulation of pancreatic secretion per se, but also as the means by which other peptides and neurotransmitters exert their actions.

## Pancreatic Polypeptide

Pancreatic polypeptide is released from specialized cells of the pancreatic islets of Langerhans after ingestion of a meal. This release occurs via a vagally dependent mechanism that involves activation of post-ganglionic muscarinic acetylcholine receptors[55]. Circulating pancreatic polypeptide then potently inhibits pancreatic exocrine secretion (reviewed in [59,130]), but not through a direct effect of pancreatic polypeptide on the pancreatic acini. Isolated *in vitro* preparations of pancreatic acini or ducts are not inhibited by pancreatic polypeptide, and there are no receptors for pancreatic polypeptide on the acinar or ductal cells[100,130]. Instead, the inhibitory effects of pancreatic polypeptide on exocrine secretion are mediated by the interaction of the peptide with receptors located in the dorsal vagal complex[30,92,100]. Despite the structural similarity with other pancreatic polypeptides, such as neuropeptide Y and peptide YY, receptors for pancreatic polypeptide can be distinguished from binding sites for neuropeptide Y and peptide YY[130] and are most likely of the Y4 subtype[84]. Microinjections of pancreatic polypeptide in the dorsal vagal complex do not affect basal plasma insulin, somatostatin, or glucagon secretion, but inhibit centrally mediated pancreatic exocrine secretion by modulating vagal cholinergic output[65,92,100].

Recent electrophysiological studies have demonstrated that approximately half of the identified pancreas-projecting DVN neurons respond to pancreatic polypeptide, either directly or through the activation of neuronal circuits between the DVN and the area postrema[23]. When challenged with glucagon-like peptide-1 (see below), these same pancreatic polypeptide-responsive neurons were unresponsive. In contrast, neurons responsive to glucagon-like peptide-1 were unresponsive to pancreatic polypeptide[128]. These pharmacological differences provide further support for the hypothesis that CNS circuits may be wired specifically according to the functions of the peripheral organ that they control. In this particular case, vagal motoneurons that respond to pancreatic polypeptide could project exclusively to the ganglionic neurons controlling exocrine secretion, while glucagon-like peptide-1 responsive DVN neurons could project exclusively to neurons controlling endocrine secretion.

## Cholecystokinin

Cholecystokinin is released from enteroendocrine cells in the small intestine in response to nutrients entering the duodenum (reviewed in [34]). Cholecystokinin then has multiple effects along the gastrointestinal tract, including increased pancreatic exocrine secretion, gastric relaxation, decreased gastric acid secretion, and reduction of food intake[32,101]. In the last two decades, a great deal of research has investigated the mechanisms of action of this peptide. Since systemic or localized perivagal administration of the toxin capsaicin significantly attenuates or abolishes the effects of cholecystokinin on pancreatic secretion (reviewed in[96]), the main site of action of cholecystokinin has been assumed to be at the level of vagal sensory neurons. The hypothesized mechanism proposes that cholecystokinin released from enteroendocrine cells acts exclusively in a paracrine manner to excite the C-type vagal afferent terminals in the intestinal wall and activate vago-vagal reflexes (reviewed in[96]). Despite its wide acceptance, this mechanism of action is open to criticism, and cholecystokinin has also been proposed to play a role in pancreatic as well as gastric control through a brainstem site of action. Cholecystokinin-1 receptors are present on neurons of the dorsal vagal complex, and these receptors are activated by exogenous administration of cholecystokinin[10,14,20,46,123,127,136]. Indeed, Viard and colleagues[123] demonstrated that intraduodenal administration of casein, a protein known to release endogenous cholecystokinin, increased pancreatic exocrine secretion even in rats in which the vagal afferent fibers were surgically removed (i.e., vagal deafferentation). Similarly, intraperitoneal administration of cholecystokinin increases Fos-immunoreactivity in NTS neurons of vagally deafferented rats[14]; and cholecystokinin excites identified pancreas-projecting DVN neurons[127] (Figure 15–3). Overall, the effects of cholecystokinin in increasing pancreatic exocrine secretion appear to occur, at least in the rat, via both a paracrine effect on the peripheral terminals of vagal afferent fibers and a hormonal effect on neurons of the dorsal vagal complex.

## Serotonin

Serotonin (5-hydroxytryptamine [5-HT]) is an important modulator of pancreatic secretion via both direct and indirect actions. The pancreas is innervated directly by serotonin-containing neurons of the stomach and small intestine[61], and serotonin has been proposed to inhibit pancreatic enzyme secretion via activation of presynaptic receptors on cholinergic neurons. The physiological role of this enteropancreatic neural reflex has still to be characterized fully.

An indirect action of serotonin to modulate pancreatic exocrine secretion via excitation of vagal afferent fibers has received more attention[70,137]. Pancreatic exocrine secretion in response to intraduodenal carbohydrates or mucosal stimulation is abolished by both vagal deafferentation and serotonin-3 receptor antagonists[70]. Recent studies from several groups have highlighted the possible synergistic actions between cholecystokinin and serotonin in the vagally mediated regulation of visceral functions, including pancreatic secretion[44,74,85]. For example, the ability of the serotonergic agonist phenylbiguanide to excite pancreatic vagal afferent fibers was attenuated by the cholecystokinin-1 receptor antagonists lorglumide or devazepide[85]. Such interactions between neurohormones and neurotransmitters that have similar actions to increase pancreatic exocrine secretion may appear, at first, inefficient or unwieldy. Ultimately, however, such interactions may provide a means for a more finely tuned and delicate regulation of the neural control of pancreatic functions.

## Thyrotropin-Releasing Hormone

Thyrotropin-releasing hormone receptors and thyrotropin-releasing hormone-immunoreactive axons originating from the medullary raphé, the parapyramidal nuclei, and the hypothalamus are present throughout the rostrocaudal extent of the dorsal vagal complex[116]. Thyrotropin-releasing hormone is a well-known activator of vagal outflow. Brainstem application of thyrotropin-releasing hormone increases gastric acid secretion and motility through direct excitation of DVN neurons[115,118]. Several studies have established that thyrotropin-releasing hormone also increases pancreatic exocrine secretion via a vagally mediated pathway, since its effects are prevented by vagotomy, ganglionic blockade with hexamethonium, blockade of post-ganglionic transmission with the muscarinic acetylcholine receptor antagonist atropine, or by a VIP antagonist[58,83,93]. Brainstem application of thyrotropin-releasing hormone also increases pancreatic blood flow via a vagally mediated effect that involves the activation of both muscarinic acetylcholine receptors and nitric oxide[135].

## Glucagon-Like Peptide-1

Glucose-sensitive neurons and axons in the dorsal vagal complex react immediately to changes in glucose levels[13,28,103,117,124,125]. *In vivo*, these changes in blood glucose are transmitted to the pancreas via the vagus to modulate insulin secretion. In response to ingestion of food, glucagon-like peptide-1 is released from intestinal cells into the circulation, where it binds to specific receptors on the pancreatic β cell and acts as a potent releaser of insulin. Glucagon-like peptide-1 also exerts major effects at the level of the CNS, decreasing food intake and increasing insulin secretion[33,47]. Glucagon-like peptide-1 is also involved in interoceptive stress, in the attenuation of toxin-induced fever, and in lithium-induced

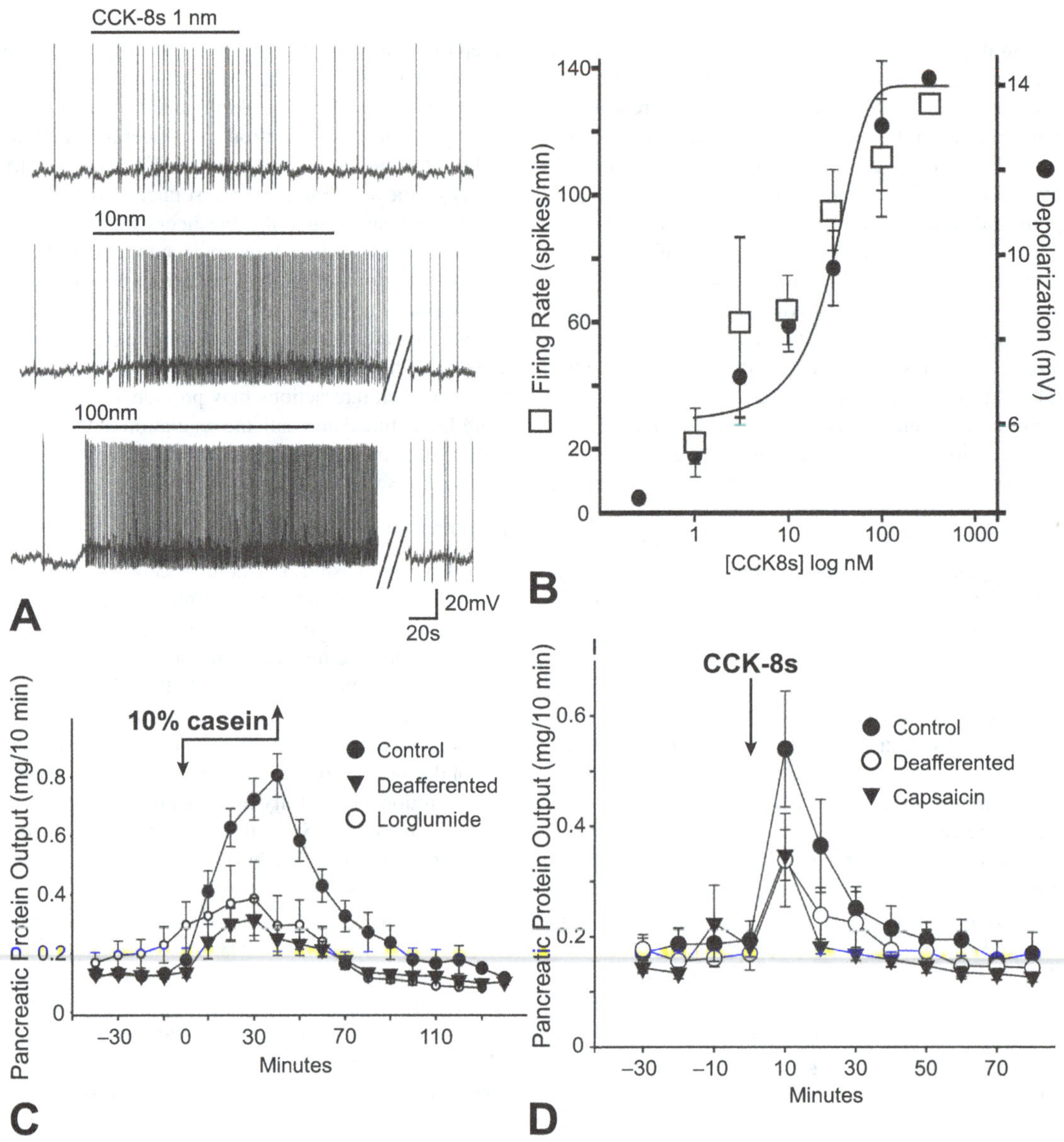


Figure 15–3 Cholecystokinin increases pancreatic protein output via excitation of pancreas-projecting DVN neurons. *A:* Cholecystokinin-8s (CCK-8s) depolarizes a subpopulation of pancreas-projecting DVN neurons. Representative traces of neuronal activity under current clamp illustrate the concentration-dependent increase in firing rate induced by perfusion of CCK-8s onto an identified pancreas-projecting DVN neuron. The neuron recovered for at least 10 minutes between successive applications. Parallel lines indicate a two-minute interval. Holding potential approximately -60mV. *B:* Concentration-response curve for the increase in firing rate induced by CCK-8s (*closed circles*; holding potential approximately -60 mV) and depolarization (*open squares*; holding potential approximately -65 mV) expressed as mean ± s.e.m. Each neuron was tested with at least three different concentrations of CCK-8s. *C:* Intraduodenal casein also increases pancreatic protein output via an effect on CCK-A receptors in the dorsal vagal complex. The graph shows the effects of duodenal infusion of casein in intact animals (control), either following pretreatment with the CCK-A receptor selective antagonist lorglumide to the fourth ventricle or following vagal deafferentation. *D:* Microinjection of CCK-8s (450 pmoles) in the dorsal vagal complex increased protein secretion; vagotomy prevented the increase in protein output induced by CCK-8s . Microinjection of vehicle (PBS) did not affect protein output. The graph shows the effects of microinjection of PBS or CCK-8s in intact animals and of CCK-8s in surgically vagotomized animals. Adapted from Viard et al. (2007)[123] and Wan et al. (2007)[127], with permission.

anorexia[33,47,66]. Glucagon-like peptide-1 also increases the impulse discharge of fibers from the hepatic branch of the vagus and increases *c-fos* expression in the NTS[91,121]. In the brainstem, the highest density of glucagon-like peptide-1 binding sites and/or mRNA is found in the dorsal vagal complex[40,67,110], whereas glucagon-like peptide-1 immunoreactive perikarya are confined to the NTS[120]. Recently, administration of glucagon-like peptide-1 has been shown to excite pancreas-projecting DVN neurons via both direct effects on the DVN neuronal membrane[128] and the modulation of NTS-DVN synaptic inputs[126]. Most importantly, glucagon-like peptide-1 does not stimulate exocrine secretion at doses that stimulate insulin secretion[3]. Glucagon-like peptide-1, then, has the potential to differentially regulate the activity of pancreas-projecting DVN neurons that control endocrine versus exocrine secretion.

### Acetylcholine

The role of the hypothalamus in the integration and processing of homeostatic information arising from the viscera, including the pancreas, cannot be overestimated. Electrical stimulation of the ventromedial anterior hypothalamus increases, whereas stimulation of the posterior hypothalamus decreases, pancreatic secretion, indicating an involvement in the regulation of efferent outflow to the pancreas. Recent studies have suggested that these "pancreas-related" hypothalamic inputs to the brainstem are themselves under cholinergic control from "higher" CNS centers. For example, microinjection of muscarinic receptor antagonists directly into either the lateral hypothalamus or the PVN inhibited basal and stimulated pancreatic exocrine secretion, and central depletion of neuronal acetylcholine stores had similar effects. In contrast, microinjection of M1 muscarinic receptor agonists into the hypothalamus significantly increased pancreatic secretion. Tract tracing in conjunction with functional studies suggest that the hypothalamus receives cholinergic inputs from the lateral septum as well as the lateral parabrachial nucleus. These nuclei have a major influence on the hypothalamic neurons that provide input to the dorsal vagal complex and thereby affect the tonic parasympathetic efferent (motor) vagal output to the pancreas[73].

### Orexin

Neurons in the brain (particularly the lateral hypothalamus, the ventral medial hypothalamus, the NTS, and the DVN) can sense changes in glucose levels directly and mount appropriate responses to minimize these changes. Electrophysiological studies demonstrate the presence of glucose-inhibited neurons (activated by hypoglycemia) and glucose-excited neurons (activated by hyperglycemia) in the lateral hypothalamic area[68]. The prominent role that the lateral hypothalamus plays in modulating the efferent (motor) outflow to the pancreas is well established[73,133]. Orexin-containing neurons in the lateral hypothalamic area project to parasympathetic and sympathetic preganglionic neurons innervating the pancreas[26], and microinjection of orexin-A antagonists into the lateral hypothalamus significantly decreases pancreatic vagal efferent nerve activity[133]. These data imply that a drop in peripheral blood glucose levels activates glucose-sensitive, orexin-containing neurons of the lateral hypothalamic area. In turn, these neurons project to, and activate, DVN neurons to stimulate pancreatic efferent outflow to regulate blood glucose levels.

## SUMMARY AND FUTURE RESEARCH

The pancreas contributes to proper control of caloric homeostasis and nutrition because of its finely tuned inputs from the sympathetic and parasympathetic branches of the autonomic nervous system, which perform as a highly integrated neural circuit. Several neuromodulators act in concert to provide adaptive responses to the ever-changing challenges necessary for proper pancreatic function.

Overwhelming evidence indicates that vagal and sympathetic motor pathways involved in pancreatic control are arranged in a manner that suggests specificity based on the unique pancreatic functions that they control. This specificity in central inputs is mirrored by the organization of pancreatic ganglion neurons, which exert specific control over the different types of pancreatic secretory elements. It is vitally important, therefore, to understand how *specific* nerve pathways regulate pancreatic secretion. The first step should be to identify the neurotransmitter phenotypes of pathways that innervate functionally distinct types of pancreatic cells. Apart from a few studies providing gross anatomical information[19,26], the autonomic innervation of the pancreas has not been mapped in detail. Currently available data stress the complexity of the system. There are functional and anatomical interactions between the parasympathetic and sympathetic nervous systems in pancreatic control as well as interactions between neuropeptide and neurohormonal mechanisms. Thus, to understand autonomic control of the pancreas, it may be necessary to adopt farsighted approaches, challenge existing dogmas, and consider neural regulation of pancreatic secretion *in toto* rather than as distinct anatomical, physiological, or pharmacological processes. Although challenging to dissect physiologically and pharmacologically, such diversity of control is likely to provide endocrinologists, neurologists, and gastroenterologists with a variety of treatment strategies aimed at correcting a variety of potential pancreatic dysfunctions.

ACKNOWLEDGEMENTS This research is supported by National Science Foundation Grant # 105-1049618.

## References

1. Ahren, B. (2000). Autonomic regulation of islet hormone secretion—implications for health and disease. *Diabetologia* 43, 393–410.
2. Ahren, B., Bottcher, G., Kowalyk, S., Dunning, B. E., Sundler, F., and Taborsky, G. J., Jr. (1990). Galanin is co-localized with noradrenaline and neuropeptide Y in dog pancreas and celiac ganglion. *Cell and Tissue Research* 261, 49–58.
3. Ahren, B., Gingerich, R. L., and Havel, P. J. (1995). Effects of cholecystokinin and glucagon-like peptide 1 on the secretion of pancreatic polypeptide in mice. *Regulatory Pepides* 59, 297–302.
4. Ahren, B., and Holst, J. J. (2001). The cephalic insulin response to meal ingestion in humans is dependent on both cholinergic and noncholinergic mechanisms and is important for postprandial glycemia. *Diabetes* 50, 1030–1038.
5. Ahren, B., Martensson, H., and Nobin, A. (1987). Effects of calcitonin gene-related peptide (CGRP) on islet hormone secretion in the pig. *Diabetologia* 30, 354–359.
6. Ahren, B., Veith, R. C., Paquette, T. L., and Taborsky, G. J., Jr. (1987). Sympathetic nerve stimulation versus pancreatic norepinephrine infusion in the dog: 2). Effects on basal release of somatostatin and pancreatic polypeptide. *Endocrinology* 121, 332–339.
7. Ahren, B., Veith, R. C., and Taborsky, G. J., Jr. (1987). Sympathetic nerve stimulation versus pancreatic norepinephrine infusion in the dog: 1). Effects on basal release of insulin and glucagon. *Endocrinology* 121, 323–331.
8. Anagnostides, A., Chadwick, V. S., Selden, A. C., and Maton, P. N. (1984). Sham feeding and pancreatic secretion. Evidence for direct vagal stimulation of enzyme output. *Gastroenterology* 87, 109–114.
9. Andersson, P. O., Holst, J., and Jarhult, J. (1982). Effects of adrenergic blockade on the release of insulin, glucagon and somatostatin from the pancreas in response to splanchnic nerve stimulation in cats. *Acta Physiologica Scandinavica* 116, 403–409.
10. Appleyard, S. M., Bailey, T. W., Doyle, M. W., Jin, Y. H., Smart, J. L., Low, M. J., and Andresen, M. C. (2005). Proopiomelanocortin neurons in nucleus tractus solitarius are activated by visceral afferents: Regulation by cholecystokinin and opioids. *Journal of Neuroscience* 25, 3578–3585.
11. Argent, B. E., Gray, M. A., Stewart, M. C., and Case, R. M. (2005). Cell physiology of pancreatic ducts. In L. R. Johnson (Ed.), *Physiology of the Gastrointestinal Tract*, pp. 1371–1396. San Diego, CA: Elsevier.
12. Aylwin, M. L., Horowitz, J. M., and Bonham, A. C. (1997). NMDA receptors contribute to primary visceral afferent transmission in the nucleus of the solitary tract. *Journal of Neurophysiology* 77, 2539–2548.
13. Ballanyi, K., Doutheil, J., and Brockhaus, J. (1996). Membrane potential and microenvironment of rat dorsal vagal cells in vitro during energy depletion. *Journal of Physiology* 495, 769–784.
14. Baptista, V., Browning, K. N., and Travagli, R. A. (2007). Effects of cholecystokinin-8s in the nucleus tractus solitarius of vagally deafferented rats. *American Journal of Physiology. Regulatory, Integrative and Comparative Physiology* 292, R1092–R1100.
15. Barlow, T. E., Greenwell, J. R., Harper, A. A., and Scratcherd, T. (1974). The influence of the splanchnic nerves on the external secretion, blood flow and electrical conductance of the cat pancreas. *Journal of Physiology* 236, 421–433.
16. Berthoud, H. R., Fox, E. A., and Powley, T. L. (1990). Localization of vagal preganglionics that stimulate insulin and glucagon secretion. *American Journal of Physiology* 258, R160–R168.
17. Berthoud, H. R., and Powley, T. L. (1987). Characteristics of gastric and pancreatic responses to vagal stimulation with varied frequencies: Evidence for different fiber calibers? *Journal of Autonomic Nervous System* 19, 77–84.
18. Berthoud, H. R., and Powley, T. L. (1990). Identification of vagal preganglionics that mediate cephalic phase insulin response. *American Journal of Physiology* 258, R523–R530.
19. Berthoud, H. R., and Powley, T. L. (1991). Morphology and distribution of efferent vagal innervation of rat pancreas as revealed with anterograde transport of DiI. *Brain Research* 553, 336–341.
20. Branchereau, P., Champagnat, J., and Denavit-Saubie, M. (1993). Cholecystokinin-gated currents in neurons of the rat solitary complex in vitro. *Journal of Neurophysiology* 70, 2584–2595.
21. Brown, M., and Vale, W. (1976). Effects of neurotensin and substance P on plasma insulin, glucagon and glucose levels. *Endocrinology* 98, 819–822.
22. Browning, K. N., Coleman, F. H., and Travagli, R. A. (2005). Characterization of pancreas-projecting rat dorsal motor nucleus of the vagus neurons.

*American Journal of Physiology. Gastrointestinal and Liver Physiology* 288, G950–G955.
23. Browning, K. N., Coleman, F. H., and Travagli, R. A. (2005). Effects of pancreatic polypeptide on pancreas-projecting rat dorsal motor nucleus of the vagus neurons. *American Journal of Physiology. Gastrointestinal and Liver Physiology* 289, G209–G219.
24. Browning, K. N., and Travagli, R. A. (2006). Short-term receptor trafficking in the dorsal vagal complex: An overview. *Autonomic Neuroscience* 126–127, 2–8.
25. Browning, K. N., Zheng, Z. L., Kreulen, D. L., and Travagli, R. A. (1999). Two populations of sympathetic neurons project selectively to mesenteric blood vessels. *American Journal of Physiology* 276, H1263–H1272.
26. Buijs, R. M., Chun, S. J., Niijima, A., Romijn, H. J., and Nagai, K. (2001). Parasympathetic and sympathetic control of the pancreas; a role for the suprachiasmatic nucleus and other hypothalamic centers that are involved in the regulation of food intake. *Journal of Comparative Neurology* 431, 405–423.
27. Cottrell, G. T., and Ferguson, A. V. (2004). Sensory circumventricular organs: Central roles in integrated autonomic regulation. *Regulatory Peptides* 117, 11–23.
28. Dallaporta, M., Perrin, J., and Orsini, J. C. (2000). Involvement of adenosine triphosphate-sensitive K+ channels in glucose-sensing in the rat solitary tract nucleus. *Neuroscience Letters* 278, 77–80.
29. Deng, X., Guarita, D. R., Wood, P. G., Kriess, C., and Whitcomb, D. C. (2001). PYY potently inhibits pancreatic exocrine secretion mediated through CCK-secretin-stimulated pathways but not 2–DG-stimulated pathways in awake rats. *Digestive Diseases and Sciences* 46, 156–165.
30. Deng, X., Wood, P. G., Sved, A. F., and Whitcomb, D. C. (2001). The area postrema lesions alter the inhibitory effects of peripherally infused pancreatic polypeptide on pancreatic secretion. *Brain Research* 902, 18–29.
31. DiMagno, E. P. (1997). Regulation of interdigestive gastrointestinal motility and secretion. *Digestion* 58 Suppl 1, 53–55.
32. Dockray, G. J. (2009). Cholecystokinin and gut-brain signalling. *Regulatory Peptides.* 155, 6–10.
33. Drucker, D. J. (2006). The biology of incretin hormones. *Cell Metabolism* 3, 153–165.
34. Dufresne, M., Seva, C., and Fourmy, D. (2006). Cholecystokinin and gastrin receptors. *Physiological Reviews* 86, 805–847.
35. Dunning, B. E., Ahren, B., Veith, R. C., and Taborsky, G. J., Jr. (1988). Nonadrenergic sympathetic neural influences on basal pancreatic hormone secretion. *American Journal of Physiology* 255, E785–E792.
36. Dunning, B. E., and Taborsky, G. J., Jr. (1991). Neural control of islet function by norepinephrine and sympathetic neuropeptides. *Advances in Experimental Medicine and Biology* 291, 107–127.
37. Edwards, A. V., and Bloom, S. R. (1994). Pancreatic endocrine responses to substance P and calcitonin gene-related peptide in conscious calves. *American Journal of Physiology* 267, E847–E852.
38. Fasanella, K. E., Christianson, J. A., Chanthaphavong, R. S., and Davis, B. M. (2008). Distribution and neurochemical identification of pancreatic afferents in the mouse. *Journal of Comparative Neurology* 509, 42–52.
39. Gilon, P., and Henquin, J. C. (2001). Mechanisms and physiological significance of the cholinergic control of pancreatic beta-cell function. *Endocrine Reviews* 22, 565–604.
40. Goke, R., Larsen, P. J., Mikkelsen, J. D., and Sheikh, S. P. (1995). Distribution of GLP-1 binding sites in the rat brain: Evidence that exendin-4 is a ligand of brain GLP-1 binding sites. *European Journal of Neuroscience* 7, 2294–2300.
41. Gorelick, F. S., and Jamieson, J. D. (2005). Structure–function relations in the pancreatic acinar cell. In L. R. Johnson (Ed.), *Physiology of the Gastrointestinal Tract*, pp. 1313–1335. San Diego, CA: Elsevier.
42. Grundy, D. (2002). Neuroanatomy of visceral nociception: Vagal and splanchnic afferent. *Gut* 51 Suppl 1, i2–i5.
43. Guarita, D. R., Deng, X., Huh, Y. B., Wood, P. G., Reeve, J. R., Jr., and Whitcomb, D. C. (2000). PYY regulates pancreatic exocrine secretion through multiple receptors in the awake rat. *Digestive Diseases and Sciences* 45, 1696–1702.
44. Hayes, M. R., Moore, R. L., Shah, S. M., and Covasa, M. (2004). 5-HT3 receptors participate in CCK-induced suppression of food intake by delaying gastric emptying. *American Journal of Physiology. Regulatory, Integrative and Comparative Physiology* 87, R817–R823.
45. Hermansen, K. (1980). Effects of substance P and other peptides on the release of somatostatin, insulin, and glucagon in vitro. *Endocrinology* 107, 256–261.
46. Holmes, G. M., Tong, M., and Travagli, R. A. (2009). Effects of brainstem cholecystokinin-8s on gastric tone and esophageal-gastric reflex. *American Journal of Physiology. Gastrointestinal and Liver Physiology* 96, G621–G631.

47. Holst, J. J. (2007). The physiology of glucagon-like peptide 1. *Physiological Reviews* 87, 1409–1439.
48. Holst, J. J., Jensen, S. L., Knuhtsen, S., and Nielsen, O. V. (1983). Autonomic nervous control of pancreatic somatostatin secretion. *American Journal of Physiology* 245, E542–E548.
49. Holst, J. J., Schaffalitzky de Muckadell, O. B., and Fahrenkrug, J. (1979). Nervous control of pancreatic exocrine secretion in pigs. *Acta Physiologica Scandinavica* 105, 33–51.
50. Holst, J. J., Schwartz, T. W., Knuhtsen, S., Jensen, S. L., and Nielsen, O. V. (1986). Autonomic nervous control of the endocrine secretion from the isolated, perfused pig pancreas. *Journal of the Autonomic Nervous Syste,* 17, 71–84.
51. Holzer, P. (1988). Local effector functions of capsaicin-sensitive sensory nerve endings: Involvement of tachykinins, calcitonin gene-related peptide and other neuropeptides. *Neuroscience* 24, 739–768.
52. Ionescu, E., Rohner-Jeanrenaud, F., Berthoud, H. R., and Jeanrenaud, B. (1983). Increases in plasma insulin levels in response to electrical stimulation of the dorsal motor nucleus of the vagus nerve. *Endocrinology* 112, 904–910.
53. Jaworek, J., Konturek, S. J., and Szlachcic, A. (1997). The role of CGRP and afferent nerves in the modulation of pancreatic enzyme secretion in the rat. *International Journal of Pancreatology* 22, 137–146.
54. Jean, A. (2001). Brainstem control of swallowing: Neuronal network and cellular mechanisms. *Physiological Reviews* 81, 929–969.
55. Jung, G., Louie, D. S., and Owyang, C. (1987). Pancreatic polypeptide inhibits pancreatic enzyme secretion via a cholinergic pathway. *American Journal of Physiology* 253, G706–G710.
56. Karlsson, S., Scheurink, A. J., Steffens, A. B., and Ahren, B. (1994). Involvement of capsaicin-sensitive nerves in regulation of insulin secretion and glucose tolerance in conscious mice. *American Journal of Physiology* 267, R1071–R1077.
57. Karlsson, S., Sundler, F., and Ahren, B. (1992). Neonatal capsaicin-treatment in mice: Effects on pancreatic peptidergic nerves and 2-deoxy-D-glucose-induced insulin and glucagon secretion. *Journal of the Autonomic Nervous System* 39, 51–59.
58. Kato, Y., and Kanno, T. (1983). Thyrotropin-releasing hormone injected intracerebroventricularly in the rat stimulates exocrine pancreatic secretion via the vagus nerve. *Regulatory Peptides* 7, 347–356.
59. Katschinski, M. (2000). Nutritional implications of cephalic phase gastrointestinal responses. *Appetite* 34, 189–196.
60. King, B. F., Love, J. A., and Szurszewski, J. H. (1989). Intracellular recordings from pancreatic ganglia of the cat. *Journal of Physiology* 419, 379–403.
61. Kirchgessner, A. L., and Gershon, M. D. (1990). Innervation of the pancreas by neurons in the gut. *Journal of Neuroscience* 10, 1626–1642.
62. Kirchgessner, A. L., and Pintar, J. E. (1991). Guinea pig pancreatic ganglia: Projections, transmitter content, and the type-specific localization of monoamine oxidase. *Journal of Comparative Neurology* 305, 613–631.
63. Kirkwood, K. S., Kim, E. H., He, X. D., Calaustro, E. Q., Domush, C., Yoshimi, S. K., Grady, E. F., Maa, J., Bunnett, N. W., and Debas, H. T. (1999). Substance P inhibits pancreatic exocrine secretion via a neural mechanism. *American Journal of Physiology* 277, G314–G320.
64. Klein, E., Salinas, A., Shemesh, E., and Dreiling, D. A. (1988). Effects of autonomic denervation on canine exocrine pancreatic secretion and blood flow. *International Journal of Pancreatology* 3, 165–170.
65. Krowicki, Z. K., and Hornby, P. J. (1995). Pancreatic polypeptide, microinjected into the dorsal vagal complex, potentiates glucose-stimulated insulin secretion in the rat. *Regulatory Peptides* 60, 185–192.
66. Lachey, J. L., D'Alessio, D. A., Rinaman, L., Elmquist, J. K., Drucker, D. J., and Seeley R. J. (2005). The role of central glucagon-like peptide-1 in mediating the effects of visceral illness: Differential effects in rats and mice. *Endocrinology* 146, 458–462.
67. Larsen, P. J., Tang-Christensen, M., Holst, J. J., and Orskov, C. (1997). Distribution of glucagon-like peptide-1 and other preproglucagon- derived peptides in the rat hypothalamus and brainstem. *Neuroscience* 77, 257–270.
68. Levin, B. E. (2007). Neuronal glucose sensing: Still a physiological orphan? *Cell Metabolism* 6, 252–254.
69. Li, Y., Hao, Y., and Owyang, C. (1997). High-affinity CCK-A receptors on the vagus nerve mediate CCK-stimulated pancreatic secretion in rats. *American Journal of Physiology* 273, G679–G685.
70. Li, Y., Hao, Y., Zhu, J., and Owyang, C. (2000). Serotonin released from intestinal enterochromaffin cells mediates luminal non-cholecystokinin-stimulated pancreatic secretion in rats. *Gastro-enterology* 118, 1197–1207.
71. Li, Y., Jiang, Y. C., and Owyang, C. (1998). Central CGRP inhibits pancreatic enzyme secretion by modulation of vagal parasympathetic outflow.

*American Journal of Physiology* 275, G957–G963.
72. Li, Y., and Owyang, C. (1993). Somatostatin inhibits pancreatic enzyme secretion at a central vagal site. *American Journal of Physiology* 265, G251–G257.
73. Li, Y., Wu, X., Zhu, J., Yan, J., and Owyang, C. (2003). Hypothalamic regulation of pancreatic secretion is mediated by central cholinergic pathways in the rat. *Journal of Physiology* 552, 571–587.
74. Li, Y., Wu, X. Y., and Owyang, C. (2004). Serotonin and cholecystokinin synergistically stimulate rat vagal primary afferent neurones. *Journal of Physiology* 559, 651–662.
75. Liddle, R. A. (2005). Regulation of pancreatic secretion. In L. R. Johnson (Ed.), *Physiology of the Gastrointestinal Tract*, pp. 1397–1435. San Diego, CA: Elsevier.
76. Lindsay, T. H., Halvorson, K. G., Peters, C. M., Ghilardi, J. R., Kuskowski, M. A., Wong, G. Y., and Mantyh, P. W. (2006). A quantitative analysis of the sensory and sympathetic innervation of the mouse pancreas. *Neuroscience* 137, 1417–1426.
77. Liu, M. T., and Kirchgessner, A. L. (1997). Guinea pig pancreatic neurons: Morphology, neurochemistry, electrical properties, and response to 5-HT. *American Journal of Physiology* 273, G1273–G1289.
78. Loewy, A. D., Franklin, M. F., and Haxihu, M. A. (1994). CNS monoamine cell groups projecting to pancreatic vagal motor neurons: A transneuronal labeling study using pseudorabies virus. *Brain Research* 638, 248–260.
79. Love, J. A. (2000). Electrical properties and synaptic potentials of rabbit pancreatic neurons. *Autonomic Neuroscience* 84, 68–77.
80. Love, J. A., and Szebeni, K. (1999). Morphology and histochemistry of the rabbit pancreatic innervation. *Pancreas* 18, 53–64.
81. Love, J. A., Yi, E., and Smith, T. G. (2007). Autonomic pathways regulating pancreatic exocrine secretion. *Autonomic Neuroscience* 133, 19–34.
82. Matthews, D. R., Lang, D. A., Burnett, M. A., and Turner, R. C. (1983). Control of pulsatile insulin secretion in man. *Diabetologia* 24, 231–237.
83. Messmer, B., Zimmerman, F. G., and Lenz, H. J. (1993). Regulation of exocrine pancreatic secretion by cerebral TRH and CGRP: Role of VIP, muscarinic, and adrenergic pathways. *American Journal of Physiology* 264, G237–G242.
84. Michel, M. C., Beck-Sickinger, A., Cox, H., Doods, H. N., Herzog, H., Larhammar, D., Quirion, R., Schwartz, T., and Westfall, T. C. (1999). XVI. International Union of Pharmacology recommendations for the nomenclature of neuropeptide Y, peptide YY, and pancreatic polypeptide receptors. *Pharmacological Reviews* 50, 143–150.
85. Mussa, B. M., Sartor, D. M., and Verberne, A. J. (2008). Activation of cholecystokinin (CCK1) and serotonin (5-HT3) receptors increases the discharge of pancreatic vagal afferents. *European Journal of Pharmacology* 601, 198–206.
86. Mussa, B. M., and Verberne, A. J. (2008). Activation of the dorsal vagal nucleus increases pancreatic exocrine secretion in the rat. *Neuroscience Letters* 433, 71–76.
87. Nathan, J. D., Peng, R. Y., Wang, Y., McVey, D. C., Vigna, S. R., and Liddle, R. A. (2002). Primary sensory neurons: A common final pathway for inflammation in experimental pancreatitis in rats. *American Journal of Physiology. Gastrointestinal and Liver Physiology* 283, G938–G946.
88. Nelson, M. T., Debas, H. T., and Mulvihill, S. J. (1993). Vagal stimulation of rat exocrine pancreatic secretion occurs via multiple mediators. *Gastroenterology* 105, 221–228.
89. Niebel, W., Eysselein, V. E., and Singer, M. V. (1987). Pancreatic polypeptide response to a meal before and after cutting the extrinsic nerves of the upper gastrointestinal tract and the pancreas in the dog. *Digestive Diseases and Sciences* 32, 1004–1009.
90. Niijima, A. (1989). Neural mechanisms in the control of blood glucose concentration. *Journal of Nutrition* 119, 833–840.
91. Nishizawa, M., Nakabayashi, H., Kawai, K., Ito, T., Kawakami, S., Nakagawa, A., Niijima, A., and Uchida, K. (2000). The hepatic vagal reception of intraportal GLP-1 is via receptor different from the pancreatic GLP-1 receptor. *Journal of the Autonomic Nervous System* 80, 14–21.
92. Okumura, T., Pappas, T. N., and Taylor, I. L. (1995). Pancreatic polypeptide microinjection into the dorsal motor nucleus inhibits pancreatic secretion in rats. *Gastroenterology* 108, 1517–1525.
93. Okumura, T., Taylor, I. L., and Pappas, T. N. (1995). Microinjection of TRH analogue into the dorsal vagal complex stimulates pancreatic secretion in rats. *American Journal of Physiology* 269, G328–G334.
94. Owyang, C. (1994). Negative feedback control of exocrine pancreatic secretion: Role of cholecystokinin and cholinergic pathway. *Journal of Nutrition* 124, 1321S–1326S.
95. Owyang, C. (1996). Physiological mechanisms of cholecystokinin action on pancreatic secretion. *American Journal of Physiology* 271, G1–G7.

96. Owyang, C., and Logsdon, C. D. (2004). New insights into neurohormonal regulation of pancreatic secretion. *Gastroenterology* 127, 957–969.
97. Pettersson, M., and Ahren, B. (1988). Insulin and glucagon secretion in rats: Effects of calcitonin gene-related peptide. *Regulatory Peptides* 23, 37–50.
98. Pettersson, M., and Ahren, B. (1990). Calcitonin gene-related peptide inhibits insulin secretion studies on ion fluxes and cyclic AMP in isolated rat islets. *Diabetes Research* 5, 9–14.
99. Pettersson, M., Ahren, B., Bottcher, G., and Sundler, F. (1986). Calcitonin gene-related peptide: Occurrence in pancreatic islets in the mouse and the rat and inhibition of insulin secretion in the mouse. *Endocrinology* 119, 865–869.
100. Putnam, W. S., Liddle, R. A., and Williams, J. A. (1989). Inhibitory regulation of rat exocrine pancreas by peptide YY and pancreatic polypeptide. *American Journal of Physiology* 256, G698–G703.
101. Raybould, H. E. (2007). Mechanisms of CCK signaling from gut to brain. *Current Opinions in Pharmacology* 7, 570–574.
102. Rinaman, L., and Miselis, R. R. (1987). The organization of vagal innervation of rat pancreas using cholera toxin-horseradish peroxidase conjugate. *Journal of Autonomic Nervous System* 21, 109–125.
103. Sakaguchi, T., Sandoh, N., and Aono, T. (1994). Glucose signal in the nucleus of the vagus nerve modulates the cyclicity of gastric motility in rats. *Brain Research* 641, 163–166.
104. Scheurink, A. J. W., Balkan, B., Strubbe, J. H., Van Dijk, G., and Steffens, A. B. (1996). Overfeeding, autonomic regulation and metabolic consequences. *Cardiovascular Drugs and Therapy* 10, 263–274.
105. Schloithe, A. C., Sutherland, K., Woods, C. M., Blackshaw, L. A., Davison, J. S., Toouli, J., and Saccone, G. T. (2008). A novel preparation to study rat pancreatic spinal and vagal mechanosensitive afferents in vitro. *Neurogastroenterology and Motility* 20, 1060–1069.
106. Schmidt, P. T., Tornoe, K., Poulsen, S. S., Rasmussen, T. N., and Holst, J. J. (2000). Tachykinins in the porcine pancreas: Potent exocrine and endocrine effects via NK-1 receptors. *Pancreas* 20, 241–247.
107. Sha, L., Ou, L. L., Miller, S. M., Ma, R., and Szurszewski, J. H. (1996). Cat pancreatic neurons: Morphology, electrophysiological properties, and responses to 5-HT. *Pancreas* 13, 111–124.
108. Sharkey, K. A., and Williams, R. G. (1983). Extrinsic innervation of the rat pancreas: Demonstration of vagal sensory neurones in the rat by retrograde tracing. *Neuroscience Letters* 42, 131–135.
109. Sharkey, K. A., Williams, R. G., and Dockray, G. J. (1984). Sensory substance P innervation of the stomach and pancreas. Demonstration of capsaicin-sensitive sensory neurons in the rat by combined immunohistochemistry and retrograde tracing. *Gastroenterology* 87, 914–921.
110. Shimizu, I., Hirota, M., Ohboshi, C., and Shima, K. (1987). Identification and localization of glucagon-like peptide-1 and its receptor in rat brain. *Endocrinology* 121, 1076–1082.
111. Streefland, C., Maes, F. W., and Bohus, B. (1998). Autonomic brainstem projections to the pancreas: A retrograde transneuronal viral tracing study in the rat. *Journal of Autonomic Nervous System* 74, 71–81.
112. Strubbe, J. H., and Steffens, A. B. (1993). Neural control of insulin secretion. *Hormones and Metabolism Research* 25, 507–512.
113. Su, H. C., Bishop, A. E., Power, R. F., Hamada, Y., and Polak, J. M. (1987). Dual intrinsic and extrinsic origins of CGRP- and NPY-immunoreactive nerves of rat gut and pancreas. *Journal of Neuroscience* 7, 2674–2687.
114. Taborsky, G. J., Jr., Dunning, B. E., Havel, P. J., Ahren, B., Kowalyk, S., Boyle, M. R., Verchere, C. B., Baskin, D. G., and Mundinger, T. O. (1999). The canine sympathetic neuropeptide galanin: A neurotransmitter in pancreas, a neuromodulator in liver. *Hormone and Metabolism Research* 31, 351–354.
115. Tache, Y., and Yang, H. (1993). Role of medullary TRH in the vagal regulation of gastric function. In Y. Tache, D. L. Wingate, and, T. F. Burks (Eds.), *Innervation of the Gut: Pathophysiological Implications*, pp. 67–80. Boca Raton, FL: CRC Press.
116. Tache, Y., Yang, H., Miampamba, M., Martinez, V., and Yuan, P. Q. (2006). Role of brainstem TRH/TRH-R1 receptors in the vagal gastric cholinergic response to various stimuli including sham-feeding. *Autonomic Neuroscience* 125, 42–52.
117. Trapp, S., Ballanyi, K., and Richter, D. W. (1994). Spontaneous activation of $K_{ATP}$ current in rat dorsal vagal neurones. *NeuroReport* 5, 1285–1288.
118. Travagli, R. A., Gillis, R. A., and Vicini, S. (1992). Effects of thyrotropin-releasing hormone on neurons in rat dorsal motor nucleus of the vagus, in vitro. *American Journal of Physiology* 263, G508–G517.

119. Travagli, R. A., Hermann, G. E., Browning, K. N., and Rogers, R. C. (2006). Brainstem circuits regulating gastric function. *Annual Review of Physiology* 68, 279–305.
120. Uttenthal, L. O., Toledano, A., and Blazquez, E., (1992). Autoradiographic localization of receptors for glucagon-like peptide-1 (7–36) amide in rat brain. *Neuropeptides* 21, 143–146.
121. Van Dijk, G., Thiele, T. E., Donahey, J. C., Campfield, L. A., Smith, F. J., Burn, P., Bernstein, I. L., Woods, S. C., and Seeley, R. J. (1996). Central infusions of leptin and GLP-1-(7–36) amide differentially stimulate c-FLI in the rat brain. *American Journal of Physiology* 271, R1096–R1100.
122. Verberne, A. J., and McInerney, K. (2006). Pancreatic vasoconstrictor responses are regulated by neurons in the rostral ventrolateral medulla. *Brain Research* 1102, 127–134.
123. Viard, E., Zheng, Z., Wan, S., and Travagli, R. A. (2007). Vagally mediated, non paracrine effects of cholecystokinin-8s on rat pancreatic exocrine secretion. *American Journal of Physiology. Gastrointestinal and Liver Physiology* 293, G494–G500.
124. Wan, S., and Browning, K. N. (2008). D-Glucose modulates synaptic transmission from the central terminals of vagal afferent fibers. *American Journal of Physiology. Gastrointestinal and Liver Physiology* 294, G757–G763.
125. Wan, S., and Browning, K. N. (2008). Glucose increases synaptic transmission from vagal afferent central nerve terminals via modulation of 5-HT3 receptors. *American Journal of Physiology. Gastrointestinal and Liver Physiology* 295, G1050–G1057.
126. Wan, S., Browning, K. N., and Travagli, R. A. (2007). Glucagon-like peptide-1 modulates synaptic transmission to identified pancreas-projecting vagal motoneurons. *Peptides* 28, 2184–2191.
127. Wan, S., Coleman, F. H., and Travagli, R. A. (2007). Cholecystokinin-8s excites identified rat pancreatic-projecting vagal motoneurons. *American Journal of Physiology. Gastrointestinal and Liver Physiology* 293, G484–G492.
128. Wan, S., Coleman, F. H., and Travagli, R. A. (2007). Glucagon-like peptide-1 (GLP-1) excites pancreas-projecting preganglionic vagal motoneurons. *American Journal of Physiology. Gastrointestinal and Liver Physiology* 292, G1474–G1482.
129. Wang, J., Zheng, H., and Berthoud, H. R. (1999). Functional vagal input to chemically identified neurons in pancreatic ganglia as revealed by Fos expression. *American Journal of Physiology* 277, E958–E964.
130. Whitcomb, D. C., and Taylor, I. L. (1992). A new twist in the brain–gut axis. *American Journal of Medical Science* 304, 334–338.
131. Won, M. H., Park, H. S., Jeong, Y. G., and Park, H. J. (1998). Afferent innervation of the rat pancreas: Retrograde tracing and immunohistochemistry in the dorsal root ganglia. *Pancreas* 16, 80–87.
132. Wood, J. D. (1987). Physiology of the enteric nervous system. In L. R. Johnson (Ed.), *Physiology of the Gastrointestinal Tract*, pp. 67–110. New York: Raven Press.
133. Wu, X., Gao, J., Yan, J., Owyang, C., and Li, Y. (2004). Hypothalamus–brain stem circuitry responsible for vagal efferent signaling to the pancreas evoked by hypoglycemia in rat. *Journal of Neurophysiology* 91, 1734–1747.
134. Yi, E., and Love, J. A. (2005). Alpha-adrenergic modulation of synaptic transmission in rabbit pancreatic ganglia. *Autonomic Neuroscience* 122, 45–57.
135. Yoneda, M., Goto, M., Nakamura, K., Yokohama, S., Kono, T., Tanamo, M., Shimada, T., and Hiraishi, H. (2005). Thyrotropin-releasing hormone in the dorsal vagal complex stimulates pancreatic blood flow in rats. *Regulatory Peptides* 131, 74–81.
136. Zheng, Z., Lewis, M. W., and Travagli, R. A. (2005). In vitro analysis of the effects of cholecystokinin (CCK) on rat brainstem motorneurons. *American Journal of Physiology. Gastrointestinal and Liver Physiology* 288, G1066–G1073.
137. Zhu, J. X., Zhu, X. Y., Owyang, C., and Li, Y. (2001). Intestinal serotonin acts as a paracrine substance to mediate vagal signal transmission evoked by luminal factors in the rat. *Journal of Physiology* 530, 431–442.
138. Zimmerman, D. W., Sarr, M. G., Smith, C. D., Nicholson, C. P., Dalton, R. R., Barr, D., Perkins, J. D., and DiMagno, E. P. (1992). Cyclic interdigestive pancreatic exocrine secretion: Is it mediated by neural or hormonal mechanisms? *Gastroenterology* 102, 1378–1384.

# 16

# Circumventricular Organs: Critical Autonomic Control Centers at the Blood–Brain Interface

ALASTAIR V. FERGUSON

The dominant role of the brain in the hierarchical control of the autonomic nervous system requires that it receive afferent information regarding not only the external environment but also the internal environment. It is now well established that the hypothalamus and medulla contain many of the essential control centers where sensory information is received and integrated. Many other chapters in this book will deal with the mechanisms through which peripheral sensory structures (e.g., baroreceptors and chemoreceptors) sense a variety of important variables and transmit this information to these centers through well-established afferent neural inputs. In addition, the central nervous system(CNS) is known to directly monitor information derived from changing concentrations of many essential constituents of the peripheral circulation. It is intriguing that the CNS is able to do this despite the fact that the majority of these substances cannot directly access autonomic control centers in the hypothalamus or medulla because these areas are protected by the blood–brain barrier.

This chapter will focus on the potential roles of a group of CNS structures known collectively as the *sensory circumventricular organs*. These specialized structures not only are able to collect and integrate such information but also are able to transmit output signals to autonomic control centers in the hypothalamus and the medulla. This chapter will commence with a description of the specialized anatomical and physiological features of the sensory circumventricular organs. Then it will review an expanding literature that suggests important roles for the sensory circumventricular organs in the regulation of diverse autonomic functions. Prior to this discussion, it must also be emphasized that there is a second group of circumventricular organs, known as the *secretory circumventricular organs*. The secretory circumventricular organs are composed primarily of axon terminals (i.e., the median eminence and neurohypophysis) or non-neuronal cell bodies (i.e., the pineal gland, subcommissural organ and choroid plexus). The primary function of these structures is secretion of chemical messengers on one side of the blood–brain barrier or the other, and they will not be discussed further in this chapter.

## BLOOD-BORNE SIGNALS AS CONTROLLERS OF AUTONOMIC OUTPUT

It is well established that the brain is able to directly sense certain constituents of the systemic circulation (e.g., osmolarity, glucose concentrations, and regulatory peptides) that provide essential feedback information to autonomic control centers in the hypothalamus and medulla. However, this conclusion ignores the problematic issue that, although autonomic control areas are highly vascular, capillaries within them demonstrate a normal blood–brain barrier. As a result, almost none of these essential signals can gain direct access to neurons within these centers. Thus, although the blood–brain barrier acts to protect and insulate the brain from large shifts in circulatory parameters, it also precludes the CNS from monitoring these same important variables. The absence of clear mechanisms through which such feedback can occur argues for the existence of additional, physiologically significant sensory centers involved in the monitoring of these variables. The sensory circumventricular organs are specialized CNS structures that lack a normal blood–brain barrier and are a potential window through which such autonomic feedback can enter the CNS. These structures, which include the subfornical organ (SFO), organum vasculosum of the lamina terminalis (OVLT), and area postrema, consist primarily of neuronal cell bodies. They receive afferent input from the circulation and communicate with other regions of the CNS through efferent neural projections to hypothalamic and medullary autonomic control centers.

## The Blood–Brain Barrier

The physical determinants of the blood–brain barrier are now well understood in that the endothelial cells of cerebral microvessels are joined together by tight junctions[1]. These tight junctions are more complex in the endothelium of brain vessels than in the periphery, and electron microscopic freeze fracture studies illustrate networks of strands formed by intramembranous particles joining adjacent cells[153]. The completeness of the blood–brain barrier effectively forces all molecular transport across cell membranes, limiting movement across the barrier to substances that either diffuse readily across the lipid bilayer or are transported across this barrier by alternative mechanisms (see below). Thus, in the absence of specialized transport systems, nearly all large hydrophilic molecules, such as peptides and proteins, are excluded. Although they do not form the barrier, astrocytes, and in particular their end feet that appear to wrap around the brain side of the endothelial cell membrane, play important roles in the development and maintenance of barrier function[1]. Barrier function is also known to be compromised in a number of pathological states, including inflammation and hypertension[1].

There are two major functional considerations associated with the existence of the barrier between the circulation and neural tissue within the CNS. First, the barrier is protective in that it not only allows preferential maintenance of the constituents of the extracellular fluid within the brain, but it also ensures that potential "toxins" in the circulation do not access the CNS and compromise CNS function. Second, by effectively creating a separate brain-fluid compartment, the barrier excludes chemical messengers used in the circulation as hormones (delivery to all accessible tissues by blood) from the CNS and thus allows these chemicals to be used separately. This compartmentalization limits the ability of regions behind the barrier to directly monitor variations in the levels of many of these important circulating indicators of physiological status.

## Mechanisms for Blood–Brain Signaling

The sections above highlight two important conclusions. The first is that autonomic control centers in the brain do obtain essential information regarding the status of physiological systems by monitoring the constituents of the circulation. Second, these control centers obtain this information even though they are located behind the blood–brain barrier and therefore cannot directly sample substances that do not cross the barrier.

There are four primary mechanisms through which substances in the circulation can access and thus potentially influence neurons within the CNS. First, lipophilic substances that can readily pass through the lipid bilayer of the cell membrane (e.g., steroids, barbiturates, and alcohol) can gain access to neural tissue behind the blood brain barrier by simple *diffusion* through the membranes of endothelial cell in the cerebral vasculature. Second, specific saturable *transporters* have been identified that have the ability to move hydrophilic substances (e.g., glucose, leptin, and cytokines) across the barrier[6]. Third, recent work has suggested that *transendothelial cell signaling* occurs when molecules act on one side of the endothelial cell and induce release of a second signaling molecule on the other side, thus signaling across the barrier[107]. Finally, there are specialized regions of the brain, the sensory circumventricular organs, where *fenestrations are found between endothelial cells* lining the blood vessels (similar to the systemic vasculature outside of the brain). These fenestrations mean that even lipophobic substances from blood can reach neural tissue without having to cross through a cell membrane. The roles of these specialized regions in sensing the constituents of the peripheral circulation and controlling autonomic output will be the focus of the remainder of this chapter.

## The Sensory Circumventricular Organs

### *Specialized Features*

The capillaries of the sensory circumventricular organs are distinct from the rest of the CNS in that they are fenestrated[53], and all lack the typical tight junctions between endothelial cells (normally indicated by immunoreactivity for ZO-1, a protein associated with the tight junctions[108]). Vascular supply of the circumventricular organs is also extensive and complex compared to other areas of the brain, resulting in a high blood volume per tissue weight, yet a slow transit time across each structure[53]. Some of these specializations include capillary loops extending to the ependymal surface, and large, perivascular spaces (Virchow-Robin spaces) surrounding the blood vessels[52]. Most of these complex specializations in the microcirculation are consistent with maximizing not only the time, but also the area for exposure of blood-borne substances to the cellular components of the circumventricular organs[52]. Finally, the sensory circumventricular organs have been demonstrated to contain exceptionally dense aggregations of a variety of different receptors for peripheral signals, including regulatory peptides (e.g., angiotensin, cholecystokinin, and ghrelin)[95,110,142] ; steroids (e.g., estradiol)[120] ; and specific ions (e.g., $Ca^{2+}$ and $Na^{+}$)[100,118]. All of these observations clearly suggest the ability of neurons in these circumventricular organs to sense circulating concentrations of these signaling molecules.

### Anatomical Description

The neuroanatomical connections between circumventricular organs and other brain centers are distinct. The forebrain and medullary circumventricular organs project to very different targets, but these targets are predictable in that nearly all of them are crucial autonomic centers in the hypothalamus and medulla. Studies with retrograde and anterograde neuroanatomical tracers have identified the efferent and afferent connections of the circumventricular organs (for a summary, see Figure 16–1); and, in many cases, the functional nature of these connections has been further clarified by additional information from electrophysiological analyses.

*Subfornical Organ (SFO)* The SFO is situated on the midline wall of the third ventricle in the dorsal region of the lamina terminalis. It protrudes slightly into the third ventricle and has a core region and peripheral outer zone with differing neuronal projections and ligand-binding abilities[89]. The SFO sends both direct (monosynaptic), and indirect (polysynaptic) efferent projections to the paraventricular nucleus (PVN) and supraoptic nucleus (SON) of the hypothalamus[81,97]. Specific excitatory projections have been found from the SFO to vasopressin- and oxytocin-secreting magnocellular neurons in the SON and PVN, as well as to parvocellular areas of the PVN that in turn project either to the median eminence, the medulla, or the spinal cord (for review, see note [38]).

The SFO also sends efferents to neurons in the anteroventral third ventricle region, specifically to the median preoptic nucleus and the OVLT[81,98], both of which in turn send additional axons to hypothalamic autonomic centers, including the SON and PVN (i.e., there are polysynaptic connections from SFO to SON and PVN)[98]. In addition, there are apparently less-dense efferent connections from the SFO to the zona incerta, raphé nuclei, infralimbic cortex, rostral and ventral portions of the bed nucleus of the stria terminalis, lateral preoptic area, lateral hypothalamus/ dorsal perifornical region, and arcuate nucleus[54,77,97].

The majority of the anatomical data suggest that SFO neurons have relatively compact dendritic trees and do not receive extensive neural inputs[28]. This observation is consistent with the suggested role for this region in receiving afferent information primarily from the systemic circulation. In most cases, the limited afferent inputs to the SFO appear to originate from the same areas that receive SFO efferents, suggesting important reciprocal communication between these regions. The SFO receives inputs from the lateral hypothalamus[80] and the median preoptic nucleus[80], as well as the lateral division of the parabrachial nucleus, nucleus of the solitary tract (NTS), midbrain raphé nuclei, and nucleus reunions of the thalamus (for review, see note [24]).

*Organum Vasculosum of the Lamina Terminalis (OVLT)* The OVLT is a midline structure in the region of the anteroventral third ventricle and is located ventral to the median preoptic nucleus and dorsal to the optic chiasm. The OVLT has been characterized as having two distinct regions: the dorsal cap and the lateral region. The neurons in these regions send efferent projections to separate target zones. The densest efferent projections of the OVLT are to the magnocellular neurons of the PVN and SON, either directly[78] or indirectly through the median preoptic nucleus[62]. Projections to neurons in the PVN that contain corticotropin-releasing hormone have also been described[125], with less-dense projections to the stria medullaris and basal ganglia.

Tracer studies indicate that most inputs to the OVLT are from the median preoptic nucleus, SFO, and NTS[5], with additional afferent inputs arising from a variety of other hypothalamic regions, including the ventromedial nucleus, arcuate nucleus, anterior and posterior hypothalamus, and dorsal hypothalamus[96].

*Area Postrema* The area postrema in mammals other than rodents and lagomorphs is a bilateral structure that protrudes into the caudal fourth ventricle on either side of the obex (for review, see note [24]). In rodents and lagomorphs, it is a single midline structure protruding into the fourth ventricle on the dorsal surface of the medulla immediately adjacent to the NTS. The area postrema contains small neurons and astrocytes, and has been divided into three regions based on neuronal morphology and projections; i.e., the mantle zone, the central zone, and the third zone. The area postrema sends efferents to and receives afferents from a variety

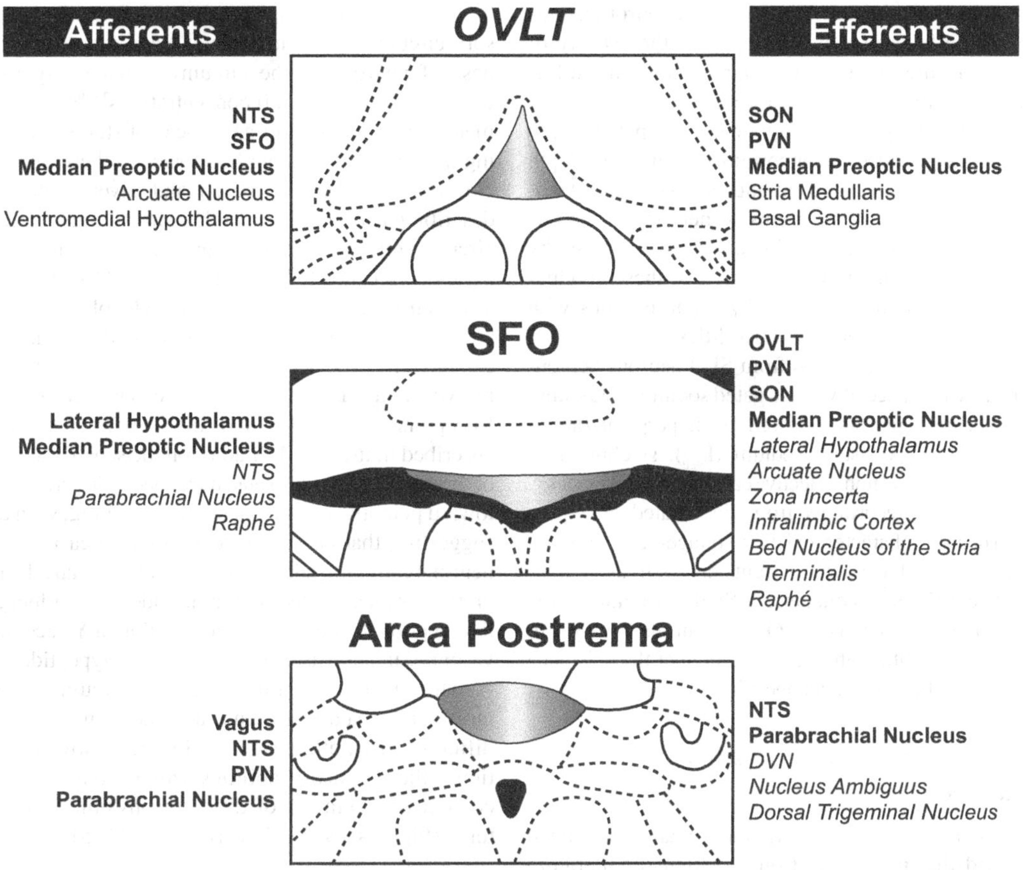


Figure 16–1 Anatomical locations of the three sensory circumventricular organs and their afferent and efferent connections. The center panels show schematic representations of the anatomical locations of the three sensory circumventricular organs, the subfornical organ (SFO), the organum vasculosum of the lamina terminals (OVLT), and the area postrema. The text on the left-hand and right-hand sides of these schematics summarizes the major (*text in bold*) and more minor (*text in italics*) anatomical inputs to (Afferent) and outputs from (Efferent) these circumventricular organs. These anatomical connections are based on data from neuroanatomical tract tracing studies. PVN, paraventricular nucleus of the hypothalamus; SON, supraoptic nucleus; NTS, nucleus of the solitary tract.

of autonomic centers in the medulla, pons, and forebrain[130,150]. The main efferent projections from the area postrema are directed to the NTS and parabrachial nucleus[130,150], with minor projections going to the A1 region in the caudal ventrolateral medulla, the dorsal motor nucleus of the vagus, and dorsal regions of the tegmental nuclei[130,150].

Similar to the other sensory circumventricular organs, the area postrema receives inputs from many of the same regions to which area postrema neurons project. The NTS and parabrachial nucleus send projections to the area postrema[105,130,150], with afferent inputs also coming from the PVN[134,150] and vagus nerve[23]. The area postrema and NTS are major sites of abdominal sensory input to the CNS (see Chapters 2 and 15)[66].

### *Intrinsic Properties of Circumventricular Organ Neurons*

Early work describing the basic firing patterns and sensitivity of neurons in the circumventricular organs came from electrophysiological studies utilizing extracellular or sharp electrode intracellular techniques. This work provided important information on the connectivity of the circumventricular organs, neuronal responses to exogenous hormones and neurotransmitters, and effects of synaptic input on the activity of neurons in the circumventricular organs. This information has already been reviewed[38,94].

In the early 1990s, the application of patch clamp techniques provided the opportunity for more in-depth analysis, using both current and voltage clamp techniques, of the activity patterns of neurons in the circumventricular organs, the ion channels expressed by these neurons, and how modulation of these conductances endows circumventricular organ neurons with their unique multi-sensory capabilities.

Patch clamp recordings from SFO neurons demonstrated the presence of voltage gated sodium, potassium, and calcium currents, as well as hyperpolarization-activated ($I_h$), persistent sodium ($I_{NaP}$), swelling-activated chloride and non-selective cationic conductances[24]. Similar patch recordings from dissociated area postrema neurons characterized their voltage-gated sodium, potassium, and calcium currents as well as a non-selective cationic conductance[24]. Studies examining the conductances expressed by OVLT neurons have yet to be published, although one would predict the existence of many of these same channels in OVLT neurons.

### *Sensory Abilities of Circumventricular Organ Neurons*

The "sensory" circumventricular organs have been assigned this name based on an extensive literature outlining the ability of these neurons to "sense" many different physiological signals, with their responses being manifested as changes in excitability. This review will not provide a detailed description of the literature related to the ability of neurons in the circumventricular organ to sense each signal but will emphasize the diversity of signals now known to influence the activity of these neurons.

A number of basic components of the systemic circulation influence the excitability of neurons in the sensory circumventricular organs (for review, see note[50]). SFO neurons express the calcium-sensing receptor in their membranes and respond to changes in extracellular calcium as a result of modulation of NSCC, $I_h$, and $I_{NaP}$ mediated by the calcium-sensing receptor. Glial cells within the SFO have also been shown to express the $Na_X$ channel and, presumably as a consequence, are sodium-sensitive[100]. SFO and OVLT neurons are also osmosensitive. In contrast to the forebrain focus on fluid balance, area postrema neurons have been reported to be sensitive to changes in glucose concentrations. Importantly, no clear information has been published to date either on the glucose responsiveness of SFO neurons or on the calcium-, sodium-, or osmosensitivity of area postrema neurons.

The presence of angiotensin II receptors in the sensory circumventricular organs[51,95] and the responsiveness of neurons in the circumventricular organs to changes in angiotensin II concentrations[36,39,106] have for many years been the primary focus of studies describing actions of circulating hormones on these neurons. Nevertheless, there is a rich and diverse literature describing actions of many other circulating factors on circumventricular organ neurons, which has been reviewed recently[50,89]. In summary, SFO neurons are also sensitive to changes in acetylcholine, amylin, atrial natriuretic peptides, calcitonin, endothelin, estrogen, ghrelin, GLP-1, interleukin 1-β, prokineticin 2, relaxin, and vasopressin (for a review, see note [50]). Receptors for amylin and interleukins have been described in the OVLT. Studies on the sensory abilities of area postrema neurons have been directed more toward potential roles in metabolic signaling, with data suggesting that certain populations of area postrema neurons can sense adrenomedullin, amylin, atrial natriuretic peptide, cholecystokinin, endothelin, glucagon like peptide-1, orexins, peptides acting at Y receptors, vasopressin and vasoactive intestinal polypeptide.

Thus, neurons within the sensory circumventricular organs area able to sense a tremendous variety of different circulating signals. In the following sections, these sensory abilities will be placed in the context of a number of different physiological systems (Figures 16–2, 16–3, 16–4 and 16–5).

## Functional Roles for the Circumventricular Organs

### *Body Fluid Homeostasis*

The sensory circumventricular organs play critical roles in the coordination of body fluid balance and cardiovascular function[38,89]. They are uniquely positioned to perform such integrative roles. Not only do they receive afferent inputs from multiple sources (Figure 16–2), but through their efferent connections to autonomic control centers, they are also able to regulate and integrate the functions of many different controllers of overall body fluid homeostasis.

*Cardiovascular Regulation* Historically, our developing recognition of the circumventricular organs as important sensory structures at the blood–brain interface probably owes more to the description of the role of SFO in sensing circulating angiotensin II in the late 1970s than any other single observation[86,133]. The roles of the renin-angiotensin system in the regulation of cardiovascular function as a result of the actions of angiotensin II in controlling vascular tone and sodium reabsorption by the kidney was already well established. However, in addition to these classical

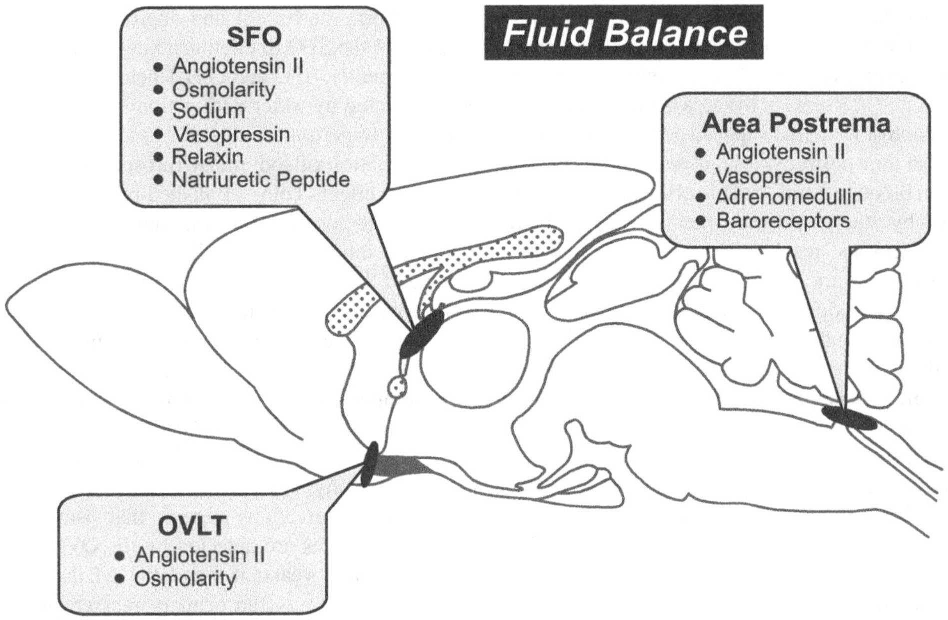


Figure 16–2 Blood-borne signals that influence body fluid homeostasis through actions at the sensory circumventricular organs. The locations of the three sensory circumventricular organs (black), the subfornical organ (SFO), the organum vasculosum of the lamina terminals (OVLT) and the area postrema, have been mapped onto a diagram of a mid-sagittal section through the rat brain. The callout boxes summarize the blood-borne signals that influence body fluid homeostasis through actions at that circumventricular organ. See text for details. Note that some signals act at more than one circumventricular organ and regulate more than one physiological function (see Figs. 16–3, 16–4, and 16–5). These data highlight the potential global interactive roles of the sensory circumventricular organs. *Dotted*, anterior and hippocampal commissure; *gray*, optic chiasm.

endocrine effects, circulating angiotensin II was shown to have behavioral (drinking), neuroendocrine (secretion of ACTH, oxytocin, and vasopressin) and autonomic (sympathetic activation) effects as a direct consequence of actions in the CNS. The densest aggregations of angiotensin II receptors are found within the sensory circumventricular organs[95], with the majority of binding occurring in the core region of the SFO[137]. SFO neurons show *c-fos* activation following intravenous angiotensin II[90]; and direct injection of angiotensin II into the SFO increases arterial pressure[86], effects that are blocked by section of the ventral stalk of the SFO[79]. At the cellular level, angiotensin II influences the excitability of SFO neurons through the combined inhibition of potassium currents, potentiation of calcium currents, and activation of a non-selective cationic conductance[38,44,103,152]. These observations suggest that the SFO is a critical relay center through which the CNS is able to monitor circulating levels of angiotensin II and influence cardiovascular function.

Activation of SFO neurons influences cardiovascular function through projections to the hypothalamus. SFO neurons activate PVN and SON neurons, which translates into the release of hormones from the pituitary gland. Inputs from the SFO also excite caudally projecting hypothalamic neurons that synapse on sympathetic preganglionic neurons in the intermediolateral cell column of the spinal cord. Consequently, chemical or electrical stimulation of the SFO results in the secretion of both vasopressin and oxytocin[41-43,61,132] and activation of sympathetic outflow[20,40]. The hypertensive effect of stimulation of the SFO is prevented by ablation of the hypothalamic PVN[46], and systemic angiotensin II acts at the SFO to control the activity of PVN neurons[47,73]. Intriguingly, the SFO neurons that project to the PVN have also been shown to utilize angiotensin II as a neurotransmitter[74]. Other regulatory peptides, including vasopressin[135,152], atrial natriuretic peptide[124], and relaxin[99], have also been shown to influence cardiovascular function as a result of actions in the SFO (Figure 16–2).

The area postrema sends efferent projections to many of the most important hindbrain cardiovascular centers, including the NTS, nucleus ambiguus, and parabrachial nucleus, and has very high densities of receptors for the cardioregulatory peptides angiotensin II, vasopressin, atrial natriuretic peptide, and endothelin[8,16,55,67]. Roles for the area postrema in cardiovascular control were first suggested by studies demonstrating that area postrema lesions resulted in a marked increase in blood pressure[156]. This observation was later supported by studies showing that activation of area postrema neurons results in rapid and reversible decreases in mean arterial pressure and heart rate in rats and rabbits[45,58]. In dogs, however, an increase in mean arterial pressure and heart rate was observed[7,48], suggesting the existence of species differences. The area postrema may also play a role in the regulation of baroreflex sensitivity since the ability of both circulating angiotensin II[49] and vasopressin[57] to control baroreflex sensitivity is dependent on an intact area postrema.

Extracellular single-unit recordings in anesthetized animals have confirmed that circulating angiotensin II increases the activity of a significant proportion (55%) of area postrema neurons, approximately half of which also receive baroreceptor input[106]. Systemic vasopressin, in contrast, inhibited 45%, and activated 38%, of area postrema neurons tested, with the majority of the latter group apparently receiving baroreceptor input[136]. *In vitro* brain slice recordings have also suggested mixed effects of these two peptides on area postrema neurons[14]. However, studies on area postrema neurons maintained in synaptic isolation suggest that both angiotensin II (40% of cells tested) and vasopressin (60% of cells tested) have predominantly direct excitatory effects on area postrema neurons[82,141] that are associated with increases in intracellular calcium[21]. Finally, such peptidergic activation of area postrema neurons has been shown to influence the excitability of single neurons in the NTS[13], identifying potential output pathways through which the area postrema may exert control over the cardiovascular system. While these studies do suggest the existence of differentially sensitive subpopulations of area postrema neurons, future work will clearly need not only to identify the innervation targets of these neurons but also to clarify whether single neurons are sensitive to more than one peptide, as might be expected.

It has also been suggested that the OVLT plays a role in cardiovascular regulation, although the evidence is less extensive than for SFO or area postrema. Studies have, however, shown that hypertensive/pressor responses to angiotensin II can be prevented by ablation of the anteroventral third ventricle region area[60] and that stimulation of the OVLT increases sympathetic nerve activity and arterial pressure[85].

*Fluid Balance* Again, initial interest in roles for the circumventricular organs in the regulation of body fluid balance originated from the demonstration that blood-borne carbachol and angiotensin II acted primarily at the SFO to elicit drinking behavior in rats[133]. Subsequently, SFO and OVLT neurons were shown to be activated by water deprivation[27], intravenous injection of hypertonic saline[102,119], sodium restriction[91], and depletion of sodium by furosemide[122], with many of these effects being abolished by the angiotensin II antagonist losartan, or the angiotensin converting enzyme inhibitor captopril[91]. The functional importance of the SFO and OVLT was confirmed by studies showing that destruction of the SFO eliminated both water and saline ingestion in rats acutely depleted of sodium[138,148]. Similarly, near-complete destruction of the lamina terminalis not only blocked drinking in both water-deprived animals and those receiving infusions of hypertonic saline[93], but also inhibited the excretion of hypertonic loads[88,92].

These observations suggest that osmotic or fluid volume changes are detected by the OVLT and SFO; and for many years; it was believed that circulating angiotensin II was the primary messenger providing this information[27]. However, it is now becoming clear that the sensory abilities of both OVLT and SFO neurons are far more sophisticated than was initially imagined. These sites appear to be sensitive to the sodium and water content of plasma[9,101,113]. Single-cell recordings have shown both OVLT[113,151] and SFO[4,56] neurons to be sensitive to both sodium and osmolarity.

Area postrema lesions have also been reported to impair osmoregulatory processes by increasing sodium intake and decreasing sodium excretion[26]. Ablation of the area postrema specifically blunts the secretion of oxytocin and vasopressin in response to injection of high-concentration saline solutions[65] and reduces *c-fos* expression in the PVN in response to an intragastric sodium load[15]. These observations can be interpreted in two ways. Area postrema neurons could be intrinsically sensitive to circulating sodium. Alternatively, they receive input regarding sodium concentration from peripheral afferents, which contribute to controlling the secretion of vasopressin and oxytocin from the posterior pituitary. Studies examining sodium- or osmo-sensitive properties of area postrema neurons have yet to be undertaken.

In addition to angiotensin II and vasopressin, the circumventricular organs are also responsive to other circulating peptides that play roles in cardiovascular control and the regulation of body fluid balance (Figure 16–2). Atrial natriuretic peptide[112], endothelin[69], orexin[154], oxytocin[64], prolactin[87], relaxin[140], and adrenomedullin[2] have all been suggested as influencing neuronal function in the circumventricular organs, indicating that there might be physiological roles for circumventricular organs that have not yet been elucidated.

### Immune Regulation

Infection leads to acute and chronic responses that result in physiological and behavioral changes. It is now well established that the immune system signals the brain to coordinate changes in body temperature, hormone release, sleep patterns, and food intake that together comprise the integrated immune response.

Systemic signaling of infection can occur directly through bacterial endotoxins, such as lipopolysaccharide, or through pyrogenic cytokines, such as the interleukins (interleukin-1β and interleukin-6). The circumventricular organs were some time ago suggested as providing an access point to the brain for circulating cytokines and endotoxins and also as having the potential to integrate the multiple components of this integrated immune response through their efferent connections to autonomic control centers in the hypothalamus and medulla. This hypothesis originally gained prominence from studies demonstrating that lesions of the OVLT (which included regions of the anteroventral third ventricle region) inhibited fever[10], although the specific role of the OVLT was later questioned following studies reporting different effects of these lesions[11,139,144]. Our own studies comparing effects of OVLT, SFO, and area postrema lesions on the febrile response to systemic lipopolysaccharide directed attention toward the SFO. We demonstrated that only SFO lesions had a significant impact on fever-generation[144], a conclusion supported by the demonstration that microinjection of an interleukin-1 receptor antagonist into the SFO also attenuated lipopolysaccharide-induced fever[17]. The area postrema has been implicated in mediating neuroendocrine responses to systemic interleukin-1β because lesions in this region attenuate increases in circulating ACTH, corticosterone[72] and noradrenaline within the PVN[72], which are normally seen in response to this stimulus.

Additional data supporting important roles for circumventricular organs in immune regulation came from the identification of interleukin-β and CD14 receptors, classic markers for endotoxin binding in all of the sensory circumventricular organs[25,35,70]. Subsequent studies supported the functional relevance to the expression of these receptors in the circumventricular organs. Peripheral administration of interleukin-1β, tumor necrosis factor-α, or lipopolysaccharide was shown to increases *c-fos* expression in the OVLT[33,34]; *c-fos* expression in SFO neurons induced by interleukin-1β[33] and interleukin-1β and lipopolysaccharide increased expression of *c-fos* and inhibitory factor kappa-B alpha in the area postrema[33,111,149]. These findings also suggest that these immune-signaling molecules play significant roles in controlling the activity of circumventricular organ neurons. This perspective is supported by recent electrophysiological studies showing that interleukin-1β depolarizes SFO neurons as a result of modulation of a non-selective cationic conductance[29]. In addition, tumor necrosis factor-α has been reported to increase the firing rate of OVLT neurons[131], although the conductances responsible for these effects have not yet been identified.

Thus, although the data suggesting sensory roles for the circumventricular organs in the regulation of immune function are not as extensive as those for fluid balance, there is strong evidence that each of the circumventricular organs may contribute to the brain's ability to initiate a coordinated immune response following increase in circulating cytokines through sensing peripheral immune signals (Figure 16–3).

### Reproduction

There is also evidence that the sensory circumventricular organs have roles in the control of reproductive functions. A number of different lesions studies suggest that removal of either the SFO, OVLT, or area postrema can have profound influence on estrous cyclicity. Steroidal, hormonal, and nutritional signals also have reproductive actions at these structures (Figure 16–4). In addition, all three sensory circumventricular organs have been found to contain significant levels of gonadotropin-releasing hormone[68], although the specific impact of this peptide is not known.

SFO lesions disrupt the estrous cycle and force rats into a prolonged state of diestrous[76]. In the SFO-lesioned rats, the surge of follicle-stimulating hormone at proestrous was absent, while the luteinizing hormone cyclicity remained unchanged[76]. In addition, studies demonstrating excitatory inputs from SFO to putative GnRH neurons[30] and the increase in circulating concentrations of luteinizing hormone upon activation of SFO neurons[31] indicate the connections through which SFO efferents may have their effects. The SFO has also been shown to have high densities of binding sites for the pregnancy hormone relaxin, which has been shown to influence the activity of SFO neurons[143]. The effects of relaxin in the SFO indicate possible roles in controlling the duration of gestation and the milk-ejection reflex. Intriguingly, relaxin can also cause hypertension as a result of actions at the SFO[140]. Finally, estrogen receptors have also been localized to the SFO[120], and it has been suggested that they modulate actions of angiotensin II in the SFO on the regulation of fluid balance[120,145,146].

Destruction of the OVLT also disrupts secretion of both luteinizing hormone and follicle-stimulating

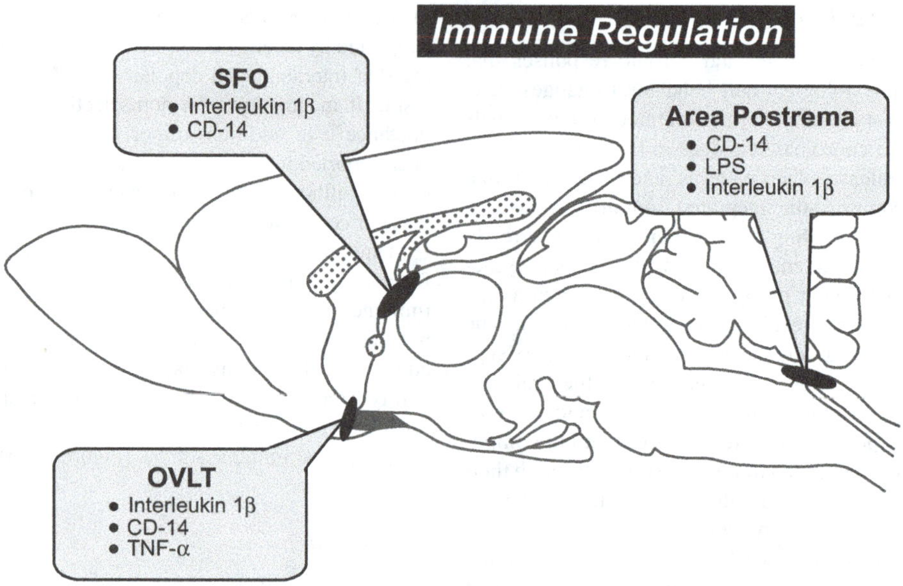


Figure 16–3 Blood-borne signals that influence immune regulation through actions at the sensory circumventricular organs. The locations of the three sensory circumventricular organs (*black*), the subfornical organ (SFO), the organum vasculosum of the lamina terminals (OVLT) and the area postrema, have been mapped onto a diagram of a mid-sagittal section through the rat brain. The callout boxes summarize the blood-borne signals that influence immune regulation through actions at that circumventricular organ. See text for details. Note that some signals act at more than one circumventricular organ and regulate more than one physiological function (see Figs. 16–2, 16–4, and 16–5). These data highlight the potential global interactive roles of the sensory circumventricular organs. *Dotted*, anterior and hippocampal commissure; *gray*, optic chiasm. LPS, lipopolysaccharide; TNF-α, tumor necrosis factor-alpha.

hormone[109]. It has also been suggested that the OVLT receives both positive and negative feedback from gonadotrophin-releasing hormone[37,126], potentially contributing to the negative feedback regulation of pulsatile gonadotrophin secretion. There is also evidence that prolactin can feed back to the OVLT to affect its own secretion[147].

The involvement of the area postrema in the control of reproduction has also been proposed. Single-cell studies have shown clear effects of estradiol on area postrema neurons[75]; but the majority of the data imply that these actions may be secondary to the role of area postrema as a feeding center. Apparently, the area postrema relays information regarding nutritional status to reproductive centers. The area postrema is also the site at which insulin-induced hypoglycemia acts to inhibit pulsatile luteinizing-hormone secretion[18]. Since lesions of the area postrema prevent suppression of estrous behavior by food-deprivation[104], this structure also appears to be the important sensory site for assessment of food availability.

## *Feeding and Metabolism*

About 30 years ago, hindbrain neuroglucoprivation induced by administration of 5-thioglucose into the fourth ventricle was found to be more effective in increasing food consumption than forebrain neuroglucoprivation induced by administration of 5-thioglucose into the lateral ventricle[117]. This observation led to a specific focus on the area postrema as a potential site for appetite control. Many lesion studies since then have demonstrated that ablation of the area postrema results in significant hypophagia and chronic depression of body weight[22,66]. It is not clear whether these effects are a result of a loss of recognition of hunger, a false feeling of satiety, or an aversion to food. Within the area postrema, there appears to be a functional link between feeding behavior, food aversions, and immune signaling. The area postrema is capable of sensing toxins in the bloodstream and triggering nausea and emesis[63]. Direct inhibition of area postrema neurons can be brought about by anti-emetic agents, such as propofol, which may be due to the

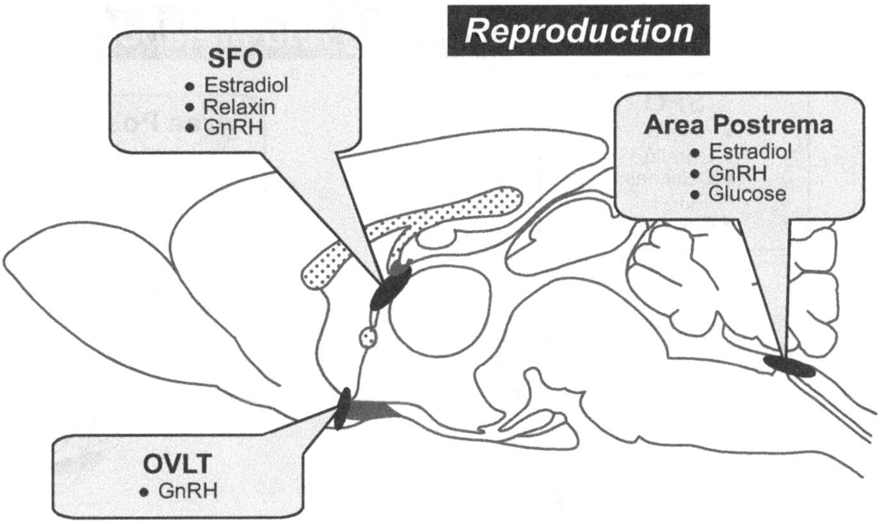


Figure 16–4 Blood-borne signals that influence reproduction through actions at the sensory circumventricular organs. The locations of the three sensory circumventricular organs (*black*), the subfornical organ (SFO), the organum vasculosum of the lamina terminals (OVLT), and the area postrema have been mapped onto a diagram of a mid-sagittal section through the rat brain. The callout boxes summarize the blood-borne signals that influence reproduction through actions at that circumventricular organ. See text for details. Note that some signals act at more than one circumventricular organ and regulate more than one physiological function (see Figs. 16–2, 16–3, and 16–5). These data highlight the potential global interactive roles of the sensory circumventricular organs. *Dotted*, anterior and hippocampal commissure; *gray*, optic chiasm. GnRH, gonadotropin releasing hormone.

inhibition of GABA currents[19]. Therefore, the area postrema can sense a toxic insult via cytokines, pathogens, and vagal inputs; trigger vomiting to remove the insult; and teach future avoidance of the toxic substance, a very sophisticated "skill set."

Recent work has also indicated that the area postrema can sense circulating concentrations of numerous blood-borne satiety signals (Figure 16–5). Amylin is secreted with insulin in response to food intake and is structurally and functionally similar to calcitonin and calcitonin gene-related peptide. Amylin administered either peripherally or centrally causes hypophagia[83] independently of vagal afferents[84]. The high density of amylin receptors in the area postrema,[128] when combined with observations that area postrema lesions reduce the effect of amylin[116,123], identifies the area postrema as one important site for the actions of this peptide. This suggestion is supported by single-cell studies showing that amylin increases the excitability of area postrema neurons through cGMP-mediated mechanisms[115]. Interestingly, the majority of neurons excited by amylin are also glucose-sensitive, implying an integrative role for these cells in transducing nutritional signals to feeding centers of the brain[116].

The area postrema is also influenced by other circulating hormones that act as signals of metabolic status, including glucagon-like peptide-1[121], cholecystokinin[32,142], and adrenomedullin[129,155]. Area postrema neurons are also activated by central injections of the orexigenic peptide ghrelin, and therefore may mediate its effects on feeding behavior[71]. The orexins/hypocretins also influence the excitability of area postrema neurons through activation of a nonselective cation conductance[154]. In combination, these data support a complex and integrative role for the area postrema in the control of feeding.

Until recently, the area postrema was thought to be the predominant circumventricular organ involved in the regulation of food intake, with dominant roles assigned to the hypothalamic arcuate nucleus in sensing circulating satiety signals. In fact, it has been suggested that the arcuate should be considered a circumventricular organ, despite the fact that there are no anatomical data reporting fenestrated capillaries in this nucleus. Perhaps some of this confusion arises from the demonstration that systemic horseradish peroxidase reaches not only the true circumventricular organs but also the arcuate nucleus[12], an observation

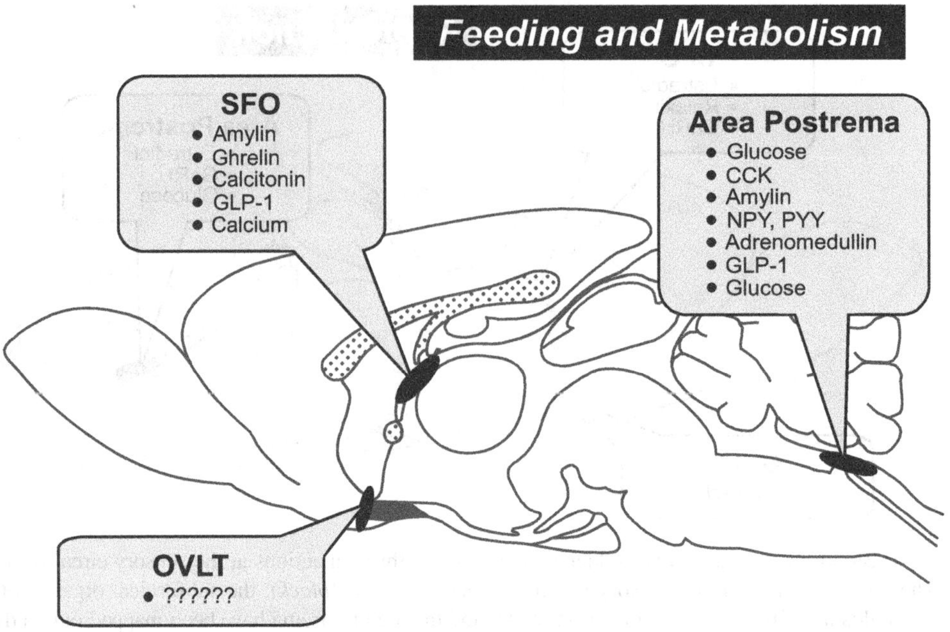


Figure 16–5 Blood-borne signals that influence feeding and metabolism through actions at the sensory circumventricular organs. The locations of the three sensory circumventricular organs (*black*), the subfornical organ (SFO), the organum vasculosum of the lamina terminals (OVLT) and the area postrema, have been mapped onto a diagram of a mid-sagittal section through the rat brain. The callout boxes summarize the blood-borne signals that influence reproduction through actions at that circumventricular organ. See text for details. Note that some signals act at more than one circumventricular organ and regulate more than one physiological function (see Figs. 16–2, 16–3, and 16–4). These data highlight the potential global interactive roles of the sensory circumventricular organs. *Dotted*, anterior and hippocampal commissure; *gray*, optic chiasm. CCK, cholecystokinin; GLP-1, glucagon-like peptide-1; NPY, neuropeptide Y; PYY, peptide YY.

that the authors of this study concluded was the result of retrograde axonal transport rather than diffusion across a leaky blood–brain barrier. Interestingly, recent work has begun to suggest roles for the true forebrain sensory circumventricular organs, the OVLT or SFO, in sensing satiety signals. Single-cell recordings have shown effects of calcitonin[127] and amylin[114,115] on SFO neurons, and our own recent work demonstrates that separate subpopulations of SFO neurons are responsive to amylin and ghrelin[110]. These data suggest potentially important roles for SFO neurons in monitoring an increasing number of satiety signals (Figure 16–5).

## Circumventricular Organs as Controllers of Integrated Autonomic Function

The information above argues persuasively that, in addition to their unique position at the blood–brain interface, the sensory circumventricular organs combine broad-ranging sensory abilities with the capability to exert control over diverse yet interrelated physiological systems. Since nearly all studies examining the sensitivity of neurons in circumventricular organ to circulating signals report that between 25% and 60% of neurons are influenced, *single neurons must have multiple sensory abilities*. This concept, at the minimal level of two signals, has been confirmed. Area postrema neurons are both glucose- and amylin-sensitive[116]. SFO neurons have been studied for their sensitivity to pairs of blood-borne signals, and individual neurons have been shown to respond to angiotensin II and osmolarity[3], to angiotensin II and atrial natriuretic peptide[59], to angiotensin II and calcitonin[127], and to angiotensin II and estrogen[146]. Whether single SFO neurons are therefore sensitive to angiotensin II, atrial natriuretic peptide, calcitonin, estradiol, and osmolarity is an intriguing and important question, as well as a somewhat daunting experimental challenge to answer.

There is to date no information regarding the ability of single circumventricular organ neurons to be more promiscuous in sensing multiple signals that would traditionally be viewed as related to different physiological systems. For example, are amylin- and glucose-sensitive area postrema neurons also sensitive to angiotensin II? Nevertheless, a picture has begun to emerge that neurons in the circumventricular organs sense multiple signals and thus could potentially control more broadly based physiological outputs in an integrated manner. Thus, although research directed toward understanding central control of fluid balance, energy homeostasis, and reproductive function remains very clearly separated into distinct fields, groups working within these separate fields clearly understand that such definitive separation seldom makes physiological sense. Humans very seldom eat without drinking; lack of available nutrients has clear inhibitory effects on reproductive function; and systemic infections not only activate the neuroimmune axis but also profoundly influence fluid and food intake.

The data presented in this chapter suggest that neurons in the sensory circumventricular organs are uniquely positioned to make important contributions to integrated control of different physiological systems. The biggest future challenge in this area will probably be the design of truly integrated experimental paradigms that can assess the real contributions of the sensory circumventricular organs to establishment of what one may call the "autonomic set-point" of the organism. The time has probably arrived when the "sensory circumventricular organs" need to be considered in a far broader context than as structures only involved in the regulation of body fluid balance.

## References


1. Abbott, N. J., Ronnback L., and Hansson, E. (2006). Astrocyte-endothelial interactions at the blood–brain barrier. *Nature Reviews Neuroscience* 7, 41–53.
2. Allen, M. A., Smith P. M., and Ferguson, A. V. (1997). Adrenomedullin microinjection into the area postrema increases blood pressure. *American Journal of Physiology* 272, R1698–R1703.
3. Anderson, J. W., Smith, P. M., and Ferguson, A. V. (2001). Subfornical organ neurons projecting to paraventricular nucleus: Whole-cell properties. *Brain Research* 921, 78–85.
4. Anderson, J. W., Washburn, D. L., and Ferguson, A. V. (2000). Intrinsic osmosensitivity of subfornical organ neurons. *Neuroscience* 100, 539–547.
5. Armstrong, W. E., Tian, M., and Wong, H. (1996). Electron microscopic analysis of synaptic inputs from the median preoptic nucleus and adjacent regions to the supraoptic nucleus in the rat. *Journal of Comparative Neurology* 373, 228–239.
6. Banks, W. A. (2005). Blood–brain barrier transport of cytokines: A mechanism for neuropathology. *Current Pharmaceutical Design* 11, 973–984.
7. Barnes, K. L., Ferrario, C. M., and Conomy, J. P. (1979). Comparison of the hemodynamic changes produced by electrical stimulation of the area postrema and nucleus tractus solitarii in the dog. *Circulation Research* 45, 136–143.
8. Bianchi, C., Gutkowska, J., Ballak, M., Thibault, G., Garcia, R., Genest, J., and Cantin, M. (1986). Radioautographic localization of 125I-atrial natriuretic factor binding sites in the brain. *Neuroendocrinology* 44, 365–372.
9. Bisley, J. W., Rees, S. M., McKinley, M. J., Hards, D. K., and Oldfield, B. J. (1996). Identification of osmoresponsive neurons in the forebrain of the rat: A fos study at the ultrastructural level. *Brain Research* 720, 25–34.
10. Blatteis, C. M., Bealer, S. L., Hunter, W. S., Llanos, -Q. J., Ahokas R. A., and Mashburn, T. A., Jr. (1983). Suppression of fever after lesions of the anteroventral third ventricle in guinea pigs. *Brain Research Bulletin* 11, 519–526.
11. Blatteis, C. M., Hales, J. R., McKinley, M. J., and Fawcett, A. A. (1987). Role of the anteroventral third ventricle region in fever in sheep. *Canadian Journal of Physiology and Pharmacology* 65, 1255–1260.
12. Broadwell, R. D., and Brightman, M. W. (1976). Entry of peroxidase into neurons of the central and peripheral nervous systems from extracerebral and cerebral blood. *Journal of Comparative Neurology* 166, 257–283.
13. Cai, Y., Hay, M., and Bishop, V. S. (1994). Stimulation of area postrema by vasopressin and angiotensin II molulates neuronal activity in the nucleus tractus solitarius. *Brain Research* 647, 242–248.
14. Cai, Y. R., and Bishop, V. S. (1995). Effects of arginine vasopressin and angiotensin II on area postrema neurons in rabbit brain slice preparation. *Neuroscience Letters* 190, 125–128.
15. Carlson, S. H., Collister J. P., and Osborn, J. W. (1998). The area postrema modulates hypothalamic fos responses to intragastric hypertonic saline in conscious rats. *American Journal of Physiology* 275, R1921–R1927.
16. Carpenter, D. O., Briggs, D. B., Knox, A. P., and Strominger, N. (1988). Excitation of area postrema neurons by transmitters, peptides, and cyclic nucleotides. *Journal of Neurophysiology* 59, 358–369.

17. Cartmell, T., Luheshi, G. N., and Rothwell, N. J. (1999). Brain sites of action of endogenous interleukin-1 in the febrile response to localized inflammation in the rat. *Journal of Physiology* 518, 585–594.
18. Cates, P. S., and O'Byrne, K. T. (2000). The area postrema mediates insulin hypoglycaemia-induced suppression of pulsatile LH secretion in the female rat. *Brain Research* 853, 151–155.
19. Cechetto, D. F., Diab, T., Gibson, C J., and Gelb, A. W. (2001). The effects of propofol in the area postrema of rats. *Anesthesia and Analgesia* 92, 934–942.
20. Cirello, J., and Gutman, M. B. (1991). Functional identification of central pressor pathways originating in the subfornical organ. *Canadian Journal of Physiology and Pharmacology* 69, 1035–1045.
21. Consolim-Colombo, F. M., Hay, M., Smith, T. C., Elizondo-Fournier M., and Bishop, V. S. (1996). Subcellular mechanisms of angiotensin II and arginine vasopressin activation of area postrema neurons. *American Journal of Physiology* 40, R34–R41.
22. Contreras, R. J., Fox, E., and Drubovich, M. L. (1982). Area postrema lesions produce feeding deficits in the rat: Effects of preoperative dieting and 2–deoxy-D-glucose. *Physiology and Behavior* 29, 875–884.
23. Contreras, R. J., Beckstead, R. M., and Norgren, R. (1982). The central projections of the trigeminal, facial, glossopharyngeal and vagus nerves: An autoradiographic study in the rat. *Journal of the Autonomic Nervous System* 6, 303–322.
24. Cottrell, G. T., and Ferguson, A. V. (2004). Sensory circumventricular organs: Central roles in integrated autonomic regulation. *Regulatory Peptides* 117, 11–23.
25. Cunningham, E. T., Jr., Wada, E., Carter, D. B., Tracey, D. E., Battey, J. F., and De Souza, E. B. (1992). In situ histochemical localization of type I interleukin-1 receptor messenger RNA in the central nervous system, pituitary, and adrenal gland of the mouse. *Journal of Neuroscience* 12, 1101–1114.
26. Curtis, K. S., Huang, W., Sved, A. F., Verbalis, J. G., and Stricker, E. M. (1999). Impaired osmoregulatory responses in rats with area postrema lesions. *American Journal of Physiology* 277, R209–R219.
27. De Luca, L. A., Jr., Xu, Z., Schoorlemmer, G. H., Thunhorst, R. L., Beltz, T. G., Menani, J. V., and Johnson, A. K. (2002). Water deprivation-induced sodium appetite: Humoral and cardiovascular mediators and immediate early genes. *American Journal of Physiology. Regulatory, Integrative and Comparative Physiology* 282, R552–R559.
28. Dellman, H. D., and Simpson, J. B. (1979). The subfornical organ. *International Review of Cytology* 58, 333–421.
29. Desson, S. E., and Ferguson, A. V. (2003). Interleukin 1beta modulates rat subfornical organ neurons as a result of activation of a non-selective cationic conductance. *Journal of Physiology* 550, 113–122.
30. Donevan, S. D., and Ferguson, A. V. (1988). Subfornical organ connections with septal neurons projecting to the median eminence. *Neuroendocrinology* 48, 67–71.
31. Donevan, S. D., Van Vugt, D. A., and Ferguson, A. V. (1989). Subfornical organ activation stimulates luteinizing hormone secretion in the rat. *Brain Research* 488, 398–402.
32. Edwards, G. L., Ladenheim, E. E., and Ritter, R. C. (1986). Dorsomedial hindbrain participation in cholecystokinin-induced satiety. *American Journal of Physiology* 251, R971–R977.
33. Elmquist, J. K., Scammell, T. E., Jacobson, C. D., and Saper, C. B. (1996). Distribution of Fos-like immunoreactivity in the rat brain following intravenous lipopolysaccharide administration. *Journal of Comparative Neurology* 371, 85–103.
34. Ericsson, A., Kovacs, K. J., and Sawchenko, P. E. (1994). A functional anatomical analysis of central pathways subserving the effects of interleukin-1 on stress-related neuroendocrine neurons. *Journal of Neuroscience* 14, 897–913.
35. Ericsson, A., Liu, C., Hart, R. P., and Sawchenko, P. E. (1995). Type 1 interleukin-1 receptor in the rat brain: Distribution, regulation, and relationship to sites of IL-1–induced cellular activation. *Journal of Comparative Neurology* 361, 681–698.
36. Felix, D. (1976). Peptide and acetylcholine action on neurones of the cat subfornical organ. *Naunyn Schmiedeberg's Archives of Pharmacology* 292, 15–20.
37. Felix, D., and Phillips, M. I. (1979). Inhibitory effects of luteinizing hormone–releasing hormone (LH-RH) on neurons in the organum vasculosum lamina terminalis (OVLT). *Brain Research* 169, 204–208.
38. Ferguson, A. V., and Bains, J. S. (1996). Electrophysiology of the circumventricular organs. *Frontiers in Neuroendocrinology* 17, 440–475.
39. Ferguson, A. V., Bicknell, R. J., Carew, M. A., and Mason, W. T. (1997). Dissociated adult rat subfornical organ neurons maintain membrane properties and angiotensin responsiveness for up to six days. *Neuroendocrinology* 66, 409–415.
40. Ferguson, A. V., Day, T. A., and Renaud, L. P. (1984). Subfornical organ stimulation excites paraventricular neurons projecting to the dorsal

medulla. *American Journal of Physiology* 247, R1088–R1092.

41. Ferguson, A. V., and Kasting, N. W. (1986). Electrical stimulation in the subfornical organ increases plasma vasopressin concentrations in the conscious rat. *American Journal of Physiology* 251, R425–R428.
42. Ferguson, A. V., and Kasting, N. W. (1987). Activation of subfornical organ efferents stimulates oxytocin secretion in the rat. *Regulatory Peptides* 18, 93–100.
43. Ferguson, A. V., and Kasting, N. W. (1988). Angiotensin acts at the subfornical organ to increase plasma oxytocin concentrations in the rat. *Regulatory Peptides* 23, 343–352.
44. Ferguson, A. V., and Li, Z. (1996). Whole-cell patch clamp recordings from forebrain slices demonstrate angiotensin II inhibits potassium currents in subfornical organ neurons. *Regulatory Peptides* 66, 55–58.
45. Ferguson, A. V., and Marcus, P. (1988). Area postrema stimulation induced cardiovascular changes in the rat. *American Journal of Physiology* 255, R855–R860.
46. Ferguson, A. V., and Renaud, L. P. (1984). Hypothalamic paraventricular nucleus lesions decrease pressor responses to subfornical organ stimulation. *Brain Research* 305, 361–364.
47. Ferguson, A. V., and Renaud, L. P. (1986). Systemic angiotensin acts at subfornical organ to facilitate activity of neurohypophysial neurons. *American Journal of Physiology* 251, R712–R717.
48. Ferrario, C. M., Barnes, K. L., Diz, D. I., Block, C. H., and Averill, D. B. (1987). Role of area postrema pressor mechanisms in the regulation of arterial pressure. *Canadian Journal of Physiology and Pharmacology* 65, 1591–1597.
49. Fink, G. D., Bruner, C. A., and Mangiapane, M. L. (1987). Area postrema is critical for angiotensin-induced hypertension in rats. *Hypertension* 9, 355–361.
50. Fry, M., Hoyda, T. D., and Ferguson A. V. (2007). Making sense of it: Roles of the sensory circumventricular organs in feeding and regulation of energy homeostasis. *Experimental Biology and Medicine* 232, 14–26.
51. Gehlert, D. R., Gackenheimer, S. L., Reel, J. K., Lin, H.-S., and Steinberg, M. I. (1990). Non-peptide angiotensin II receptor antagonists discriminate subtypes of 125I-angiotensin II binding sites in the rat brain. *European Journal of Pharmacology* 187, 123–126.
52. Gross, P. M. (1991). Morphology and physiology of capillary systems in subregions of the subfornical organ and area postrema. *Canadian Journal of Physiology and Pharmacology* 69, 1010–1025.
53. Gross, P. M. (1992). Circumventricular organ capillaries. *Progress in Brain Research* 91, 219–233.
54. Gruber, K., McRae-Degueurce, A., Wilkin, L. D., Mitchell, L. D., and Johnson, A. K. (1987). Forebrain and brainstem afferents to the arcuate nucleus in the rat: Potential pathways for the modulation of hypophyseal secretions. *Neuroscience Letters* 75, 1–5.
55. Guan, J. L., Wang, Q. P., and Shioda, S. (2000). Observation of the ultrastructure and synaptic relationships of angiotensin II-like immunoreactive neurons in the rat area postrema. *Synapse* 38, 231–237.
56. Gutman, M. B., Ciriello, J., and Mogenson, G. J. (1988). Effects of plasma angiotensin II and hypernatremia on subfornical organ neurons. *American Journal of Physiology* 254, R746–R754.
57. Hasser, E. M., and Bishop, V. S. (1990). Reflex effect of vasopressin after blockade of $V_1$ receptors in the area postrema. *Circulation Research* 67, 265–271.
58. Hasser, E. M., Nelson, D. O., Haywood, J. R., and Bishop, V. S. (1987). Inhibition of renal sympathetic nervous activity by area postrema stimulation in rabbits. *American Journal of Physiology* 253, H91–H99.
59. Hattori, Y., Kasai, M., Uesugi, S., Kawata, M., and Yamashita, H. (1988). Atrial natriuretic polypeptide depresses angiotensin II induced excitation of neurons in the rat subfornical organ in vitro. *Brain Research* 443, 355–359.
60. Haywood, J. R., Fink, G. D., Buggy, J., Boutelle, S., Johnson, A. K., and Brody, M. J. (1983). Prevention of two-kidney, one clip renal hypertension in rat by ablation of AV3V tissue. *American Journal of Physiology* 245, H683–H689.
61. Holmes, M. C., Catt, K. J., and Aguilera, G. (1987). Involvement of vasopressin in the down-regulation of pituitary corticotropin-releasing factor receptors after adrenalectomy. *Endocrinology* 121, 2093–2098.
62. Honda, K., Negoro, H., Higuchi, T., and Takano, S. (1990). Activation of supraoptic neurosecretory cells by osmotic stimulation of the median preoptic nucleus. *Neuroscience Letters* 119, 167–170.
63. Hornby, P. J. (2001). Central neurocircuitry associated with emesis. *American Journal of Medicine* 111 Suppl 8A, 106S–112S.
64. Hosono, T., Schmid, H. A., Kanosue, K., and Simon, E. (1999). Neuronal actions of oxytocin on the subfornical organ of male rats. *American Journal of Physiology* 276, E1004–E1008.

65. Huang, W., Sved, A. F., and Stricker, E. M. (2000). Vasopressin and oxytocin release evoked by NaCl loads are selectively blunted by area postrema lesions. *American Journal of Physiology. Regulatory, Integrative and Comparative Physiology* 278, R732–R740.
66. Hyde, T. M., and Miselis, R. R. (1983). Effects of area postrema/caudal medial nucleus of solitary tract lesions on food intake and body weight. *American Journal of Physiology* 244, R577–R587.
67. Jones, C. R., Hiley, C. R., Pelton, J. T., and Mohr, M. (1989). Autoradiographic visualization of the binding sites for [125I] endothelin in rat and human brain. *Neuroscience Letters* 97, 276–279.
68. Kizer, J. S., Palkovits, M., and Brownstein, M. J. (1976). Releasing factors in the circumventricular organs of the rat brain. *Endocrinology* 98, 311–317.
69. Koseki, C., Imai, M., Hirata, Y., Yanagisawa, M., and Masaki, T. (1989). Autoradiographic localization of [125I]-endothelin-1 binding sites in rat brain. *Neuroscience Research* 6, 581–585.
70. Laflamme, N., and Rivest, S. (2001). Toll-like receptor 4: The missing link of the cerebral innate immune response triggered by circulating gram-negative bacterial cell wall components. *FASEB Journal* 15, 155–163.
71. Lawrence, C. B., Snape, A. C., Baudoin, F. M., and Luckman, S. M. (2002). Acute central ghrelin and GH secretagogues induce feeding and activate brain appetite centers. *Endocrinology* 143, 155–162.
72. Lee, H. Y., Whiteside, M. B., and Herkenham, M. (1998). Area postrema removal abolishes stimulatory effects of intravenous interleukin-1beta on hypothalamic-pituitary-adrenal axis activity and c-Fos mRNA in the hypothalamic paraventricular nucleus. *Brain Research Bulletin* 46, 495–503.
73. Li, Z., and Ferguson, A. V. (1993). Angiotensin II responsiveness of rat paraventricular and subfornical organ neurons *in vitro*. *Neuroscience* 55, 197–207.
74. Li, Z., and Ferguson, A. V. (1993). Subfornical organ efferents to the paraventricular nucleus utilize angiotensin as a neurotransmitter. *American Journal of Physiology* 265, R302–R309.
75. Li, Z., and Hay, M. (2000). 17-beta-estradiol modulation of area postrema potassium currents. *Journal of Neurophysiology* 84, 1385–1391.
76. Limonta, P., Maggi, R., Giudici, D., Martini, L., and Piva, F. (1981). Role of the subfornical organ (SFO) in the control of gonadotropin secretion. *Brain Research* 229, 75–84.
77. Lind, R. W. (1986). Bi-directional, chemically specified neural connections between the subfornical organ and the midbrain raphé system. *Brain Research* 384, 250–261.
78. Lind, R. W. (1988). Angiotensin and the lamina terminalis: Illustrations of a complex unity. *Clinical and Experimental Hypertension* 10, 79–105.
79. Lind, R. W., Ohman, L. E., Lansing, M. B., and Johnson, A. K. (1983). Transection of subfornical organ neural connections diminishes the pressor response to intravenously infused angiotensin II. *Brain Research* 275, 361–364.
80. Lind, R. W., Swanson, L. W., and Ganten, D. (1984). Angiotensin II immunoreactivity in the neural afferents and efferents of the subfornical organ of the rat. *Brain Research* 321, 209–215.
81. Lind, R. W., Van Hoesen, G. W., and Johnson, A. K. (1982). An HRP study of the connections of the subfornical organ of the rat. *Journal of Comparative Neurology* 210, 265–277.
82. Lowes, V. L., Sun, K., Li, Z., and Ferguson, A. V. (1995). Vasopressin actions on area postrema neurons *in vitro*. *American Journal of Physiology* 269, R463–R468.
83. Lutz, T. A., Del Prete, E., and Scharrer, E. (1994). Reduction of food intake in rats by intraperitoneal injection of low doses of amylin. *Physiology and Behavior* 55, 891–895.
84. Lutz, T. A., Del Prete, E., and Scharrer, E. (1995). Subdiaphragmatic vagotomy does not influence the anorectic effect of amylin. *Peptides* 16, 457–462.
85. Mangiapane, M. L., and Brody, M. J. (1987). Vasoconstrictor and vasodilator sites within anteroventral third ventricle region. *American Journal of Physiology* 253, R827–R831.
86. Mangiapane, M. L., and Simpson, J. B. (1980). Subfornical organ lesions reduce the pressor effect of systemic angiotensin II. *Neuroendocrinology* 31, 380–384.
87. Mangurian, L. P., Jurjus, A. R., and Walsh, R. J. (1999). Prolactin receptor localization to the area postrema. *Brain Research* 836, 218–220.
88. May, C. N., McAllen, R. M., and McKinley M. J. (2000). Renal nerve inhibition by central NaCl and ANG II is abolished by lesions of the lamina terminalis. *American Journal of Physiology. Regulatory, Integrative and Comparative Physiology* 279, R1827–R1833.
89. McKinley, M. J., Allen, A. M., Burns, P., Colvill, L. M., and Oldfield, B. J. (1998). Interaction of circulating hormones with the brain: The roles of the subfornical organ and the organum vasculosum of the lamina terminalis. *Clinical and Experimental Pharmacology and Physiology* Suppl 25, S61–S67.

90. McKinley, M. J., Badoer, E., and Oldfield, B. J. (1992). Intravenous angiotensin II induces Fos-immunoreactivity in circumventricular organs of the lamina terminalis. *Brain Research* 594, 295–300.
91. McKinley, M. J., Colvill, L. M., Giles, M. E., and Oldfield, B. J. (1997). Distribution of Fos-immunoreactivity in rat brain following a dipsogenic dose of captopril and effects of angiotensin receptor blockade. *Brain Research* 747, 43–51.
92. McKinley, M. J., Lichardus, B., McDougall, J. G., and Weisinger, R. S. (1992). Periventricular lesions block natriuresis to hypertonic but not isotonic NaCl loads. *American Journal of Physiology* 262, F98–F107.
93. McKinley, M. J., Mathai, M. L., Pennington, G., Rundgren, M., and Vivas, L. (1999). Effect of individual or combined ablation of the nuclear groups of the lamina terminalis on water drinking in sheep. *American Journal of Physiology* 276, R673–R683.
94. McKinley, M. J., McAllen, R. M., Davern, P., Giles, M. E., Penschow, J., Sunn, N., Uschakov, A., and Oldfield, B. J. (2003). The sensory circumventricular organs of the mammalian brain. *Advances in Anatomy, Embryology and Cell Biology* 172, III–XII, 1–122.
95. Mendelsohn, F. A., Quirion, R., Saavedra, J. M., Aguilera, G., and Catt, K. J. (1984). Autoradiographic localization of angiotensin II receptors in rat brain. *Proceedings of the National Academy of Sciences USA* 81, 1575–1579.
96. Merchenthaler, I., and Liposits, Z. (1994). Mapping of thyrotropin-releasing hormone (TRH) neuronal systems of rat forebrain projecting to the median eminence and the OVLT. Immunocytochemistry combined with retrograde labeling at the light and electron microscopic levels. *Acta Biologica Hungarica* 45, 361–374.
97. Miselis, R. R. (1982). The subfornical organ's neural connections and their role in water balance. *Peptides* 3, 501–502.
98. Miselis, R. R., Shapiro, R. E., and Hand, P. J. (1979). Subfornical organ efferents to neural systems for control of body water. *Science* 205, 1022–1025.
99. Mumford, A. D., Parry, L. J., and Summerlee, A. J. (1989). Lesion of the subfornical organ affects the haemotensive response to centrally administered relaxin in anaesthetized rats. *Journal of Endocrinology* 122, 747–755.
100. Noda, M. (2006). The subfornical organ, a specialized sodium channel, and the sensing of sodium levels in the brain. *The Neuroscientist* 12, 80–91.
101. Oldfield, B. J., Badoer, E., Hards, D. K., and McKinley, M. J. (1994). Fos production in retrogradely labelled neurons of the lamina terminalis following intravenous infusion of either hypertonic saline or angiotensin II. *Neuroscience* 60, 255–262.
102. Oldfield, B. J., Bicknell, R. J., McAllen, R. M., Weisinger, R. S., and McKinley, M. J. (1991). Intravenous hypertonic saline induces Fos immunoreactivity in neurons throughout the lamina terminalis. *Brain Research* 561, 151–156.
103. Ono, K., Honda, E., and Inenaga, K. (2001). Angiotensin II induces inward currents in subfornical organ neurones of rats. *Journal of Neuroendocrinology* 13, 517–523.
104. Panicker, A. K., and Wade, G. N. (1998). Insulin-induced repartitioning of metabolic fuels inhibits hamster estrous behavior: Role of area postrema. *American Journal of Physiology* 43, R1094–R1098.
105. Papas, S., and Ferguson, A. V. (1990). Electrophysiological characterization of reciprocal connections between the parabrachial nucleus and the area postrema in the rat. *Brain Research Bulletin* 24, 577–582.
106. Papas, S., Smith, P., and Ferguson, A. V. (1990). Electrophysiological evidence that systemic angiotensin influences rat area postrema neurons. *American Journal of Physiology* 258, R70–R76.
107. Paton, J. F., Waki, H., Abdala, A. P., Dickinson, J., and Kasparov, S. (2007). Vascular-brain signaling in hypertension: Role of angiotensin II and nitric oxide. *Current Hypertension Reports* 9, 242–247.
108. Petrov, T., Howarth, A. G., Krukoff, T. L., and Stevenson, B. R. (1994). Distribution of the tight junction-associated protein ZO-1 in circumventricular organs of the CNS. *Molecular Brain Research* 21, 235–246.
109. Piva, F., Limonta, P., and Martini, L. (1982). Role of the organum vasculosum laminae terminalis in the control of gonadotrophin secretion in rats. *Journal of Endocrinology* 93, 355–364.
110. Pulman, K. J., Fry, W. M., Cottrell, G. T., and Ferguson, A. V. (2006). The subfornical organ: A central target for circulating feeding signals. *Journal of Neuroscience* 26, 2022–2030.
111. Quan, N., Whiteside, M., Kim, L., and Herkenham M. (1997). Induction of inhibitory factor kappa B alpha mRNA in the central nervous system after peripheral lipopolysaccharide administration: An in situ hybridization

histochemistry study in the rat. *Proceedings of the National Academy of Sciences USA* 94, 10985–10990.

112. Richard, D., and Bourque, C. W. (1996). Atrial natriuretic peptide modulates excitatory transmission from osmoreceptor afferents to the supraoptic nucleus. *Journal of Neuroscience* 16, 7526–7532.
113. Richard, D., and Bourque, C. W. (1995). Synaptic control of rat supraoptic neurones during osmotic stimulation of the organum vasculosum lamina terminalis in vitro. *Journal of Physiology* 489, 567–577.
114. Riediger, T., Rauch, M., and Schmid, H. A. (1999). Actions of amylin on subfornical organ neurons and on drinking behavior in rats. *American Journal of Physiology* 276, R514–R521.
115. Riediger, T., Schmid, H. A., Lutz, T., and Simon, E. (2001). Amylin potently activates AP neurons possibly via formation of the excitatory second messenger cGMP. *American Journal of Physiology. Regulatory, Integrative and Comparative Physiology* 281, R1833–R1843.
116. Riediger, T., Schmid, H. A., Lutz, T. A., and Simon, E. (2002). Amylin and glucose co-activate area postrema neurons of the rat. *Neuroscience Letters* 328, 121–124.
117. Ritter, R. C., Slusser, P. G., and Stone, S. (1981). Glucoreceptors controlling feeding and blood glucose: Location in the hindbrain. *Science* 213, 451–452.
118. Rogers, K. V., Dunn, C. K., Hebert, S. C., and Brown, E. M. (1997). Localization of calcium receptor mRNA in the adult rat central nervous system by in situ hybridization. *Brain Research* 744, 47–56.
119. Rohmeiss, P., Beyer, C., Hocher, B., Qadri, F., Gretz, N., Strauch, M., and Unger, T. (1995). Osmotically induced natriuresis and blood pressure response involves angiotensin $AT_1$ receptors in the subfornical organ. *Journal of Hypertension* 13, 1399–1404.
120. Rosas-Arellano, M. P., Solano-Flores, L. P., and Ciriello, J. (1999). Co-localization of estrogen and angiotensin receptors within subfornical organ neurons. *Brain Research* 837, 254–262.
121. Rowland, N. E., Crews, E. C., and Gentry, R. M. (1997). Comparison of Fos induced in rat brain by GLP-1 and amylin. *Regulatory Peptides* 71, 171–174.
122. Rowland, N. E., Fregly, M. J., Han, L., and Smith, G. (1996). Expression of Fos in rat brain in relation to sodium appetite: Furosemide and cerebroventricular renin. *Brain Research* 728, 90–96.
123. Rowland, N. E., and Richmond, R. M. (1999). Area postrema and the anorectic actions of dexfenfluramine and amylin. *Brain Research* 820, 86–91.
124. Saavedra, J. M., Israel, A., Kurihara, M., and Fuchs, E. (1986). Decreased number and affinity of rat atrial natriuretic peptide (6–33) binding sites in the subfornical organ of spontaneously hypertensive rats. *Circulation Research* 58, 389–392.
125. Saper, C. B., and Levisohn, D. (1983). Afferent connections of the median preoptic nucleus in the rat: Anatomical evidence for a cardiovascular integrative mechanism in the anteroventral third ventricular (AV3V) region. *Brain Research* 288, 21–31.
126. Sayer, R. J., Hubbard, J. I., and Sirett, N. E. (1984). Rat organum vasculosum laminae terminalis in vitro: Responses to transmitters. *American Journal of Physiology* 247, R374–R379.
127. Schmid, H. A., Rauch, M., and Koch, J. (1998). Effect of calcitonin on the activity of ANG II-responsive neurons in the rat subfornical organ. *American Journal of Physiology* 274, R1646–R1652.
128. Sexton, P. M., Paxinos, G., Kenney, M. A., Wookey, P. J., and Beaumont, K. (1994). *In vitro* autoradiographic localization of amylin binding sites in rat brain. *Neuroscience* 62, 553–567 .
129. Shan, J., and Krukoff, T. L. (2000). Area postrema ablation attenuates activation of neurones in the paraventricular nucleus in response to systemic adrenomedullin. *Journal of Neuroendocrinology* 12, 802–810.
130. Shapiro, R. E., and Miselis, R. R. (1985). The central neural connections of the area postrema of the rat. *Journal of Comparative Neurology* 234, 344–364.
131. Shibata, M., and Blatteis, C. M. (1991). Differential effects of cytokines on thermosensitive neurons in guinea pig preoptic area slices. *American Journal of Physiology* 261, R1096–R1103.
132. Simpson, J. B. (1981). The circumventricular organs and the central actions of angiotensin. *Neuroendocrinology* 32, 248–256.
133. Simpson, J. B., and Routtenberg, J. B. (1975). Subfornical organ lesions reduce intravenous angiotensin-induced drinking. *Brain Research* 88, 154–161.
134. Smith, P. M., and Ferguson, A. V. (1996). Paraventricular nucleus efferents influence area postrema neurons. *American Journal of Physiology* 270, R342–R347.

135. Smith, P. M., and Ferguson, A. V. (1997). Vasopressin acts in the subfornical organ to decrease blood pressure. *Neuroendocrinology* 66, 130–135.
136. Smith, P. M., Lowes, V. L., and Ferguson, A. V. (1994). Circulating vasopressin influences area postrema neurons. *Neuroscience* 59, 185–194.
137. Song, K., Allen, A. M., Paxinos, G., and Mendelsohn, F. A.O. (1992). Mapping of angiotensin II receptor subtype heterogeneity in rat brain. *Journal of Comparative Neurology* 316, 467–484.
138. Starbuck, E. M., and Fitts, D. A. (1998). Influence of salt intake, ANG II synthesis and SFO lesion on thirst and blood pressure during sodium depletion. Subfornical organ. *Appetite* 31, 309–331.
139. Stitt, J. T. (1985). Evidence for the involvement of the organum vasculosum laminae terminalis in the febrile response of rabbits and rats. *Journal of Physiology* 368, 501–511.
140. Summerlee, A. J. S., and Wilson, B. C. (1994). Role of the subfornical organ in the relaxin induced prolongation of gestation in the rat. *Endocrinology* 134, 2115–2120.
141. Sun, K., and Ferguson, A. V. (1996). Angiotensin II and glutamate influence area postrema neurons in rat brain slices. *Regulatory Peptides* 63, 91–98.
142. Sun, K., and Ferguson, A. V. (1997). Cholecystokinin activates area postrema neurons in rat brain slices. *American Journal of Physiology* 272, R1625–R1630.
143. Sunn, N., Egli, M., Burazin, T. C., Burns, P., Colvill, L., Davern, P., Denton, D. A., Oldfield, B. J., Weisinger, R. S., Rauch, M., Schmid H. A., and McKinley, M. J. (2002). Circulating relaxin acts on subfornical organ neurons to stimulate water drinking in the rat. *Proceedings of the National Academy of Sciences USA* 99, 1701–1706.
144. Takahashi, Y., Smith, P. M., Ferguson, A. V., and Pittman, Q. J. (1997). Circumventricular organs and fever. *American Journal of Physiology* 273, R1690–R1695.
145. Tanaka, J., Kariya, K., Miyakubo, H., Sakamaki, K., and Nomura, M. (2002). Attenuated drinking response induced by angiotensinergic activation of subfornical organ projections to the paraventricular nucleus in estrogen-treated rats. *Neuroscience Letters* 324, 242–246.
146. Tanaka, J., Miyakubo, H., Okumura, T., Sakamaki, K., and Hayashi, Y. (2001). Estrogen decreases the responsiveness of subfornical organ neurons projecting to the hypothalamic paraventricular nucleus to angiotensin II in female rats. *Neuroscience Letters* 307, 155–158.
147. Thompson, S. A. (1982). Localization of immunoreactive prolactin in ependyma and circumventricular organs of rat brain. *Cell and Tissue Research* 225, 79–93.
148. Thunhorst, R. L., Beltz, T. G., and Johnson, A. K. (1999). Effects of subfornical organ lesions on acutely induced thirst and salt appetite. *American Journal of Physiology* 277, R56–R65.
149. Vallieres, L., and Rivest, S. (1997). Regulation of the genes encoding interleukin-6, its receptor, and gp130 in the rat brain in response to the immune activator lipopolysaccharide and the proinflammatory cytokine interleukin-1 beta. *Journal of Neurochemistry* 69, 1668–1683.
150. van der Kooy, D., and Koda, L. Y. (1983). Organization of the projections of a circumventricular organ: The area postrema in the rat. *Journal of Comparative Neurology* 219, 328–338.
151. Vivas, L., Chiaraviglio, E., and Carrer, H. F. (1990). Rat organum vasculosum laminae terminalis in vitro responses to changes in sodium concentration. *Brain Research* 519, 294–300.
152. Washburn, D. L. S., Beedle, A. M., and Ferguson, A. V. (1999). Inhibition of subfornical organ neuronal potassium channels by vasopressin. *Neuroscience* 93, 349–359.
153. Wolburg, H., Liebner, S., and Lippoldt, A. (2003). Freeze-fracture studies of cerebral endothelial tight junctions. *Methods in Molecular Medicine* 89, 51–66.
154. Yang, B., and Ferguson, A. V. (2002). Orexin-A depolarizes dissociated rat area postrema neurons through activation of a nonselective cationic conductance. *Journal of Neuroscience* 22, 6303–6308.
155. Yang, B., and Ferguson, A. V. (2003). Adrenomedullin influences dissociated rat area postrema neurons. *Regulatory Peptides* 112, 9–17.
156. Ylitalo, P., Karppanen, H., and Paasonen, M. K. (1974). Is the area postrema a control centre of blood pressure? *Nature* 274, 58–59 .

# 17

# Central Autonomic Control of Energy Homeostasis

BARRY E. LEVIN AND ALISON M. STRACK

The term *energy homeostasis* is a modification of the first law of thermodynamics by which the amount of energy intake as food equals the amount of energy expended as work plus the amount expended as heat (thermogenesis). When intake exceeds expenditure, the excess is stored primarily as glycogen and fat, which are used to supply fuel when food is in short supply. This process is regulated over very different time frames and by many different physiological and metabolic systems; dysregulation of either intake or expenditure can lead to obesity. Early studies using hypothalamic lesions pointed to the brain as the primary regulator of energy homeostasis and the importance of the autonomic nervous system in this process. Ventromedial hypothalamic lesions produce increased food intake (hyperphagia) and obesity[77], which are also associated with defective autonomic control of organs involved in the regulation of energy expenditure[75,88]. On the other hand, electrical stimulation of the ventromedial hypothalamus leads to generalized sympathoadrenal activation[78] with increased activity in thermogenic tissues[68]. Lesions of the lateral hypothalamic area reduce food intake and increase sympathetic activity until a new, lower defended body weight is reached[7,68,88]. While these and other studies led to the conclusion that the hypothalamus was the central controller of energy homeostasis, we now know that control resides in a much broader, distributed network of specialized "metabolic-sensing" neurons that occur throughout the brain. These neurons monitor and respond to a complex set of inputs, including those from a variety of sensory, metabolic, behavioral, and hormonal signals from the external and internal environments (Figure 17–1). The autonomic nervous system is a critical component of both the afferent and efferent control mechanisms, regulating all aspects of energy homeostasis, including food intake, absorption, and assimilation, the mobilization and storage of nutrients and thermogenesis.

## GENERAL CONCEPTS OF ENERGY HOMEOSTASIS

The autonomic nervous system acts as one of many interfaces between the brain and periphery in the control of energy homeostasis (Figures 17.1 and 17.2). In addition to inputs through their sympathetic and parasympathetic afferents, organs release hormones (e.g., leptin and insulin), peptides (e.g., amylin, peptide YY, glucagon-like peptide-1, cholecystokinin, and ghrelin) and metabolites (e.g., glucose, free fatty acids, lactate, and ketone bodies). These substances are either actively transported across the blood–brain barrier or interact with viscerosensory afferents within the organs from which they are released (Figures 17.1 and 17.2). These signals from the periphery converge upon and are integrated by specialized metabolic-sensing neurons located in a variety of interconnected brain regions involved in autonomic control. These include the nucleus of the solitary tract (NTS), rostral (RVLM) and caudal ventrolateral medulla (CVLM), raphé pallidus and obscurus, the hypothalamic paraventricular, arcuate, ventromedial and dorsomedial nuclei, and lateral

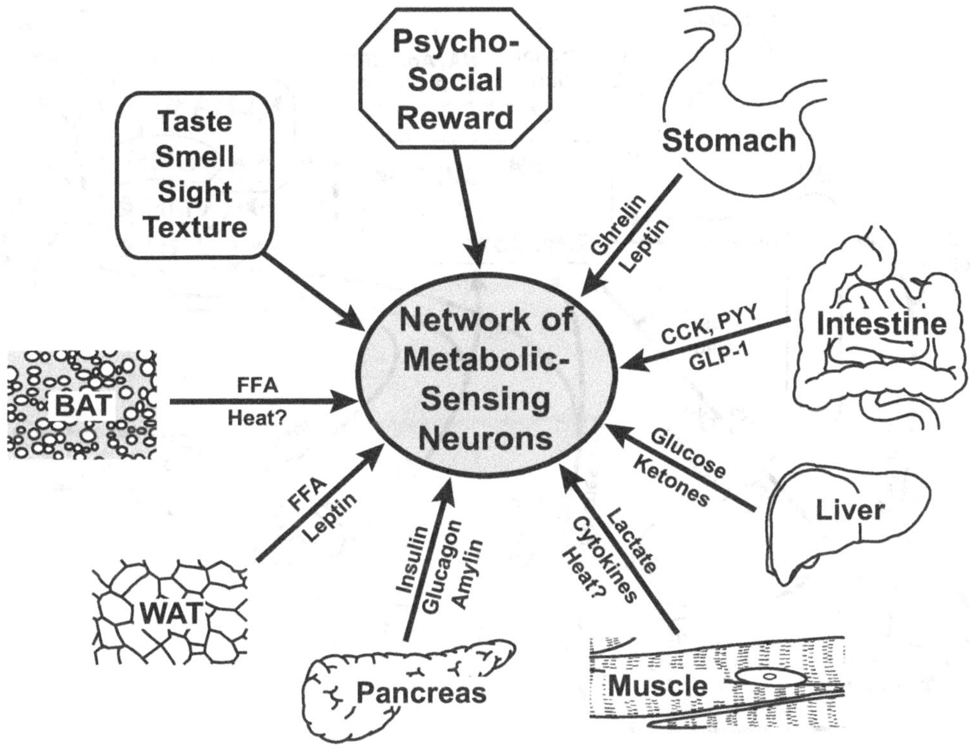


Figure 17–1 Inputs to the network of metabolic-sensing neurons. The network of metabolic-sensing neurons distributed throughout the brain receives multiple inputs. These inputs include metabolic substrates and end-products (glucose, free fatty acid [FFA)], lactate, ketone bodies, heat), hormones (leptin, insulin, glucagon, amylin) and neuropeptides related to energy metabolism (ghrelin, cholecystokinin [CCK], peptide YY [PYY], glucagon-related peptide-1 [GLP-1]), cytokines and adipokines. In addition to these hormonal and metabolic outputs of the peripheral neurons, sensory information is also provided to the brain via visceral afferent nerves. Metabolic-sensing neurons also integrate information about the oro-sensory properties of food (taste, smell, sight, and texture of food) and the psychosocial and rewarding properties of food and food-related events.

hypothalamic area, as well as other non-autonomic areas, such as the substantia nigra and ventral tegmental area (Figures 17.2 and 17.3)[35]. Output from these brain regions regulates autonomic and hormonal systems that control the physiological and metabolic functions of organs involved in energy homeostasis.

Metabolic-sensing neurons were first identified by their ability to use ambient glucose concentrations to control their firing rate. When ambient glucose levels rise, one class of these neurons is excited, while another is inhibited. A host of other metabolic substrates, including fatty acids, lactate or ketone bodies, and hormones such as leptin and insulin, have subsequently been shown to be additional signaling molecules that alter the firing rates of glucose-sensing neurons[35]. The combined input from neural, hormonal, and metabolic signals from the periphery summate to regulate membrane potential, metabolic function, and gene transcription in glucose-sensing neurons, thereby causing changes in neuronal activity and in the release of neuroactive substances.

Because of historical precedents, a majority of early studies focused on hypothalamic neurons as regulators of energy homeostasis. Researchers soon realized that most manipulations of the "ventromedial hypothalamus" actually altered function in both the ventromedial and arcuate nuclei. Later, the arcuate nucleus was shown to contain two sets of neurons whose primary function appears to be the regulation of energy homeostasis. Neurons that express neuropeptide Y and are located medially in the arcuate nucleus are classed as anabolic. Release of neuropeptide Y onto target neurons in the PVN and lateral hypothalamic area potently stimulates food intake and inhibits

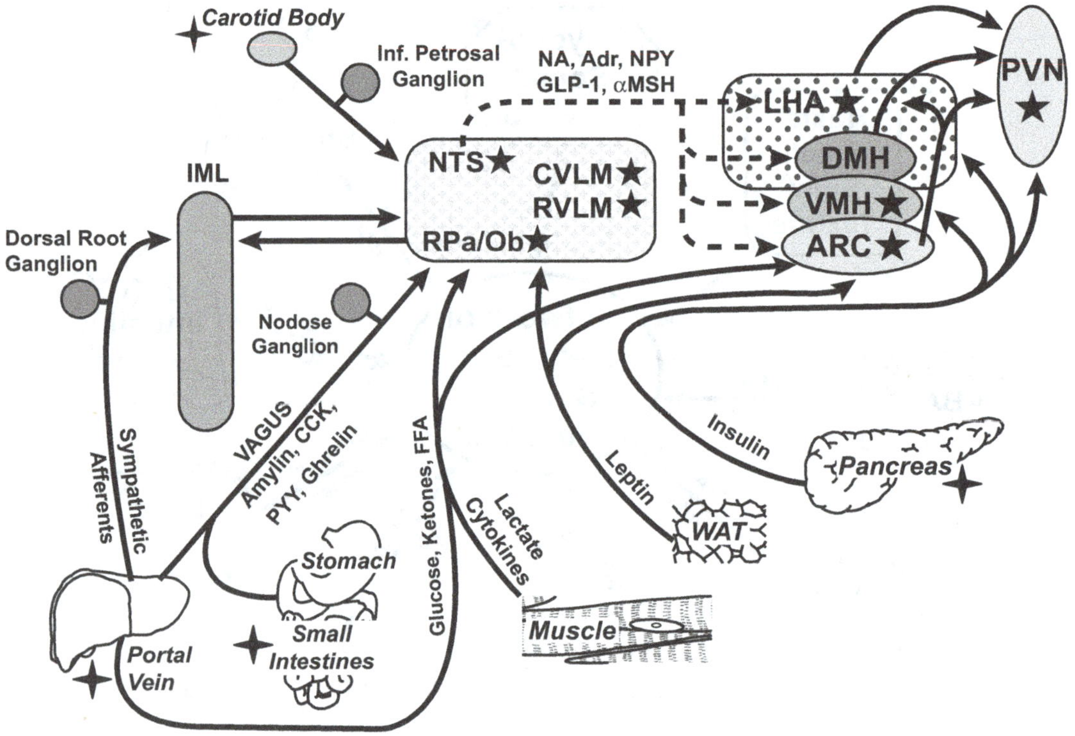


Figure 17–2 Convergence of viscerosensory afferent information onto metabolic-sensing neurons. Vagal, glossopharyngeal and sympathetic afferents from metabolic sensors (denoted by *four-pointed stars*) in the portal vein, carotid body, stomach, and small intestines converge on metabolic-sensing neurons (denoted by *five-pointed stars*) in the nucleus of the solitary tract (NTS) in the dorsal medulla. These signals are integrated along with metabolic and hormonal signals from the periphery, which are transported across the blood–brain barrier or cross through the fenestrated barrier in the area postrema adjacent to the NTS. In addition to the NTS, metabolic-sensing neurons in the caudal (CVLM) and rostral ventrolateral medulla (RVLM) that contain noradrenaline, adrenaline, neuropeptide Y (NPY), glucagon-like peptide (GLP-1), and/or α-melanocyte stimulating hormone (α-MSH) also integrate these incoming signals. The medullary metabolic-sensing neurons project to various hypothalamic nuclei (arcuate [ARC], ventromedial [VMH], dorsomedial [DMH], paraventricular [PVN]), and lateral hypothalamic area (LHA). Metabolic-sensing serotonin neurons in the raphé pallidus and obscurus (RPa/Ob) project to sympathetic preganglionic neurons in the intermediolateral (IML) cell column of the spinal cord. Metabolites and hormones also interact with metabolic-sensing neurons in the hypothalamus. Neurons in the arcuate nucleus project to additional metabolic-sensing neurons in the PVN and lateral hypothalamic area. The lateral hypothalamic area also projects to the PVN, which, along with the lateral hypothalamic area, gives rise to descending projections to autonomic centers in the medulla and spinal cord. *Dotted lines* denote polysynaptic pathways.

energy expenditure by decreasing sympathetic activity in thermogenic organs. Laterally located arcuate neurons produce proopiomelanocortin, a pro-hormone for α-melanocyte stimulating hormone. This catabolic peptide interacts with melanocortin-3 and -4 receptors to inhibit food intake and stimulate sympathetic nerve activity, including to the brown adipose tissue, thus increasing thermogenesis by acting on some of the same PVN and lateral hypothalamic neurons that are targeted by the neuropeptide Y-containing arcuate neurons. Some proopiomelanocortin neurons in the arcuate nucleus also project to the intermediolateral cell column of the spinal cord so they are positioned to modulate the activity of sympathetic preganglionic neurons[15]. Arcuate neuropeptide Y neurons also produce and co-release agouti-related peptide, a unique peptide that acts as a functional antagonist of melanocortin-3 and -4 receptors. Thus, activation of arcuate neuropeptide Y neurons releases a strong anabolic peptide and an equally potent inhibitor of catabolic

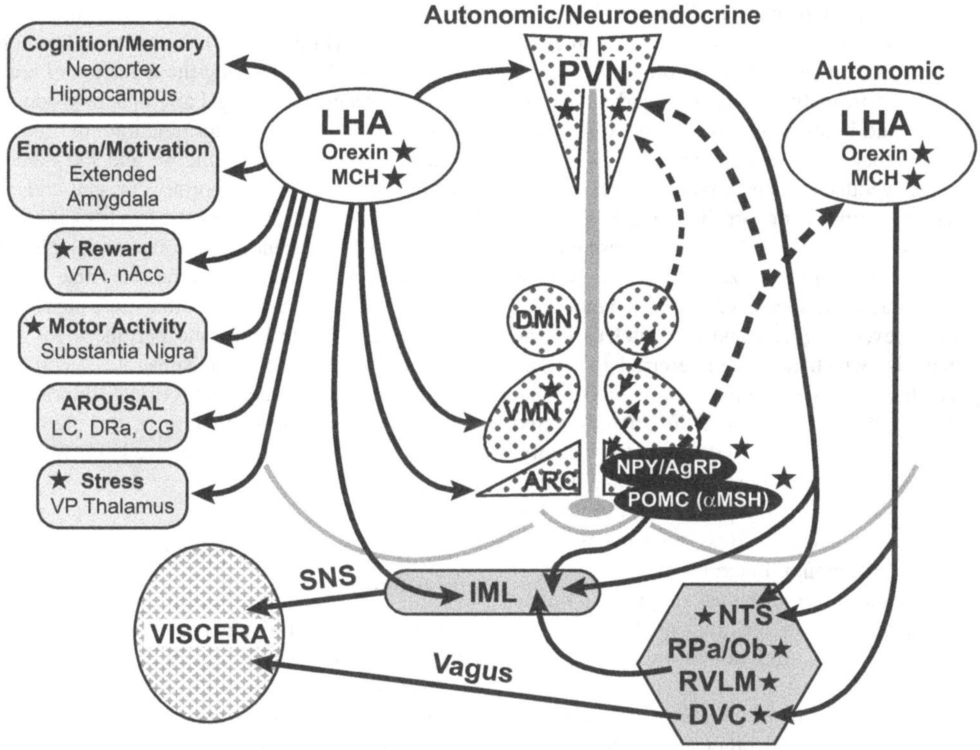


Figure 17–3 CNS projections of metabolic-sensing neurons. Metabolic-sensing neurons (*stars*) are localized throughout the hypothalamus and brainstem as well as other areas, including the substantia nigra and ventral tegmental area (VTA). Neuropeptide Y (NPY) and proopiomelanocortin (α-MSH) neurons in the arcuate nucleus are prototypic metabolic-sensing neurons. They project to the PVN and to metabolic-sensing neurons in the lateral hypothalamic area (*heavy dotted lines*) that synthesize orexin and melanin concentrating hormone (MCH). Proopiomelanocortin neurons in the arcuate nucleus also express cocaine-amphetamine related transcript and project to sympathetic preganglionic neurons in the intermediolateral cell column (IML) of the spinal cord. Metabolic-sensing neurons in the PVN send axons to the median eminence and pituitary to modulate neuroendocrine outputs; other projections go to sympathetic and parasympathetic premotor neurons in the medulla that control visceral functions related to energy homeostasis. Unlike the relatively restricted output of neuropeptide Y and proopiomelanocortin neurons in the arcuate nucleus, lateral hypothalamic neurons that produce orexin and melanin concentrating hormone project widely to brain areas that regulate many behavioral and physiological functions, some of which are involved in the regulation of various aspects of energy homeostasis. DVC, dorsal vagal complex.

pathways. Importantly, arcuate neuropeptide Y and proopiomelanocortin neurons are prototypic metabolic-sensing neurons. Neuropeptide Y neurons are inhibited and proopiomelanocortin neurons are excited by glucose, while both leptin and insulin inhibit neuropeptide Y and stimulate proopiomelanocortin gene transcription. Insulin and leptin acutely inhibit neuropeptide Y neuronal activity and stimulate proopiomelanocortin neuronal activity[35].

Two other important groups of metabolic-sensing neurons occur in the lateral hypothalamic area. These neurons produce the anabolic peptides, either orexin (hypocretin) or melanocyte-concentrating hormone. Unlike neurons in the arcuate nucleus that contain neuropeptide Y and proopiomelanocortin, the neurons in the lateral hypothalamic area are involved in a much wider spectrum of metabolic, physiological, and behavioral processes[69,83] (Figure 17–3). Orexin neurons are inhibited and melanin-concentrating hormone neurons are excited by glucose[8]; both express leptin receptors and both receive inputs from arcuate neurons that release neuropeptide Y and proopiomelanocortin[16].

The metabolic-sensing neurons in the lateral hypothalamic area receive inputs from thalamic regions involved in nociception, from limbic and striatal regions involved in motivation and reward, and from hypothalamic and brainstem networks that coordinate foraging, gustatory, feeding, and defensive behaviors. In turn, lateral hypothalamic neurons containing melanin-concentrating hormone or orexin project to brain regions with a wide variety of functions. These include areas involved in non-homeostatic reward systems (i.e., the nucleus accumbens, ventral tegmental area, prefrontal cortex, amygdala, and bed nucleus of the stria terminalis, which are often referred to collectively as the "extended amygdala"); neocortical and hippocampal areas involved in cognition and memory; striatal areas involved in motor activity; hindbrain areas involved in consciousness and arousal (i.e., locus coeruleus, dorsal raphé, central gray); and thalamic areas involved in stress responsivity (i.e., ventroposterior thalamus). Lateral hypothalamic neurons also project to regions that supply autonomic efferents, including the central nucleus of the amygdala, PVN, NTS, and dorsal vagal complex[12] (Figure 17–3).

In addition to neurons in the arcuate nucleus and lateral hypothalamic area, other metabolic-sensing neurons include γ-aminobutyric acid–containing neurons in the ventromedial hypothalamic nucleus; dopaminergic neurons in the substantia nigra and ventral tegmental area; adrenergic and noradrenergic neurons in the NTS, RVLM, and CVLM; serotonergic neurons in the raphé pallidus and obscurus[35,65]; and cholinergic neurons in the dorsal vagal complex[3]. There are likely to be other collections of metabolic-sensing neurons scattered in other brain sites that remain to be discovered.

In summary, all of the known collections of metabolic-sensing neurons are located in brain areas that are known to play critical regulatory roles in energy homeostasis. In addition to receiving direct or indirect inputs from autonomic visceral afferents, the metabolic-sensing neurons are also connected to intrinsic systems involved in non-homeostatic control of ingestion, reward, and motivation, as well as areas involved in primary sensing of the oro-sensory, gustatory, and olfactory properties of food (Figures 17.1 and 17.3).

## VISCEROSENSORY AFFERENTS INVOLVED IN ENERGY HOMEOSTASIS

Many of the same metabolic and hormonal signals that affect metabolic-sensing neurons in the brain are also sensed at sites in the periphery that provide input to the central metabolic-sensing neurons via viscerosensory afferents (Figure 17–2). A variety of hormones is released from the gut during the ingestion of nutrients and act on receptors in vagal afferents to produce satiation, which leads to termination of individual meals[76,79]. Nutrients like glucose and fatty acids are also sensed in the hepatic portal vein, gut, and carotid body, and information about the levels of these nutrients is transmitted centrally through vagal, glossopharyngeal, and sympathetic afferents that terminate primarily in the NTS. The fact that there are redundant systems in both the brain and periphery for sensing many of the same metabolic substrates, peptides, and hormones demonstrates the critical importance of these signals for the regulation of the physiological and metabolic functions involved in maintaining energy homeostasis.

### Hepatic and Hepatic Portal Sensors and Afferents

In addition to central glucose-sensing neurons, glucose sensors occur within the hepatic portal vein. The route by which these sensors convey information to the brain depends upon the level of glucose in the portal vein. Raising portal glucose levels decreases the vagal afferent discharge that impinges upon NTS neurons, many of which are also inhibited by direct application of glucose. Increased afferent discharge results in increased activity in adrenal, hepatic, splanchnic, and pancreatic sympathetic outflows and reduced vagal activity to the pancreas[1,51]. On the other hand, lowering glucose levels in the portal vein by producing systemic hypoglycemia activates sensors in the portal vein that transmit signals to the hindbrain via sympathetic afferents. These signals initiate a marked counterregulatory release of adrenaline from the adrenal medulla, noradrenaline from sympathetic nerves, and glucagon from the pancreatic alpha cells, which act to return glucose levels to normal by increasing hepatic glycogenolysis and gluconeogenesis[21]. Thus, the hepatic portal vein, like the brain, may have different glucose sensors that respond to either high or low glucose levels.

In addition to glucose, sensors in either the portal vein or the liver respond to alterations in levels of individual amino acids, such as leucine or alanine[81], and alterations in ATP levels in the liver by transmitting signals to the brainstem via hepatic vagal afferents[18]. Several peptides that are released in response to the absorption of nutrients from the gut, including somatostatin[47] and glucagon-like peptide-1[48], can be detected by portal sensors and alter the activity of hepatic vagal afferents.

### Intestinal Sensors and Afferents

In addition to glucose-sensing elements in the myenteric plexus of the small intestine that detect changes in absorbed glucose[40], a host of gut peptides released during the absorption of nutrients acts on receptors in vagal afferents to alter meal size and duration. Cholecystokinin was the first well-described example of such a gut-satiety peptide. It is released from the duodenum during gastric distention and the entry of fat into the duodenum. It acts on vagal cholecystokinin-1 receptors to augment afferent vagal activity, which also increases in the presence of a gastric load[76]. These afferent volleys converge on NTS neurons, which then inhibit gastric emptying and thus contribute to the satiating effects of cholecystokinin[71,72]. Peptide YY is another gut peptide that is released from the distal small intestine and acts through vagal afferents to produce satiation[26]. Ghrelin is a notable exception to the "rule" that gut peptides produce satiety. It is synthesized and released from the stomach as a consequence of sympathetic activation[27,46] and interacts with its receptors on vagal afferents to activate neurons in the NTS and stimulate food intake[11].

Leptin was first identified as a hormone synthesized in and released from white adipose tissue in proportion to the size of white adipose fat stores. Leptin is transported into the brain to produce a catabolic drive when adipose stores increase, and a strong anabolic drive when they decrease (see below)[89]. Leptin also interacts with peripheral sensors to regulate energy homeostasis. Leptin acts directly in white adipose tissue to produce reflex sympathetic activation in white and brown adipose tissue, the pancreas, the liver and adrenal medulla, and also activates vagal outflow to the pancreas and liver[52]. Leptin is also synthesized and released from the stomach, where it interacts with its receptors on gastric vagal afferents to inhibit food intake either independently or synergistically with cholecystokinin[2,55,56].

In summary, both peripheral and central sensors detect a number of metabolic substrates, hormones, and peptides involved in the regulation of energy homeostasis. The redundancy of these multiple feedback systems provides both backup for control of energy homeostasis and also a network by which various signals related to energy status are sensed with different temporal, qualitative, and quantitative patterns. Afferent inputs from peripheral sensors terminate in various brain sites and are integrated by metabolic-sensing neurons that also directly sense some of the same signals. The integrated output of the distributed network of metabolic-sensing neurons leads to a coordinated autonomic, neurohumoral, and behavioral activation that allows the individual to regulate its energy homeostasis within relatively narrow limits under most circumstances.

## METABOLIC-SENSING NEURONS AS INTEGRATORS AND REGULATORS OF AUTONOMIC ACTIVITY AND ENERGY HOMEOSTASIS

The distributed network of metabolic-sensing neurons receives multiple inputs from the periphery. Each input is integrated as a function of the temporal pattern, strength, and number of sites at which the signal is received. The net impact of these inputs on each neuron is in turn influenced by whether the individual is in homeostatic equilibrium or a state of negative or positive energy balance. Metabolic and hormonal signals from the periphery affect metabolic-sensing neurons both indirectly through afferent inputs, and directly via the circumventricular organs, which do not have a blood–brain barrier, or by the active transport of circulating signals across the blood–brain barrier. The circulating concentrations of molecules that produce short-term signals (glucose and fatty acids, and hormones such as insulin and gut-satiety peptides) vary markedly as a function of meal-taking. Longer-term signals reflecting the overall state of adipose stores (e.g., leptin) also undergo considerable phasic variations, but their tonic baseline levels vary more slowly over periods of days. Tonic variations in these long-term signals affect the background "gain" of membrane potential and gene transcription in metabolic-sensing neurons. Phasic variations in long-term signals are summated together with other typically phasic short-term signals (glucose, fatty acids, neurotransmitters, and neuropeptides from neural afferents) to produce rapid changes in metabolic activity, membrane potential, neuronal activity, and transmitter release. Thus, individual metabolic-sensing neurons will be influenced differentially by incoming signals depending upon their anatomical location, their complement of receptors, and the specific metabolic pathways and neural afferents with which they are connected. Despite their anatomical and physiological diversity, the efferent outputs of the metabolic-sensing neurons are collectively summed from the various parts of the distributed network of metabolic sensors to alter autonomic function and energy homeostasis. The temporal pattern with which various signals impinge upon individual components of this integrated network of metabolic sensors is a major driving force for maintaining energy balance.

### Temporal Patterns of Afferent Signals and Resultant Autonomic Function

#### *Short-term signals*

Glucose is the prototypical and best studied of the short-term metabolic signals. It is sensed both peripherally and centrally by specialized sensors. Central glucose-sensing neurons are either excited or inhibited depending upon their complement of various transporters, intracellular metabolic pathways, and ion channels[35]. Glucose injected through the carotid artery acts directly on spinally projecting neurons in the dorsal cap and ventral tier of the PVN (as well as other forebrain areas) to produce generalized sympathetic activation and an increase in activity of efferent vagal nerves to the pancreas[30,50]. The arcuate and ventromedial nuclei of the hypothalamus contain relatively large populations of glucose-sensing neurons (up to 10%–30% of neurons[35]), which play a critical role in the regulation of glucose homeostasis. The marked counterregulatory response that occurs during systemic hypoglycemia can be blocked by simultaneous focal infusion of glucose into the ventromedial hypothalamus[4] (i.e., both ventromedial hypothalamic and arcuate nuclei). On the other hand, selective inhibition of intracellular glucose metabolism in ventromedial hypothalamic neurons with the competitive inhibitor of glucose metabolism, 2-deoxyglucose, produces comparable levels of activation of the sympathoadrenal system to that produced by systemic hypoglycemia[5]. Similar counterregulatory responses can be elicited by directly inhibiting glucose metabolism in brainstem areas, including the CVLM and raphé pallidus and obscurus[64]. Changes in brain glucose availability also affect parasympathetic function. Injection of 2-deoxyglucose into the carotid artery, a manipulation that competitively decreases cellular glucose metabolism in the forebrain, increases activity in the gastric branch of the vagus[22]; and this is mimicked by direct injection of 2-deoxyglucose into the lateral hypothalamic area[53]. Neurons in the ventromedial hypothalamus also sense fatty acids[85]. Slow infusion of fatty acids into this region inhibits hepatic glucose production through inhibition of vagal input to the liver[28]. While interesting, these and similar studies must be interpreted with caution, because it is not known how the doses of glucose and fatty acids injected directly into the brain compare to actual physiological levels. Nevertheless, data from such studies support the idea that the cellular responses of metabolic-sensing neurons to alterations in ambient substrate levels play an important role in the central autonomic control of energy homeostasis.

### *Leptin: a Long- and Short-Term Signal*

Leptin is at least one of the long-sought "lipostatic" signals that are produced in adipose tissue and inform the brain of the size of adipose stores[24,89]. The sympathetic nervous system controls leptin production in adipose tissue via inhibitory feedback[62]. After its release into the blood, leptin is transported into the brain where it interacts with neurons that express leptin receptor-b, the signaling form of the leptin receptor that is a member of the JAK-STAT family of cytokine receptors[82]. Leptin receptor-b is expressed by neuropeptide Y/agouti-related peptide neurons in the arcuate nucleus and by proopiomelanocortin neurons, as well as other neurons in the ventromedial and dorsomedial hypothalamic nuclei, ventral tegmental area and NTS[17]. Leptin acts as a long-term signal, increasing transcription and production of proopiomelanocortin and decreasing transcription and production of neuropeptide Y and agouti-related peptide. Leptin also acts as a short-term regulator of neuronal function and autonomic activity. Direct leptin injection into the ventromedial hypothalamic nucleus markedly increases plasma levels of noradrenaline and adrenaline[70]. Intracerebroventricular injection of leptin increases sympathetic outflow to brown adipose tissue, muscle, kidney, heart, blood vessels, pancreas, and liver. This increased outflow leads to increased thermogenesis[14,44], elevated heart rate and blood pressure[20,60], reduced insulin secretion[42,84], acute stimulation of hepatic gluconeogenesis and glycogenolysis[13,39], and a reduction in leptin production by white adipocytes[58].

## INTEGRATED PHYSIOLOGICAL FUNCTIONS INVOLVED IN AUTONOMIC REGULATION OF ENERGY HOMEOSTASIS

### Control of Individual Meals

Humans eat for a number of reasons. These include hypoglycemia, being in a state of negative energy balance, altered day length, circadian and ultradian rhythms of hormones, peptides and metabolites, withdrawal of short-term satiety factors, habit, and psycho-social factors. A given meal begins with behavioral arousal followed by increased sympathetic activity, which increases cardiac output in support of the physical activity needed to forage for food. When food is ingested, both parasympathetic and sympathetic efferents activate salivation, swallowing, gastric acid secretion, and motility in the esophagus, stomach, and bowel. As nutrients move down the gastrointestinal tract, they inhibit the release of the orexigenic peptide ghrelin from the stomach and stimulate the release of satiety peptides, such as cholecystokinin, peptide YY, glucagon-like peptide-1, enterostatin, and leptin. These peptides act primarily on vagal afferents. In concert with inputs from gastric stretch receptors and peripheral metabolic sensors, these peptides alter the activity of metabolic-sensing neurons in the NTS as well as other hindbrain neurons that contain noradrenaline, adrenaline, glucagon-like peptide-1, and α-melanocyte-stimulating hormone. These hindbrain neurons then send information to various forebrain sites that also contain metabolic-sensing neurons (Figure 17–2). These indirect signals from the periphery and the direct effects of metabolites and hormones are integrated within the distributed network of metabolic-sensing neurons. The result is modulation of the ongoing activity of sympathoadrenal and parasympathetic efferents involved in the absorption and assimilation of nutrients. Under the influence of long-term, tonic signals such as leptin, this sequence of events regulates the size and duration of the individual meal as well as the timing of the onset of the next meal.

## Control of Energy Assimilation and Storage

As nutrients are absorbed, they raise blood levels of glucose, fatty acids, and amino acids. Rising glucose levels directly stimulate insulin release from the β-cells of the pancreas, and this release is enhanced by activation of parasympathetic excitatory and withdrawal of sympathetic inhibitory inputs to the β-cells[59]. Insulin stimulates glucose uptake and metabolism in muscle, liver, and other organs. Insulin also acts centrally to stimulate sympathetic outflow[36], causing an increase in blood flow to organs required for digestion and assimilation of nutrients[67]. Insulin acts directly on the liver to inhibit hepatic glucose production by promoting hepatic glycogen storage. Insulin also has indirect effects on the liver through its actions on ventromedial hypothalamic glucose-sensing neurons, so that glycogen storage is enhanced through the action of hepatic vagal afferents[57,74]. Glucose acts on central metabolic-sensing neurons to produce sympathetic activation, increasing heat production in brown adipose tissue (in rodents and other small animals) and in muscle[54,61]. This so-called diet-induced thermogenesis helps to maintain energy balance during times of excess caloric intake.

## Homeostatic Versus Non-Homeostatic Controls of Ingestion

When intake chronically exceeds expenditure, adipose stores increase and tonic levels of leptin rise, inhibiting the production of the anabolic peptides, neuropeptide Y, and agouti-related peptide, and stimulating production of the catabolic peptide, α-melanocyte-stimulating hormone, in the brain[73]. These changes in peptide levels decrease food intake and increase sympathetic activity to thermogenic tissues. Leptin acts to increase thermogenesis both directly through its action in muscle and indirectly by central activation of muscle sympathetic nerve activity; both effects increase fatty acid oxidation[44]. Thus, under the influence of this negative feedback system in situations where food supplies are readily available, most individuals maintain their body weight and adipose mass within relatively narrow limits. Because it takes several days for adipose stores to increase when intake consistently exceeds expenditure, this regulatory mechanism occurs over a time frame of several days[34].

Negative feedback inhibition by leptin is an example of the homeostatic control of intake and expenditure. However, this negative feedback system has either a reduced or no effect on intake when individuals are eating more than their metabolic needs in preparation for times when food is scarce. Thus, most feral animals increase their food intake when the amount of daylight and ambient temperatures start to decrease in the fall. This ability to eat beyond one's metabolic needs is enhanced by the development of resistance to the normal inhibitory central feedback provided by leptin and insulin. An increase in dietary fat content enhances this resistance[9], as does increasing the palatability of the diet. The intake of highly palatable foods, while influenced by leptin and insulin, is largely dependent upon the extended amygdala (Figure 17–3), a system of interconnected brain areas involved in reward and motivation in the context of food intake. Intake governed by the extended amygdala is non-homeostatic because it is regulated by the rewarding properties of food and is largely, but not completely, independent of inhibitory feedback from homeostatic signals such as leptin and insulin. Consequently, animals will ingest large quantities of highly palatable foods even in the face of massive enlargement of adipose stores and large increases in blood levels of leptin and insulin[33]. This mechanism helps to promote the intake and storage of excess calories in preparation for the oncoming winter when food supplies are limited.

## Negative Energy Balance and the Defended Body Weight

A shortage, rather than excess, of food supplies poses the most important threat to the survival of the individual and the species. While leptin acts to inhibit intake and increase expenditure during periods of excess energy availability, falling leptin levels, which occur during periods of reduced nutrient availability, ensure that the individual will be driven to seek food and that existing energy stores will be conserved (Figure 17–4). During short periods of energy deficit, sympathetic activity to the liver increases, stimulating glycogenolysis and transiently increasing blood glucose levels[80]. However, glycogen stores are quickly depleted, resulting in falling glucose levels and reduced insulin secretion. Sympathetic activation in adipose stores mobilizes fatty acids as a secondary source of metabolic substrate[43]. Increased adipose sympathetic activity and falling glucose levels also inhibit leptin production, causing a precipitous fall in blood leptin[32,63]. Consequently, leptin no longer inhibits anabolic pathways (e.g., arcuate neurons that release neuropeptide Y/agouti-related peptide) and no longer stimulates catabolic pathways (e.g., arcuate neurons that release pro-opiomelanocortin)[45]. This shift towards anabolism is reinforced by sympathetic release of the orexigenic peptide ghrelin from the stomach during fasting[46] and by falling blood-glucose levels, which stimulate hepatic portal vein sympathetic afferents and central glucose-sensing neurons (Figure 17–2). These additional factors increase the drive to eat by reinforcing the feeling of hunger that is unmasked by withdrawal of leptin and insulin. Hunger leads to arousal and drives the animal to forage for food. Sympathoadrenal activation increases cardiac output and further mobilizes glucose and fatty acids to fuel the metabolic processes upon which physical activity depends.

The powerful drive to seek and ingest food stimulated by the reduction in leptin and insulin levels occurs simultaneously with sympathetically mediated mobilization of energy stores from the liver and adipose tissue. At the same time, sympathetic activity is reduced in thermogenic tissues, such as muscle and brown adipose tissue. In these tissues, sympathetic input is necessary to stimulate fatty acid oxidation, which produces ATP and/or heat by activation of 5'-AMP-activated kinase[44] and uncoupling of oxidative phosphorylation[19], respectively (Figure 17–4). Thus, falling leptin levels result in decreased sympathetic activity in thermogenic tissues, leading to reduced resting metabolic rate and conservation of existing energy stores. This reduced metabolic rate is

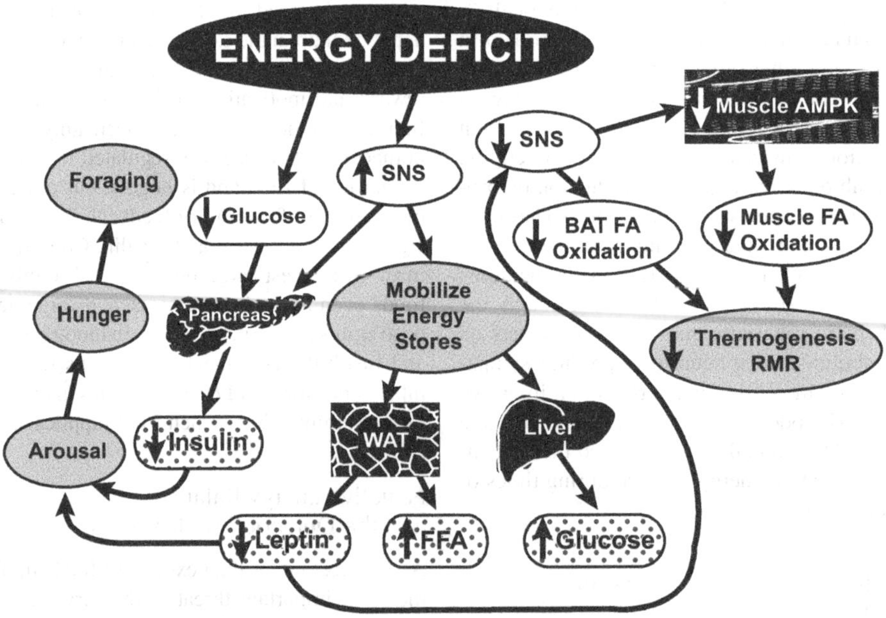


Figure 17–4 Physiological sequelae of energy restriction. When food supplies are limited, the individual goes into negative energy balance. This state triggers a sequence of events to preserve energy. Substrates to fuel metabolic functions (first glucose from hepatic glycogen stores and then fatty acids from adipose stores) are mobilized; metabolic rate declines to conserve existing stores, and the individual is driven to seek new food sources. Energy deficit increases sympathetic outflow to the liver and adipose stores to mobilize substrates. However, in so doing, adipose production of leptin decreases and insulin secretion decreases. Reduced plasma levels of insulin and leptin disinhibit central anabolic and inhibit catabolic neuronal networks, driving the individual to seek food. Withdrawal of leptin causes a reduction in sympathetic drive to thermogenic tissues (brown adipose tissue [BAT] in rodents and human infants) and muscle leading to reduced thermogenesis and the resting metabolic rate (RMR). In muscle, direct withdrawal of leptin and indirect withdrawal of sympathetic input reduces the activity of 5' AMP activated kinase, which reduces fatty acid oxidation and lowers metabolic rate.

a function of lowering the amount of metabolically active lean body mass and persists as long as energy intake is restricted[2941]. However, there is a metabolic memory or "set-point" that is determined by the level of existing adipose stores when energy restriction begins. This "defended adipose mass" is restored almost exactly when food again becomes readily available[32,41]. The level at which defended adipose mass is set is a function of a host of factors, including genetic background, perinatal environment, dietary content, and palatability. The idea that this set-point resides within the brain is bolstered by the observations that lesions within the distributed network of metabolic-sensing neurons at sites such as the ventromedial hypothalamus and lateral hypothalamic area markedly alter its level[23].

## Obesity and the Autonomic Nervous System

Obesity has reached epidemic proportions in both the developed and developing worlds[86]. The metabolic and pathological consequences of obesity (type 2 diabetes, hyperlipidemia, hypertension, cardiovascular disease, and stroke) and its psychosocial stigmata produce a severe affliction that affects up to 20% to 30% of the population in the United States. Current evidence suggests that those who become obese have an underlying "thrifty genotype." This genotype protects them and their relatives during periods of famine by allowing them to eat well beyond their metabolic needs to increase adipose stores in preparation for periods of low food availability[49]. About 60% of obesity is inherited, and most of such inheritance is polygenic in origin. Hence, there will be many different factors that predispose one to obesity[6]. A reduction in leptin signaling in one form or another is a common feature of several animal models of obesity. Most of these models also show reduced sympathetic activity in a number of metabolically critical organs, such as the heart, liver, brown adipose tissue, and/or the pancreas[25,31,38]. These observations suggest a link between defective leptin signaling, sympathetic function, and the predisposition to develop obesity. A reduction in sensitivity to leptin would provide affected individuals with a competitive advantage during times of impending food shortage since they would be able to ingest and store more calories despite rising leptin levels associated with expanding adiposity[34]. However, obesity is the major negative consequence of reduced leptin sensitivity, because individuals become obese when they are exposed to highly palatable, energy-dense food that can be acquired with little expenditure of calories.

Once obesity-prone individuals become obese, their new, elevated body weight set-point is avidly defended against all attempts to lower it by restricting caloric intake. When food is again readily available, they quickly return to their previous level of adiposity[10,29,32,41]. Thus, the set-point can be moved upward but rarely downward in most obese individuals. This upward resetting suggests that new permanent neural connections may form with each upward movement of the body weight set-point. In clinical practice, this means that about 80% to 90% of obese individuals will eventually regain any weight lost by dieting. Only regular vigorous exercise appears to normalize the reduced metabolic rate that accompanies weight loss and promotes regaining of lost weight[87]. Although metabolic rate remains depressed in the absence of regular vigorous exercise, some measures of generalized sympathetic function do normalize with prolonged caloric restriction. This finding suggests that depressed sympathetic function is not required for the persistent decrease in metabolic rate that follows weight loss[37]. Importantly, administration of exogenous leptin can normalize both the reduced metabolic rate and the reduced sympathetic activity that occur during caloric restriction[66]. Thus, an underlying defect in sympathetic function may predispose some individuals to obesity, and reduced sympathetic activity may contribute to the lowered metabolic rate associated with chronic caloric restriction.

## SUMMARY

The autonomic nervous system plays a critical role in the regulation of energy homeostasis. It is involved in virtually all phases of energy intake, assimilation, expenditure, and storage. Signals relayed from the periphery through viscerosensory afferents act synergistically with hormonal and metabolic signals on a network of specialized metabolic-sensing neurons that are distributed throughout the brain. Each of these signals impinges on the metabolic-sensing neurons with different temporal patterns. Integration of these signals is key in controlling neuronal activity, metabolism, and gene transcription. The output of these metabolic-sensing neurons activates autonomic efferent pathways that control metabolism and hormone secretion. Critical hormones, including leptin and insulin, reflect the size of adipose stores and act centrally to inhibit further food intake, to increase thermogenesis, and to reduce insulin secretion via sympathetic activation. When food supply is limited, adipose stores become depleted, reducing the levels of leptin and insulin. These reductions lead to a net anabolic balance in central regulatory systems, stimulate hunger, reduce sympathetically mediated thermogenesis, and increase sympathetic activity in the liver and adipose stores to mobilize metabolic substrates. By acting on the distributed network of metabolic-sensing neurons in the brain, a variety of neural, metabolic, and hormonal signals from the periphery usually maintains autonomic function and the regulation of energy homeostasis within narrow limits so that the system remains in homeostatic balance. However, individuals with a reduced sensitivity to the negative feedback effects of signals, such as leptin and insulin, often have altered autonomic function, These reduced responses provide these individuals with a competitive advantage when food is scarce but predispose them to become obese when food is readily available at low energetic cost.

## References


1. Adachi, A., Shimizu, N., Oomura, Y., and Kobashi, M. (1984). Convergence of hepatoportal glucose-sensitive afferent signals to glucose-sensitive units within the nucleus of the solitary tract. *Neuroscience Letters* 46, 215–218.
2. Bado, A., Levasseur, S., Attoub, S., Kermorgant, S., Laigneau, J. P., Bortoluzzi, M. N., Moizo, L., Lehy, T., Guerre-Millo, M., Marchand-Brustel, Y., and Lewin, M. J. (1998). The stomach is a source of leptin. *Nature* 394, 790–793.
3. Balfour, R. H., Hansen, A. M. K., and Trapp, S. (2006). Neuronal responses to transient hypoglycaemia in the dorsal vagal complex of the rat brainstem. *Journal of Physiology* 570, 469–484.
4. Borg, M. A., Sherwin, R. S., Borg, W. P., Tamborlane, W. V., and Shulman, G. I. (1997). Local ventromedial hypothalamus glucose perfusion blocks counterregulation during systemic hypoglycemia in awake rats. *Journal of Clinical Investigation* 99, 361–365.
5. Borg, W. P., Sherwin, R. S., During, M. J., Borg, M. A., and Shulman, G. I. (1995). Local ventromedial hypothalamic glucopenia triggers counterregulatory hormone release. *Diabetes* 44, 180–184.
6. Bouchard, C., and Tremblay, A. (1997). Genetic influences on the response of body fat and fat distribution to positive and negative energy balances in human identical twins. *Journal of Nutrition* 127, 943S–947S.
7. Boyle, P. C., and Keesey, R. E. (1975). Chronically reduced body weight in rats sustaining lesions of the lateral hypothalamus and maintained on palatable diets and drinking solutions. *Journal of Comparative Physiology and Psychology* 88, 218–223.
8. Burdakov, D., Gerasimenko, O., and Verkhratsky, A. (2005). Physiological changes in glucose differentially modulate the excitability of hypothalamic melanin-concentrating hormone and orexin neurons in situ. *Journal of Neuroscience* 25, 2429–2433.
9. Clegg, D. J., Benoit, S. C., Reed, J. A., Woods, S. C., and Levin, B. E. (2005). Reduced anorexic effects of insulin in obesity-prone rats and rats fed a moderate fat diet. *American Journal of Physiology. Regulatory, Integrative and Comparative Physiology* 288, R981–R986.
10. Corbett, S. W., Stern, J. S., and Keesey, R. E. (1986). Energy expenditure in rats with diet-induced obesity. *American Journal of Clinical Nutrition* 44, 173–180.
11. Date, Y., Murakami, N., Toshinai, K., Matsukura, S., Niijima, A., Matsuo, H., Kangawa, K., and Nakazato, M. (2002). The role of the gastric afferent vagal nerve in ghrelin-induced feeding and growth hormone secretion in rats. *Gastroenterology* 123, 1120–1128.
12. Date, Y., Ueta, Y., Yamashita, H., Yamaguchi, H., Matsukura, S., Kangawa, K., Sakurai, T., Yanagisawa, M., and Nakazato, M. (1999). Orexins, orexigenic hypothalamic peptides, interact with autonomic, neuroendocrine and neuroregulatory systems. *Proceedings of the National Academy of Sciences USA* 96, 748–753.
13. Dobbins, R. L., Szczepaniak, L. S., Zhang, W., and McGarry, J. D. (2003). Chemical sympathectomy alters regulation of body weight during prolonged ICV leptin infusion. *American Journal of Physiology. Endocrinology and Metabolism* 284, E778–E787.
14. Egawa, M., Yoshimatsu, H., and Bray, G. A. (1991). Neuropeptide Y suppresses sympathetic activity to interscapular brown adipose tissue in rats. *American Journal of Physiology* 260, R328–R334.
15. Elias, C. F., Lee, C., Kelly, J., Aschkenasi, C., Ahima, R. S., Couceyro, P. R., Kuhar, M. J., Saper, C. B., and Elmquist, J. K. (1998). Leptin activates hypothalamic CART neurons projecting to the spinal cord. *Neuron* 21, 1375–1385.
16. Elias, C. F., Saper, C. B., Maratos-Flier, E., Tritos, N. A., Lee, C., Kelly, J., Tatro, J. B., Hoffman, G. E., Ollmann, M. M., Barsh, G. S., Sakurai, T., Yanagisawa, M., and Elmquist, J. K. (1998). Chemically defined projections linking the mediobasal hypothalamus and the lateral hypothalamic area. *Journal of Comparative Neurology* 402, 442–459.
17. Elmquist, J. K., Bjorbaek, C., Ahima, R. S., Flier, J. S., and Saper, C. B. (1998). Distributions of leptin receptor mRNA isoforms in the rat brain. *Journal of Comparative Neurology* 395, 535–547.
18. Friedman, M. I. (1995). Control of energy intake by energy metabolism. *American Journal of Clinical Nutrition* 62, 1096S–1100S.
19. Haynes, W. G. (2000). Interaction between leptin and sympathetic nervous system in hypertension. *Current Hypertension Reports* 2, 311–318.
20. Haynes, W. G., Morgan, D. A., Sivitz, W. I., and Mark, A. L. (1999). Interactions between the

melanocortin system and leptin in control of sympathetic nerve traffic. *Hypertension* 33, 542–547.
21. Jackson, P. A., Cardin, S., Coffey, C. S., Neal, D. W., Allen, E. J., Penaloza, A. R., Snead, W. L., and Cherrington, A. D. (2000). Effect of hepatic denervation on the counterregulatory response to insulin-induced hypoglycemia in the dog. *American Journal of Physiology. Endocrinology and Metabolism* 279, E1249–E1257.
22. Kadekaro, M., Timo-Iaria, C., Valle, L. E., and Velha, L. P. (1972). Site of action of 2-deoxy-D-glucose mediating gastric secretion in the cat. *Journal of Physiology* 221, 1–13.
23. Keesey, R. E., Mitchell, J. S., and Kemnitz, J. W. (1979). Body weight and body composition of male rats following hypothalamic lesions. *American Journal of Physiology* 237, R68–R73.
24. Kennedy, G. C. (1953). The role of depot fat in the hypothalamic control of food intake in the rat. *Proceedings of Royal Society of London: B Biological Sciences* 611, 221–235.
25. Knehans, A. W., and Romsos, D. R. (1983). Norepinephrine turnover in obese (ob/ob) mice: Effects of age, fasting, and acute cold. *American Journal of Physiology* 244, E567–E574.
26. Koda, S., Date, Y., Murakami, N., Shimbara, T., Hanada, T., Toshinai, K., Niijima, A., Furuya, M., Inomata, N., Osuye, K., and Nakazato, M. (2005). The role of the vagal nerve in peripheral PYY3-36-induced feeding reduction in rats. *Endocrinology* 146, 2369–2375.
27. Kojima, M., Hosoda, H., Date, Y., Nakazato, M., Matsuo, H., and Kangawa, K. (1999). Ghrelin is a growth-hormone-releasing acylated peptide from stomach. *Nature* 402, 656–660.
28. Lam, T. K., Pocai, A., Gutierrez-Juarez, R., Obici, S., Bryan, J., Aguilar-Bryan, L., Schwartz, G. J., and Rossetti, L. (2005). Hypothalamic sensing of circulating fatty acids is required for glucose homeostasis. *Nature Medicine* 11, 320–327.
29. Leibel, R. L., Rosenbaum, M., and Hirsch, J. (1995). Changes in energy expenditure resulting from altered body weight. *New England Journal of Medicine* 332, 621–628.
30. Levin, B. E. (1992). Intracarotid glucose-induced norepinephrine response and the development of diet-induced obesity. *International Journal of Obesity* 16, 451–457.
31. Levin, B. E. (1995). Reduced norepinephrine turnover in organs and brains of obesity-prone rats. *American Journal of Physiology* 268, R389–R394.
32. Levin, B. E., and Dunn-Meynell, A. A. (2000). Defense of body weight against chronic caloric restriction in obesity-prone and -resistant rats. *American Journal of Physiology. Regulatory, Integrative and Comparative Physiology* 278, R231–R237.
33. Levin, B. E., and Dunn-Meynell, A. A. (2002). Defense of body weight depends on dietary composition and palatability in rats with diet-induced obesity. *American Journal of Physiology. Regulatory, Integrative and Comparative Physiology* 282, R46–R54.
34. Levin, B. E., Dunn-Meynell, A. A., Ricci, M. R., and Cummings, D. E. (2003). Abnormalities of leptin and ghrelin regulation in obesity-prone juvenile rats. *American Journal of Physiology. Endocrinology and Metabolism* 285, E949–E957.
35. Levin, B. E., Routh, V. H., Kang, L., Sanders, N. M., and Dunn-Meynell, A. A. (2004). Neuronal glucosensing: What do we know after 50 years? *Diabetes* 53, 2521–2528.
36. Levin, B. E., and Sullivan, A. C. (1987). Glucose, insulin and sympathoadrenal activation. *Journal of the Autonomic Nervous System* 20, 233–242.
37. Levin, B. E., Triscari, J., Hogan, S., and Sullivan, A. C. (1987). Resistance to diet-induced obesity: Food intake, pancreatic sympathetic tone and insulin. *American Journal of Physiology* 252, R471–R478.
38. Levin, B. E., Triscari, J., and Sullivan, A. C. (1982). Sympathetic activity in thyroid-treated Zucker rats. *American Journal of Physiology* 243, R170–R178.
39. Liu, L., Karkanias, G. B., Morales, J. C., Hawkins, M., Barzilai, N., Wang, J., and Rossetti, L. (1998). Intracerebroventricular leptin regulates hepatic but not peripheral glucose fluxes. *Journal of Biological Chemistry* 273, 31160–31167.
40. Liu, M., Seino, S., and Kirchgessner, A. L. (1999). Identification and characterization of glucoresponsive neurons in the enteric nervous system. *Journal of Neuroscience* 19, 10305–10317.
41. Maclean, P. S., Higgins, J. A., Johnson, G. C., Fleming-Elder, B. K., Peters, J. C., and Hill, J. O. (2004). Metabolic adjustments with the development, treatment, and recurrence of obesity in obesity-prone rats. *American Journal of Physiology. Regulatory, Integrative and Comparative Physiology* 287, R288–R297.
42. Marks, J. L., and Waite, K. (1996). Some acute effects of intracerebroventricular neuropeptide Y on insulin secretion and glucose metabolism in the rat. *Journal of Neuroendocrinology* 8, 507–513.
43. Migliorini, R. H., Garofalo, M. A., and Kettelhut, I. C. (1997). Increased sympathetic activity in rat white adipose tissue during prolonged fasting. *American Journal of Physiology* 272, R656–R661.
44. Minokoshi, Y., Kim, Y. B., Peroni, O. D., Fryer, L. G., Muller, C., Carling, D., and Kahn, B. B. (2002). Leptin stimulates fatty-acid oxidation by

activating AMP-activated protein kinase. *Nature* 415, 339–343.

45. Mizuno, T. M., Kleopoulos, S. P., Bergen, H. T., Roberts, J. L., Priest, C. A., and Mobbs, C. V. (1998). Hypothalamic pro-opiomelanocortin mRNA is reduced by fasting in ob/ob and db/db mice, but is stimulated by leptin. *Diabetes* 47, 294–297.
46. Mundinger, T. O., Cummings, D. E., and Taborsky, G. J., Jr. (2006). Direct stimulation of ghrelin secretion by sympathetic nerves. *Endocrinology* 147, 2893–2901.
47. Nakabayashi, H. (1997). Neural monitoring system for circulating somatostatin in the hepatoportal area. *Nutrition* 13, 225–229.
48. Nakabayashi, H., Nishizawa, M., Nakagawa, A., Takeda, R., and Niijima, A. (1996). Vagal hepatopancreatic reflex effect evoked by intraportal appearance of tGLP-1. *American Journal of Physiology* 271, E808–E813.
49. Neel, J. V., Weder, A. B., and Julius, S. (1998). Type II diabetes, essential hypertension, and obesity as "syndromes of impaired genetic homeostasis": the "thrifty genotype" hypothesis enters the 21st century. *Perspectives in Biology and Medicine* 42, 44–74.
50. Niijima, A. (1975). The effect of glucose on the activity of the adrenal nerve and pancreatic branch of the vagus nerve in the rabbit. *Neuroscience Letters* 1, 159–162.
51. Niijima, A. (1984). Reflex control of the autonomic nervous system activity from the glucose sensors in the liver in normal and midpontinc-transected animals. *Journal of the Autonomic Nervous System* 10, 279–285.
52. Niijima, A. (1999). Reflex effects from leptin sensors in the white adipose tissue of the epididymis to the efferent activity of the sympathetic and vagus nerve in the rat. *Neuroscience Letters* 262, 125–128.
53. Niijima, A., Kannan, H., and Yamashita, H. (1988). Neural control of blood glucose homeostasis: Effect of microinjection of glucose into hypothalamic nuclei on efferent activity of pancreatic branch of vagus nerve in the rat. *Brain Research Bulletin* 20, 811–816.
54. Perkins, M. N., Rothwell, N. J., Stock, M. J., and Stone, T. W. (1981). Activation of brown adipose tissue thermogenesis by the ventromedial hypothalamus. *Nature* 289, 401–402.
55. Peters, J. H., Karpiel, A. B., Ritter, R. C., and Simasko, S. M. (2004). Cooperative activation of cultured vagal afferent neurons by leptin and cholecystokinin. *Endocrinology* 145, 3652–3657.
56. Peters, J. H., McKay, B. M., Simasko, S. M., and Ritter, R. C. (2005). Leptin-induced satiation mediated by abdominal vagal afferents. *American Journal of Physiology. Regulatory, Integrative and Comparative Physiology* 288, R879–R884.
57. Pocai, A., Lam, T. K., Gutierrez-Juarez, R., Obici, S., Schwartz, G. J., Bryan, J., Aguilar-Bryan, L., and Rossetti, L. (2005). Hypothalamic K(ATP) channels control hepatic glucose production. *Nature* 434, 1026–1031.
58. Pocai, A., Morgan, K., Buettner, C., Gutierrez-Juarez, R., Obici, S., and Rossetti, L. (2005). Central leptin acutely reverses diet-induced hepatic insulin resistance. *Diabetes* 54, 3182–3189.
59. Porte, D., Jr. and Robertson, R. P. (1973). Control of insulin secretion by catecholamines, stress, and the sympathetic nervous system. *Federation Proceedings* 32, 1792–1796.
60. Rahmouni, K., Haynes, W. G., Morgan, D. A., and Mark, A. L. (2003). Role of melanocortin-4 receptors in mediating renal sympathoactivation to leptin and insulin. *Journal of Neuroscience* 23, 5998–6004.
61. Ravussin, E., and Bogardus, C. (1982). Thermogenic response to insulin and glucose infusions in man: A model to evaluate the different components of the thermic effect of carbohydrate. *Life Sciences* 31, 2011–2018.
62. Ricci, M. R., and Fried, S. K. (1999). Isoproterenol decreases leptin expression in adipose tissue of obese humans. *Obesity Research* 7, 233–240.
63. Ricci, M. R., Lee, M.-J., Russell, C. D., Wang, Y., Sullivan, S., Schneider, S. H., Brolin, R. E., and Fried, S. K. (2005). Isoproterenol decreases leptin release from rat and human adipose tissue through posttranscriptional mechanisms. *American Journal of Physiology. Endocrinology and Metabolism* 288, E798–E804.
64. Ritter, S., Dinh, T. T., and Zhang, Y. (2000). Localization of hindbrain glucoreceptive sites controlling food intake and blood glucose. *Brain Research* 856, 37–47.
65. Roper, J., and Ashcroft, F. M. (1995). Metabolic inhibition and low internal ATP activate K-ATP channels in rat dopaminergic substantia nigra neurones. *Pflügers Archiv* 430, 44–54.
66. Rosenbaum, M., Goldsmith, R., Bloomfield, D., Magnano, A., Weimer, L., Heymsfield, S., Gallagher, D., Mayer, L., Murphy, E., and Leibel, R. L. (2005). Low-dose leptin reverses skeletal muscle, autonomic, and neuroendocrine adaptations to maintenance of reduced weight. *Journal of Clinical Investigation* 115, 3579–3586.
67. Rowe, J. W., Young, J. B., Minaker, K. L., Stevens, A. L., Pallotta, J., and Landsberg, L. (1981). Effect of insulin and glucose infusions on sympathetic nervous system activity in normal man. *Diabetes* 30, 219–225.

68. Saito, M., Minokoshi, Y., and Shimazu, T. (1987). Ventromedial hypothalamic stimulation accelerates norepinephrine turnover in brown adipose tissue of rats. *Life Sciences* 41, 193–197.
69. Sakurai, T., Amemiya, A., Ishii, M., Matsuzaki, I., Chemelli, R. M., Tanaka, H., Williams, S. C., Richardson, J. A., Kozlowski, G. P., Wilson, S., Arch, J. R., Buckingham, R. E., Haynes, A. C., Carr, S. A., Annan, R. S., McNulty, D. E., Liu, W. S., Terrett, J. A., Elshourbagy, N. A., Bergsma, D. J., and Yanagisawa, M. (1998). Orexins and orexin receptors: A family of hypothalamic neuropeptides and G protein-coupled receptors that regulate feeding behavior. *Cell* 92, 573–585.
70. Satoh, N., Ogawa, Y., Katsuura, G., Numata, Y., Tsuji, T., Hayase, M., Ebihara, K., Masuzaki, H., Hosoda, K., Yoshimasa, Y., and Nakao, K. (1999). Sympathetic activation of leptin via the ventromedial hypothalamus: Leptin-induced increase in catecholamine secretion. *Diabetes* 48, 1787–1793.
71. Schwartz, G. J., McHugh, P. R., and Moran, T. H. (1991). Integration of vagal afferent responses to gastric loads and cholecystokinin in rats. *American Journal of Physiology* 261, R64–R69.
72. Schwartz, G. J., and Moran, T. H. (2002). Leptin and neuropeptide y have opposing modulatory effects on nucleus of the solitary tract neurophysiological responses to gastric loads: Implications for the control of food intake. *Endocrinology* 143, 3779–3784.
73. Schwartz, M. W., and Niswender, K. D. (2004). Adiposity signaling and biological defense against weight gain: Absence of protection or central hormone resistance? *Journal of Clinical Endocrinology and Metabolism* 89, 5889–5897.
74. Shimazu, T. (1981). Central nervous system regulation of liver and adipose tissue metabolism. *Diabetologia* 20 Suppl, 343–356.
75. Smith, F. J., and Campfield, L. A. (1986). Pancreatic adaptation in VMH obesity: In vivo compensatory response to altered neural input. *American Journal of Physiology* 251, R70–R76.
76. Smith, G. P., and Gibbs, J. (1984). Gut peptides and postprandial satiety. *Federation Proceedings* 43, 2889–2892.
77. Smith, P. E. (1927). The disabilities caused by hypophysectomy and their repair. The tuberal (hypothalamic) syndrome in the rat. *Journal of the American Medical Association* 88, 158–161.
78. Stoddard-Apter, S. L., Bergdall, V. K., Townsend, D. W., and Levin, B. E. (1986). Plasma catecholamines associated with hypothalamically elicited defense behavior. *Physiology and Behavior* 36, 867–873.
79. Strader, A. D., and Woods, S. C. (2005). Gastrointestinal hormones and food intake. *Gastroenterology* 128, 175–191.
80. Takahashi, A., Ishimaru, H., Ikarashi, Y., Kishi, E., and Maruyama, Y. (1997). Effects of ventromedial hypothalamus stimulation on glycogenolysis in rat liver using in vivo microdialysis. *Metabolism* 46, 897–901.
81. Tanaka, K., Inoue, S., Nagase, H., Takamura, Y., and Niijima, A. (1990). Amino acid sensors sensitive to alanine and leucine exist in the hepatoportal system in the rat. *Journal of the Autonomic Nervous System* 31, 41–46.
82. Tartaglia, L. A., Dembski, M., Weng, X., Deng, N., Culpepper, J., Devos, R., Richards, G. J., Campfield, L. A., Clark, F. T., Deeds, J., Muir, C., Sanker, S., Moriarity, A., Moore, K. J., Smutko, J. S., Mays, G. G., Woolf, E. A., Monroe, C. A., and Tepper, R. I. (1995). Identification and expression cloning of a leptin receptor, OB-R. *Cell* 83, 1263–1271.
83. Tritos, N. A., Vicent, D., Gillette, J., Ludwig, D. S., Flier, E. S., and Maratos-Flier, E. (1998). Functional interactions between melanin-concentrating hormone, neuropeptide Y, and anorectic neuropeptides in the rat hypothalamus. *Diabetes* 47, 1687–1692.
84. Van Dijk, G., Bottone, A. E., Strubbe, J. H., and Steffens, A. B. (1994). Hormonal and metabolic effects of paraventricular hypothalamic administration of neuropeptide Y during rest and feeding. *Brain Research* 660, 96–103.
85. Wang, R., Cruciani-Guglielmacci, C., Migrenne, S., Magnan, C., Cotero, V., and Routh, V. H. (2006). The effects of oleic-acid (OA) on distinct populations of neurons in the hypothalamic arcuate nucleus (ARC) are dependent on extracellular glucose levels. *Journal of Neurophysiology* 95, 1491–1498.
86. Wang, Y. (2001). Cross-national comparison of childhood obesity: The epidemic and the relationship between obesity and socioeconomic status. *International Journal of Epidemiology* 30, 1129–1136.
87. Wing, R. R., and Hill, J. O. (2001). Successful weight loss maintenance. *Annual Review of Nutrition* 21, 323–341.
88. Yoshimatsu, H., Niijima, A., Oomura, Y., Yamabe, K., and Katafuchi, T. (1984). Effects of hypothalamic lesion on pancreatic autonomic nerve activity in the rat. *Brain Research* 303, 147–152.
89. Zhang, Y., Proenca, R., Maffei, M., Barone, M., Leopold, L., and Friedman, J. M. (1994). Positional cloning of the mouse obese gene and its human homologue. *Nature* 372, 425–432.

# 18

# Central Nervous System Regulation of Body Temperature

SHAUN F. MORRISON AND WILLIAM W. BLESSING

## BRAIN TEMPERATURE AND THE MYTH OF A SINGLE BODY TEMPERATURE

In mammals, alert consciousness and normally patterned motor activities only occur when the temperature of the brain and spinal cord (the central nervous system [CNS]) is approximately 36°C to 39°C. If brain temperature is above this range, alert consciousness is altered and the normal patterning of both behavioral and physiological responses is impaired. As brain temperature approaches 45°C, both the brain and peripheral organs suffer tissue damage due to protein denaturation. Below-normal brain temperatures are also associated with reduced alertness and with behavioral and physiological disorganization. However, in contrast to the hyperthermic state, hypothermia, per se, does not physically damage the CNS or peripheral tissues. Indeed, with appropriate medical support, the temperature of the anesthetized individual may be reduced to 15°C to20°C without harm. In hibernating mammals, body and brain temperatures fall to even lower levels. Hypothermia is associated with torpor and inactivity; but normal consciousness and behavior resume when the body and CNS are rewarmed. That moderate hypothermia does not damage bodily tissues, including peripheral nerves, is also evident in normal life when the temperature of acral regions (feet, hands, etc.) falls substantially during exposure to a cold environment. Axons still conduct; muscles still contract, and sensory receptors still function.

The temperature of any region of the body depends on the current metabolic activity of the region, on the amount and temperature of blood flowing through the region, and on the temperature gradients to surrounding tissues. Consequently, there is no single "true" body or core temperature. Measured rectal temperature may, itself, vary by as much as 0.9°C, depending on the closeness of the thermometer tip to veins carrying blood from the cool buttocks and legs[41]. Nevertheless, the concept of body temperature or core temperature is useful as a generalization and as a guide to brain temperature.

## EQUILIBRIUM RATHER THAN SET-POINT

Engineering theory provided a controlled-system set-point model that became the classic framework for describing body temperature regulation. In this model, defended changes in body temperature arise from changes in the set-point of the neural "thermostat." Thus, during fever, pyrogens produce an elevated set-point for body temperature that "causes" the increase in sympathetic outflow to thermoregulatory cutaneous vascular beds contributing to the febrile rise in body temperature. In contrast, during exercise, for example, the thermal set-point is not changed, and the increase in body temperature, due to the excess heat generated during muscle metabolism, is reflexly countered by an inhibition of cutaneous vasoconstrictor sympathetic outflow. Beyond the regulation of individual thermal effectors, myriad interactions among the non-thermoregulatory physiological parameters can also influence body temperature. If the set-point deviations of individual parameters were corrected independently, these interactions would indirectly produce a cascade of subsequent set-point deviations. The validity and utility of the set-point model have been increasingly criticized, leading to the more useful concept of body temperature as the outcome of an equilibrium or balance among the activities of the available thermoregulatory effector mechanisms and the physiological parameters that influence them[98,114].

The set-point model has not proven to be a rich source of testable hypotheses concerning the actual neural pathways that regulate body temperature, mainly because a neuron-based set-point mechanism in the mammalian brain has been difficult to conceptualize, let alone discover. By emphasizing body temperature as the endpoint, the set-point model has discouraged the "deconstruction" of temperature into its constituent contributing elements; namely, heat production within the body and heat transfer between the body and the environment. In contrast, by its very nature, a model based on an equilibrium among effector processes focuses on the anatomy, physiology, and pharmacology of the CNS control of specific thermoeffectors, suggesting hypotheses concerning the mechanisms that govern thermoregulation.

## CENTRAL COMMAND, BODY TEMPERATURE, AND BODILY HOMEOSTASIS

Regulation of body temperature involves so many physiological systems that an overall understanding of the process presupposes a framework for understanding overall bodily homeostasis. For the latter, it is helpful to adopt a "central command" view of bodily homeostasis, rather than a "perturbation from the periphery" view that envisions the brain as restoring various set-points in response to inputs from the external or internal environments. Neural circuitry within the brain and spinal cord can be viewed as computer-style programs, generating patterns of activity in somatic motor nerves, autonomic nerves, and pituitary hormone secretion. These patterns coordinate the psychological, behavioral, and physiological effector systems responsible for maintaining body temperature, as well as the other sequential activities of daily life that maintain the integrity of the individual and the species. Rudimentary programs are genetically coded, but are modified by life experiences so that patterned regulatory commands coordinate the distinct somatic, autonomic, and endocrine effector mechanisms in a unified functionally efficient manner. In natural life, activities occur in a sequential fashion (hunting, eating, waste elimination, grooming, sleeping, etc.), so that correction of regional deficits or excesses (including excess heat) may be "postponed" because the next activity cycle involves different tissue effector systems.

For the regulation of body temperature in natural life, as for all homeostatic functions, inputs from the external and internal environments are best thought of as triggers, signals, or releasing stimuli for eliciting patterned behaviors, in the ethological sense described by Lorenz and Tinbergen[33]. In anesthetized animal preparations, output responses may be quantitatively related to the magnitude of input stimuli. However, in conscious animals, complexly patterned responses occur as a result of inputs that may seem minor unless considered in context. Such triggered responses are state-dependent, varying not only with the status of other homeostatic variables (e.g., osmotic balance, blood glucose, blood volume, and tissue oxygenation) but also with circadian and seasonal rhythms, with arousal state, and with social situation.

Complex responses can occur as a result of apparently minor environmental inputs (triggers) because, in the natural homeostatic process, feedforward is often more important than feedback in the modification of centrally patterned responses. Thus, when an alert rat is introduced into a cold environment, detection of the cold air triggers feedforward, heat-conservation responses *before* body temperature falls. In Figure 18–1, for example, introduction to a cold environment is associated with both major increases in heat production by activation of the sympathetic outflow to brown adipose tissue and major decreases in heat loss by activation of the sympathetic outflow to the tail vasculature. There may even be a slight increase in body temperature because the cold air also triggers piloerection, shivering, nest building, curled-up body posture, etc.

A focus on the equilibrium among the factors contributing to both sides of the heat equation can clarify and enrich many research issues. For instance, rather than distinguishing fever and hyperthermia according to whether or not the set-point is readjusted, a focus on the afferent process that triggers the increase in body temperature suggests that fever arises from an afferent process involving cytokine-prostaglandin pathways that are acetylsalicylate-sensitive; other increases in body temperature can be classified as hyperthermia.

## RHYTHMS IN BODY TEMPERATURE CIRCADIAN RHYTHM, SLEEP, AND THE MENSTRUAL CYCLE

An hour or so before an individual awakens, body temperature begins to increase so that body temperature is approximately 0.5°C higher (in humans) during waking than during sleeping, it declines again with sleep onset. The nocturnal fall in temperature is due

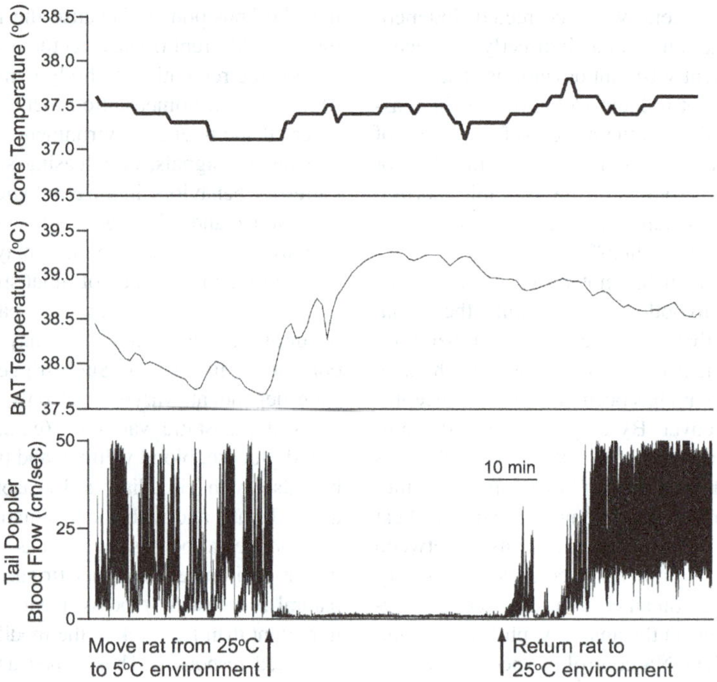


Figure 18–1 Thermoregulation during sudden exposure to cold in a conscious rat. Core (rectal) temperature remains stable or increases a little as brown adipose tissue (BAT) temperature increases and tail artery blood flow falls in a conscious rat moved from a cage at room temperature to new cage at 5°C. Modified from Blessing et al. (2006)[13], with permission.

both to increased heat loss to the environment and to reduced heat production[54], with the heat loss component reflected in vasodilation of the thermoregulatory cutaneous circulation (Figure 18–2A). The circadian temperature rhythm is superimposed on an ultradian temperature and metabolic rhythm, which, in rats, includes periodic thermogenesis in brown adipose tissue (Figure 18–2B).

The biological function of the circadian and ultradian temperature cycles is not understood. The increases in temperature are associated with other physiological and metabolic events that prepare the individual for action. It may be that, just as fever assists in defense against infectious agents in the internal environment, physiologically increased temperatures improve body and brain efficiency for the period when the active individual faces challenges in the external environmental. Studies in humans show that the circadian temperature fall still occurs when sleep is prohibited, so that it is not a consequence of sleep per se[54]. Thus, the circadian rhythms in both sleep and body temperature appear to reflect an integration of the pattern generation for these two behaviors. The suprachiasmatic nucleus, containing the neurons responsible for circadian rhythmicity, projects strongly to the more dorsally located subparaventricular zone[25], which projects, in turn, to the dorsomedial hypothalamic nucleus. Lesions of the ventral subparaventricular zone and the dorsomedial hypothalamic nucleus markedly reduce circadian rhythms of sleep, with only small effects on body temperature, whereas the circadian rhythm in body temperature (but not in sleep) is substantially reduced by dorsal subparaventricular zone lesions. The neuronal networks controlling the circadian and ultradian rhythmicities in thermal effector activity and in body temperature remain to be determined, as do their interactions with similar rhythms in behaviors such as motor activity and sleep.

Body temperature increases by approximately 0.5°C in the post-ovulatory luteal phase of the human menstrual cycle. Mechanisms underlying the temperature increase have not been extensively investigated. Mediation via a brain central-command process is likely, but little is known concerning relevant brain neurotransmitters and pathways. Women in the luteal phase of the cycle have a higher metabolic rate, feel the cold more, put on thicker clothing, and have more constricted thermoregulatory vascular beds[5,51].

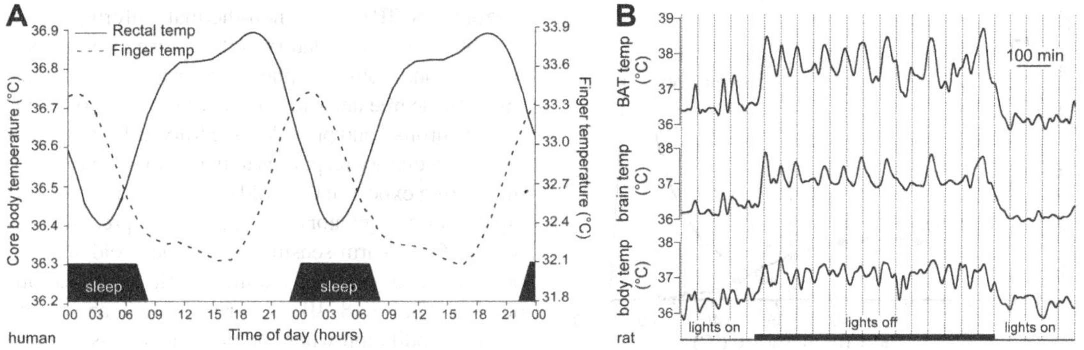


Figure 18–2 Circadian and ultradian rhythms in body temperature. *A:* During the circadian cycle, body temperature is inversely related to finger temperature, an index of the amount of blood flowing to the thermoregulatory circulation in humans. Modified from Eus and Van Someren (2004)[36], with permission. *B:* Increases in BAT thermogenesis contribute to ultradian increases in body and brain temperature during the dark (active) period in conscious unrestrained rats. Modified from Ootsuka et al. (2009)[91], with permission.

Thus, the thermoregulatory effector mechanisms are similar to those activated during the febrile response, although luteal phase hyperthermia is not acetylsalicylate-sensitive[17].

## AFFERENT SIGNALS FOR THERMOREGULATION

Information about the local environmental temperature is conveyed to central thermoregulatory circuits through the activation of thermoreceptors, consisting of unencapsulated nerve terminals in the skin. The axons of thermoreceptors make up a significant fraction of the axons in peripheral nerves. Warm receptors are unmyelinated C fibers, activated between 30°C and 50°C. Cold receptors are lightly myelinated Aδ fibers, active between 10°C and 40°C. At temperatures between 30°C and 35°C, both warm and cold thermoreceptors will be discharging (Figure 18–3A). As skin temperature falls, cold receptors increase their firing frequency, and warm receptor discharge declines. Increases in skin temperature produce the opposite response. Although thermoreceptors are very sensitive to localized changes in skin temperature, particularly if the changes occur rapidly, their individual outputs do not accurately indicate absolute skin temperature.

Cutaneous thermal afferents project to the superficial laminae of the spinal dorsal horn or to the spinal nucleus of the trigeminal nerve. Neurons in lamina I of the spinal dorsal horn project extensively to brainstem, pontine, and mesencephalic sites[30], as well as to the spinal intermediolateral cell column[29] (IML), where the cell bodies of sympathetic preganglionic neurons are located. Spinothalamic neurons in lamina I that respond specifically to innocuous cutaneous warming[1] or cooling[32] provide discrete ascending sensory pathways for temperature sensation and localization, while projections from lamina I to the lateral parabrachial nucleus mediate thermoregulatory autonomic and somatic reflex responses[76] (Figure 18–3B). In a cold environment, for example, feedforward cold defense of body and brain temperatures is accomplished when neurons in the external lateral subnucleus of the lateral parabrachial nucleus receive glutamate-mediated skin-cooling signals from second-order sensory neurons in the dorsal horn. These neurons, in turn, project to the median preoptic nucleus to excite GABAergic interneurons that reduce the discharge of warm-sensitive medial preoptic area neurons whose activity inhibits the elaboration of cold defense effector responses, such as shivering and brown adipose tissue thermogenesis and cutaneous vasoconstriction[75,76].

Central thermosensitive neurons are most concentrated in the preoptic area and anterior hypothalamus, where warm-sensitive neurons (Figure 18–4A2) outnumber cold-sensitive neurons. The basis for the inherent thermal sensitivity of neurons in the preoptic area is a temperature-related alteration in the rate of rise of the depolarizing prepotential (Figures 18–4A2, 18–4A4) that leads to action-potential generation[38]. Temperature does not affect the prepotentials of temperature-insensitive neurons (Figures 18–4A1, 18–4A3). Neurons in the preoptic area that sense local temperature integrate signals from skin and deep-body thermal afferents

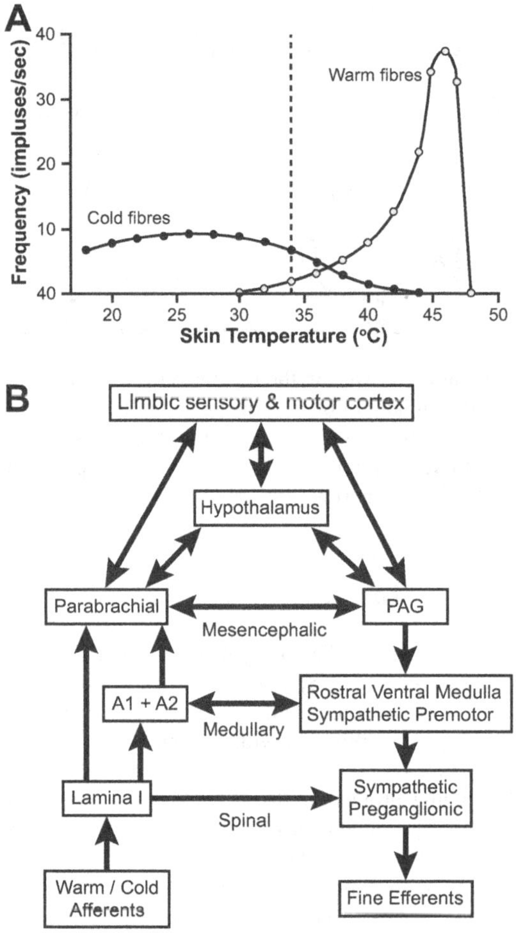


Figure 18–3 Afferent signals activate efferent thermoregulatory pathways. *A:* Response properties of skin thermal receptors. Modified from Hensel and Kenshalo (1969)[44], with permission. *B:* Schematic of the thermal afferent and brown adipose tissue (BAT) and cutaneous vasoconstrictor (CVC) thermoregulatory efferent pathways providing the basis for thermoregulatory autonomic reflex responses. Dorsal horn sensory neurons activated by cutaneous warm and cold receptors transmit thermal sensory information to parabrachial neurons, as well as to the cortical areas that provide perception, localization and the emotional context of thermal sensation. Parabrachial neurons provide cutaneous thermal input to the preoptic hypothalamic thermoregulatory networks, including thermoresponsive neurons in the preoptic area. Descending hypothalamic efferents control the outputs from dorsomedial hypothalamic (DMH) and medullary (raphé) sites that determine the level of activation of autonomic pathways controlling thermal effector tissues.

(Figure 18–3B) with non-thermal information to mediate thermoregulatory reflex responses. Under normal conditions, peripheral thermal afferents determine the degree and range of thermosensitivity in preoptic neurons[14] and provide a feedforward activation of thermoregulatory responses to maintain brain temperature during exposure to a cold environment[15]. The principal thermoregulatory output of the preoptic area derives from warm-sensitive rather than cold-sensitive neurons[24] and produces a tonic inhibition of heat production (Figure 18–4B) in normothermia, and a cutaneous vasodilation when the preoptic area is warmed. Evidence is accumulating for the independent control of different thermoregulatory effector mechanisms by preoptic area neurons[71], including markedly different sensitivities of thermogenic and cutaneous vasoconstrictor sympathetic outflows to changes in skin versus core temperatures[90].

## AFFERENT SIGNALS FOR FEVER

Thermoregulatory changes are common manifestations of systemic inflammation and infection. The defended increase in core temperature characteristic of fever, a component of the acute-phase response to infection, is thought to support immune system responses and reduce the viability of invading organisms. The integrated febrile response is mediated by the brain and includes psychological, behavioral, and physiological components that result in increased heat production and decreased heat loss to the environment (see below).

Lipopolysaccharide, a glycolipid in the bacterial cell wall, has been used in many experimental studies of fever. When administered intravenously or intraperitoneally, lipopolysaccharide causes a fever similar to that seen in natural infections. Detection of peripherally administered lipopolysaccharide by the immune surveillance system activates production of pro-inflammatory cytokines, including interleukin-1β, interleukin-6, and tumor necrosis factor-α. These blood-borne cytokines, as well as other potential pro-inflammatory compounds, including anaphylatoxic component C5a of the complement cascade and perhaps platelet-activating factor, cause prostaglandin synthesis (especially prostaglandin $E_2$) by inducing expression of cyclooxygenase-2 and other prostaglandin synthases. Targeted disruption of genes affecting the synthesis and receptor interactions of prostaglandin $E_2$ emphasizes its crucial role in initiating the febrile response[100].

Receptors for prostaglandin $E_2$ are located in various parts of the CNS. There is a high concentration of prostaglandin E subtype 3 receptors ($EP_3$ receptors) in the preoptic area[73], and prostaglandin $E_2$-mediated activation of these receptors is critical for the occurrence of the fever response[55]. Although activation of $EP_3$ receptors is thought to inhibit neuronal discharge, systemic administration of lipopolysaccharide or cytokines increases expression of Fos protein in an as-yet-unidentified population of neurons in the preoptic area. The relationship between "thermoregulatory" and "fever-related" neurons in the preoptic area is yet to be determined (see below).

Several sites have been proposed for the production of the prostaglandin $E_2$ that activates fever-related mechanisms in the preoptic area. Pro-inflammatory cytokines act on cells associated with intracerebral blood vessels, perhaps macrophages or endothelial cells, to induce prostaglandin $E_2$-synthesizing enzymes in

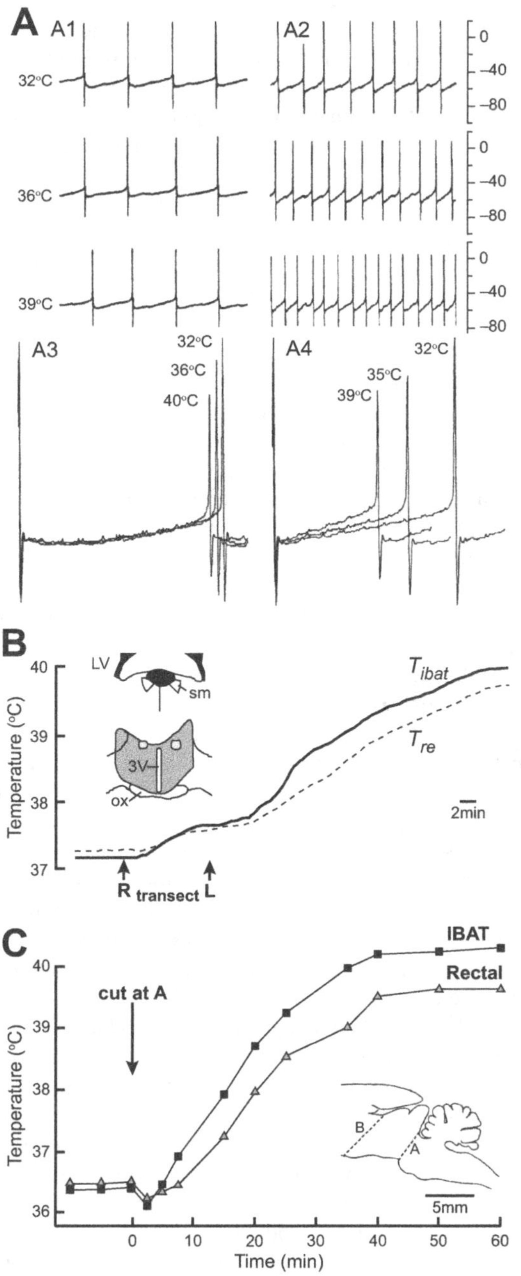


Figure 18–4 Preoptic area contains neurons with intrinsic thermal sensitivity and provides a descending inhibitory influence on bat thermogenesis. *A:* The effect of lowering local temperature on the discharge of a temperature-insensitive neuron (*A1*) and a warmth-sensitive neuron (*A2*) in the preoptic hypothalamus. Reducing the local temperature has no effect on the membrane potential or the rate of rise of the depolarizing prepotential in the temperature-insensitive neuron (*A3*) but markedly reduces the rate of rise of the prepotential in the warmth-sensitive neuron, resulting in a decreased firing rate (*A2*). Modified from Griffin et al. (1996)[38], with permission. *B:* Transection of the neuraxis caudal to the preoptic area stimulates brown adipose thermogenesis, producing an increase in brown adipose tissue temperature ($T_{bat}$) and in core temperature ($T_{re}$). Modified from Chenet al. (1998)[24], with permission. *C:* Precollicular transection of the neuraxis (*A in the inset*) elicits a large increase in the temperature of interscapular brown adipose tissue (Ibat) and in rectal temperature, whereas a similar transection at the level of the superior colliculus (*B in the inset*) had no effect on these temperatures (data not shown). Modified from Rothwell et al. (1983)[101], with permission.

these cells[34,63,115]. The prostaglandin $E_2$ produced in these cells diffuses into the parenchyma and acts on the $EP_3$ receptors on preoptic area neurons to stimulate CNS thermoregulatory pathways and thereby cause fever. Even peripherally produced, circulating prostaglandin $E_2$ is thought to cross the blood–brain barrier and contribute to fever development through the same central action and activation of the same thermal effector pathways[88]. Although an action of pro-inflammatory cytokines or prostaglandin $E_2$ itself on the distal processes of vagal afferent neurons is an additional potential pathway whereby fever signals could reach brain thermoregulatory centers, its physiological importance remains to be established, and the issue is controversial[6,35,88,99]. Separate mechanisms of infection signaling to the brain might provoke the temporally different phases of fever that are commonly observed after systemic infection.

## EFFECTOR SYSTEMS FOR THERMOREGULATION

The central nervous system engages a variety of physiological mechanisms in strategies to maintain an optimal core and brain temperature. These are employed in a sequence that appears to optimize energy conservation. For example, as the environment cools, it would be optimal from the perspective of energy consumption to reduce heat loss to the environment through cutaneous vasoconstriction before engaging highly metabolic thermogenic processes. This is seen in experimental paradigms involving skin cooling: the threshold for activation of the sympathetic outflow to the cutaneous circulation is reached before that for stimulation of thermogenesis. These responses can be preceded by behavioral compensation, such as adding insulating clothing in anticipation of exposure to a low environmental temperature. These behavioral adaptations may be triggered as a learned response or from a non-thermal sensory input (seeing frost on the lawn or hearing a weather report).

## HEAT TRANSFER BETWEEN THE BODY AND THE ENVIRONMENT

The CNS controls the level of heat transfer to the environment through autonomic and somatic neural pathways that determine (a) thermoregulatory cutaneous blood flow; (b) evaporative heat loss via panting, saliva spreading, and sweating; (c) piloerection; and (d) behavioral measures. Evaporative heat loss is the only mechanism effective in reducing body temperature if the environmental temperature is greater than core temperature.

Panting consists of an increased respiratory frequency that can be driven by increases in local temperature in the preoptic area[94]. Although the pathway from the preoptic area mediating the augmented respiratory frequency is not understood, it probably involves stimulation of the respiratory rhythm–generating network in the pre-Bötzinger region of the rostral ventrolateral medulla (RVLM) and is accompanied by an increase in fluid secretion within the respiratory tract. Saliva spreading would be ineffective if not accompanied by increased saliva production, which is mediated primarily through increased parasympathetic outflow to the salivary glands. Salivary secretion is facilitated by warming the skin or local warming of the preoptic area[49]. Parasympathetic post-ganglionic neurons controlling salivation receive their preganglionic drive from the salivatory nuclei in the rostral medulla and caudal pons. Neurons in the salivatory nucleus are synaptically connected to neurons in the lateral hypothalamic area, paraventricular nucleus, preoptic area, and lamina terminalis[46], likely sites for the integration of thermoregulatory, body fluid, and osmolarity signals necessary to balance the drives for increased evaporative heat loss and for the maintenance of body fluid homeostasis during heat stress.

Increased production and secretion from sweat glands is mediated primarily by axons of cholinergic sympathetic post-ganglionic neurons that release acetylcholine onto muscarinic receptors on the glands. Sudomotor post-ganglionic neurons receive input from sudomotor preganglionic neurons within the IML. These preganglionic neurons are located at spinal levels appropriate for the post ganglionic neurons that they innervate and, in cats, are characterized by their content of corticotrophin-releasing factor–like immunoreactivity[105]. The location of sudomotor sympathetic premotor neurons controlling thermoregulatory sweating and the pathways through which increases in preoptic hypothalamic temperature stimulate these premotor pathway have not been determined. The principal populations of premotor neurons exciting sympathetic preganglionic neurons controlling piloerection and the pathways through which these preganglionic neurons are activated by a cold stimulus are also unknown.

Behavioral thermoregulation is exhibited by even the simplest animals. Amoebae will move along a temperature gradient to an optimal temperature for cellular function. Moving to an environment with a different temperature and changing body posture (curled up to conserve heat, splayed to increase heat loss) are among the most common thermoregulatory behaviors employed by both poikilothermic and endothermic animals. The human capacity to alter the environment has resulted in an advanced repertoire of thermoregulatory behaviors ranging from engineered systems to control the temperature of our living, working, and traveling environments, to disposable, chemically powered hand warmers. A key element in behavioral thermoregulation is motivation, which appears to be driven by the interaction of peripheral (and perhaps central) information from thermal afferents with the limbic system, including the reward circuit involving dopaminergic inputs to the nucleus accumbens. The deviations from normothermic thermal sensation produced by excessively hot or cold environments elicit negative emotions, are perceived as uncomfortable, and provide a drive to initiate behavioral thermoregulation.

## CNS CONTROL OF CUTANEOUS HEAT LOSS TO THE ENVIRONMENT

Regulation of cutaneous blood flow is an important mechanism determining heat exchange between the body and the environment. The rat tail and the pinna of the rabbit ear have provided important model systems for elucidating the relevant CNS pathways and transmitter systems controlling cutaneous blood flow via sympathetic vasoconstrictor neurons. For the rabbit ear and for human forearm skin, there is physiological evidence for cutaneous vasodilator sympathetic nerves, but identification of a neuroanatomical substrate is lacking. There is no parasympathetic innervation of the rabbit pinna, nor is the tissue innervated by sympathetic neurons that synthesize acetylcholine or vasoactive intestinal peptide, the neurotransmitters that commonly mediate vasodilator responses[66]. Appropriate immunohistochemical studies in humans must distinguish postulated sympathetic vasodilator fibers from sympathetic sudomotor fibers. Excellent summaries of peripheral autonomic control of the skin vasculature[48,65] provide information about the neurochemical characteristics of cutaneous sympathetic post-ganglionic neurons and on the discharge patterns and reflex responses of the sympathetic innervation of the skin.

Neuroanatomical and physiological studies indicate that the raphé nuclei and parapyramidal region of the rostral medulla oblongata contain premotor neurons regulating sympathetic outflow to the tail vasculature. Neurons in this region are prominently infected (Figure 18–5A, 18–5B) at short time intervals after injection of the transneuronal tracer, pseudorabies virus, into the tails of rats[72,109,113]. Excitation of neurons in this region increases vasoconstrictor sympathetic discharge to the rat tail[97] and reduces cutaneous blood flow (Figure 18–5D)[12], with less effect on other regional sympathetic vasoconstrictor discharges (Figure 18–5C). Conversely, inhibition of rostral raphé and/or parapyramidal neuronal discharge reduces the basal cutaneous vasoconstrictor sympathetic discharge to the rat tail[96], reverses the increases in skin sympathetic outflow evoked by cooling the skin[87], and dilates the cutaneous bed (Figure 18–5D)[9,84]. Functional magnetic resonance imaging suggests that, in humans, activity of neurons in the medullary raphé increases during cold exposure[64]. Interestingly, inhibition of neurons in either the rostral raphé or the RVLM is capable of blocking the stimulation of cutaneous vasoconstriction by mild skin cooling, suggesting a cutaneous vasoconstrictor sympathetic premotor pathway from the RVLM[89]. These data, along with those supporting multiple cardiac-specific premotor pathways from the RVLM and the rostral raphé[21], indicate an important role for spinal integration of diverse premotor inputs for target tissues with both thermoregulatory and cardiovascular functions.

Differences in the latencies of sympathetic responses evoked from raphé and from spinal sites indicate that the axonal conduction velocities of raphé-spinal sympathetic premotor neurons controlling cutaneous sympathetic outflow[83] and those controlling thermogenesis in brown adipose tissue[70] are less than 1 m/s, in the range for unmyelinated axons (Figure 18–6A). Detailed characterization, including the neurotransmitter phenotypes, of cutaneous and of brown adipose tissue sympathetic premotor neurons with such slowly conducting axons remains an elusive goal. Transneuronal viral tracing studies from either the rat tail or brown adipose tissue show that a proportion of the neurons contains markers for 5-HT synthesis[19,109,113] and that there is a mostly non-overlapping population containing vesicular glutamate transporter 3[72]. Spinal glutamatergic transmission is necessary for activation of brown adipose tissue[72] and cutaneous (Figure 18–6B) sympathetic outflows. Spinal application of 5-HT, possibly acting through 5-$HT_{2A}$ receptors, has an excitatory effect on cutaneous sympathetic outflow (Figure 18–6B)[62,83]. Interaction of exogenously applied spinal 5-HT with 5-$HT_{1A}$/5-$HT_7$ receptors in the IML can excite the sympathetic outflow to brown adipose tissue and potentiates the increases in brown adipose tissue sympathetic nerve activity elicited by activation of glutamate receptors in the IML[60,61]. Activation of 5-$HT_{1A}$ receptors in the rostral raphé and parapyramidal region reverses cold-induced cutaneous vasoconstriction[82,85] and leptin-evoked increases in brown adipose tissue thermogenesis[68], presumably by inhibiting the discharge of local neurons, including those containing 5-HT. However, the normal thermoregulatory role of the raphé-spinal 5-HT pathway and its interaction with the descending glutamatergic pathway in the control of cutaneous vasoconstriction and thermogenesis in brown adipose tissue is not yet established. The puzzling presence of markers for neurotransmission by γ-aminobutyric acid (GABA) in

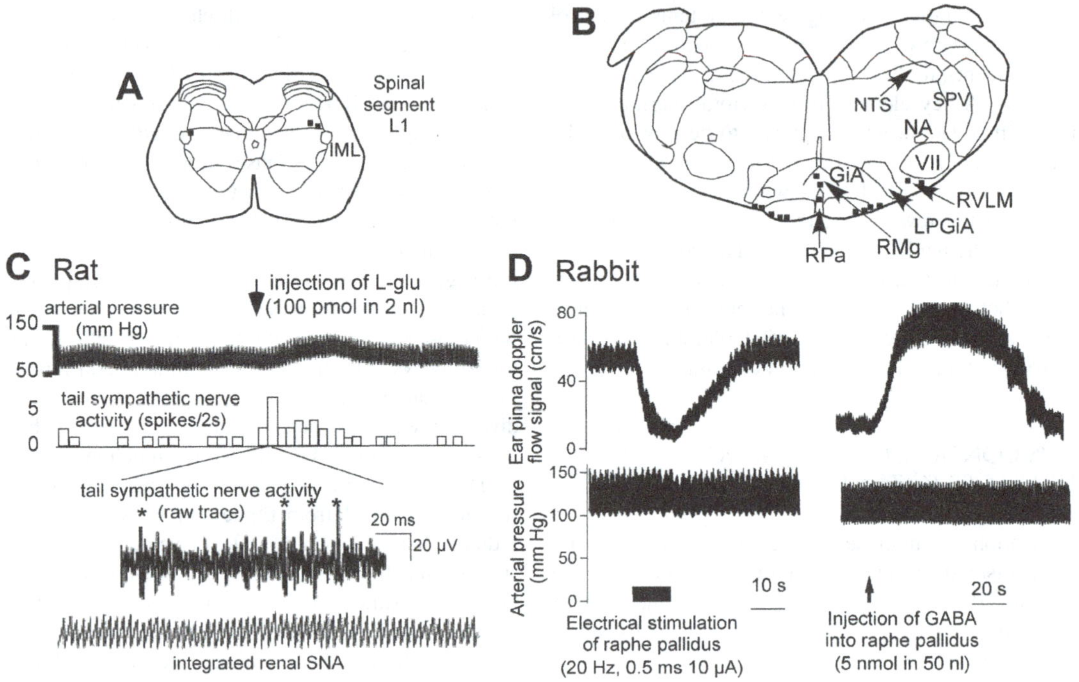


Figure 18–5 Rostral medullary raphé nuclei control blood flow to thermoregulatory cutaneous vascular beds. Distribution in the spinal cord (*A*) and in the medulla oblongata (*B*) of virus-containing neurons at a short survival time after injection of pseudorabies virus into the tail of the rat. Modified from Smith et al. (1998)[109], with permission. *C:* Excitation of neurons in the medullary raphé with L-glutamate increases sympathetic discharge to the tail more than to the kidney in the anesthetized rat. Modified from Rathner and McAllen (1999)[97], with permission. *D:* In the anesthetized rabbit, electrical stimulation of the medullary raphé vigorously constricts the vascular bed of the rabbit ear pinna without substantially affecting arterial pressure, whereas inhibition of raphé neurons dilates the vasculature of the pinna. Modified from Blessing and Nalivaiko (1999)[12], with permission.

some rostral raphé and parapyramidal 5-HT neurons[110] suggests that there may also be an inhibitory pathway to these spinal outflows.

As with other thermoregulatory effectors, the thermal sensitivity of cutaneous vasoconstriction appears to arise primarily from neurons in the preoptic area that also receive peripheral thermal sensory inputs. Warming the preoptic area inhibits thermoregulatory cutaneous vasoconstrictor tone, presumably through increased discharge of warm-sensitive inhibitory neurons in the preoptic area[122]. Electrical stimulation of the dorsomedial hypothalamic nucleus constricts the cutaneous bed in the pinna of the rabbit ear[78], and disinhibition of neurons in the dorsomedial hypothalamic nucleus activates the sympathetic outflow to the rat tail[96]. Although dorsomedial hypothalamic nucleus neurons can activate cutaneous vasoconstrictor sympathetic outflow, the activity of these neurons is not necessary for the cold-evoked discharge of postganglionic vasoconstrictor neurons innervating the rat tail[96]. The inhibitory influence of preoptic area projection neurons controlling cutaneous vasoconstriction may target neurons in the ventral tegmental area, which provide an important excitatory drive necessary to maintain the discharge of cutaneous vasoconstrictor sympathetic premotor neurons in the rostral raphé[121]. Alternatively, it may directly target the cutaneous vasoconstrictor sympathetic premotor neurons[45,73]. Excitation of neurons in a region between the caudal lateral hypothalamus and ventrolateral periaqueductal gray (PAG) inhibits cutaneous vasoconstriction and may contribute to the vasodilatory response to warming the preoptic area[121].

## HEAT PRODUCTION

Heat production is critical for prevention of hypothermia and for survival during exposure to a cold environment in which the rate of heat generation by

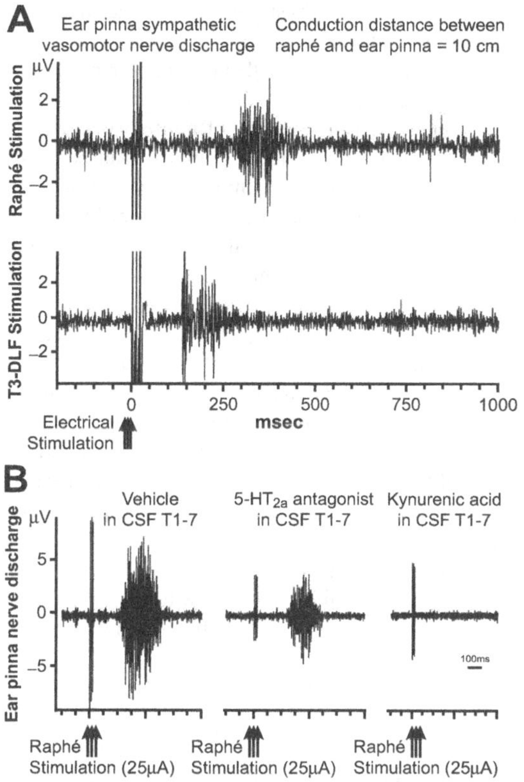


Figure 18–6 Spinal application of 5-HT2A receptor antagonist reduces ear pinna sympathetic vasomotor discharge. Sympathetic discharge to the pinna of the ear in the anesthetized rabbit in response to electrical stimulation of the rostral raphé and parapyramidal region or the dorsolateral funiculus in the T3 spinal cord (*A*) and before and after sequential application of SR46349B (5-$HT_{2A}$ antagonist) and kynurenic acid (glutamate receptor antagonist) to the cerebrospinal fluid around the upper thoracic spinal cord (*B*). Modified from Ootsuka and Blessing (2005)[83], with permission.

basic metabolic processes is insufficient to compensate for that lost to the environment, despite maximal cutaneous vasoconstriction. Heat production also contributes to the increase in body temperature during fever. Thermogenesis is of greatest thermoregulatory significance for animals with a large surface area (for heat loss) to body mass (for generating metabolic heat) ratio, such as rodents and the young of larger mammals, including human infants. In larger homeotherms, including adult humans, with a smaller surface area to body mass ratio, heat generated as a byproduct of basal tissue metabolism (in combination with cutaneous vasoconstriction, with the insulating properties of both subcutaneous adipose and piloerection, and with behavioral responses) is usually sufficient for survival in all but the coldest environments. Nonetheless, although its functional significance remains to be determined, significant depots of sympathetically regulated brown adipose tissue have been identified in adult humans, and their activation is reduced when body temperature in increased[79]. Thermogenesis can arise either from the rapid muscle contractions of shivering or from the increased metabolic oxidation of energy substrates such as that occurring during the stimulation of uncoupling protein 1 in brown adipose tissue.

## CNS CONTROL OF SHIVERING THERMOGENESIS

The rapid contractions of skeletal muscles (i.e., involuntary tremor) that define shivering are generated by an oscillatory instability in spinal circuits producing increased alpha and gamma (fusimotor) motor neuronal activity to skeletal muscle[104] in response to augmented cold signals from central and peripheral cold receptors[108]. The supraspinal premotor pathway necessary to drive shivering has not been established, although reticulospinal neurons responsive to cold stimuli have been identified[2] in the vicinity of the red nucleus, where cold-evoked shivering responses can be facilitated. The thermal sensitivity for shivering is primarily within the preoptic area and appears to be consistent with the regulation of other effector responses to cold (cutaneous vasoconstriction and thermogenesis in brown adipose tissue), since shivering is inhibited by glutamate activation of neurons in the preoptic area or by local warming of the preoptic area[122]. Although early lesion and electrical stimulation studies led to a proposed role for the posterior hypothalamus[40,43] in the descending neural circuit for shivering, recent data implicating neurons in the dorsomedial hypothalamus in skin cooling–evoked shivering suggest the need for a detailed anatomical mapping of this region using cell-specific agents to activate shivering or inhibit cold-induced shivering. Consistent with the pathway proposed for cold-induced activation of brown adipose tissue thermogenesis[69,74], neurons in the caudal hypothalamus that drive shivering may receive a tonic inhibitory input from warm-sensitive neurons in the preoptic area. Relief of this inhibition during cold exposure would allow descending activation of the spinal oscillatory circuits that induce shivering. Paralleling other cold-defense responses, neurons in the rostral medullary raphé play an essential role in shivering responses[16,111].

## CNS CONTROL OF NON-SHIVERING THERMOGENESIS

The principal effector of non-shivering thermogenesis in small mammals is brown adipose tissue. This tissue is composed of adipocytes replete with mitochondria containing uncoupling protein 1, which shunts the energy obtained from the oxidation of free fatty acids into heat. The heat is then conducted to the blood circulating through the brown adipose tissue vasculature, which dilates during brown adipose tissue activation, and is thus distributed throughout the body. Cold stimuli activate brain circuits that increase the sympathetic outflow to brown adipose tissue and increase the release of noradrenaline from sympathetic post-ganglionic terminals onto $\beta_3$-adrenoceptors on brown adipocytes. Transmitter release regulates the level of heat production in brown adipose tissue by (a) augmenting the activity of the lipase that determines the amount of cytoplasmic free fatty acids available for mitochondrial oxidation, and by (b) increasing the content of uncoupling protein 1 in the mitochondria through increased transcription[18].

Considerable progress has been made in recent years in our understanding of the functional pathway through which cold stimuli (Figure 18–7B) elicit increases in sympathetic nerve activity and thermogenesis in brown adipose tissue. Activation of glutamate receptors within the IML of spinalized rats is sufficient to elicit synchronized discharge of sympathetic preganglionic neurons supplying brown adipose tissue, as reflected in the burst discharges in post-ganglionic sympathetic nerve activity to brown adipose tissue. However, under normal conditions, activation of sympathetic outflow to brown adipose tissue results from increased discharge of supraspinal sympathetic premotor pathways that control the thermogenic activity of brown adipose tissue. Viral retrograde tracing[3,19,81,116] (Figure 18–7B) and pharmacological studies involving activation or inactivation of local neuronal populations (Figure 18–7A)[20,22,67,68,70,73,74] have shown that the principal sympathetic premotor neurons regulating metabolism and thermogenesis in brown adipose tissue lie within the rostral raphé pallidus region (Figure 18–7B) and neighboring parapyramidal nucleus, and include raphé-spinal neurons expressing the vesicular glutamate transporter 3[72]. Indeed, inhibition of neurons in rostral raphé pallidus reverses the activation of brown adipose tissue sympathetic nerve activity and thermogenesis (Figure 18–7C) elicited by all of the physiological and pharmacological approaches tested.

The discharge of sympathetic premotor neurons in circuits controlling brown adipose tissue is determined by the integration of a variety of inhibitory and excitatory inputs to the rostral raphé pallidus. Transections at the pontomedullary border, immediately rostral to the rostral raphé pallidus, produce a prominent increase in brown adipose tissue thermogenesis (Figure 18–4C)[101,106]. Thus, there must be a source of potent excitation of brown adipose tissue sympathetic premotor neurons from within the medulla, as well as a source of significant inhibitory control of brown adipose tissue sympathetic nerve activity from neurons rostral to the transection, probably from within the midbrain retrorubral field[107]. Disinhibition of neurons in a restricted region of the dorsomedial hypothalamic nucleus excites sympathetic nerve activity to brown adipose tissue (Figure 18–8A) through stimulation of brown adipose tissue sympathetic premotor neurons in rostral raphé pallidus[20,119]. Thus, there must be a tonic, GABAergic inhibitory restraint of a dorsomedial hypothalamic nucleus projection pathway (Figure 18–8C) that is capable of activating brown adipose tissue sympathetic premotor neurons. Cooling the preoptic area[4,47], microinjection of $GABA_A$ agonists into the preoptic area[93], or transections immediately caudal to the preoptic area[24] elicit large increases in brown adipose tissue thermogenesis (Figure 18–4B). These data indicate that, at normal core temperatures, tonically active projection neurons in the preoptic area, potentially warm-sensitive neurons[24,122], provide an important inhibitory regulation of brown adipose tissue sympathetic nerve activity. Thus, current evidence strongly supports the following model of the cold-evoked activation of sympathetically mediated brown adipose tissue thermogenesis. Stimulation of peripheral cold receptors by skin cooling activates an ascending pathway involving neurons in the lateral parabrachial nucleus. These neurons inhibit tonically active, warm-sensitive, GABAergic neurons in preoptic area which project to neurons in the dorsomedial hypothalamic nucleus. Finally, these hypothalamic neurons activate brown adipose tissue sympathetic premotor neurons (Figure 18–7B) through direct[45,77,103] or indirect[69] projections to the rostral raphé pallidus. The potential role of a direct GABAergic inhibition of brown adipose tissue sympathetic premotor neurons from neurons in the preoptic area[73] remains to be determined.

## CNS MECHANISMS AND PATHWAYS MEDIATING FEVER

Release of prostaglandin $E_2$ within the preoptic area and its activation of local $EP_3$ receptors, potentially on

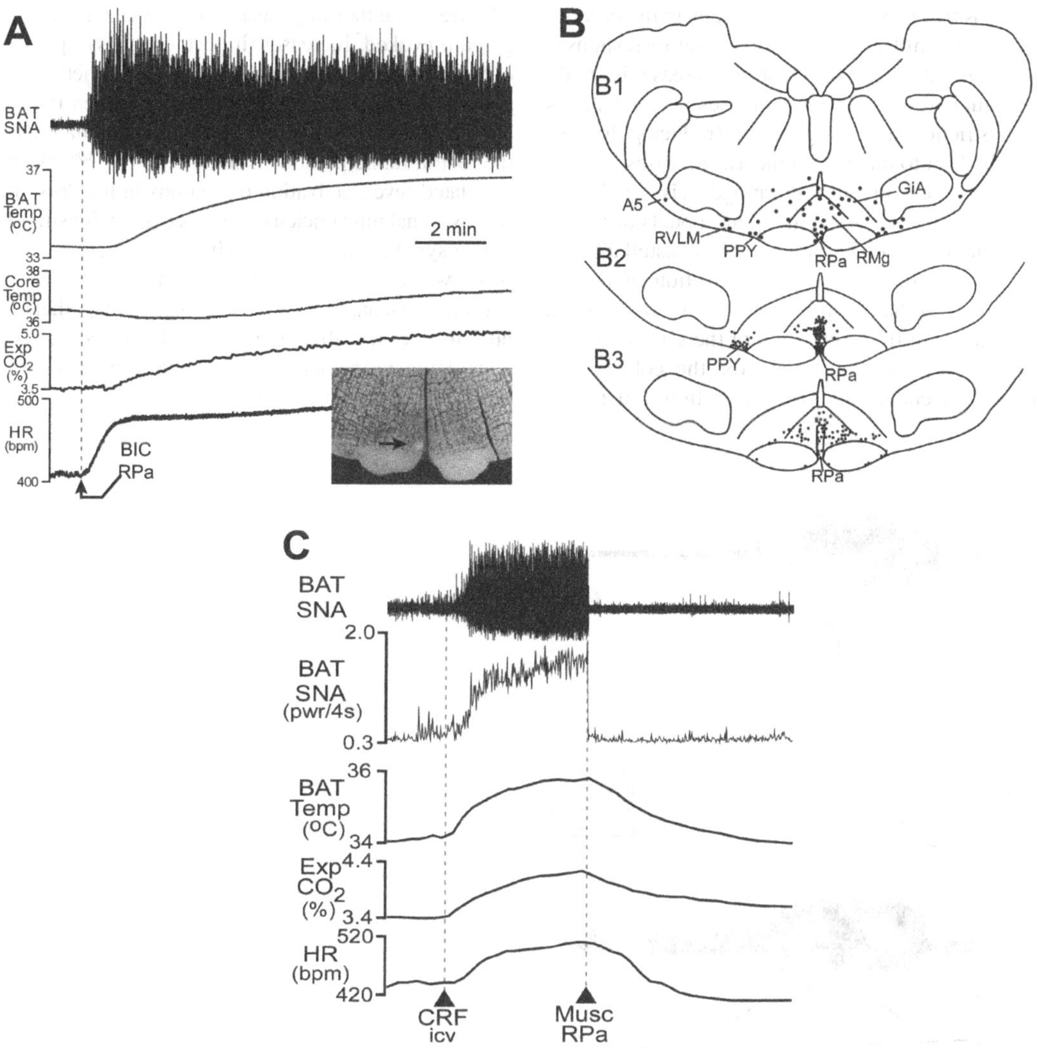


Figure 18–7 Rostral raphé pallidus contains sympathetic premotor neurons essential for activation of brown adipose tissue thermogenesis. *A:* Disinhibition of neurons in the rostral raphé pallidus (RPa, *arrow in inset*) with microinjection of the $GABA_A$ antagonist, bicuculline (BIC), elicits a potent increase in brown adipose tissue (BAT) sympathetic nerve activity (SNA), BAT temperature, expired $CO_2$ and heart rate (HR). Modified from Morrison et al. (1999)[70], with permission. *B:* Locations of neurons in the rostral raphé pallidus and parapyramidal areas (*B1*) retrogradely infected following pseudorabies virus (PRV) injections into BAT, modified from Yoshida et al. (2003)[116], with permission; (*B2*) expressing Fos following cold exposure, modified from Cano et al. (2003)[19], with permission; and (*B3*) infected following PRV into BAT and expressing vesicular glutamate transporter 3 (VGLUT3), modified from Nakamura et al. (2004)[72], with permission. *C:* Inhibition of neurons in the RPa with a microinjection of the $GABA_A$ agonist, muscimol (Musc), reverses the increases in BAT SNA, BAT thermogenesis, expired $CO_2$ and HR elicited by intracerebroventricular (icv) injection of corticotrophin releasing factor (CRF). Modified from Cerri and Morrison (2006)[23], with permission.

warm-sensitive neurons[95], are key steps in the production of fever. Similar to the thermoregulatory responses during cold defense, the febrile increase in body temperature results from increases in cutaneous vasoconstriction and piloerection (reducing loss of metabolic heat to the environment), increases in shivering and non-shivering thermogenesis (including from brown adipose tissue in rodent models of fever), and an inhibition of sweating. This constellation of responses is mimicked by microinjection of prostaglandin $E_2$ into the preoptic area (Figure 18–8B) and appears to result from activation of the same descending pathways described above for the cold-evoked responses in cutaneous vasoconstriction and brown adipose tissue thermogenesis. In particular, the prostaglandin-evoked increases in cutaneous sympathetic outflow and in brown adipose tissue sympathetic nerve activity (Figure 18–8B) are eliminated when the discharge of their sympathetic premotor populations in the rostral raphé pallidus is inhibited[53,58,67,73,96]. During simulated fever, activation of neurons in the dorsomedial hypothalamic nucleus is also necessary for stimulation of sympathetic nerve activity to, and thermogenesis in, brown adipose tissue[59,77,118]. In contrast, inhibition of neuronal discharge in the dorsomedial hypothalamic nucleus does not affect the increase in cutaneous vasoconstrictor sympathetic outflow evoked by prostaglandin $E_2$ injection into the preoptic area[96].

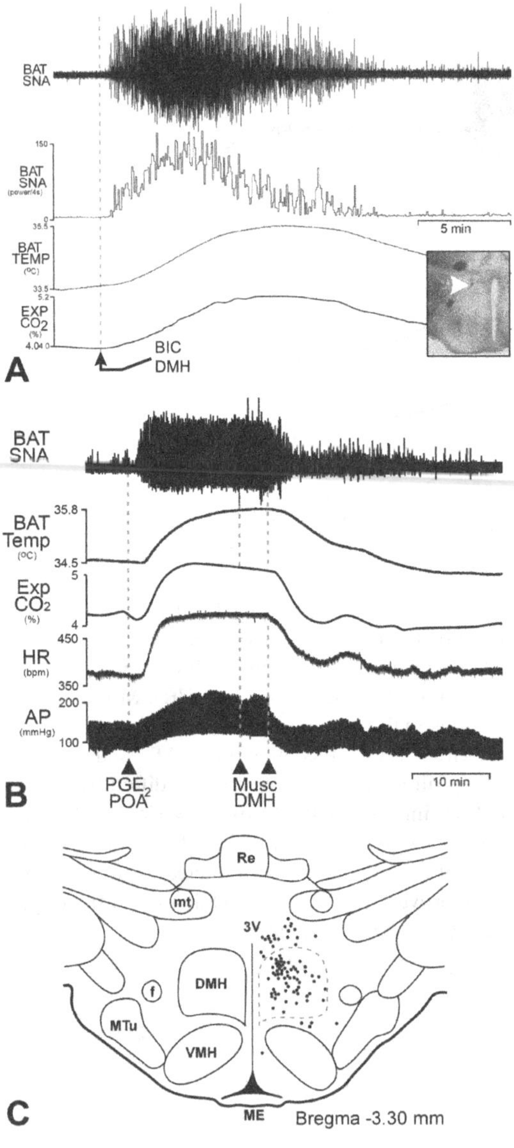


Figure 18–8 Activity of neurons in the dorsomedial hypothalamus is required for febrile activation of brown adipose tissue thermogenesis. *A:* Disinhibition of neurons in the dorsomedial hypothalamus (DMH, *arrow in inset*) with microinjection of the $GABA_A$ antagonist, bicuculline (Bic) elicits a vigorous increase in brown adipose tissue (BAT) sympathetic nerve activity (SNA), BAT temperature and expired $CO_2$. Modified from Cao et al. (2004)[20], with permission. *B:* Inhibition of neurons in the DMH with microinjections of the $GABA_A$ agonist, muscimol (Musc), reversed the stimulation of BAT SNA, BAT thermogenesis, expired $CO_2$, HR and arterial pressure (AP) produced by microinjection of prostaglandin $E_2$ ($PGE_2$) into the preoptic area (POA). Modified from Madden and Morrison (2004)[59], with permission. *C:* Sites of neurons in DMH retrogradely infected following pseudorabies virus injection into BAT. Modified from Cao et al. (2004)[20], with permission.

## CNS NEUROTRANSMITTERS AND RECEPTORS ALTERING BODY TEMPERATURE

Several studies of CNS pathways and neurotransmitters involved in thermoregulation were published before recognition of the multiple receptor subtypes mediating neurotransmitter action. In the case of serotonin, for example, stimulation of 5-$HT_{1A}$ receptors in the CNS lowers body temperature, and stimulation of 5-$HT_{2A}$ receptors raises body temperature[31,39]. Hence, the "temperature effect of serotonin" is not a very useful concept because of the difficulty of interpreting many of the earlier studies of the effects of serotonin on body temperature referred to in early reviews[27,57].

An important subclass of 5-$HT_{1A}$ receptors (autoreceptors) occurs on the perikarya and dendrites of 5-HT-synthesizing neurons in the midbrain, pontine, and medullary raphé nuclei[112]. However, since post-synaptic 5-$HT_{1A}$ receptors are present on non-5-HT-synthesizing neurons and can hyperpolarize them[42,50,52], the effects of 5-$HT_{1A}$ agonists cannot be automatically attributed to 5-HT-synthesizing neurons. Direct injection of 8-hydroxy-2-(di-n-propylamino) tetralin (8-OH-DPAT) into the rostral medullary raphé and parapyramidal region inhibits evoked sympathetic activity to both brown adipose tissue and thermoregulatory cutaneous beds[68,74,82,85]. Injection of the 5-$HT_{1A}$ receptor antagonist WAY 100635 into the same region reverses the effects of systemically administered 8-OH-DPAT on cutaneous blood flow and on brown adipose tissue thermogenesis, indicating that neurons within the rostral medullary raphé and parapyramidal region are an important site of action for systemically administered drugs that act on 5-$HT_{1A}$ receptors.

Drugs that stimulate 5-$HT_{2A}$ receptors increase body temperature by reducing heat loss and increasing heat production[10,86]. Systemic administration of a 5-$HT_{2A}$ receptor antagonist causes a slight decrease in the temperature of brown adipose tissue and an increase in tail blood flow in rats, as well as a reduction in sympathetic discharge to the pinna of the rabbit ear. These data suggest that activity of endogenous 5-HT neurons in both rabbits and rats tends to increase thermoregulatory sympathetic outflow by activation of post-synaptic 5-$HT_{2A}$ receptors at CNS sites that may include the spinal cord[62,83,92]. The hyperthermia that occurs in the serotonin syndrome, which is associated with the use of selective serotonin reuptake inhibitors, presumably reflects net stimulation of 5-$HT_{2A}$ receptors[102].

Apomorphine lowers body temperature by acting as an agonist at receptors of the dopamine D2 family[28,80]. The hypothermic effect of stimulation of these receptors is not blocked by domperidone, a dopamine D2–like antagonist that does not cross the blood–brain barrier. The preoptic area is one candidate region for the effect of apomorphine, since stimulation of dopamine receptors in the preoptic area increases heat loss via mechanisms that include increased blood flow to the cutaneous beds[28].

## SALIENT/EMOTIONAL ENVIRONMENTAL STIMULI MODIFY CNS CONTROL OF HEAT EXCHANGE

Blood flow to thermoregulatory cutaneous vascular beds suddenly falls when an individual detects a salient, possibly threatening, but not necessarily noxious environmental event (Figure 18–9). These sympathetic cutaneous vasomotor alerting responses occur in association with alerting-related changes in the hippocampal electroencephalogram (Figure 18–9) and are mediated by vasoconstrictor drive that is selective for the cutaneous bed[8,10], rather than by the more generalized vasoconstriction that would be part of the "fight or flight response" or the "defense reaction" proposed by Walter Cannon. Indeed, the change in regional distribution of blood flow that occurs with simple alerting stresses is similar to that occurring during exposure to cold or during the acute febrile response. Sustained sympathetic cutaneous vasomotor alerting responses to stressful stimuli could reduce heat loss to the environment and thus contribute, along with increased heat production in brown adipose tissue[13], to stress-induced hyperthermia[120].

## PSYCHOTROPIC DRUGS AND BODY TEMPERATURE

Many drugs with major effects on psychological functioning in humans have marked effects on body temperature in experimental animals[102]. Amphetamine and related compounds, including 3,4-methylenedioxymethamphetamine (MDMA or "Ecstasy"), activate thermoregulatory sympathetic outflows, causing hyperthermia in rats through both increased heat production by brown adipose tissue and decreased heat loss due to cutaneous vasoconstriction[11,13,37]. The hyperthermic effect of MDMA is dependent on ambient temperature, such that, paradoxically, the drug decreases body temperature in a cold environment, possibly due to the evoked release of several monoamines with effects on a variety of receptors. Cocaine also causes hyperthermia, but the mechanisms have not been extensively studied. The hallucinogens lysergic acid diethylamide and mescaline cause vigorous hyperthermia in experimental animals[26], presumably by net stimulation of 5-$HT_{2A}$ receptors.

Chlorpromazine, the first conventional antipsychotic agent, vigorously lowers body temperature

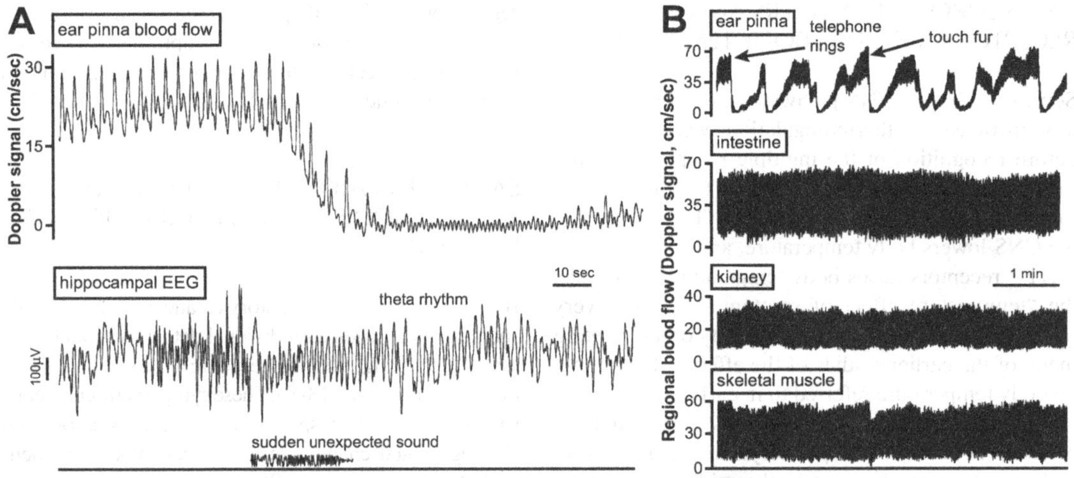


Figure 18–9 Salient stimuli cause sudden decreases in blood flow to the thermoregulatory cutaneous vascular bed. *A:* In the conscious rabbit, an unexpected sound that alerts the animal, as documented by the appearance of theta (5–9 Hz) rhythm in the hippocampal electroencephalogram (EEG), causes a sudden fall in blood flow to the pinna of the ear (sympathetic cutaneous vasomotor alerting response, SCVAR). This response to a salient stimulus is selective for the cutaneous vascular bed (*A*) and does not occur in intestinal, renal or skeletal muscle blood flow (*B*). Modified from Yu and Blessing (1997)[117], with permission.

("artificial hibernation"), reflecting both increased heat loss and decreased metabolic heat production[56]. Cannabinoids also lower body temperature[26]. Clozapine, the first atypical antipsychotic agent, has a robust hypothermic action, reversing the physiological responses of cutaneous vasoconstriction and sympathetically mediated thermogenesis that normally support body temperature during cold exposure or cause hyperthermia during the acute febrile response[7] or in response to administration of MDMA[13] (Figure 18–10). Thus, there are a number of circumstances in which CNS control of arousal and emotional state is integrated with CNS control of thermoregulation.

## SUMMARY

Thermoregulation is one of many interacting homeostatic systems controlled by the CNS. Body temperature reflects an equilibrium or balance point among the differentially controlled activities of the various thermoregulatory effector mechanisms, including heat loss through the cutaneous circulation, which may be aided by evaporation or reduced by piloerection, and heat production either through shivering or sympathetically regulated thermogenesis. Cutaneous thermal afferent signals are conveyed via the dorsal horn (and trigeminal nucleus) and lateral parabrachial nucleus to the preoptic area, where they are integrated with the activity of local thermoresponsive neurons to influence the discharge of neurons in specific efferent pathways to different thermoregulatory effector tissues (Figure 18–3B). Neurons in the preoptic area, dorsomedial hypothalamus, PAG, RVLM, parapyramidal nucleus, and rostral medullary raphé nucleus play prominent roles in the pathways controlling thermoregulatory effector function. The output of projection neurons from these regions is determined by the relative balance of tonically active glutamatergic excitatory inputs and GABAergic inhibitory ones. Aminergic and peptidergic signals can influence body temperature by modulating the synaptic integration of these primary amino acid transmitters at many sites in the central thermoregulatory network.

Although significant recent research progress has enhanced our understanding of the central mechanisms underlying the control of body temperature, several areas remain poorly understood. As with the circuits controlling other autonomic functions, the sources and mechanisms responsible for the tonic discharge and the synchronous bursting that characterizes the sympathetic outflow to thermoregulatory effectors remain to be delineated. The neural basis for tremor-like discharge in somatic motor neurons during shivering is not known. The sites and mechanisms underlying the critical integration of thermoregulation with other

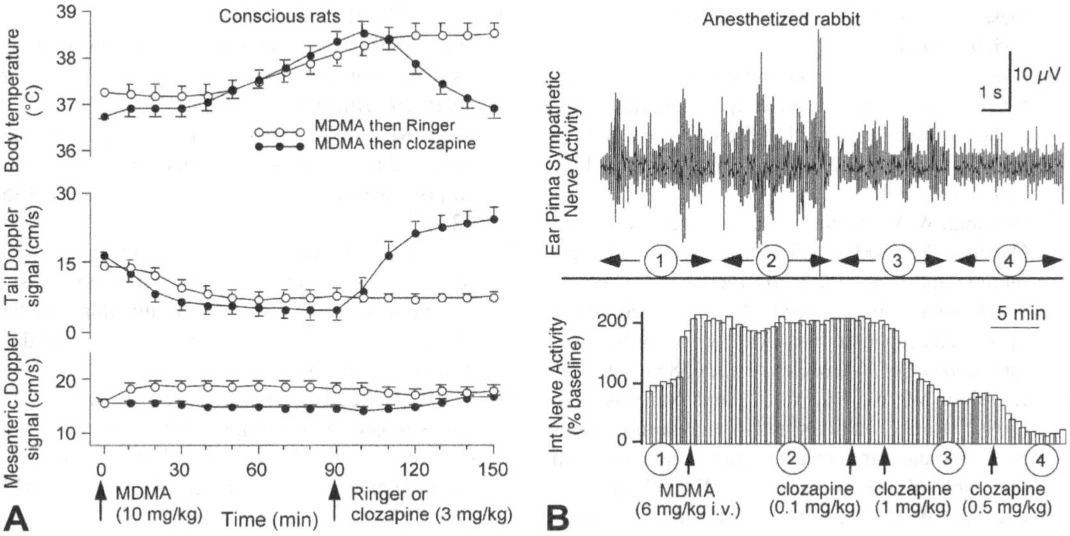


Figure 18–10 Clozapine, a drug used to treat schizophrenia, reverses hyperthermia and vasoconstriction of thermoregulatory cutaneous vessels elicited by Ecstasy. *A:* The increase in body temperature elicited by administration of 3,4-methylenedioxy-methamphetamine (MDMA or Ecstasy) in a rat is associated with tail artery constriction without a change in mesenteric blood flow. Clozapine reversed these effects. *B:* Clozapine reverses MDMA-elicited increases in sympathetic nerve activity to the pinna of the ear in anesthetized rabbits. Modified from Blessing et al. (2003)[11], with permission.

homeostatic systems, such as water and salt balance, regulation of blood volume and arterial pressure, and control of metabolism and energy balance, have not yet been investigated. The projection neurons connecting important regions in the central thermoregulatory pathways (Figure 18–3B) remain to be characterized, including the inhibitory output neurons of the preoptic area, the excitatory output neurons in the dorsomedial hypothalamus, and the sympathetic premotor neurons in the rostral raphé and parapyramidal regions of the medulla. The microcircuitry of the preoptic area and the role and regulation of the pontine inhibitory area for thermogenesis also represent significant gaps in our understanding of central thermoregulation.

## References

1. Andrew, D., and Craig, A. D. (2001). Spinothalamic lamina I neurones selectively responsive to cutaneous warming in cats. *Journal of Physiology* 537, 489–495.
2. Asami, T., Hori, T., Kiyohara, T., and Nakashima, T. (1988). Convergence of thermal signals on the reticulospinal neurons in the midbrain, pons and medulla oblongata. *Brain Research Bulletin* 20, 581–596.
3. Bamshad, M., Song, C. K., and Bartness, T. J. (1999). CNS origins of the sympathetic nervous system outflow to brown adipose tissue. *American Journal of Physiology* 276, R1569–R1578.
4. Banet, M., Hensel, H., and Liebermann, H. (1978). The central control of shivering and non-shivering thermogenesis in the rat. *Journal of Physiology* 283, 569–584.
5. Bartelink, M. L., Wollersheim, H., Theeuwes, A., Van Duren, D., and Thien, T. (1990). Changes in skin blood flow during the menstrual cycle: The influence of the menstrual cycle on the peripheral circulation in healthy female volunteers. *Clinical Science* 78, 527–532.
6. Blatteis, C. M. (2007). The onset of fever: New insights into its mechanism. *Progress in Brain Research* 162, 3–14.
7. Blessing, W. W. (2004). Clozapine and olanzapine, but not haloperidol, reverse cold-induced and lipopolysaccharide-induced cutaneous vasoconstriction. *Psychopharmacology (Berlin)* 175, 487–493.
8. Blessing, W. W. (2005). Clozapine increases cutaneous blood flow and reduces sympathetic cutaneous vasomotor alerting responses (SCVARs) in rats: Comparison with effects of haloperidol. *Psychopharmacology (Berlin)* 181, 518–528.
9. Blessing, W. W., and Nalivaiko, E. (2001). Raphé magnus/pallidus neurons regulate tail but not

mesenteric arterial blood flow in rats. *Neuroscience* 105, 923–929.

10. Blessing, W. W., and Seaman, B. (2003). 5-hydroxytryptamine(2A) receptors regulate sympathetic nerves constricting the cutaneous vascular bed in rabbits and rats. *Neuroscience* 117, 939–948.
11. Blessing, W. W., Seaman, B., Pedersen, N. P., and Ootsuka, Y. (2003). Clozapine reverses hyperthermia and sympathetically mediated cutaneous vasoconstriction induced by 3,4-methylenedioxymethamphetamine (Ecstasy) in rabbits and rats. *Journal of Neuroscience* 23, 6385–6391.
12. Blessing, W. W., Yu, Y. H., and Nalivaiko, E. (1999). Raphé pallidus and parapyramidal neurons regulate ear pinna vascular conductance in the rabbit. *Neuroscience Letters* 270, 33–36.
13. Blessing, W. W., Zilm, A., and Ootsuka, Y. (2006). Clozapine reverses increased brown adipose tissue thermogenesis induced by 3,4-methylenedioxymethamphetamine and by cold exposure in conscious rats. *Neuroscience* 141, 2067–2073.
14. Boulant, J. A., and Hardy, J. D. (1974). The effect of spinal and skin temperatures on the firing rate and thermosensitivity of preoptic neurones. *Journal of Physiology* 240, 639–660.
15. Bratincsak, A., and Palkovits, M. (2005). Evidence that peripheral rather than intracranial thermal signals induce thermoregulation. *Neuroscience* 135, 525–532.
16. Brown, J. W., Sirlin, E. A., Benoit, A. M., Hoffman, J. M., and Darnall, R. A. (2008). Activation of 5-HT1A receptors in medullary raphé disrupts sleep and decreases shivering during cooling in the conscious piglet. *American Journal of Physiology. Regulatory, Integrative and Comparative Physiology* 294, R884–R894.
17. Cagnacci, A., Arangino, S., Tuveri, F., Paoletti, A. M., and Volpe, A. (2002). Regulation of the 24h body temperature rhythm of women in luteal phase: Role of gonadal steroids and prostaglandins. *Chronobiology International* 19, 721–730.
18. Cannon, B., and Nedergaard, J. (2004). Brown adipose tissue: Function and physiological significance. *Physiological Reviews* 84, 277–359.
19. Cano, G., Passerin, A. M., Schiltz, J. C., Card, J. P., Morrison, S. F., and Sved, A. F. (2003). Anatomical substrates for the central control of sympathetic outflow to interscapular adipose tissue during cold exposure. *Journal of Comparative Neurology* 460, 303–326.
20. Cao, W. H., Fan, W., and Morrison, S. F. (2004). Medullary pathways mediating specific sympathetic responses to activation of dorsomedial hypothalamus. *Neuroscience* 126, 229–240.
21. Cao, W. H., and Morrison, S. F. (2003). Disinhibition of rostral raphé pallidus neurons increases cardiac sympathetic nerve activity and heart rate. *Brain Research* 980, 1–10.
22. Cerri, M., and Morrison, S. F. (2005). Activation of lateral hypothalamic neurons stimulates brown adipose tissue thermogenesis. *Neuroscience* 135, 627–638.
23. Cerri, M., and Morrison, S. F. (2006). Corticotropin releasing factor increases in brown adipose tissue thermogenesis and heart rate through dorsomedial hypothalamus and medullary raphé pallidus. *Neuroscience* 140, 711–721.
24. Chen, X. M., Hosono, T., Yoda, T., Fukuda, Y., and Kanosue, K. (1998). Efferent projection from the preoptic area for the control of non-shivering thermogenesis in rats. *Journal of Physiology* 512, 883–892.
25. Chou, T. C., Scammell, T. E., Gooley, J. J., Gaus, S. E., Saper, C. B., and Lu, J. (2003). Critical role of dorsomedial hypothalamic nucleus in a wide range of behavioral circadian rhythms. *Journal of Neuroscience* 23, 10691–10702.
26. Clark, W. G. (1987). Changes in body temperature after administration of antipyretics, LSD, delta 9–THC and related agents: II. *Neuroscience and Biobehavioral Reviews* 11, 35–96.
27. Clark, W. G., and Lipton, J. M. (1986). Changes in body temperature after administration of adrenergic and serotonergic agents and related drugs including antidepressants: II. *Neuroscience and Biobehavioral Reviews* 10, 153–220.
28. Cox, B., Kerwin, R., and Lee, T. F. (1978). Dopamine receptors in the central thermoregulatory pathways of the rat. *Journal of Physiology* 282, 471–483.
29. Craig, A. D. (1993). Propriospinal input to thoracolumbar sympathetic nuclei from cervical and lumbar lamina I neurons in the cat and the monkey. *Journal of Comparative Neurology* 331, 517–530.
30. Craig, A. D. (1995). Distribution of brainstem projections from spinal lamina I neurons in the cat and the monkey. *Journal of Comparative Neurology* 361, 225–248.
31. Cryan, J. F., Kelliher, P., Kelly, J. P., and Leonard, B. E. (1999). Comparative effects of serotonergic agonists with varying efficacy at the 5-HT(1A) receptor on core body temperature: Modification by the selective 5-HT(1A) receptor antagonist WAY 100635. *Journal of Psychopharmacology* 13, 278–283.
32. Dostrovsky, J. O., and Craig, A. D. (1996). Cooling-specific spinothalamic neurons in the monkey. *Journal of Neurophysiology* 76, 3656–3665.

33. Eibl-Eibesfeldt, E. (1970). *Ethology: The Biology of Behavior*. New York: Holt, Rinehart and Winston.
34. Elmquist, J. K., Breder, C. D., Sherin, J. E., Scammell, T. E., Hickey, W. F., Dewitt, D., and Saper, C. B. (1997). Intravenous lipopolysaccharide induces cyclooxygenase 2–like immunoreactivity in rat brain perivascular microglia and meningeal macrophages. *Journal of Comparative Neurology* 381, 119–129.
35. Elmquist, J. K., E., S. T., and Saper, C. B. (1997). Mechanisms of CNS response to systemic immune challenge: The febrile response. *Trends in Neurosciences* 20, 565–570.
36. Eus, J. W., and Van Someren, E. J. (2004). Sleep propensity is modulated by circadian and behavior-induced changes in cutaneous temperature. *Journal of Thermal Biology* 29, 437–444.
37. Gordon, C. J., Watkinson, W. P., O'Callaghan, J. P., and Miller, D. B. (1991). Effects of 3,4-methylenedioxymethamphetamine on autonomic thermoregulatory responses of the rat. *Pharmacology, Biochemistry, and Behavior* 38, 339–344.
38. Griffin, J. D., Kaple, M. L., Chow, A. R., and Boulant, J. A. (1996). Cellular mechanisms for neuronal thermosensitivity in the rat hypothalamus. *Journal of Physiology* 492, 231–242.
39. Gudelsky, G. A., Koenig, J. I., and Meltzer, H. Y. (1986). Thermoregulatory responses to serotonin (5-HT) receptor stimulation in the rat. Evidence for opposing roles of 5-HT2 and 5-HT1A receptors. *Neuropharmacology* 25, 1307–1313.
40. Halvorson, I., and Thornhill, J. (1993). Posterior hypothalamic stimulation of anesthetized normothermic and hypothermic rats evokes shivering thermogenesis. *Brain Research* 610, 208–215.
41. Hardy, J. D., and Bard, P. (1974). Body Temperature Regulation. In V. B. Mountcastle (Ed.), *Medical Physiology*, pp. 1305–1342. St Louis, MO: The C.V. Mosby Company,.
42. Helke, C. J., Capuano, S., Tran, N., and Zhuo, H. (1997). Immunocytochemical studies of the 5-HT(1A) receptor in ventral medullar neurons that project to the intermediolateral cell column and contain serotonin or tyrosine hydroxylase immunoreactivity. *Journal of Comparative Neurology* 379, 261–270.
43. Hemingway, A. (1963). Shivering. *Physiological Reviews* 43, 397–422.
44. Hensel, H., and Kenshalo, D. R. (1969). Warm receptors in the nasal region of cats. *Journal of Physiology* 204, 99–112.
45. Hermann, D. M., Luppi, P. H., Peyron, C., Hinckel, P., and Jouvet, M. (1997). Afferent projections to the rat nuclei raphé magnus, raphé pallidus and reticularis gigantocellularis pars alpha demonstrated by iontophoretic application of choleratoxin (subunit b). *Journal of Chemical Neuroanatomy* 13, 1–21.
46. Hubschle, T., McKinley, M. J., and Oldfield, B. J. (1998). Efferent connections of the lamina terminalis, the preoptic area and the insular cortex to submandibular and sublingual gland of the rat traced with pseudorabies virus. *Brain Research* 806, 219–231.
47. Imai-Matsumura, K., and Nakayama, T. (1987). The central efferent mechanism of brown adipose tissue thermogenesis induced by preoptic cooling. *Canadian Journal of Physiology and Pharmacology* 65, 1299–1303.
48. Jänig, W. (1990). Functions of the sympathetic innervation of the skin. In A. D. Loewy and K. M. Spyer (Eds.), *Central Regulation of Autonomic Functions*, pp. 334–348. New York: Oxford University Press.
49. Kanosue, K., Nakayama, T., Tanaka, H., Yanase, M., and Yasuda, H. (1990). Modes of action of local hypothalamic and skin thermal stimulation on salivary secretion in rats. *Journal of Physiology* 424, 459–471.
50. Kia, H. K., Miquel, M. C., Brisorgueil, M. J., Daval, G., Riad, M., El Mestikawy, S., Hamon, M., and Verge, D. (1996). Immunocytochemical localization of serotonin1A receptors in the rat central nervous system. *Journal of Comparative Neurology* 365, 289–305.
51. Kim, H. E., and Tokura, H. (1995). Effects of the menstrual cycle on dressing behavior in the cold. *Physiology and Behavior* 58, 699–703.
52. Kirby, L. G., Pernar, L., Valentino, R. J., and Beck, S. G. (2003). Distinguishing characteristics of serotonin and non-serotonin-containing cells in the dorsal raphé nucleus: Electrophysiological and immunohistochemical studies. *Neuroscience* 116, 669–683.
53. Korsak, A., and Gilbey, M. P. (2004). Rostral ventromedial medulla and the control of cutaneous vasoconstrictor activity following i.c.v. prostaglandin E(1). *Neuroscience* 124, 709–717.
54. Krauchi, K., and Wirz-Justice, A. (1994). Circadian rhythm of heat production, heart rate, and skin and core temperature under unmasking conditions in men. *American Journal of Physiology* 267, R819–R829.
55. Lazarus, M., Yoshida, K., Coppari, R., Bass, C. E., Mochizuki, T., Lowell, B. B., and Saper, C. B. (2007). EP3 prostaglandin receptors in the median preoptic nucleus are critical for fever responses. *Nature Neuroscience* 10, 1131–1133.
56. Leblanc, J. (1958). Chlorpromazine hypothermia in rats. *Journal of Applied Physiology* 13, 237–238.

57. Lomax, P. (1970). Drugs and body temperature. *International Review of Neurobiology* 12, 1–43.
58. Madden, C. J., and Morrison, S. F. (2003). Excitatory amino acid receptor activation in the raphé pallidus area mediates prostaglandin-evoked thermogenesis. *Neuroscience* 122, 5–15.
59. Madden, C. J., and Morrison, S. F. (2004). Excitatory amino acid receptors in the dorsomedial hypothalamus mediate prostaglandin-evoked thermogenesis in brown adipose tissue. *American Journal of Physiology. Regulatory, Integrative and Comparative Physiology* 286, R320–R325.
60. Madden, C. J., and Morrison, S. F. (2006). Serotonin potentiates sympathetic responses evoked by spinal NMDA. *Journal of Physiology* 577, 525–537.
61. Madden, C. J., and Morrison, S. F. (2008). Brown adipose tissue sympathetic nerve activity is potentiated by activation of 5-hydroxytryptamine (5-HT)1A/5-HT7 receptors in the rat spinal cord. *Neuropharmacology* 54, 487–496.
62. Marina, N., Taheri, M., and Gilbey, M. P. (2006). Generation of a physiological sympathetic motor rhythm in the rat following spinal application of 5-HT. *Journal of Physiology* 571, 441–450.
63. Matsumura, K., Cao, C., Ozaki, M., Morii, H., Nakadate, K., and Watanabe, Y. (1998). Brain endothelial cells express cyclooxygenase-2 during lipopolysaccharide-induced fever: Light and electron microscopic immunocytochemical studies. *Journal of Neuroscience* 18, 6279–6289.
64. McAllen, R. M., Farrell, M., Johnson, J. M., Trevaks, D., Cole, L., McKinley, M. J., Jackson, G., Denton, D. A., and Egan, G. F. (2006). Human medullary responses to cooling and rewarming the skin: A functional MRI study. *Proceedings of the National Academy of Sciences USA* 103, 809–813.
65. Morris, J. L., and Gibbins, I. L., ed. (1997). *Autonomic Innervation of the Skin*, vol. 12. Amsterdam, Netherlands: Harwood Academic Publishers.
66. Morris, J. L., Zhu, B. S., Gibbins, I. L., and Blessing, W. W. (1999). Subpopulations of sympathetic neurons project to specific vascular targets in the pinna of the rabbit ear. *Journal of Comparative Neurology* 412, 147–160.
67. Morrison, S. F. (2003). Raphé pallidus neurons mediate prostaglandin E2–evoked increases in brown adipose tissue thermogenesis. *Neuroscience* 121, 17–24.
68. Morrison, S. F. (2004). Activation of 5-HT1A receptors in raphé pallidus inhibits leptin-evoked increases in brown adipose tissue thermogenesis. *American Journal of Physiology. Regulatory, Integrative and Comparative Physiology* 286, R832–R837.
69. Morrison, S. F. (2004). Central pathways controlling brown adipose tissue thermogenesis. *News in Physiological Sciences* 19, 67–74.
70. Morrison, S. F., Sved, A. F., and Passerin, A. M. (1999). GABA-mediated inhibition of raphé pallidus neurons regulates sympathetic outflow to brown adipose tissue. *American Journal of Physiology.* 276, R290–R297.
71. Nagashima, K., Nakai, S., Tanaka, M., and Kanosue, K. (2000). Neuronal circuitries involved in thermoregulation. *Autonomic Neuroscience* 85, 18–25.
72. Nakamura, K., Matsumura, K., Hubschle, T., Nakamura, Y., Hioki, H., Fujiyama, F., Boldogkoi, Z., Konig, M., Thiel, H. J., Gerstberger, R., Kobayashi, S., and Kaneko, T. (2004). Identification of sympathetic premotor neurons in medullary raphé regions mediating fever and other thermoregulatory functions. *Journal of Neuroscience* 24, 5370–5380.
73. Nakamura, K., Matsumura, K., Kaneko, T., Kobayashi, S., Katoh, H., and Negishi, M. (2002). The rostral raphé pallidus nucleus mediates pyrogenic transmission from the preoptic area. *Journal of Neuroscience* 22, 4600–4610.
74. Nakamura, K., and Morrison, S. F. (2007). Central efferent pathways mediating skin cooling-evoked sympathetic thermogenesis in brown adipose tissue. *American Journal of Physiology. Regulatory, Integrative and Comparative Physiology* 292, R127–R136.
75. Nakamura, K., and Morrison, S. F. (2008). Preoptic mechanism for cold-defensive responses to skin cooling. *Journal of Physiology* 586, 2611–2620.
76. Nakamura, K., and Morrison, S. F. (2008). A thermosensory pathway that controls body temperature. *Nature Neuroscience* 11, 62–71.
77. Nakamura, Y., Nakamura, K., Matsumura, K., Kobayashi, S., Kaneko, T., and Morrison, S. F. (2005). Direct pyrogenic input from prostaglandin EP3 receptor-expressing preoptic neurons to the dorsomedial hypothalamus. *European Journal of Neuroscience* 22, 3137–3146.
78. Nalivaiko, E., and Blessing, W. W. (2001). Raphé region mediates changes in cutaneous vascular tone elicited by stimulation of amygdala and hypothalamus in rabbits. *Brain Research* 891, 130–137.
79. Nedergaard, J., Bengtsson, T., and Cannon, B. (2007). Unexpected evidence for active brown adipose tissue in adult humans. *American Journal of Physiology. Endocrinology and Metabolism* 293, E444–E452.
80. Ögren, S. O., and Fuxe, K. (1988). Apomorphine and pergolide induce hypothermia by stimulation

of dopamine D-2 receptors. *Acta Physiologica Scandinavica* 133, 91–95.

81. Oldfield, B. J., Giles, M. E., Watson, A., Anderson, C., Colvill, L. M., and McKinley, M. J. (2002). The neurochemical characterisation of hypothalamic pathways projecting polysynaptically to brown adipose tissue in the rat. *Neuroscience* 110, 515–526.
82. Ootsuka, Y., and Blessing, W. W. (2003). 5-Hydroxytryptamine 1A receptors inhibit cold-induced sympathetically mediated cutaneous vasoconstriction in rabbits. *Journal of Physiology* 552, 303–314.
83. Ootsuka, Y., and Blessing, W. W. (2005). Activation of slowly conducting medullary raphé-spinal neurons, including serotonergic neurons, increases cutaneous sympathetic vasomotor discharge in rabbit. *American Journal of Physiology. Regulatory, Integrative and Comparative Physiology* 288, R909–R918.
84. Ootsuka, Y., and Blessing, W. W. (2005). Inhibition of medullary raphé/parapyramidal neurons prevents cutaneous vasoconstriction elicited by alerting stimuli and by cold exposure in conscious rabbits. *Brain Research* 1051, 189–193.
85. Ootsuka, Y., and Blessing, W. W. (2006). Activation of 5-HT1A receptors in rostral medullary raphé inhibits cutaneous vasoconstriction elicited by cold exposure in rabbits. *Brain Research* 1073–1074, 252–261.
86. Ootsuka, Y., and Blessing, W. W. (2006). Thermogenesis in brown adipose tissue: Increase by 5-HT2A receptor activation and decrease by 5-HT1A receptor activation in conscious rats. *Neuroscience Letters* 395, 170–174.
87. Ootsuka, Y., Blessing, W. W., and McAllen, R. M. (2004). Inhibition of rostral medullary raphé neurons prevents cold-induced activity in sympathetic nerves to rat tail and rabbit ear arteries. *Neuroscience Letters* 357, 58–62.
88. Ootsuka, Y., Blessing, W. W., Steiner, A. A., and Romanovsky, A. A. (2008). Fever response to intravenous prostaglandin E2 is mediated by the brain but does not require afferent vagal signaling. *American Journal of Physiology. Regulatory, Integrative and Comparative Physiology* 294, R1294–R1303.
89. Ootsuka, Y., and McAllen, R. M. (2005). Interactive drives from two brain stem premotor nuclei are essential to support rat tail sympathetic activity. *American Journal of Physiology. Regulatory, Integrative and Comparative Physiology* 289, R1107–R1115.
90. Ootsuka, Y., and McAllen, R. M. (2006). Comparison between two rat sympathetic pathways activated in cold-defense. *American Journal of Physiology. Regulatory, Integrative and Comparative Physiology* 291, R589–R595.
91. Ootsuka, Y., Menezes, R., Alimoradian, A., Zaretsky, D., Hunt, J., Stephanidis, A., Oldfield, B. J., and Blessing, W. W. (2009). Brown adipose tissue thermogenesis heats brain and body as part of the brain-coordinated ultradian basic rest-activity cycle. *Neuroscience* 164, 849–861.
92. Ootsuka, Y., Nalivaiko, E., and Blessing, W. W. (2004). Spinal 5-HT2A receptors regulate cutaneous sympathetic vasomotor outflow in rabbits and rats; relevance for cutaneous vasoconstriction elicited by MDMA (3,4–methylenedioxymethamphetamine, "Ecstasy") and its reversal by clozapine. *Brain Research* 1014, 34–44.
93. Osaka, T. (2004). Cold-induced thermogenesis mediated by GABA in the preoptic area of anesthetized rats. *American Journal of Physiology. Regulatory, Integrative and Comparative Physiology* 287, R306–R313.
94. Pleschka, K., and Wang, S. C. (1975). The activity of respiratory neurons before and during panting in the cat. *Pflügers Archiv* 353, 303–315.
95. Ranels, H. J., and Griffin, J. D. (2005). Effects of prostaglandin E2 on the electrical properties of thermally classified neurons in the ventromedial preoptic area of the rat hypothalamus. *BMC Neuroscience* 6, 14.
96. Rathner, J. A., Madden, C. J., and Morrison, S. F. (2008). Central pathway for spontaneous and prostaglandin E2–evoked cutaneous vasoconstriction. *American Journal of Physiology. Regulatory, Integrative and Comparative Physiology* 295, R343–R354.
97. Rathner, J. A., and McAllen, R. M. (1999). Differential control of sympathetic drive to the rat tail artery and kidney by medullary premotor cell groups. *Brain Research* 834, 196–199.
98. Romanovsky, A. A. (2004). Do fever and anapyrexia exist? Analysis of set point-based definitions. *American Journal of Physiology. Regulatory, Integrative and Comparative Physiology* 287, R992–R995.
99. Romanovsky, A. A. (2004). Signaling the brain in the early sickness syndrome: Are sensory nerves involved? *Frontiers in Bioscience* 9, 494–504 .
100. Romanovsky, A. A., Almeida, M. C., Aronoff, D. M., Ivanov, A. I., Konsman, J. P., Steiner, A. A., and Turek, V. F. (2005). Fever and hypothermia in systemic inflammation: Recent discoveries and revisions. *Frontiers in Bioscience* 10, 2193–2216.
101. Rothwell, N. J., Stock, M. J., and Thexton, A. J. (1983). Decerebration activates thermogenesis in the rat. *Journal of Physiology* 342, 15–22.

102. Rusyniak, D. E., and Sprague, J. E. (2006). Hyperthermic Syndromes Induced by Toxins. *Clinics in Laboratory Medicine* 26, 165–184.
103. Samuels, B. C., Zaretsky, D. V., and Dimicco, J. A. (2004). Dorsomedial hypothalamic sites where disinhibition evokes tachycardia correlate with location of raphé-projecting neurons. *American Journal of Physiology. Regulatory, Integrative and Comparative Physiology* 287, R472–R478.
104. Schafer, S. S., and Schafer, S. (1973). The behavior of the proprioceptors of the muscle and the innervation of the fusimotor system during cold shivering. *Experimental Brain Research* 17, 364–380.
105. Shafton, A. D., Oldfield, B. J., and McAllen, R. M. (1992). CRF-like immunoreactivity selectively labels preganglionic sudomotor neurons in cat. *Brain Research* 599, 253–260.
106. Shibata, M., Benzi, R. H., Seydoux, J., and Girardier, L. (1987). Hyperthermia induced by pre-pontine knife-cut: Evidence for a tonic inhibition of non-shivering thermogenesis in anaesthetized rat. *Brain Research* 436, 273–282.
107. Shibata, M., Iriki, M., Arita, J., Kiyohara, T., Nakashima, T., Miyata, S., and Matsukawa, T. (1996). Procaine microinjection into the lower midbrain increases brown fat and body temperatures in anesthetized rats. *Brain Research* 716, 171–179.
108. Simon, E. (1974). Temperature regulation: The spinal cord as a site of extrahypothalamic thermoregulatory functions. *Reviews of Physiology, Biochemistry and Pharmacology* 71, 1–76.
109. Smith, J. E., Jansen, A. S., Gilbey, M. P., and Loewy, A. D. (1998). CNS cell groups projecting to sympathetic outflow of tail artery: Neural circuits involved in heat loss in the rat. *Brain Research* 786, 153–164.
110. Stornetta, R. L., Mcquiston, T. J., and Guyenet, P. G. (2004). GABAergic and glycinergic presympathetic neurons of rat medulla oblongata identified by retrograde transport of pseudorabies virus and in situ hybridization. *Journal of Comparative Neurology* 479, 257–270.
111. Tanaka, M., Owens, N. C., Nagashima, K., Kanosue, K., and McAllen, R. M. (2006). Reflex activation of rat fusimotor neurons by body surface cooling, and its dependence on the medullary raphé. *Journal of Physiology* 572, 569–583.
112. Thor, K. B., Blitz-Siebert, A., and Helke, C. J. (1990). Discrete localization of high-density 5-HT1A binding sites in the midline raphé and parapyramidal region of the ventral medulla oblongata of the rat. *Neuroscience Letters* 108, 249–254.
113. Toth, I. E., Toth, D. E., Boldogkoi, Z., Hornyak, A., Palkovits, M., and Blessing, W. W. (2006). Serotonin-synthesizing neurons in the rostral medullary raphé/parapyramidal region transneuronally labelled after injection of pseudorabies virus into the rat tail. *Neurochemical Research* 31, 277–286.
114. Werner, J. (1980). The concept of regulation of human body temperature. *Journal of Thermal Biology* 5, 75–82.
115. Yamagata, K., Matsumura, K., Inoue, W., Shiraki, T., Suzuki, K., Yasuda, S., Sugiura, H., Cao, C., Watanabe, Y., and Kobayashi, S. (2001). Coexpression of microsomal-type prostaglandin E synthase with cyclooxygenase-2 in brain endothelial cells of rats during endotoxin-induced fever. *Journal of Neuroscience* 21, 2669–2677.
116. Yoshida, K., Nakamura, K., Matsumura, K., Kanosue, K., Konig, M., Thiel, H. J., Boldogkoi, Z., Toth, I., Roth, J., Gerstberger, R., and Hubschle, T. (2003). Neurons of the rat preoptic area and the raphé pallidus nucleus innervating the brown adipose tissue express the prostaglandin E receptor subtype EP3. *European Journal of Neuroscience* 18, 1848–1860.
117. Yu, Y. H., and Blessing, W. W. (1997). Cutaneous vasoconstriction in conscious rabbits during alerting responses detected by hippocampal theta-rhythm. *American Journal of Physiology* 272, R208–R216.
118. Zaretskaia, M. V., Zaretsky, D. V., and Dimicco, J. A. (2003). Role of the dorsomedial hypothalamus in thermogenesis and tachycardia caused by microinjection of prostaglandin E2 into the preoptic area in anesthetized rats. *Neuroscience Letters* 340, 1–4.
119. Zaretskaia, M. V., Zaretsky, D. V., Shekhar, A., and Dimicco, J. A. (2002). Chemical stimulation of the dorsomedial hypothalamus evokes nonshivering thermogenesis in anesthetized rats. *Brain Research* 928, 113–125.
120. Zethof, T. J., Van Der Heyden, J. A., Tolboom, J. T., and Olivier, B. (1995). Stress-induced hyperthermia as a putative anxiety model. *European Journal of Pharmacology* 294, 125–135.
121. Zhang, Y. H., Hosono, T., Yanase-Fujiwara, M., Chen, X. M., and Kanosue, K. (1997). Effect of midbrain stimulations on thermoregulatory vasomotor responses in rats. *Journal of Physiology* 503, 177–186.
122. Zhang, Y. H., Yanase-Fujiwara, M., Hosono, T., and Kanosue, K. (1995). Warm and cold signals from the preoptic area: Which contribute more to the control of shivering in rats? *Journal of Physiology* 485, 195–202 .

19

# Autonomic Regulation of the Urinary Bladder and Urethra

WILLIAM C. DE GROAT

The functions of the lower urinary tract to store and periodically release urine are dependent upon neural circuitry in the brain and spinal cord[31,67]. This dependence on central nervous control distinguishes the lower urinary tract from many other visceral organs that maintain a certain level of activity even after elimination of extrinsic neural input. The lower urinary tract is also unusual because of the complexity of its neural regulation. For example, micturition depends on the integration of autonomic and somatic efferent mechanisms within the lumbosacral spinal cord. This integration is necessary to coordinate the activity of visceral organs (i.e., the bladder and urethra) with that of the striated muscles of the urethra. In addition, micturition is under voluntary control and depends upon learned behavior that develops during maturation of the nervous system. In contrast, many other visceral functions are regulated involuntarily. This chapter will review the central neural mechanisms controlling the lower urinary tract.

## INNERVATION OF THE LOWER URINARY TRACT

Storage and elimination of urine is dependent upon the coordinated activity of two functional units in the lower urinary tract: (1) a reservoir (the urinary bladder), and (2) an outlet, consisting of bladder neck, urethra, and striated muscles of the urethral sphincter[46]. These structures are, in turn, controlled by three sets of peripheral nerves: sacral parasympathetic (pelvic nerves), thoracolumbar sympathetic (hypogastric nerves and sympathetic chain), and sacral somatic nerves (pudendal nerves) (Figure 19–1).

## SACRAL PARASYMPATHETIC PATHWAYS

The sacral parasympathetic outflow provides the major excitatory input to the urinary bladder. Cholinergic parasympathetic preganglionic neurons located in the intermediolateral region of the sacral spinal cord[68] send axons via the pelvic nerves to ganglion cells in the pelvic plexus and in the wall of the bladder. Transmission in bladder ganglia is mediated by a nicotinic cholinergic mechanism, which can be modulated by activation of various receptors, including muscarinic cholinoceptors, adrenoceptors, purinoceptors, and peptide receptors[29]. The ganglion cells in turn excite bladder smooth muscle via the release of cholinergic (acetylcholine) and non-adrenergic, non-cholinergic transmitters. Cholinergic excitatory transmission in the bladder is mediated by muscarinic cholinoceptors; whereas non-cholinergic excitatory transmission is mediated by adenosine triphosphate (ATP), acting on P2X-type purinoceptors[17]. Muscarinic inhibitory and facilitatory receptors are also present on parasympathetic nerve terminals[87]. Inhibitory input to the urethral smooth muscle is mediated by nitric oxide released by parasympathetic nerves[46]. Both $M_2$ and $M_3$ muscarinic receptor subtypes are expressed in bladder smooth muscle. However, the $M_3$ subtype is the principal receptor involved in excitatory transmission in

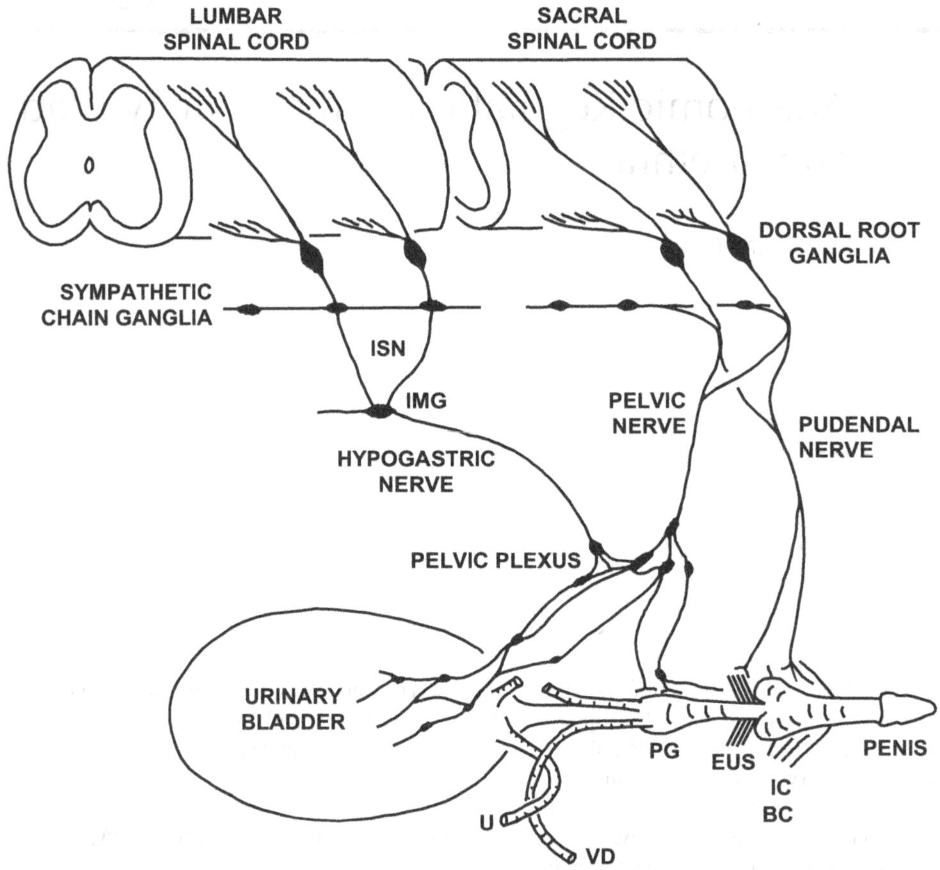


Figure 19–1 Sympathetic, parasympathetic and somatic innervation of the urogenital tract of the male cat. Axons of sympathetic preganglionic neurons emerge from the lumbar spinal cord and pass to the sympathetic chain ganglia and then via the inferior splanchnic nerves (ISN) to the inferior mesenteric ganglia (IMG). Preganglionic and post-ganglionic sympathetic axons travel in the hypogastric nerve to the pelvic plexus and the urogenital organs. Parasympathetic preganglionic axons, which originate in the sacral spinal cord, pass in the pelvic nerve to ganglion cells in the pelvic plexus and to distal ganglia in urogenital organs. Sacral somatic pathways travel via the pudendal nerve, which provides an innervation to the penis, the ischiocavernosus (IC), bulbocavernosus (BC) and external urethral sphincter (EUS) muscles. The pudendal and pelvic nerves also contain post-ganglionic axons from the caudal sympathetic chain ganglia. These three sets of nerves also contain afferent axons from the lumbosacral dorsal root ganglia. Ureter, U; prostate gland, PG; vas deferens, VD.

normal bladders[60]. In certain disease states, such as neurogenic bladder in humans, a functional role for $M_2$ receptors can emerge.

## THORACOLUMBAR SYMPATHETIC AND SACRAL SOMATIC EFFERENT PATHWAYS

Sympathetic pathways to the lower urinary tract, which originate in the lumbosacral sympathetic chain ganglia as well as in the prevertebral inferior mesenteric ganglia, pass to the bladder via the hypogastric and pelvic nerves. Sympathetic efferent pathways elicit various effects, including: (1) inhibition of the detrusor muscle via β-adrenoceptors; (2) excitation of the bladder base and urethra via $\alpha_1$-adrenoceptors[46]; and (3) inhibition and facilitation in bladder parasympathetic ganglia via $\alpha_2$- and $\alpha_1$-adrenoceptors, respectively[29,53].

The efferent innervation of the urethral striated muscles originates from neurons in a circumscribed region of the lateral ventral horn that is termed "Onuf's nucleus.' Sphincter motor neurons send their axons into the pudendal nerve and excite sphincter muscles via the release of acetylcholine that stimulates postjunctional nicotinic receptors on the muscle cells.

## AFFERENT PATHWAYS

Afferent axons innervating the urinary tract are present in the three sets of nerves[39,67]. The most important afferents for initiating micturition are those passing in the pelvic nerve to the sacral spinal cord. These afferents are small myelinated (Aδ) and unmyelinated (C) fibers, which convey information from receptors in the bladder wall to second-order neurons in the spinal cord. Aδ bladder afferents in the cat respond in a graded manner to passive distension as well as to active contraction of the bladder and exhibit pressure thresholds in the range of 5 mmHg to 15 mmHg, which are similar to the pressures at which humans report the first sensation of bladder filling. The Aδ fibers also code for noxious stimuli in the bladder. In contrast, unmyelinated C-fiber bladder afferents in the cat are insensitive to mechanical stimuli and commonly do not respond to even high levels of intravesical pressure. However, activity in these C-fiber afferents is unmasked by chemical irritation of the bladder mucosa. These findings indicate that C-fiber afferents in the cat have specialized functions, such as the signaling of inflammatory or noxious events in the lower urinary tract. In the rat, A-fiber and C-fiber bladder afferents cannot be distinguished on the basis of stimulus modality. Thus, both types of afferents consist of mechanosensitive and chemosensitive populations[39,67,85].

C-fiber bladder afferent neurons synthesize and release various neuropeptides, including calcitonin-gene-related peptide, vasoactive intestinal polypeptide, pituitary-adenylate cyclase-activating polypeptide, tachykinins (substance P and neurokinin A), galanin, and endothelin[67], and express receptors for some of these peptides. The C-fiber afferent neurons also express receptors for other substances, including acetylcholine, ATP, prostaglandins, and neurotrophic factors, that are released in the bladder by urothelial cells, efferent nerves, and inflammatory cells[2,75,110]. These substances modulate afferent nerve excitability and change the response of afferents to mechanical stimulation. Peptide-containing afferent axons project into the lumbosacral parasympathetic nucleus in the spinal cord. Since application of various neuropeptides to the spinal cord influences bladder activity, neuropeptides may be transmitters in the afferent pathways from the lower urinary tract[33,37]. The C-fiber afferents also express transient receptor potential (TRP) receptors [39,41,42,45], such as TRPV1[2], and therefore are sensitive to the neurotoxins capsaicin and resiniferatoxin[67,81].

The properties of lumbosacral dorsal root ganglion cells innervating the bladder, urethra, and external urethral sphincter in the rat and cat have been studied with patch clamp recording techniques[103–106]. Based on responsiveness to capsaicin, approximately 70% of bladder afferent neurons in the rat are likely to be of the C-fiber type. These neurons have high threshold tetrodotoxin-resistant sodium channels[103,105] and produce action potentials and phasic firing (one to two spikes) in response to prolonged depolarizing current pulses[80,81,104]. A-fiber afferent neurons are resistant to capsaicin, have low-threshold tetrodotoxin-sensitive sodium channels, and produce action potentials and tonic firing (multiple spikes) to depolarizing current pulses. Approximately 90% of the bladder afferent neurons also are excited by ATP, which induces depolarization and firing through activation of $P2X_3$ or $P2X_{2/3}$ receptors[111].

## UROTHELIUM

The urothelium, which has been traditionally viewed as a passive barrier, also has specialized sensory and signaling properties that allow it to respond to chemical and mechanical stimuli and to engage in reciprocal chemical communication with neighboring nerves in the bladder wall[9,26,67] (Figure 19–2). These properties include: (1) expression of adrenoceptors as well as nicotinic, muscarinic, tachykinin, and capsaicin (TRPV1) receptors[6,9–11]; (2) responsiveness to transmitters released from sensory nerves; (3) close physical association with afferent nerves; and (4) ability to release chemical mediators, such as ATP[43], acetylcholine[49,101], and nitric oxide, that can regulate the activity of adjacent nerves and thereby trigger local vascular changes and/or reflex bladder contractions.

The role of ATP in communication between the urothelium and afferent nerves has attracted considerable attention because bladder distension releases ATP from the urothelium[43], and intravesical administration of ATP induces bladder hyperactivity by stimulating purinergic $P2X_3$ or $P2X_{2/3}$ receptors on afferent nerves [45,67,71,76,110]. Mice in which the $P2X_3$ receptor is knocked out exhibit hypoactive bladders and inefficient voiding, suggesting that normal bladder function depends upon activation of $P2X_3$ receptors on bladder afferent nerves by ATP released from the urothelium[21]. In humans and cats with interstitial cystitis, a painful bladder condition, ATP release from urothelial cells is enhanced[7,94]. Higher levels of ATP may induce abnormal firing of afferent nerves, and pain.

The presence of muscarinic and nicotinic cholinoceptors in the urothelium has focused attention on the role of acetylcholine as a chemical mediator of interactions between nerves and the urothelium.

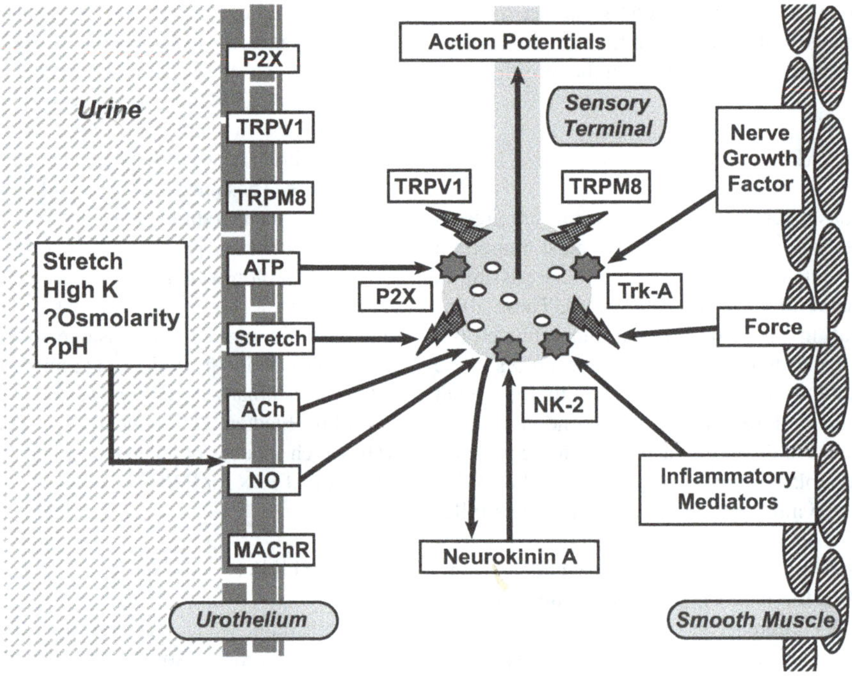


Figure 19–2 Receptors on urothelium and sensory nerve endings in the bladder mucosa and chemical mediators that can modulate the excitability of mucosal sensory nerves. Urothelial cells and sensory nerves express common receptors (P2X, TRPV1, and TRPM8). Distension of the bladder activates stretch receptors and triggers the release of urothelial transmitters, such as ATP, acetylcholine (ACh), and nitric oxide (NO), that may interact with adjacent nerves. Receptors in afferent nerves or the urothelium can respond to changes in pH, osmolality, high K+ concentration, chemicals in the urine, or inflammatory mediators released in the bladder wall. Neuropeptides (neurokinin A) released from sensory nerves in response to distension or chemical stimulation can act on NK-2 autoreceptors to sensitize the mechanosensitive nerve endings. The smooth muscle can generate force which may influence some mucosal endings. Nerve growth factor released from muscle or urothelium can exert an acute and chronic influence on the excitability of sensory nerves via an action on Trk-A receptors. ACh, acetylcholine; MAChR, muscarinic receptor; TRPV1, transient receptor potential vanilloid receptor 1 that is sensitive to capsaicin; TRPM8, menthol/cold receptor; NO, nitric oxide, Trk-A, tyrosine kinase A receptor.

Urothelial cells express the various proteins necessary for the synthesis and storage of acetylcholine, including the plasma membrane choline transporter, choline acetyltransferase, and the vesicular acetylcholine transporter, as well as the enzyme responsible for the metabolism of acetylcholine (acetylcholinesterase). Chemical or mechanical stimuli have also been reported to release acetylcholine from the bladder urothelium in rats and humans[26,27,49,101], and experiments using the reverse transcriptase polymerase chain reaction have revealed the expression of multiple subtypes of nicotinic ($\alpha 7$, $\alpha 3$, $\beta 4$, and $\beta 5$)[6] and muscarinic cholinoceptors ($M_1$–$M_5$) in rat urothelial cells[51,55]. In addition, exogenous muscarinic and nicotinic agonists applied to cultured urothelial cells elicit an increase in the concentration of intracellular $Ca^{+2}$ and evoke the release of nitric oxide and ATP. Intravesical administration of muscarinic as well as nicotinic receptor agonists or anticholinesterase agents that increase the levels of endogenous acetylcholine facilitates reflex bladder activity in rats and cats[6,27,56]. Thus, the clinical effect of antimuscarinic agents to decrease sensory symptoms in overactive bladder may be related to blockade of muscarinic receptors in the urothelium or afferent nerves.

## ANATOMY OF CENTRAL NERVOUS PATHWAYS CONTROLLING THE LOWER URINARY TRACT

The reflex circuitry controlling micturition consists of four basic components: primary afferent neurons, spinal efferent neurons, spinal interneurons, and neurons in the brain that modulate spinal reflex pathways.

## Pathways in the Spinal Cord

### Afferent Projections in the Spinal Cord

Afferent pathways from the bladder project into Lissauer's tract at the apex of the dorsal horn and then send collaterals laterally and medially around the dorsal horn into spinal cord laminae V–VII and X at the base of the dorsal horn (Figure 19–3A)[31,88]. The lateral pathway terminates in the region of the sacral parasympathetic nucleus, and some axons also travel to the dorsal commissure (Figure 19–3A).

### Efferent Neurons

Parasympathetic preganglionic neurons are located in the intermediolateral gray matter (laminae V–VII) in the sacral segments of the spinal cord (Figure 19–4)[68], whereas sympathetic preganglionic neurons are located in medial (lamina X) and lateral sites (laminae V–VII) in the rostral lumbar spinal cord. Motor neurons supplying the external urethral sphincter are located in lamina IX in Onuf's nucleus in the cat and in the dorsolateral motor nucleus in the rat (Figure 19–4).

Parasympathetic preganglionic neurons are commonly spindle-shaped with dendrites projecting to four major areas: (1) the lateral and dorsolateral funiculus, (2) lamina I on the lateral edge of the dorsal horn, (3) the dorsal gray commissure, and (4) the gray matter and lateral funiculus ventral to the sacral parasympathetic nucleus (Figure 19–4)[66]. These dendritic projections may be the location of the major synaptic inputs to the preganglionic neurons; i.e., lamina I dendrites receiving primary afferent projections, dendrites in the lateral funiculus receiving bulbospinal projections[64], and medial dendrites receiving interneuronal

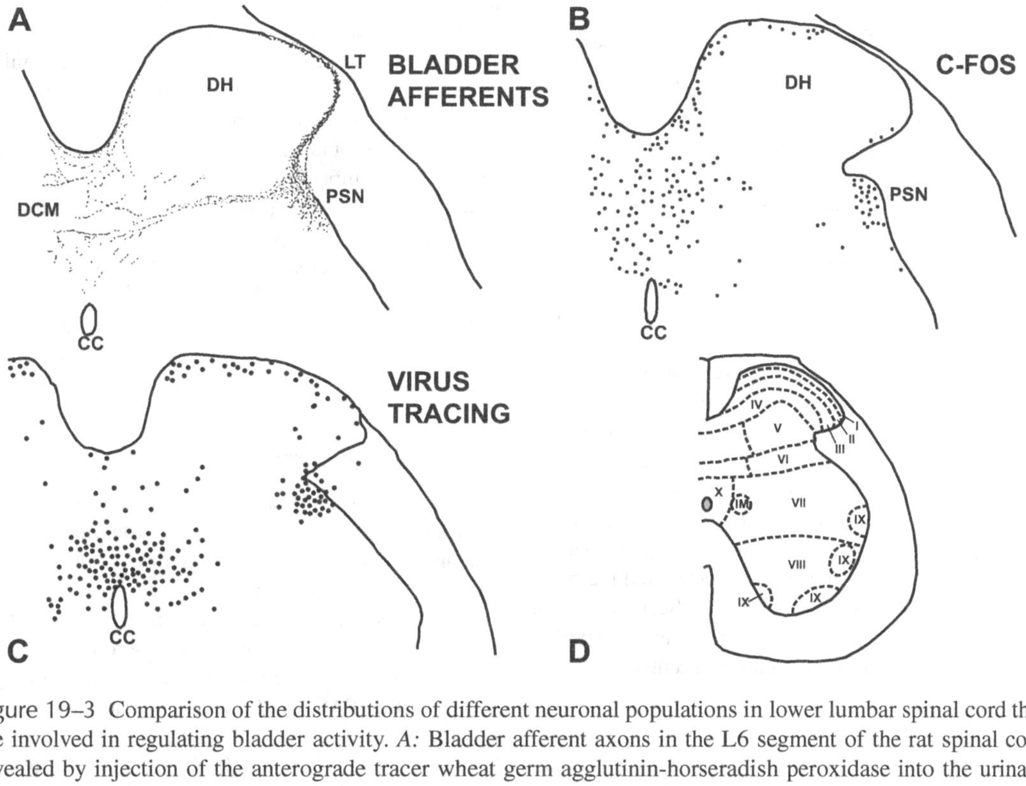


Figure 19–3 Comparison of the distributions of different neuronal populations in lower lumbar spinal cord that are involved in regulating bladder activity. *A:* Bladder afferent axons in the L6 segment of the rat spinal cord revealed by injection of the anterograde tracer wheat germ agglutinin-horseradish peroxidase into the urinary bladder, which labels the central processes of sensory neurons that innervate the bladder. *B:* Distribution of neurons in the L6 segment of the rat spinal cord that show Fos-immunoreactivity in their nuclei following chemical irritation of the lower urinary tract. *C:* Distribution of interneurons in the L6 segment of the rat spinal cord that were labeled by transneuronal transport of pseudorabies virus injected into the urinary bladder. *D:* Diagram showing the laminar organization of the cat spinal cord. DH, dorsal horn; PSN, sacral parasympathetic nucleus; CC, central canal; DCM, dorsal gray commissure.

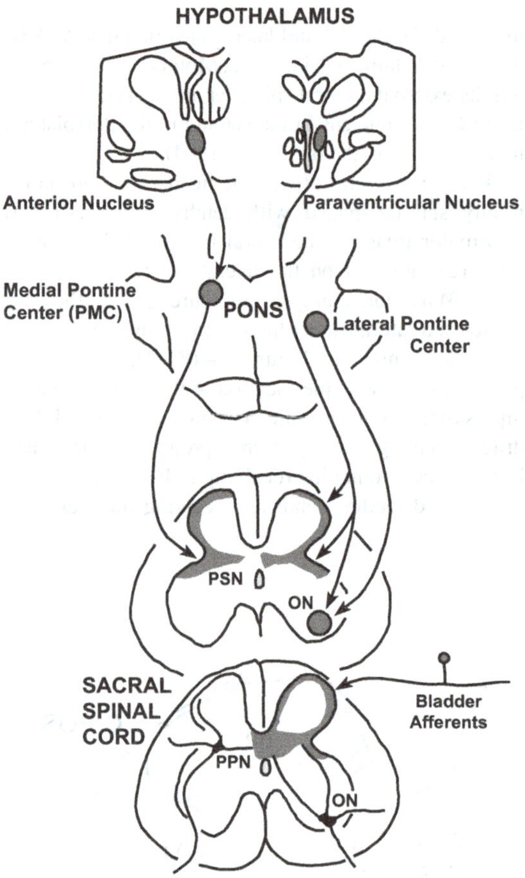


Figure 19–4 Neural connections between the brain and the sacral spinal cord that may regulate the lower urinary tract in the cat. Lower section showing the sacral spinal cord shows the location and morphology of a preganglionic neuron in the sacral parasympathetic nucleus (PSN), a sphincter motor neuron in Onuf's nucleus (ON), and the sites of central termination of afferent projections (*shaded area*) from the urinary bladder. Upper section of the sacral cord shows the sites of termination (*shaded areas*) of descending pathways arising from the medial pontine micturition center (PMC), the lateral pontine sphincter or urine storage center, and the paraventricular nuclei of the hypothalamus. Section through the pons shows the projection from the anterior hypothalamic nuclei to the pontine micturition center.

projections from the dorsal commissure and inputs from the contralateral side of the spinal cord. Motor neurons controlling the external urethral sphincter have a similar dendritic pattern (Figure 19–4).

The most striking feature of the sacral preganglionic neurons in the cat is an extensive axon collateral system that projects bilaterally to various regions of the dorsal and ventral horns, including the area around the central canal, the intermediolateral gray matter, the dorsal commissure, and the lateral dorsal horn[66]. These axon collaterals activate interneurons that are involved in a bilateral recurrent inhibitory pathway that provides negative feedback control of the parasympathetic outflow to the bladder[23].

## *Spinal Interneurons*

Interneurons retrogradely labeled by injection of pseudorabies virus into the urinary bladder or urethra of the rat (Figure 19–3C) are located in regions of the spinal cord receiving afferent input from the bladder. Large populations of interneurons are located just dorsal and medial to the preganglionic neurons as well as in the dorsal commissure and lamina I[69,93,99]. Interneurons in these locations make excitatory and inhibitory synaptic connections with parasympathetic preganglionic neurons[3,4,28,65].

The spinal neurons involved in processing afferent input from the lower urinary tract have been identified by the expression of the immediate early gene, *c-fos* (Figure 19–3B). In the rat, chemical or mechanical stimulation of the bladder and urethra increases the levels of Fos protein primarily in the dorsal commissure, the superficial dorsal horn, and the area of the sacral parasympathetic nucleus (Figure 19–3B)[8]. Some of these interneurons make local connections in the spinal cord and participate in segmental spinal reflexes[3,4,28,65]; whereas others send long projections to supraspinal centers, such as the periaqueductal gray (PAG), Barrington's nucleus, the hypothalamus and thalamus, that are involved in the control of micturition[12,50].

## *Pathways in the Brain*

In the rat, transneuronal virus tracing methods have identified many populations of neurons in the brain that are involved in the control of the bladder, urethra, and urethral sphincter. These areas include Barrington's nucleus (the pontine micturition center), medullary raphé nuclei that contain serotonergic neurons, the locus coeruleus that contains noradrenergic neurons, the PAG, and the A5 noradrenergic cell group (Figure 19–5)[69,93,99]. Several regions in the hypothalamus and the cerebral cortex also contained virus-infected neurons. Trans-synaptically labeled cortical neurons were located primarily in the medial frontal cortex.

Other anatomical studies in which anterograde tracers were injected into brain areas and then identified in terminals in the spinal cord (Figure 19–4) are

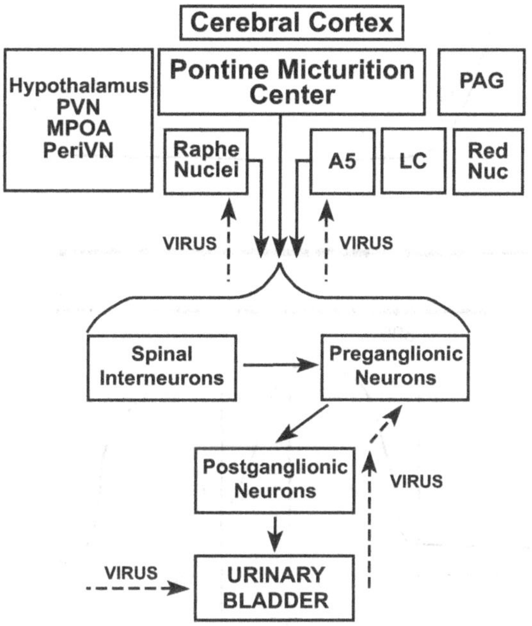


Figure 19–5 Trans-synaptic labeling of central neurons after injection of pseudorabies virus into the urinary bladder or the urethra Virus is transported transneuronally in a retrograde direction (*dashed arrows*). Normal synaptic connections are indicated by *solid arrows*. The pattern of trans-synaptic viral labeling is the same in neonatal and adult rats. At long survival times, the virus can be detected in neurons at specific sites in the spinal cord and brain, extending to the pontine micturition center in the pons (i.e., Barrington's nucleus) and to the cerebral cortex. Other sites in the brain labeled by the virus are: (*1*) the paraventricular nucleus (PVN), medial preoptic area (MPOA) and periventricular nucleus (Peri.V.N.) of the hypothalamus, (*2*) periaqueductal gray (PAG), (*3*) locus coeruleus (LC) and subcoeruleus, (*4*) red nucleus, (*5*) medullary raphé nuclei, and (*6*) the noradrenergic cell group designated as A5.

consistent with the virus tracing data. Tracer injected into the paraventricular nucleus of the hypothalamus labeled axons in the sacral parasympathetic nucleus as well as axons within Onuf's nucleus[50]. On the other hand, neurons in the anterior hypothalamus project to the pontine micturition center. Neurons in the pontine micturition center in turn project primarily to the sacral parasympathetic nucleus, the lateral edge of the dorsal horn, and the dorsal commissure. These areas contain the dendrites of parasympathetic preganglionic neurons, sphincter motor neurons (Onuf's nucleus), and the central processes of primary afferent neurons innervating the bladder (Figure 19.4). Conversely, projections from neurons in the lateral pons in the cat, an area implicated in the control of the urethral sphincter, terminate rather selectively in the Onuf's nucleus. Thus, the sites of termination of descending projections from the pons are optimally located to regulate reflex mechanisms at the spinal level.

## CENTRAL NERVOUS SYSTEM CONTROL OF THE LOWER URINARY TRACT

### Activity of the Lower Urinary Tract During Storage and Voiding

The neural pathways controlling lower urinary tract function are organized as simple on–off switching circuits (Figures 19.6 and 19.7) that maintain an inverse relationship between the urinary bladder and urethral outlet[22]. Intravesical pressure measurements during bladder filling in both humans and animals reveal low and relatively constant bladder pressures when bladder volume is below the threshold for inducing voiding (Figure 19–6). The accommodation of the bladder to increasing volumes of urine is primarily a passive phenomenon dependent upon the intrinsic properties of the vesical smooth muscle and quiescence of the parasympathetic efferent pathway. In some species, urine storage is also facilitated by sympathetic reflexes that inhibit bladder activity, close the bladder neck, and contract the proximal urethra (Figure 19–7A). During bladder filling, the activity of the sphincter muscle (as indicated by the sphincter electromyogram) also increases (Figure 19–6), reflecting an increase in efferent firing in the pudendal nerve and an increase in outlet resistance that contributes to the maintenance of urinary continence.

Urine storage can be switched to voiding either involuntarily (Figure 19–6A) or voluntarily. Involuntary voiding is readily demonstrated in the human infant (Figure 19–6A) and is initiated when the volume of urine exceeds the pressure threshold for a micturition reflex. At this point, increased afferent firing from tension receptors in the bladder produces firing in the sacral parasympathetic pathways and inhibition of sympathetic and somatic pathways. The expulsion phase consists of an initial relaxation of the urethral sphincter (Figure 19–6A) followed by a contraction of the bladder, an increase in bladder pressure and a flow of urine. Relaxation of the urethral outlet is mediated by activation of a parasympathetic reflex pathway to the urethra that triggers the release of an inhibitory transmitter, nitric oxide[46], as well as by removal of adrenergic and somatic excitatory inputs to the urethra that are mediated by lumbar sympathetic and sacral pudendal nerves, respectively[67].

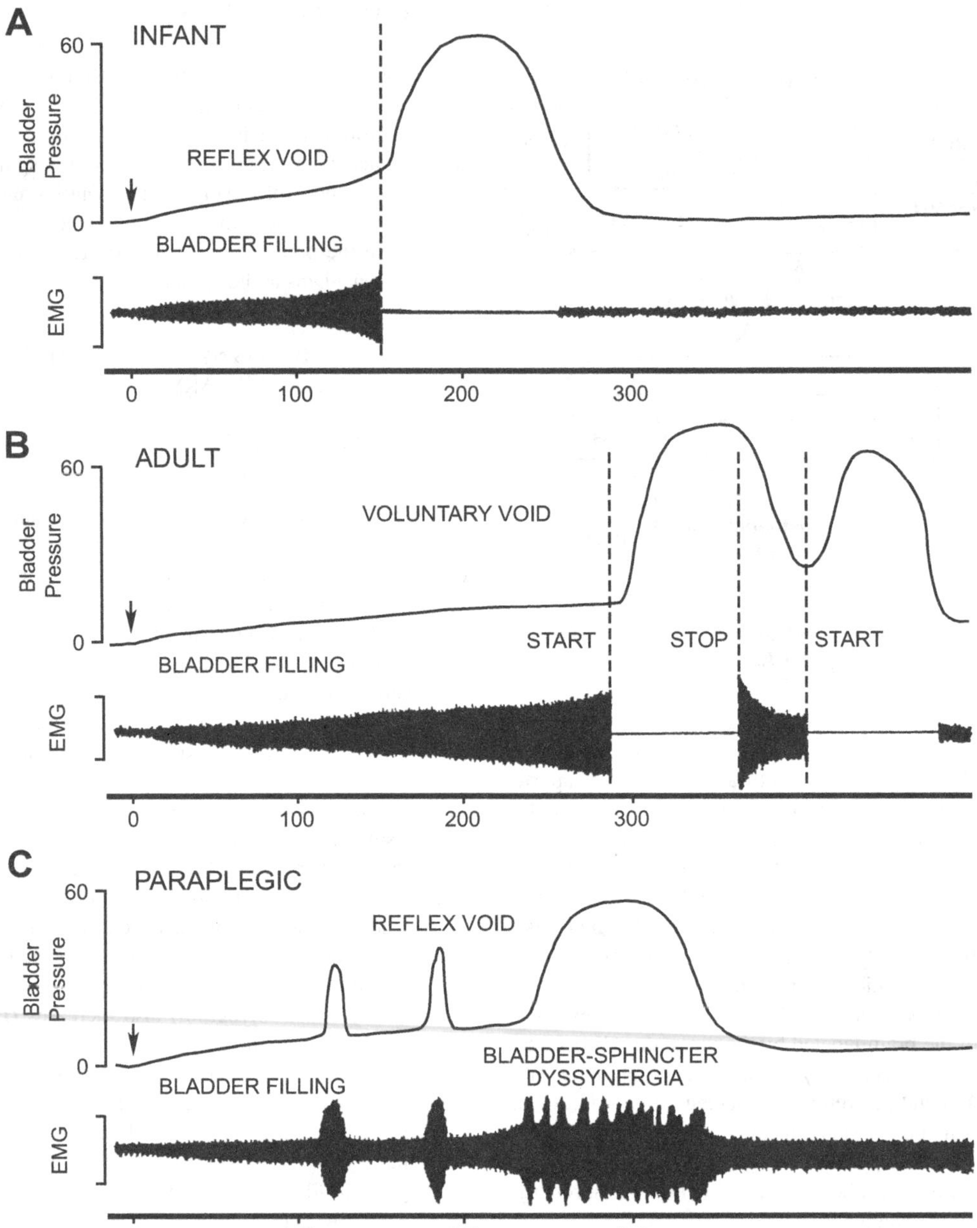


Figure 19–6 Comparison of voiding responses in an infant, an adult with an intact spinal cord, and an adult with a spinal cord injury Cystometrograms and sphincter electromyograms from an infant. (*A*), and adult with an intact spinal cord (*B*) and a paraplegic adult (*C*). The abscissa in all records represents bladder volume in milliliters; the ordinates represent bladder pressure in cm $H_2O$ and electrical activity of the electromyogram recording (EMG). On the *left side* of each trace, the *arrows* indicate the start of a slow infusion of fluid into the bladder (bladder filling). *Vertical dashed lines* indicate the start of sphincter relaxation, which precedes by a few seconds the bladder contraction in *A* and *B*. In an infant (*A*), increasing bladder pressure triggers reflex voiding, which is accompanied by sphincter relaxation as indicated by cessation of EMG activity. In an adult (*B*), voluntary cessation of voiding (stop) is associated with an initial increase in sphincter EMG followed by a reciprocal relaxation of the bladder. A resumption of voiding is again associated with sphincter relaxation and a delayed increase in bladder pressure. In the paraplegic patient (*C*), the reciprocal relationship between bladder and sphincter is abolished. During bladder filling, transient uninhibited bladder contractions occur in association with sphincter activity. Further filling leads to more prolonged and simultaneous contractions of the bladder and sphincter (bladder-sphincter dyssynergia). Loss of the reciprocal relationship between bladder and sphincter in paraplegic patients interferes with bladder emptying.

## Storage Mechanisms

### *Sympathetic Storage Reflex*

Although the integrity of the sympathetic input to the lower urinary tract is not essential for micturition, it does contribute to the storage function of the bladder. Surgical interruption or pharmacological blockade of the sympathetic innervation can reduce urethral outflow resistance, reduce bladder capacity, and increase the frequency and amplitude of bladder contractions recorded under constant-volume conditions[31].

Sympathetic reflex activity is elicited by a sacrolumbar intersegmental spinal reflex pathway that is triggered by vesical afferent activity in the pelvic nerves (Figure 19–7A)[34]. The reflex pathway is inhibited when bladder pressure is raised to the threshold for producing micturition (Figure 19–7B). This inhibitory response is abolished by transection of the spinal cord at the lower thoracic level, indicating that it originates at a supraspinal site, possibly the pontine micturition center. Thus, the vesicosympathetic reflex represents a negative feedback mechanism (Figure 19–7A); it allows the bladder to accommodate larger volumes during bladder filling but is turned off during voiding to allow the bladder to empty completely.

### *Urethral Sphincter Storage Reflex*

Motor neurons innervating the striated muscles of the external urethral sphincter exhibit a tonic discharge that increases during bladder filling. This activity is mediated in part by a spinal reflex pathway activated by low-level afferent input from the bladder (Figure 19–7A). Studies in cats have suggested that neurons in the ventrolateral region of the pontine reticular formation provide a tonic excitatory input to the motor neurons supplying the external urethral sphincter[50]. Electrical stimulation in this region (termed the *pontine urine storage center*, Figure 19–7A) excites the external urethral sphincter motor neurons. During micturition, the firing of sphincter motor neurons is inhibited (Figure 19–7B). This inhibition is dependent in part on supraspinal mechanisms since it is less prominent in animals with chronic spinal cord injuries[32].

## Voiding Mechanisms

### *Spinobulbospinal Micturition Reflex Pathway*

Voiding, which can be initiated voluntarily or reflexively, is mediated by activation of the sacral parasympathetic efferent pathway to the bladder and urethra as well as reciprocal inhibition of the somatic pathway to the urethral sphincter (Figure 19–7B). In contrast to storage mechanisms that are dependent on spinal reflex pathways, voiding is dependent on neural circuitry in the brain and spinal cord[22,36]. Studies in cats using brain lesioning and electrophysiological techniques have revealed that reflex micturition is mediated by a spinobulbospinal pathway that passes through the pontine micturition center in the rostral brainstem (Figures 19.5 and 19.7B). In the cat, the ascending limb of the reflex originates from spinal tract neurons in the sacral spinal cord that are activated by afferent input from the bladder[12,35,62]. These neurons send information via axons in the lateral funiculus to a relay station in the PAG that in turn provides an excitatory input to the pontine micturition center[13,50]. In the rat, ascending projections from the spinal cord also terminate directly in the pontine micturition center[40]. Additional bladder sensory inputs to the brain are carried by the spinothalamic tract, the spinohypothalamic tract, and dorsal column pathways to the gracile nucleus.

Single-unit recordings in the pontine micturition center of the cat and rat revealed several populations of neurons with firing patterns that correlate with reflex bladder contractions[28,78,79,91,92,96], including: (1) neurons that are silent in the absence of bladder activity but fire prior to and during reflex bladder contractions (called *direct neurons*), (2) neurons that are active during the period between bladder contractions and are inhibited during contractions (called *inverse neurons*), and (3) neurons that fire transiently at the beginning and end of bladder contractions (called *on-off neurons*). Subpopulations of direct and inverse neurons were also identified based on slow changes in firing during and between bladder contractions[78]. A large percentage of direct neurons project to the lumbosacral spinal cord; whereas only a small percentage of inverse neurons send axons to the cord. Thus, inverse neurons may function as local inhibitory neurons in the pontine micturition center. Both direct and inverse neurons exhibit excitatory synaptic responses to electrical stimulation of afferent axons in the pelvic nerve[28].

Pharmacological and electrophysiological studies indicate that circuitry in the pontine micturition center allows the spinobulbospinal micturition reflex pathway to function as a switch that is either in a completely "off" mode (storage) or maximally "on" mode (voiding). During bladder filling, the parasympathetic efferent pathway to the bladder, including the population of direct neurons in the pontine micturition center, is turned off; but at a critical level of bladder distension, afferent activity arising from tension receptors in the bladder switches the pathway to maximal activity[28,30,91]. Drugs injected into the pontine micturition center can change the set-point (bladder volume threshold) for activation of the switch without altering the magnitude of the micturition reflex measured as the amplitude of voiding contractions[59]. Similarly, lesions in the brain rostral to the pons

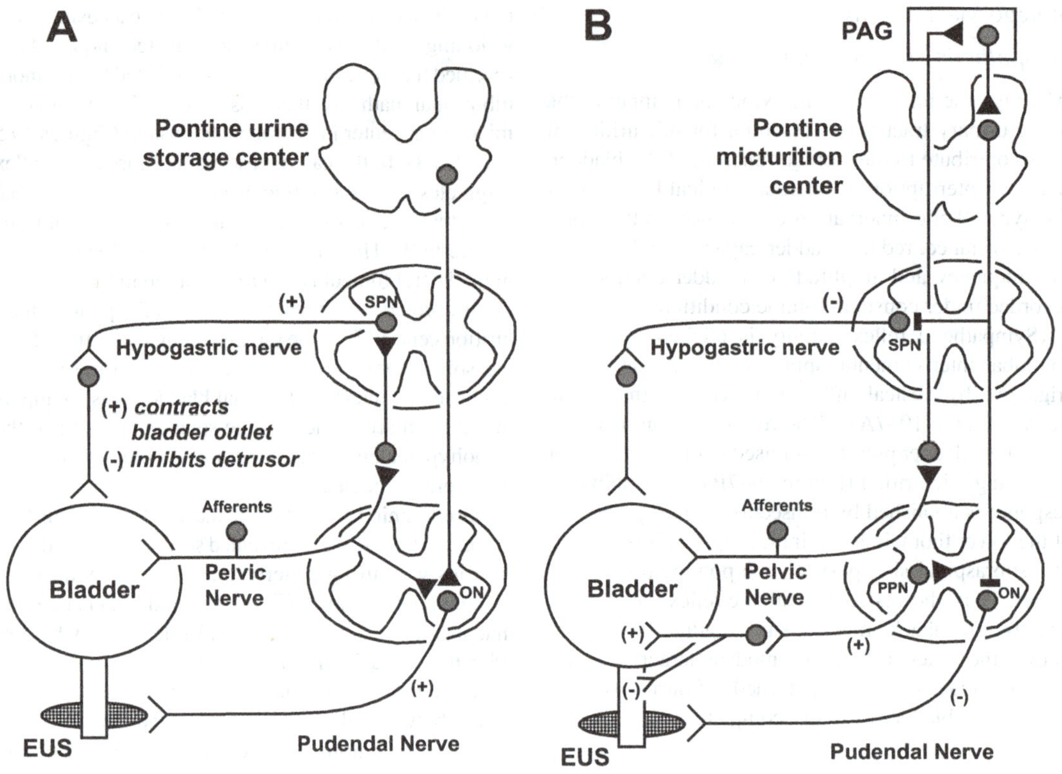


Figure 19–7 Nerve pathways controlling urine storage and voiding. *A:* Urine storage. During the storage of urine, distention of the bladder produces a low level of firing in vesical afferent axons, which in turn stimulates (1) the sympathetic outflow to the bladder outlet (base and urethra) and (2) pudendal outflow to the external urethral sphincter (EUS). These responses occur by spinal reflex pathways and represent guarding reflexes, which promote continence. Sympathetic firing also inhibits the detrusor muscle and modulates transmission in bladder ganglia. A region in the rostral pons (the pontine urine storage center) increases activity of the EUS. *B:* Voiding reflexes. During elimination of urine, intense firing of bladder afferents activates spinobulbospinal reflex pathways passing through the pontine micturition center, resulting in stimulation of the parasympathetic outflow to the bladder and urethral smooth muscle and inhibition of the sympathetic and pudendal outflows to the urethral outlet. Ascending afferent input from the spinal cord may pass through relay neurons in the periaqueductal gray (PAG) before reaching the pontine micturition center. (+) or ▶, excitatory mechanisms or synapses; (-) or ⊢, inhibitory mechanisms or synapses. ON, motor neurons in Onuf's nucleus; PPN, parasympathetic preganglionic neurons; SPN, sympathetic preganglionic neurons

(e.g., diencephalon and cerebral cortex) can alter the set-point of the micturition reflex, indicating that the switching circuit in the pontine micturition center is tonically modulated by inhibitory and excitatory influences from the forebrain.

Analysis of reflex bladder contractions and electrical activity in bladder post-ganglionic nerves has provided strong support for the view that the micturition reflex is mediated by a pathway passing through a switching center in the rostral pons (Figure 19–7B). Reflex micturition can be elicited in adult cats and rats with an intact neuraxis or following supracollicular decerebration but not following lesions in the pontine micturition center or acute transection of the neuraxis at any point caudal to the pontine micturition center[22,35,36]. Stimulation of bladder afferents evokes long latency discharges (120 ms–150 ms) in bladder post-ganglionic nerves; these discharges persist after supracollicular decerebration but are eliminated by spinal cord transection. Afferent nerve stimulation also evokes neuronal firing in the pontine micturition center at latencies from 30 ms to 40 ms, and electrical stimulation in the pontine micturition center evokes bladder contractions and post-ganglionic nerve firing at latencies of 60 ms to 75 ms [22,72]. The sum of the latencies of the putative ascending (afferent-pontine) and descending limbs (pontine-efferent) of the reflex approximate the latency of the entire reflex pathway. Electrical stimulation of afferent axons in the pelvic nerve evokes potentials in the PAG at shorter latency than the evoked potentials in the pontine micturition center[72]. These data support the conclusion from axonal tracing studies in the cat[50] suggesting that the ascending limb of the micturition reflex passes through a relay center in the PAG prior to reaching the pontine micturition center.

### *Suprapontine Control of Micturition*

Lesioning and electrical stimulation studies indicate that voluntary control of micturition depends on connections between the frontal cortex, hypothalamus, and other forebrain structures, including the anterior cingulate gyrus, amygdala, bed nucleus of the stria terminalis, and septal nuclei, where electrical stimulation elicits excitatory bladder responses[1,31]. Damage to the cerebral cortex, due to tumors, aneurysms, or cerebrovascular disease, appears to remove inhibitory control of the pontine micturition center, resulting in bladder overactivity. Pharmacological studies in rats indicate that decerebration or brain damage induced by occlusion of the middle cerebral artery induces bladder overactivity, in part by eliminating tonic glutamatergic and dopaminergic inhibitory mechanisms and unmasking a dopaminergic excitatory mechanism[100].

Human brain-imaging studies (Figure 19–8) using single photon emission computed tomography, positron emission tomography, and functional magnetic resonance imaging have examined the areas of the brain involved in the control of micturition[5,15,44,48,52]. Some studies evaluated the brain areas responsible for the perception of bladder fullness and the sensation of the desire to void during bladder filling[5]. Others have examined brain activity during micturition[15,16,73], voluntary contractions of the pelvic floor during urine withholding[14], or during cold stimulation of the bladder[61]. Studies using positron emission tomography revealed that two cortical areas, the dorsolateral prefrontal cortex and the anterior cingulate gyrus, were active during voiding (i.e., exhibited increased blood flow). The hypothalamus, including the preoptic area, as well as the pons and the PAG, also showed activity in concert with voluntary micturition. Other positron emission tomography studies that examined the changes in brain activity during filling of the bladder revealed that increased activity occurred in the PAG, the midline pons, the mid-cingulate gyrus, and bilaterally in the frontal lobes. These results are consistent with the notion that the PAG receives information about bladder fullness and then relays this information to other brain areas involved in the control of urine storage.

The prefrontal cortex is thought to be the seat of planning of complex behaviors. Its role in micturition may be to make a decision as to whether or not micturition should take place at a particular time or place[44,52]. On the other hand, the anterior cingulate is a part of the limbic system and is thought to be involved in cognitive processes requiring attention and executive control. Thus, the anterior cingulate cortex may influence how much attention one pays to signals coming from the bladder and how one reacts to them: such as deciding to void or activating mechanisms (e.g., urethral sphincter contraction) to postpone voiding. Single photon emission computed tomography in patients with urgency incontinence revealed hypoperfusion of the anterior cingulate gyrus as well as other frontal lobe regions, such as the prefrontal cortex[44,45]. This may reflect weaker activation of inhibitory circuits in these regions, leading to symptoms of overactive bladder.

### *Spinal Micturition Reflex Pathways*

Spinal-cord injury rostral to the lumbosacral level eliminates voluntary and supraspinal control of voiding. This loss of control leads initially to an areflexic bladder and complete urinary retention, followed by a slow development of automatic micturition and bladder hyperactivity (Figure 19–6C) mediated by spinal reflex pathways. However, voiding is commonly inefficient due to simultaneous contractions of the bladder and urethral sphincter (bladder-sphincter dyssynergia) (Figure 19–6C). Electrophysiological studies in animals have shown that the spinal micturition reflex is mediated by a spinal segmental pathway that has a short central delay of approximately 5 ms and is triggered by a C-fiber afferent limb (Figure 19–9). This fast reflex contrasts with the spinobulbospinal micturition reflex in normal animals that occurs after a much longer central delay (60 ms–70 ms) and in response to myelinated Aδ afferent input from the bladder (Figure 19–9). In normal cats, capsaicin, a neurotoxin known to disrupt the function of C-fiber afferents, did not block reflex contractions of the bladder or the bladder reflex evoked by Aδ fibers. However, in cats with chronic spinal injury, capsaicin completely blocked bladder reflexes evoked by C fibers[20,33]. Evidence of the contribution of C-fiber bladder afferents to bladder hyperactivity and involuntary voiding in humans has been obtained from studies in which capsaicin or resiniferatoxin, another C-fiber afferent neurotoxin, were administered intravesically to patients with neurogenic detrusor overactivity due to multiple sclerosis or spinal cord injuries[44]. In these patients the toxins increased bladder capacity and reduced the frequency of incontinence.

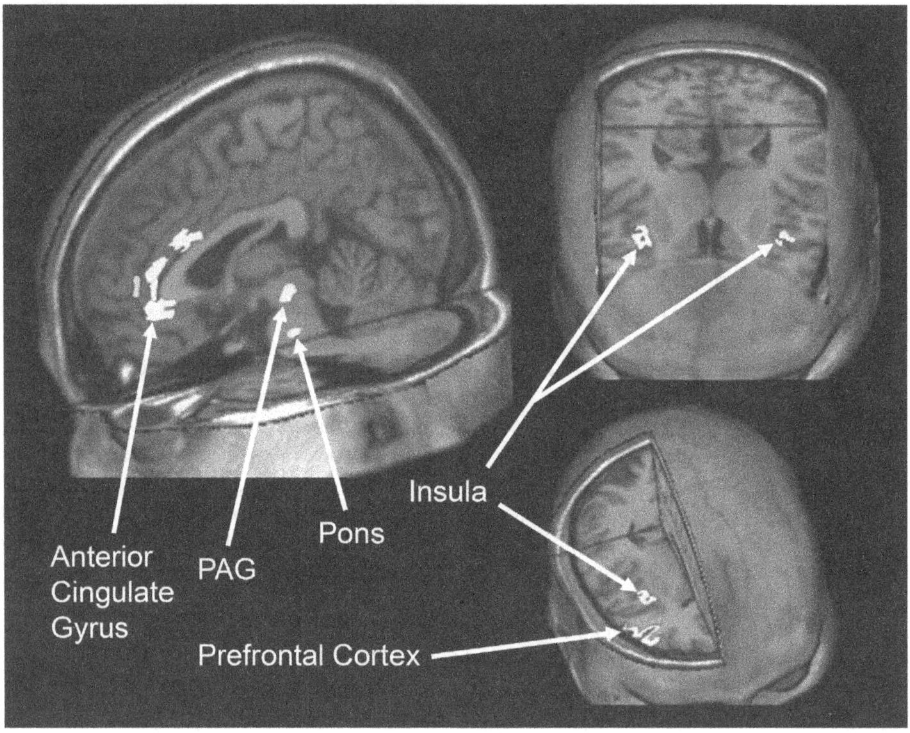


Figure 19–8 Summary of regions of interest comparing "full vs. empty" bladder conditions in humans. Based on the five studies using positron emission tomography[5,15,16,61,73]. Figure created using MRIcro software (www.mricro.com77). PAG, periaqueductal gray. Reproduced from Kavia et al. (2005)[52], with permission.

Several mechanisms seem to underlie the emergence of bladder reflexes mediated by C-fibers. These mechanisms include changes in central synaptic connections and alterations in the properties of the peripheral afferent receptors that lead to sensitization of the "silent" C fibers and the unmasking of responses to mechanical stimuli[38,98]. In rats, bladder afferent neurons undergo both morphological (i.e., neuronal hypertrophy)[88] and physiological changes (i.e., up-regulation of tetrodotoxin-sensitive $Na^+$ channels and down-regulation of tetrodotoxin-resistant $Na^+$ channels) following spinal cord injury or urethral outlet obstruction[103]. This neuronal plasticity may be mediated by the actions of neurotrophic factors, such as nerve growth factor released within the spinal cord or the urinary bladder[58,89,90,98]. The production of neurotrophic factors, including nerve growth factor, increases in the bladder after spinal cord injury[98], and chronic administration of nerve growth factor into the bladder of rats induces bladder hyperactivity and increases the firing frequency of dissociated bladder afferent neurons[38,102]. On the other hand, intrathecal application of antibodies against nerve growth factor, which bind nerve growth factor and neutralize its actions in the spinal cord, suppresses detrusor hyperreflexia and detrusor-sphincter dyssynergia in spinal-cord-injured rats[83,84].

Spinal cord injury in cats and rats also causes the reemergence of a neonatal exteroceptive micturition reflex that is activated by tactile stimulation of cutaneous afferent axons in the perineum (i.e., the perineal-to-bladder reflex)[25]. In neonatal animals, this reflex is activated by the mother licking the perineal region of the young animal. The stimulation is essential for survival of the neonate, because isolation of the newborn from its mother leads to urinary retention. The adult form of reflex voiding, which is triggered by bladder distension, does not become functional until several weeks after birth. As the adult reflex is appearing, the neonatal perineal-to-bladder reflex becomes progressively weaker and eventually disappears[35]. Thus, postnatal maturation of voiding function is associated with a prominent reorganization of synaptic connections in bladder reflex pathways, leading to down-regulation of primitive spinal mechanisms and up-regulation of mature supraspinal mechanisms.

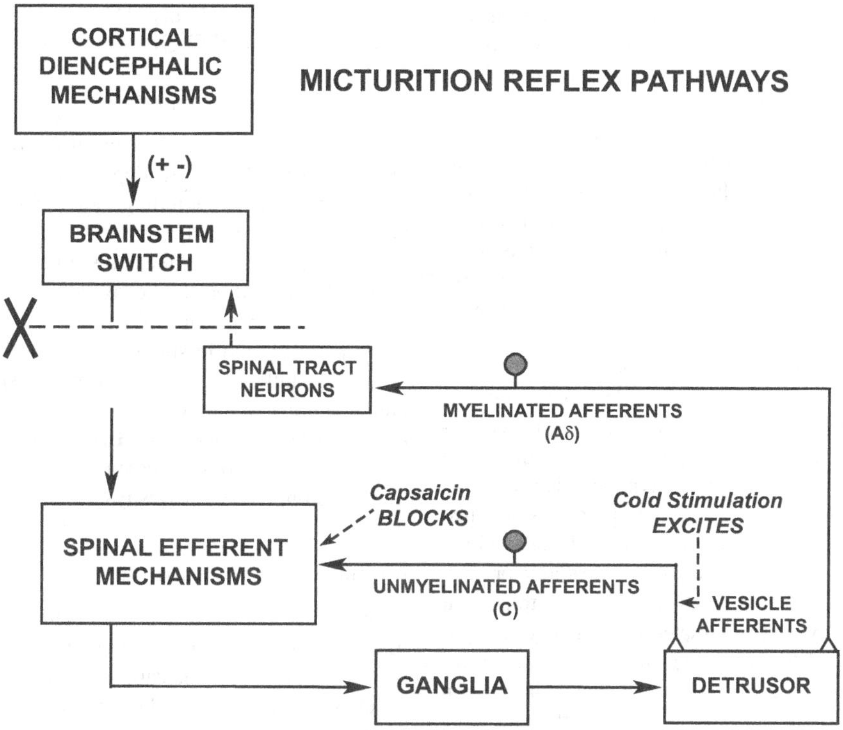


Figure 19–9 Organization of the parasympathetic excitatory reflex pathway to the detrusor muscle This scheme is based on electrophysiological studies in cats. In cats with an intact spinal cord, micturition is initiated by a supraspinal reflex pathway passing through a center in the brainstem. The pathway is triggered by myelinated afferents (A-δ fibers), which are connected to the tension receptors in the bladder wall. Injury to the spinal cord above the sacral segments (*X*) interrupts the connections between the brain and spinal autonomic centers and initially blocks micturition. However, over a period of several weeks following cord injury, a spinal reflex mechanism emerges, which is triggered by unmyelinated vesical afferents (C-fibers); the A-fiber afferent inputs are ineffective. The C-fiber reflex pathway is usually weak or undetectable in animals with an intact nervous system. Stimulation of the C-fiber bladder afferents by instillation of ice water into the bladder (cold stimulation) activates voiding responses in patients with spinal cord injury or in infants. Capsaicin (20–30 mg, subcutaneously) blocks the C-fiber reflex in cats with chronic spinal cord injuries but does not block micturition reflexes in cats with intact cords. Intravesical capsaicin also suppresses detrusor hyper-reflexia and cold-evoked reflexes in patients with neurogenic bladder dysfunction.

It seems likely that this developmental switching mechanism is dependent upon competition between brain and spinal pathways because spinal cord injury in adult animals and humans, which interrupts brain–spinal cord connections, causes the reemergence of the neonatal perineal-to-bladder reflex[25,38]. Spinal cord injury in humans also unmasks a bladder reflex elicited by instillation of cold water into the bladder[45,47]. This cold-evoked bladder reflex, which is activated by C-fiber afferents (Figure 19–9), is not present in normal adults but occurs in neonates and is then suppressed during postnatal maturation of the nervous system.

The changes in neural circuitry underlying developmental and injury-induced plasticity in parasympathetic pathways to the urinary bladder have been studied with tract tracing techniques and electrophysiological methods[25]. Although the spinobulbospinal micturition reflex is nonfunctional in young kittens and rat pups, the pathway seems to be "wired-up" and can be activated under certain conditions. Thus, injection of pseudorabies virus into the bladders of neonatal rats labeled neurons in the same brain regions that were labeled in adult rats[93]. Furthermore in 50% of two-day-old rats and 100% of six-–nine-day-old rats, removal of the forebrain by decerebration unmasked reflex bladder activity *in vivo* in response to bladder distension[25]. This activity was abolished by transection of the spinal cord rostral to the lumbar level, indicating that it was mediated by a supraspinal pathway. Similar reflexes could be unmasked in kittens after the administration of general anesthetics, indicating that supraspinal bladder-to-bladder reflexes are organized relatively soon after birth but are tonically suppressed in young, awake animals by inhibitory mechanisms in the brain. It has been proposed that suppression of these inhibitory mechanisms during postnatal development leads to the emergence of the latent reflex pathway and the appearance of mature voiding mechanisms[25].

The mechanisms underlying the developmental suppression of the perineal-to-bladder reflex and its reemergence after spinal cord injury have been studied with patch clamping methods of parasympathetic preganglionic neurons in spinal cord slice preparations obtained from 6- to 28-day-old rats[4]. Interneurons located within 100 micrometers dorsal to the parasympathetic preganglionic neurons were stimulated with extracellular micropipettes to elicit glutamatergic excitatory postsynaptic currents (EPSCs) in the preganglionic neurons. The interneurons receive excitatory synaptic input from primary afferent axons and therefore are thought to be part of a disynaptic parasympathetic reflex pathway (Figure 19–10) that might underlie the perineal-to-bladder and cold-evoked bladder reflexes. In preparations removed from one- and two–week-old rats, the EPSCs evoked by stimulation of the interneurons were large and of constant amplitude. However, in preparations from three-week-old rats, an age when the spinobulbospinal micturition has emerged, the amplitude of the EPSCs declined by 50%. Transection of the spinal cord between one and two weeks of age prevented the reduction in synaptic transmission that occurred at three weeks of age. These changes were attributed to remodeling of synapses in the sacral parasympathetic nucleus (Figure 19–10). These observations led to the proposal that the bulbospinal pathways to the parasympathetic preganglionic neurons mature during the second to third postnatal week, at the same time when the mature bladder-to-bladder spinobulbospinal reflex is emerging. As a result of this process, the excitatory inputs from interneurons onto parasympathetic preganglionic neurons are down-regulated, possibly because competition from descending axons causes elimination of interneuronal synapses[4]. Transection of the spinal cord, which causes degeneration of descending axons, blocks this synaptic reorganization and maintains the primitive neonatal reflex pathway. A similar degeneration of descending axons in adult animals could stimulate axonal sprouting in interneuronal pathways and cause the reemergence of the neonatal perineal-to-bladder reflex in chronic spinal animals.

## NEUROTRANSMITTERS IN CENTRAL MICTURITION REFLEX PATHWAYS

### Excitatory Neurotransmitters

Excitatory transmission in central pathways controlling the lower urinary tract depends on several types of neurotransmitters, including glutamate, neuropeptides, nitric oxide, and ATP[37,63,82,108]. Pharmacological experiments in rats have revealed that glutamate is an essential transmitter in the ascending, pontine, and descending limbs of the spinobulbospinal micturition reflex pathway and in spinal reflex pathways controlling the bladder and external urethral sphincter[18,107]. Glutamatergic synaptic mechanisms involving both *N*-methyl-D-aspartate (NMDA) and non-NMDA receptors appear to interact synergistically to mediate transmission in these pathways

### Inhibitory Neurotransmitters

Several types of inhibitory transmitters, including inhibitory amino acids (GABA, glycine) and opioid peptides (enkephalins), can suppress the micturition reflex when applied in the central nervous system. Experimental evidence in anesthetized animals indicates that GABA and enkephalins exert a tonic inhibitory control in the pontine micturition center and regulate bladder capacity[31,59,67]. These substances also have inhibitory actions in the spinal cord. Glycine or GABA has been implicated in (1) recurrent inhibition in the sacral parasympathetic pathway to the bladder of the cat, (2) inhibition of reflex bladder activity by stimulation of the distal bowel in the rat, (3) inhibition of motor neurons innervating the external urethral sphincter during micturition, and (4) inhibition of bladder activity induced by electrical stimulation of the rostral pontine reticular formation[23,37,86,91].

### Transmitters with Mixed Excitatory and Inhibitory Actions

Some transmitters, including dopamine, serotonin (5-hydroxytryptamine, 5-HT), noradrenaline (NA), acetylcholine, and non-opioid peptides such as vasoactive intestinal polypeptide and corticotropin-releasing factor, have both inhibitory and excitatory effects on reflex bladder activity[1,31,54,57,70,74,95,109]. In some instances, different effects are mediated by different types of receptors. For example, the inhibitory effects of dopamine are mediated by $D_1$-like ($D_1$ and $D_5$) receptor subtypes; and the facilitative effects, by $D_2$-like ($D_2$, $D_3$ and $D_4$) subtypes. Loss of forebrain dopaminergic inhibitory mechanisms after middle cerebral artery occlusion in rats[100] or in patients with

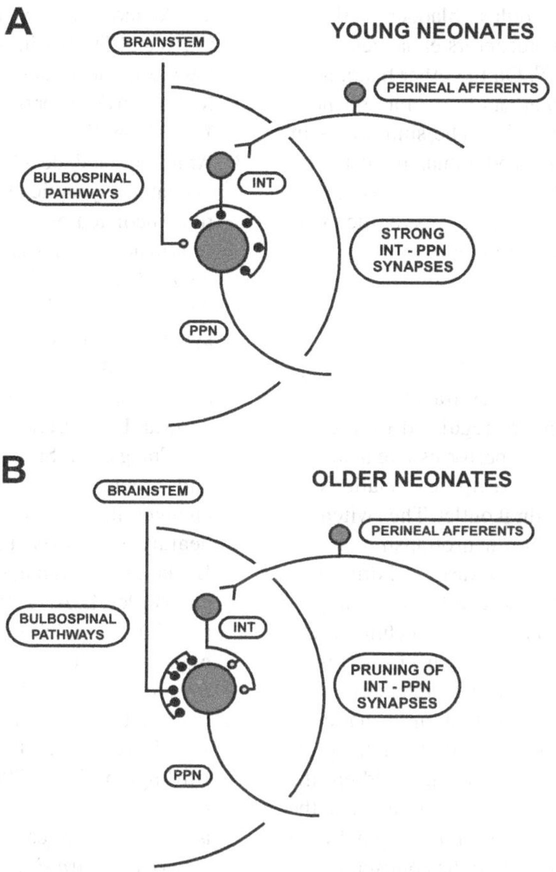


Figure 19–10 Synaptic reorganization in the sacral parasympathetic nucleus that might underlie the change in bladder reflexes during postnatal development. *A:* In young neonates (birth to two weeks of age), interneurons (INT) located immediately dorsal to the sacral parasympathetic nucleus make strong synaptic connections with the parasympathetic preganglionic neurons (PPN). These INT receive synaptic inputs from primary afferent neurons, some of which are likely to innervate the perineal region. This disynaptic reflex pathway is hypothesized to mediate the perigenital-to-bladder reflex, which produces voiding in the neonatal rat. Inputs to the sacral parasympathetic nucleus from bulbospinal axons originating in the pontine micturition center make weak synaptic connections with the preganglionic neurons in young neonates. *B:* In older neonates (3– 4 weeks of age), bulbospinal inputs to the parasympathetic preganglionic neurons increase at the time when the spinobulbospinal micturition reflex emerges. At the same time, synapses that preganglionic neurons receive from segmental interneurons are eliminated (synaptic pruning), contributing to the down-regulation of the perigenital-to-bladder reflex. In the spinal slice preparation, quantal analysis of unitary excitatory post-synaptic currents evoked in preganglionic neurons by the stimulation of single interneurons revealed that interneuronal synapses on preganglionic neurons release 50% fewer quanta of the excitatory transmitter glutamate during the third postnatal week compared to the first two postnatal weeks. This change is prevented by spinal cord transection during the second postnatal week, suggesting that it is due to the influence of descending pathways from the brain on synapses from interneurons onto preganglionic neurons.

idiopathic Parkinson's disease is associated with bladder hyperactivity[37].

Interest in the role of 5-HT in the central control of micturition has increased following the introduction of duloxetine, a 5-HT-noradrenaline reuptake inhibitor, for the treatment of stress urinary incontinence[97]. 5-HT has complex effects on the lower urinary tract that vary in different species[24]. In the cat, activation of central

$5\text{-}HT_{1A}$ receptors inhibits reflex bladder activity; whereas activation of $5\text{-}HT_2$ receptors enhances activity of the urethral sphincter[97]. On the other hand, activation of central $5\text{-}HT_{1A}$ receptors in the rat enhances bladder and sphincter reflexes[18,19]. The similarities in the effects of duloxetine in cat and human indicate that micturition in the cat may be a useful model for developing centrally acting serotonergic agents for the treatment of lower urinary tract dysfunction.

## SUMMARY

The functions of the lower urinary tract to store and periodically eliminate urine are regulated by a complex neural control system that performs like a simple switching circuit to maintain a reciprocal relationship between the bladder and urethral outlet. The switching circuit is modulated by several neurotransmitter systems and is therefore sensitive to a variety of drugs and neurological diseases. Further research is needed, particularly in humans using brain imaging techniques, to identify the pathways in the forebrain that exert voluntary control over primitive micturition reflex circuitry in the brainstem and spinal cord. More information is required about the neuroplasticity underlying the postnatal development of bladder control in children, the loss of that control in adults after neural injury, and the partial recovery of bladder function after spinal cord injury. It is also important to define the contribution of neurotrophic factors released in the bladder or in the central nervous system to neuroplasticity. Detailed studies of peripheral afferent pathways, including the role of the urothelial cells in bladder sensory transduction mechanisms, are necessary in order to explore the pathophysiology of urinary urgency sensations and urgency incontinence. A more complete understanding of the peripheral and central neural mechanisms involved in bladder and urethral control will no doubt facilitate the development of new diagnostic methods and therapies for lower urinary tract dysfunction.

ACKNOWLEDGEMENTS This research is supported by National Institutes of Health grants # DK49430 and DK077783.

## References

1. Andersson, K. E., and Pehrson, R. (2003). CNS involvement in overactive bladder: Pathophysiology and opportunities for pharmacological intervention. *Drugs* 63, 2595–2611.
2. Apostolidis, A., Popat, R., Yiangou, Y., Cockayne, D., Ford, A. P., Davis, J. B., Dasgupta, P., Fowler, C. J., and Anand, P. (2005). Decreased sensory receptors P2X3 and TRPV1 in suburothelial nerve fibers following intradetrusor injections of botulinum toxin for human detrusor overactivity. *Journal of Urology* 174, 977–982;.
3. Araki, I., and de Groat, W. C. (1996). Unitary excitatory synaptic currents in preganglionic neurons mediated by two distinct groups of interneurons in neonatal rat sacral parasympathetic nucleus. *Journal of Neurophysiology* 76, 215–226.
4. Araki, I., and de Groat, W. C. (1997). Developmental synaptic depression underlying reorganization of visceral reflex pathways in the spinal cord. *Journal of Neuroscience* 17, 8402–8407.
5. Athwal, B. S., Berkley, K. J., Hussain, I., Brennan, A., Craggs, M., Sakakibara, R., Frackowiak, R. S., and Fowler, C. J. (2001). Brain responses to changes in bladder volume and urge to void in healthy men. *Brain* 124, 369–377.
6. Beckel, J. M., Kanai, A., Lee, S. J., de Groat, W. C., and Birder, L. A. (2006). Expression of functional nicotinic acetylcholine receptors in rat urinary bladder epithelial cells. *American Journal of Physiology. Renal Physiology* 290, F103–F110.
7. Birder, L. A., Barrick, S. R., Roppolo, J. R., Kanai, A. J., de Groat, W. C., Kiss, S., and Buffington, C. A. (2003). Feline interstitial cystitis results in mechanical hypersensitivity and altered ATP release from bladder urothelium. *American Journal of Physiology. Renal Physiology* 285, F423–F429.
8. Birder, L. A., and de Groat, W. C. (1993). Induction of c-fos expression in spinal neurons by nociceptive and nonnociceptive stimulation of LUT. *American Journal of Physiology* 265, R326–R333.
9. Birder, L. A., de Groat, W. C., and Apodaca, G. (2008). Physiology of the urothelium. In E. Shick and J. Corcos (Eds.), *Textbook of the Neurogenic Bladder*, pp. 19–39. London: Taylor and Francis.
10. Birder, L. A., Kanai, A. J., de Groat, W. C., Kiss, S., Nealen, M. L., Burke, N. E., Dineley, K. E., Watkins, S., Reynolds, I. J., and Caterina, M. J. (2001). Vanilloid receptor expression suggests a sensory role for urinary bladder epithelial cells. *Proceedings of the National Academy of Sciences USA* 98, 13396–13401.
11. Birder, L. A., Nakamura, Y., Kiss, S., Nealen, M. L., Barrick, S., Kanai, A. J., Wang, E., Ruiz, G., de Groat, W. C., Apodaca, G., Watkins, S., and Caterina, M. J. (2002). Altered urinary bladder function in mice lacking the vanilloid receptor TRPV1. *Nature Neuroscience* 5, 856–860.
12. Birder, L. A., Roppolo, J. R., Erickson, V. L., and de Groat, W. C. (1999). Increased c-Fos expression

in spinal lumbosacral projection neurons and preganglionic neurons after irritation of the lower urinary tract in the rat. *Brain Research* 834, 55–65.
13. Blok, B. F., De Weerd, H., and Holstege, G. (1995). Ultrastructural evidence for a paucity of projections from the lumbosacral cord to the pontine micturition center or M-region in the cat: A new concept for the organization of the micturition reflex with the periaqueductal gray as central relay. *Journal of Comparative Neurology* 359, 300–309.
14. Blok, B. F., Sturms, L. M., and Holstege, G. (1997). A PET study on cortical and subcortical control of pelvic floor musculature in women. *Journal of Comparative Neurology* 389, 535–544.
15. Blok, B. F., Sturms, L. M., and Holstege, G. (1998). Brain activation during micturition in women. *Brain* 121 (Pt 11), 2033–2042.
16. Blok, B. F., Willemsen, A. T., and Holstege, G. (1997). A PET study on brain control of micturition in humans. *Brain* 120 (Pt 1), 111–121.
17. Burnstock, G. (2001). Purinergic signaling in the lower urinary tract. In M. P. Abbracchio and M. Williams (Eds.), *Handbook of Experimental Pharmacology*, pp. 423–515. Berlin: Springer Verlag,.
18. Chang, H. Y., Cheng, C. L., Chen, J. J., and de Groat, W. C. (2006). Roles of glutamatergic and serotonergic mechanisms in reflex control of the external urethral sphincter in urethane-anesthetized female rats. *American Journal of Physiology. Regulatory, Integrative and Comparative Physiology* 291, R224–R234.
19. Chang, H. Y., Cheng, C. L., Chen, J. J., and de Groat, W. C. (2007). Serotonergic drugs and spinal cord transections indicate that different spinal circuits are involved in external urethral sphincter activity in rats. *American Journal of Physiology. Renal Physiology* 292, F1044–F1053.
20. Cheng, C. L., Liu, J. C., Chang, S. Y., Ma, C. P., and de Groat, W. C. (1999). Effect of capsaicin on the micturition reflex in normal and chronic spinal cord-injured cats. *American Journal of Physiology* 277, R786–R794.
21. Cockayne, D. A., Hamilton, S. G., Zhu, Q. M., Dunn, P. M., Zhong, Y., Novakovic, S., Malmberg, A. B., Cain, G., Berson, A., Kassotakis, L., Hedley, L., Lachnit, W. G., Burnstock, G., McMahon, S. B., and Ford, A. P. (2000). Urinary bladder hyporeflexia and reduced pain-related behaviour in P2X3-deficient mice. *Nature* 407, 1011–1015.
22. de Groat, W. C. (1975). Nervous control of the urinary bladder of the cat. *Brain Research* 87, 201–211.
23. de Groat, W. C. (1976). Mechanisms underlying recurrent inhibition in the sacral parasympathetic outflow to the urinary bladder. *Journal of Physiology* 257, 503–513.
24. de Groat, W. C. (2002). Influence of central serotonergic mechanisms on lower urinary tract function. *Urology* 59, 30–36.
25. de Groat, W. C. (2002). Plasticity of bladder reflex pathways during postnatal development. *Physiology and Behavior* 77, 689–692.
26. de Groat, W. C. (2004). The urothelium in overactive bladder: Passive bystander or active participant? *Urology* 64, 7–11.
27. de Groat, W. C. (2006). Integrative control of the lower urinary tract: Preclinical perspective. *British Journal of Pharmacology* 147 Suppl 2, S25–S40.
28. de Groat, W. C., Araki, I., Vizzard, M. A., Yoshiyama, M., Yoshimura, N., Sugaya, K., Tai, C., and Roppolo, J. R. (1998). Developmental and injury induced plasticity in the micturition reflex pathway. *Behavioural Brain Research* 92, 127–140.
29. de Groat, W. C., and Booth, A. M. (1993). Synaptic transmission in pelvic ganglia. In C. A. Maggi (Ed.), *The Autonomic Nervous System, vol. 3*, pp. 291–347. London: Harwood Academic Publishers.
30. de Groat, W. C., Booth, A. M., Milne, R. J., and Roppolo, J. R. (1982). Parasympathetic preganglionic neurons in the sacral spinal cord. *Journal of the Autonomic Nervous System* 5, 23–43.
31. de Groat, W. C., Booth, A. M., and Yoshimura, N. (1993). Neurophysiology of micturition and its modification in animal models of human disease. In C. A. Maggi (Ed.), *The Autonomic Nervous System, vol. 3*, pp. 227–289.London: Harwood Academic Publishers.
32. de Groat, W. C., Fraser, M. O., Yoshiyama, M., Smerin, S., Tai, C., Chancellor, M. B., Yoshimura, N., and Roppolo, J. R. (2001). Neural control of the urethra. *Scandinavian Journal of Urology and Nephrology* Suppl, 35–43; discussion, 106–125.
33. de Groat, W. C., Kawatani, M., Hisamitsu, T., Cheng, C. L., Ma, C. P., Thor, K., Steers, W., and Roppolo, J. R. (1990). Mechanisms underlying the recovery of urinary bladder function following spinal cord injury. *Journal of the Autonomic Nervous System* 30 Suppl, S71–S77.
34. de Groat, W. C., and Lalley, P. M. (1972). Reflex firing in the lumbar sympathetic outflow to activation of vesical afferent fibres. *Journal of Physiology* 226, 289–309.
35. de Groat, W. C., Nadelhaft, I., Milne, R. J., Booth, A. M., Morgan, C., and Thor, K. (1981). Organization of the sacral parasympathetic reflex pathways to the urinary bladder and large intestine. *Journal of the Autonomic Nervous System* 3, 135–160.

36. de Groat, W. C., and Ryall, R. W. (1969). Reflexes to sacral parasympathetic neurones concerned with micturition in the cat. *Journal of Physiology* 200, 87–108.
37. de Groat, W. C., and Yoshimura, N. (2001). Pharmacology of the lower urinary tract. *Annual Review of Pharmacology and Toxicology* 41, 691–721.
38. de Groat, W. C., and Yoshimura, N. (2006). Mechanisms underlying the recovery of lower urinary tract function following spinal cord injury. *Progress in Brain Research* 152, 59–84.
39. de Groat, W. C., and Yoshimura, N. (2009). Afferent nerve regulation of bladder function in health and disease. In Canning B. J. and Spina D. (Eds.), *Pharmacology of Sensory Nerves, Handbook of Experimental Pharmacology 194, pp. 91–138.* Heidelberg, Germany: Springer.
40. Ding, Y. Q., Zheng, H. X., Gong, L. W., Lu, Y., Zhao, H., and Qin, B. Z. (1997). Direct projections from the lumbosacral spinal cord to Barrington's nucleus in the rat: A special reference to micturition reflex. *Journal of Comparative Neurology* 389, 149–160.
41. Du, S., Araki, I., Yoshiyama, M., Nomura, T., and Takeda, M. (2007). Transient receptor potential channel A1 involved in sensory transduction of rat urinary bladder through C-fiber pathway. *Urology* 70, 826–831.
42. Everaerts, W., Gevaert, T., Nilius, B., and De Ridder, D. (2008). On the origin of bladder sensing: Tr(i)ps in urology. *Neurourology and Urodynamics* 27, 264–273.
43. Ferguson, D. R., Kennedy, I., and Burton, T. J. (1997). ATP is released from rabbit urinary bladder epithelial cells by hydrostatic pressure changes—a possible sensory mechanism? *Journal of Physiology* 505, 503–511.
44. Fowler, C. J. (2006). Integrated control of lower urinary tract—clinical perspective. *British Journal of Pharmacology* 147 Suppl 2, S14–S24.
45. Fowler, C. J., Griffiths, D., and de Groat, W. C. (2008). The neural control of micturition. *Nature Reviews Neuroscience* 9, 453–466.
46. Fry, C. H., Brading, A. F., Hussain, M., and Al, E. (2005). Cell biology. In P. Abrams, L. Cardozo, S. Khoury and A. Wein (Eds.), *Incontinence*, pp. 313–362. Paris, France: Health Publications.
47. Geirsson, G., Fall, M., and Lindstrom, S. (1993). The ice-water test—a simple and valuable supplement to routine cystometry. *British Journal of Urology* 71, 681–685.
48. Griffiths, D., Tadic, S. D., Schaefer, W., and Resnick, N. M. (2007). Cerebral control of the bladder in normal and urge-incontinent women. *Neuroimage* 37, 1–7.
49. Hanna-Mitchell, A. T., Beckel, J. M., Barbadora, S., Kanai, A. J., de Groat, W. C., and Birder, L. A. (2007). Non-neuronal acetylcholine and urinary bladder urothelium. *Life Sciences* 80, 2298–2302.
50. Holstege, G., and Mouton, L. J. (2003). Central nervous system control of micturition. *International Review of Neurobiology* 56, 123–145.
51. Kanai, A., Roppolo, J., Ikeda, Y., Zabbarova, I., Tai, C., Birder, L., Griffiths, D., de Groat, W., and Fry, C. (2007). Origin of spontaneous activity in neonatal and adult rat bladders and its enhancement by stretch and muscarinic agonists. *American Journal of Physiology. Renal Physiology* 292, F1065–F1072.
52. Kavia, R. B., Dasgupta, R., and Fowler, C. J. (2005). Functional imaging and the central control of the bladder. *Journal of Comparative Neurology* 493, 27–32.
53. Keast, J. R., Kawatani, M., and de Groat, W. C. (1990). Sympathetic modulation of cholinergic transmission in cat vesical ganglia is mediated by alpha 1- and alpha 2-adrenoceptors. *American Journal of Physiology* 258, R44–R50.
54. Klausner, A. P., Streng, T., Na, Y. G., Raju, J., Batts, T. W., Tuttle, J. B., Andersson, K. E., and Steers, W. D. (2005). The role of corticotropin releasing factor and its antagonist, astressin, on micturition in the rat. *Autonomic Neuroscience: Basic and Clinical* 123, 26–35.
55. Kullmann, F. A., Artim, D., Beckel, J., Barrick, S., de Groat, W. C., and Birder, L. A. (2008). Heterogeneity of muscarinic receptor-mediated Ca2+ responses in cultured urothelial cells from rat. *American Journal of Physiology. Renal Physiology* 294, F971–F981.
56. Kullmann, F. A., Artim, D. E., Birder, L. A., and de Groat, W. C. (2008). Activation of muscarinic receptors in rat bladder sensory pathways alters reflex bladder activity. *Journal of Neuroscience* 28, 1977–1987.
57. Lee, S. J., Nakamura, Y., and de Groat, W. C. (2003). Effect of (+/-)-epibatidine, a nicotinic agonist, on the central pathways controlling voiding function in the rat. *American Journal of Physiology. Regulatory, Integrative and Comparative Physiology* 285, R84–R90.
58. Liu, H. T., and Kuo, H. C. (2008). Urinary nerve growth factor levels are increased in patients with bladder outlet obstruction with overactive bladder symptoms and reduced after successful medical treatment. *Urology* 72, 104–108; discussion, 108.
59. Mallory, B. S., Roppolo, J. R., and de Groat, W. C. (1991). Pharmacological modulation of the

pontine micturition center. *Brain Research* 546, 310–320.

60. Matsui, M., Motomura, D., Fujikawa, T., Jiang, J., Takahashi, S., Manabe, T., and Taketo, M. M. (2002). Mice lacking M2 and M3 muscarinic acetylcholine receptors are devoid of cholinergic smooth muscle contractions but still viable. *Journal of Neuroscience* 22, 10627–10632.
61. Matsuura, S., Kakizaki, H., Mitsui, T., Shiga, T., Tamaki, N., and Koyanagi, T. (2002). Human brain region response to distention or cold stimulation of the bladder: A positron emission tomography study. *Journal of Urology* 168, 2035–2039.
62. McMahon, S. B., and Morrison, J. F. (1982). Spinal neurones with long projections activated from the abdominal viscera of the cat. *Journal of Physiology* 322, 1–20.
63. Miura, A., Kawatani, M., and de Groat, W. C. (2001). Effects of pituitary adenylate cyclase activating polypeptide on lumbosacral preganglionic neurons in the neonatal rat spinal cord. *Brain Research* 895, 223–232.
64. Miura, A., Kawatani, M., and de Groat, W. C. (2001). Excitatory synaptic currents in lumbosacral parasympathetic preganglionic neurons elicited from the lateral funiculus. *Journal of Neurophysiology* 86, 1587–1593.
65. Miura, A., Kawatani, M., and de Groat, W. C. (2003). Excitatory synaptic currents in lumbosacral parasympathetic preganglionic neurons evoked by stimulation of the dorsal commissure. *Journal of Neurophysiology* 89, 382–389.
66. Morgan, C. W., de Groat, W. C., Felkins, L. A., and Zhang, S. J. (1993). Intracellular injection of neurobiotin or horseradish peroxidase reveals separate types of preganglionic neurons in the sacral parasympathetic nucleus of the cat. *Journal of Comparative Neurology* 331, 161–182.
67. Morrison, J. F., Birder, L. A., Craggs, M., de Groat, W. C., Downie, J. W., Drake, M., Fowler, C. J., and Thor, K. (2005). Neural control. In P. Abrams, L. Cardozo, S. Khoury and A. Wein (Eds.), *Incontinence*, pp. 363–422. Paris, France Health Publications.
68. Nadelhaft, I., de Groat, W. C., and Morgan, C. (1980). Location and morphology of parasympathetic preganglionic neurons in the sacral spinal cord of the cat revealed by retrograde axonal transport of horseradish peroxidase. *Journal of Comparative Neurology* 193, 265–281.
69. Nadelhaft, I., Vera, P. L., Card, J. P., and Miselis, R. R. (1992). Central nervous system neurons labeled following the injection of pseudorabies virus into the rat urinary bladder. *Neuroscience Letters* 143, 271–274.
70. Nakamura, Y., Ishiura, Y., Yokoyama, O., Namiki, M., and de Groat, W. C. (2003). Role of protein kinase C in central muscarinic inhibitory mechanisms regulating voiding in rats. *Neuroscience* 116, 477–484.
71. Nishiguchi, J., Hayashi, Y., Chancellor, M. B., De Miguel, F., de Groat, W. C., Kumon, H., and Yoshimura, N. (2005). Detrusor overactivity induced by intravesical application of adenosine 5'-triphosphate under different delivery conditions in rats. *Urology* 66, 1332–1337.
72. Noto, H., Roppolo, J. R., Steers, W. D., and de Groat, W. C. (1989). Excitatory and inhibitory influences on bladder activity elicited by electrical stimulation in the pontine micturition center in the rat. *Brain Research* 492, 99–115.
73. Nour, S., Svarer, C., Kristensen, J. K., Paulson, O. B., and Law, I. (2000). Cerebral activation during micturition in normal men. *Brain* 123, 781–789.
74. Pavcovich, L. A., and Valentino, R. J. (1995). Central regulation of micturition in the rat the corticotropin-releasing hormone from Barrington's nucleus. *Neuroscience Letters* 196, 185–188.
75. Rong, W., and Burnstock, G. (2004). Activation of ureter nociceptors by exogenous and endogenous ATP in guinea pig. *Neuropharmacology* 47, 1093–1101.
76. Rong, W., Spyer, K. M., and Burnstock, G. (2002). Activation and sensitisation of low and high threshold afferent fibres mediated by P2X receptors in the mouse urinary bladder. *Journal of Physiology* 541, 591–600.
77. Rorden, C., and Brett, M. (2000). Stereotaxic display of brain lesions. *Behavioural Neurology* 12, 191–200.
78. Sasaki, M. (2004). Feed-forward and feedback regulation of bladder contractility by Barrington's nucleus in cats. *Journal of Physiology* 557, 287–305.
79. Sasaki, M. (2005). Properties of Barrington's neurones in cats: Units that fire inversely with micturition contraction. *Brain Research* 1033, 41–50.
80. Sculptoreanu, A., de Groat, W. C., Buffington, C. A., and Birder, L. A. (2005). Abnormal excitability in capsaicin-responsive DRG neurons from cats with feline interstitial cystitis. *Experimental Neurology* 193, 437–443.
81. Sculptoreanu, A., de Groat, W. C., Buffington, C. A., and Birder, L. A. (2005). Protein kinase C contributes to abnormal capsaicin responses in DRG neurons from cats with feline interstitial cystitis. *Neuroscience Letters* 381, 42–46.
82. Seki, S., Erickson, K. A., Seki, M., Nishizawa, O., Igawa, Y., Ogawa, T., de Groat, W. C.,

Chancellor, M. B., and Yoshimura, N. (2005). Elimination of rat spinal neurons expressing neurokinin 1 receptors reduces bladder overactivity and spinal c-Fos expression induced by bladder irritation. *American Journal of Physiology. Renal Physiology* 288, F466–F473.

83. Seki, S., Sasaki, K., Fraser, M. O., Igawa, Y., Nishizawa, O., Chancellor, M. B., de Groat, W. C., and Yoshimura, N. (2002). Immunoneutralization of nerve growth factor in lumbosacral spinal cord reduces bladder hyperreflexia in spinal cord injured rats. *Journal of Urology* 168, 2269–2274.
84. Seki, S., Sasaki, K., Igawa, Y., Nishizawa, O., Chancellor, M. B., de Groat, W. C., and Yoshimura, N. (2004). Suppression of detrusor-sphincter dyssynergia by immunoneutralization of nerve growth factor in lumbosacral spinal cord in spinal cord injured rats. *Journal of Urology* 171, 478–482.
85. Shea, V. K., Cai, R., Crepps, B., Mason, J. L., and Perl, E. R. (2000). Sensory fibers of the pelvic nerve innervating the rat's urinary bladder. *Journal of Neurophysiology* 84, 1924–1933.
86. Shefchyk, S. J. (2001). Sacral spinal interneurones and the control of urinary bladder and urethral striated sphincter muscle function. *Journal of Physiology* 533, 57–63.
87. Somogyi, G. T., and de Groat, W. C. (1999). Function, signal transduction mechanisms and plasticity of presynaptic muscarinic receptors in the urinary bladder. *Life Sciences* 64, 411–418.
88. Steers, W. D., Ciambotti, J., Etzel, B., Erdman, S., and de Groat, W. C. (1991). Alterations in afferent pathways from the urinary bladder of the rat in response to partial urethral obstruction. *Journal of Comparative Neurology* 310, 401–410.
89. Steers, W. D., Kolbeck, S., Creedon, D., and Tuttle, J. B. (1991). Nerve growth factor in the urinary bladder of the adult regulates neuronal form and function. *Journal of Clinical Investigation* 88, 1709–1715.
90. Steers, W. D., and Tuttle, J. B. (2006). Mechanisms of disease: The role of nerve growth factor in the pathophysiology of bladder disorders. *Nature Clinical Practice. Urology* 3, 101–110.
91. Sugaya, K., Nishijima, S., Miyazato, M., and Ogawa, Y. (2005). Central nervous control of micturition and urine storage. *Journal of Smooth Muscle Research* 41, 117–132.
92. Sugaya, K., Ogawa, Y., Hatano, T., Nishijima, S., Matsuyama, K., and Mori, S. (2003). Ascending and descending brainstem neuronal activity during cystometry in decerebrate cats. *Neurourology and Urodynamics* 22, 343–350.
93. Sugaya, K., Roppolo, J. R., Yoshimura, N., Card, J. P., and de Groat, W. C. (1997). The central neural pathways involved in micturition in the neonatal rat as revealed by the injection of pseudorabies virus into the urinary bladder. *Neuroscience Letters* 223, 197–200.
94. Sun, Y., Keay, S., De Deyne, P. G., and Chai, T. C. (2001). Augmented stretch activated adenosine triphosphate release from bladder uroepithelial cells in patients with interstitial cystitis. *Journal of Urology* 166, 1951–1956.
95. Tai, C., Miscik, C. L., Ungerer, T. D., Roppolo, J. R., and de Groat, W. C. (2006). Suppression of bladder reflex activity in chronic spinal cord injured cats by activation of serotonin 5-HT1A receptors. *Experimental Neurology* 199, 427–437.
96. Tanaka, Y., Koyama, Y., Kayama, Y., Kawauchi, A., Ukimura, O., and Miki, T. (2003). Firing of micturition center neurons in the rat mesopontine tegmentum during urinary bladder contraction. *Brain Research* 965, 146–154.
97. Thor, K. B. (2003). Serotonin and norepinephrine involvement in efferent pathways to the urethral rhabdosphincter: Implications for treating stress urinary incontinence. *Urology* 62, 3–9.
98. Vizzard, M. A. (2006). Neurochemical plasticity and the role of neurotrophic factors in bladder reflex pathways after spinal cord injury. *Progress in Brain Research* 152, 97–115.
99. Vizzard, M. A., Erickson, V. L., Card, J. P., Roppolo, J. R., and de Groat, W. C. (1995). Transneuronal labeling of neurons in the adult rat brainstem and spinal cord after injection of pseudorabies virus into the urethra. *Journal of Comparative Neurology* 355, 629–640.
100. Yokoyama, O., Yoshiyama, M., Namiki, M., and de Groat, W. C. (2002). Changes in dopaminergic and glutamatergic excitatory mechanisms of micturition reflex after middle cerebral artery occlusion in conscious rats. *Experimental Neurology* 173, 129–135.
101. Yoshida, M., Miyamae, K., Iwashita, H., Otani, M., and Inadome, A. (2004). Management of detrusor dysfunction in the elderly: Changes in acetylcholine and adenosine triphosphate release during aging. *Urology* 63, 17–23.
102. Yoshimura, N., Bennett, N. E., Hayashi, Y., Ogawa, T., Nishizawa, O., Chancellor, M. B., de Groat, W. C., and Seki, S. (2006). Bladder overactivity and hyperexcitability of bladder afferent neurons after intrathecal delivery of nerve growth factor in rats. *Journal of Neuroscience* 26, 10847–10855.
103. Yoshimura, N., and de Groat, W. C. (1997). Plasticity of $Na^+$ channels in afferent neurones innervating rat urinary bladder following spinal cord injury. *Journal of Physiology* 503, 269–276.

104. Yoshimura, N., and de Groat, W. C. (1999). Increased excitability of afferent neurons innervating rat urinary bladder after chronic bladder inflammation. *Journal of Neuroscience* 19, 4644–4653.
105. Yoshimura, N., Seki, S., Novakovic, S. D., Tzoumaka, E., Erickson, V. L., Erickson, K. A., Chancellor, M. B., and de Groat, W. C. (2001). The involvement of the tetrodotoxin-resistant sodium channel Na(v)1.8 (PN3/SNS) in a rat model of visceral pain. *Journal of Neuroscience* 21, 8690–8696.
106. Yoshimura, N., White, G., Weight, F. F., and de Groat, W. C. (1996). Different types of $Na^+$ and A-type $K^+$ currents in dorsal root ganglion neurones innervating the rat urinary bladder. *Journal of Physiology* 494, 1–16.
107. Yoshiyama, M., and de Groat, W. C. (2005). Supraspinal and spinal alpha-amino-3-hydroxy-5-methylisoxazole-4-propionic acid and N-methyl-D-aspartate glutamatergic control of the micturition reflex in the urethane-anesthetized rat. *Neuroscience* 132, 1017–1026.
108. Yoshiyama, M., and de Groat, W. C. (2008). The role of vasoactive intestinal polypeptide and pituitary adenylate cyclase-activating polypeptide in the neural pathways controlling the lower urinary tract. *Journal of Molecular Neuroscience* 36, 227–240.
109. Yoshiyama, M., Kakizaki, H., and de Groat, W. C. (2003). Suppression of the micturition reflex in urethane-anesthetized rats by intracerebroventricular injection of WAY100635, a 5-HT(1A) receptor antagonist. *Brain Research* 980, 281–287.
110. Yu, Y., and de Groat, W. C. (2008). Sensitization of pelvic afferent nerves in the in vitro rat urinary bladder-pelvic nerve preparation by purinergic agonists and cyclophosphamide pretreatment. *American Journal of Physiology. Renal Physiology* 294, F1146–F1156.
111. Zhong, Y., Banning, A. S., Cockayne, D. A., Ford, A. P., Burnstock, G., and McMahon, S. B. (2003). Bladder and cutaneous sensory neurons of the rat express different functional P2X receptors. *Neuroscience* 120, 667–675.

20

# Autonomic Regulation of Sexual Function

LESLEY MARSON

Reproductive function encompasses many behavioral components, such as sexual desire, arousal, motor behavior, and reward. In males, specific physiological responses i.e., penile erection, seminal emission, and ejaculation, are representative of the various stages of sexual function. In females, sexual responses consist of vaginal and clitoral vasocongestion, changes in tactile sensitivity and orgasm/climax. Cognitive cues also accompany sexual behavior. The autonomic and somatic nervous systems regulate sexual function and the concomitant changes that occur, including increases in blood pressure, heart rate, and respiration, and changes in specific circulating hormones. The major goal of engaging in sexual behavior is related to the successful propagation of the species, which is associated with a positive-feedback activation of central reward pathways.

A number of factors influence control of reproductive function by the central nervous system (Figure 20–1). Sensory and cognitive inputs lead to desire, arousal, climax, and reward. Hormone levels in the brain and circulation influence the amount of sensory stimulation that leads to desire and arousal, and brain feedback systems may enhance or minimize sexual reflexes. Peripheral genital stimulation enhances excitability within sensory afferents and the spinal cord. The brain perceives and modulates sexual function; but the spinal cord contains the neural circuits for erection, ejaculation, vasocongestion, and climax.

This chapter will focus on the brain, spinal cord, and peripheral nerves that mediate sexual function in the male and female. While some valuable insights have been gained from studies in humans, much of what we know about the anatomy, physiology, and pharmacology of the CNS pathways that regulate sexual function has come from the rat. Sexual responses (e.g., penile erection, vaginal vasocongestion, and ejaculation/climax) are primarily mediated by reflex mechanisms at the spinal cord level. Sensory inputs (e.g., olfactory, visual) and the levels of circulating gonadal steroid hormones may act to inhibit or facilitate these spinal reflex pathways. A strong degree of interconnection exists within the forebrain, midbrain, and hindbrain; these pathways receive afferent information and relay efferent information to spinal circuits that mediate the pelvic reflexes through peripheral autonomic and somatic nerve that control sexual function. Sexual responses are under both voluntary and involuntary control, and significant changes occur during sexual maturation that depend on the type and plasma levels of gonadal steroid hormones.

The prime objective of sexual behavior is to maintain reproduction of the species. While the specific functions vary between males and females (e.g., sperm production and delivery by the male; receipt of sperm coordinated with egg transport and fertilization in females), there is substantial similarity between the CNS mechanisms mediating sexual desire, arousal, and orgasm in males and females. These include mechanisms involved in genital and psychological arousal; vasodilatation in the penis, clitoris, and vagina; smooth and skeletal muscle contractions; and reward.

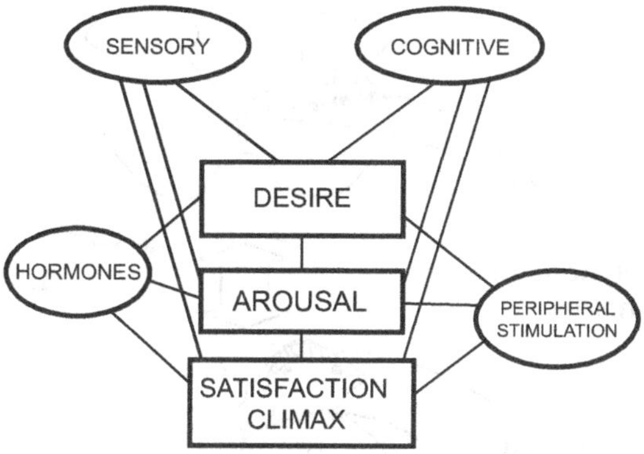


Figure 20–1 Factors influencing sexual function. Diagram illustrating several factors that influence the autonomic control of reproductive function. Sensory and cognitive inputs from the brain and genitalia may trigger desire and arousal responses. Peripheral stimulation may also influence the amount of sensory input that is perceived or involuntarily generated. Desire leads to arousal responses that may trigger climax/ejaculation, which is perceived as rewarding. Each level is influenced by central and peripheral hormone levels.

Many diseases affect normal functioning of sexual responses, such as peripheral neuropathy (as in diabetes and multiple sclerosis) and hypertension. Central diseases and their treatment may also alter arousal and the ability to ejaculate or achieve orgasm (e.g., Parkinson's disease, spinal cord injury, stroke, and treatment with antidepressants).

## PERIPHERAL AND SPINAL INNERVATION

### Peripheral Innervation

The internal reproductive organs and external genitalia are primarily regulated by three branches of the nervous system: parasympathetic, sympathetic, and somatic. The pelvic nerve supplies parasympathetic input; the hypogastric nerve, sympathetic input; and the pudendal nerve, motor input. However, sympathetic (noradrenergic) fibers that participate in penile erection have been reported to travel in the pudendal nerve[36]. In addition, the vagus nerve innervates the uterus/cervix and may relay viscerosensory inputs during sexual function after spinal cord injury. The autonomic and somatic innervation of the pelvic organs, including detailed examination of rodent major pelvic ganglia, have been studied in detail by several authors[54–58,62,65,79,96] and thus will only be briefly summarized in this chapter.

### Sensory Mechanisms

The pelvic and hypogastric nerves convey sensory information primarily from the internal pelvic organs, while the sensory innervation from the genitals and skeletal muscles is provided by the pudendal nerve. The sensory afferents synapse onto many interneurons within the spinal cord. These interneurons relay information locally to preganglionic neurons and motoneurons that mediate the appropriate reflexes and to interneurons that project to the brain, where sensory and hormonal information is processed.

The hypogastric, pelvic, and pudendal nerve afferents are sensitive to levels of circulating gonadal steroid hormones and relay sensory and noxious information from the internal genital organs, vagina, and skin[9,96]. The pudendal inputs regulate the level of sexual receptivity in response to peripheral stimulation and can trigger erection and ejaculation in males and lordosis in females[2,61,77]. Branches of the pudendal nerve innervate the penis/clitoris, perineal skin, skeletal muscles, and the urethra. The distribution of the sensory afferents allows them to transmit considerable information relevant to mating, such as initiation and strength of sexual arousal, the location and movement of the penis, and climax. The glans penis contains numerous specialized nerve endings that become very sensitive during erection. The inputs carried by the pelvic nerve initiate the luteinizing hormone and prolactin surge that occurs after mating or cervical stimulation in female rodents, which often accompanies pregnancy or pseudo-pregnancy[32]. Vagal afferents may also be involved in pregnancy or pseudo-pregnancy[24].

### Spinal Pathways

Intrinsic spinal pathways are vital for relaying and translating the peripheral sensory inputs to the appropriate efferent output (e.g., genital stimulation leading to genital arousal and the associated mood changes). In addition, psychogenic erections are initiated by thought processes in the cortex and limbic system that then relay to the arousal and erectile centers in the spinal cord. Evidence in humans and animals suggests that the sympathetic spinal regions (lower thoracolumbar regions) mediate psychogenic arousal[90,107]. As outlined above, sexual response comprises a coordinated activation of sympathetic, parasympathetic, and somatic output; and the spinal cord pathways function as the spinal pattern generator for these responses.

A number of neuroanatomical and electrophysiological studies have examined the location of spinal interneurons involved in genital function. These studies have shown that pelvic afferents synapse on multiple interneurons in the spinal cord, which then relay through a spinal pattern generator, the preganglionic and post-ganglionic neurons, and motoneurons to mediate the appropriate output (Figure 20–2).

Electrophysiological studies have identified field potentials and synaptically activated neurons in the medial portions of the lumbosacral spinal gray matter after stimulation of the pudendal nerve and pelvic viscera[34,51]. Putative spinal interneurons activated with genital stimuli have been identified using immunoreactivity for Fos, the protein product of the immediate early gene, *c-fos*, which allows visualization of activated neurons[64,68,69]. Stimulation of genital afferents resulted in labeled neurons in the medial dorsal horn, the dorsal gray commissure, and the intermediate and lateral gray matter. The distribution of interneurons is consistent with the distribution of pelvic sensory terminals and is similar in males and females (Figures 20.2 and 20.3). Neurotrophic viruses that are transported transneuronally through several synapses (for example, pseudorabies virus) have also been used to map CNS neurons that innervate the penis, perineal muscles, clitoris, vagina, or uterus[67,74,92]. The majority of labeled neurons in the spinal cord were located in the dorsal gray commissure and in the vicinity of the intermediolateral cell column of the lower thoracic, upper and lower lumbar, and sacral cord (T13–L2 and L5–S1), similar to the locations of labeled neurons in the Fos studies (Figure 20–3). Transganglionic labeling of clitoral, pudendal, and pelvic afferents has shown that they terminate in the same regions as the virus-labeled neurons and the Fos-positive neurons (see also Chapter 7). This complex system allows coordination of sexual reflexes and inhibition of bladder function. Further research is required to understand the spinal mechanisms and how brain inputs modulate spinal neural activity regulating sexual function.

One group of neurons in the medial gray has been shown to be critical for ejaculation in rats[111]. A neurotoxin based on a substance P analogue that has high affinity for the neurokinin 1 receptor, specifically reduced the occurrence of ejaculation when administered into the lumbar cord. The reduced ejaculatory behavior was associated with a loss of cells in the medial cord (L3–L4) that stained for galanin, cholecystokinin, and enkephalin. These neurons (termed *lumbar spinothalamic* or LSt cells) project to the thalamus[25]. Galanin-immunoreactive neurons in the medial gray matter are also activated specifically with ejaculatory behavior and with the urethrogenital reflex[69,111]. These studies suggest that the activated

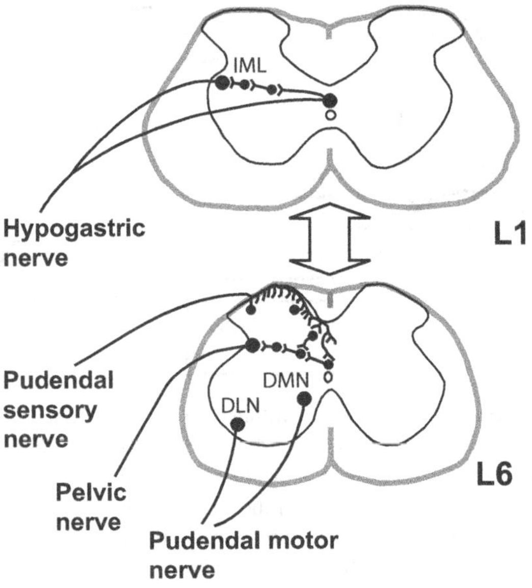


Figure 20–2 Spinal pathways activated by the urethrogenital reflex. Diagram showing one possible pathway for activation of the spinal circuitry controlling the urethrogenital reflex. The diagram is based on immunohistochemical studies of Fos induced by activation of the reflex following brief distension of the urethra. The urethrogenital reflex is mediated via pudendal sensory nerve afferents that terminate in the dorsal horn and dorsal gray commissure of the fifth lumbar to first sacral segments in the rat (*bottom section*). Interneurons immunoreactive for Fos occur in the dorsal horn and dorsal gray commissure (shown at L6). After relaying via spinal interneurons in the medial, intermediate, and lateral gray matter, the efferent components of the urethrogenital reflex were activated, resulting in firing of the hypogastric, pelvic, and pudendal motor nerves. *Large arrow* between L1 and L6 sections indicates the presence of activated interneurons in lumbar segments 2–5 that were found especially in the medial gray matter. The pudendal motor neurons did not stain for Fos. However, these motoneurons have many dendritic branches that project into the vicinity of the neurons with Fos-immunoreactive nuclei. DLN, dorsolateral nucleus, DMN, dorsomedial nucleus; IML, intermediolateral cell column. Modified from Marson et al. (2003)[68] with permission.

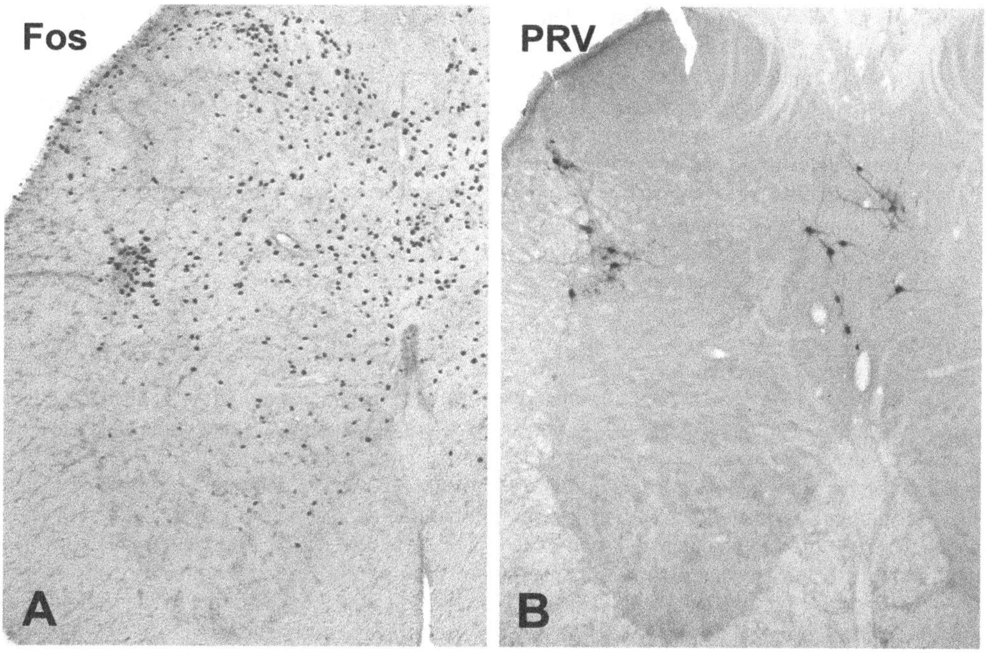


Figure 20–3 Interneurons involved in sexual responses in the sixth lumbar and first sacral segment in the rat. *A:* Fos-immunoreactive nuclei after stimulation of the urethrogenital reflex in the female rat. *B:* neurons labeled with pseudorabies virus four days after injection of the virus into the bulbospongiosus muscle of a male rat. Fos-immunoreactive neurons and virus-labeled neurons both occur in the vicinity of the sacral parasympathetic nucleus, where the cell bodies of parasympathetic preganglionic neurons are located.

neurons may be part of the spinal pattern generator involved in ejaculation. Descending regulation of sexual reflexes in both genders involves inhibition and facilitation of spinal reflexes by the brain. While some new insights on brain regulation have been discovered over the past 50 years, there is still a lack of understanding of the brain pathways and neurotransmitters and how they regulate specific components of reproductive function.

The peripheral nerves, preganglionic neurons, spinal, and brain structures (e.g., pudendal motor neurons, medial preoptic area, and ventromedial nucleus of the hypothalamus) that regulate sexual behavior are sensitive to androgens and estrogens. During development, the level of gonadal steroid hormones determines their survival into sexual dimorphic structures as well as coding their mechanisms of action. More information about sexual dimorphic nuclei can be found in reviews focusing on this topic[76,87,88,102,112].

For more details about spinal neurons involved in regulating the pelvic viscera generally and the reproductive organs in particular, Chapters 6, 7, and 8 should be consulted.

## ASCENDING SENSORY PATHWAYS

Sensory information is relayed to supraspinal sites via the spinothalamic and spinoreticular pathways. The spinothalamic pathways primarily travel in the dorsal columns and consist of myelinated fast-conducting axons. These axons terminate in the posterolateral nucleus of the thalamus and also project to the medial thalamus. Spinoreticular fibers cross the midline and travel in the lateral spinal columns and terminate in the brainstem reticular formation. Vagal axons may also convey sensory information from female pelvic structures to sensory nuclei in the brainstem[60]. These nuclei, in turn, project to specific areas of the cortex.

Cortical evoked potentials in the sensory cortex were found following electrical stimulation of the dorsal nerve of the penis/clitoris[38,45]. In humans, positron emission tomography and functional magnetic resonance imaging have been used to examine brain regions that show an increase in cerebral blood flow during specific activities related to sexual function[35,49,60]. These studies have largely used visual sexual stimuli to map out brain areas activated during arousal. However, a few studies have examined brain areas specifically activated with vaginocervical stimulation and ejaculation/orgasm[49,60]. Areas commonly activated with arousing visual stimuli included the anterior cingulate and insular cortex, striatum, amygdala, and hypothalamus. These pathways may also be important in psychogenically mediated sexual arousal and nocturnal erections. Additional areas activated with vaginocervical stimulation or ejaculation include the cerebellum, ventral tegmental area, and thalamus. Many of these brain regions have been shown to be involved in the descending motor control of sexual reflexes in animals.

Activation of many brain sites can evoke sexual responses; and these areas receive genital sensory information, indicating that the CNS pathways mediating sexual responses are influenced by peripheral stimuli. For example, the nucleus paragigantocellularis, the paraventricular nucleus (PVN), and ventromedial nuclei of the hypothalamus, and the periaqueductal gray (PAG), medial preoptic area, and medial amygdala have all been shown to contain neurons with activity that is modulated by pelvic sensory input. These areas, in turn, regulate autonomic and motor output that is involved in controlling sexual behavior.

## REFLEX MECHANISMS MEDIATING MALE SEXUAL FUNCTION

Components of sexual behavior in males, i.e. arousal, penile erection, emission, and ejaculation, all require coordination of the sympathetic, parasympathetic, and somatic nerves that arise from multiple segments of the spinal cord. While erection and ejaculation are spinally mediated reflexes, brain inputs tonically inhibit or facilitate these reflexes and in turn receive rewarding sensations.

### Penile Erection

Full penile erection requires activation of and balance between autonomic and somatic activity. Parasympathetic nerves regulate vasodilatation (engorgement and erection), and sympathetic inputs to the penile smooth muscle and arteries contribute to the vasoconstrictor tone that keeps the penis flaccid (see Figure 1 in reference [101]). Activation of sympathetic pathways outside the penis also contributes to blood retention in the penis, and contraction of the perineal muscles maintains penile rigidity. Relaxation of the erectile tissue, i.e., corpus cavernosum and corpus spongiosum, and vasodilatation of the penile arteries via activation of the cavernous nerve (a mixed sympathetic and parasympathetic nerve) and the dorsal nerve of the penis, leads to increased blood flow into the penis. The erectile tissue is surrounded by a rigid structure, the tunica albuginea; and distension of the penile smooth muscle obstructs venous outflow. This results in an increase in pressure within the penis, and penile erection. The increase in intracavernous pressure that occurs during erection is frequently monitored as an index of erection in animal models[10].

The major neurotransmitter that mediates penile erection is nitric oxide[3,19]. Nitric oxide released from parasympathetic nerves and endothelial cells mediates vascular and smooth muscle relaxation via production of cyclic guanosine monophosphate (cGMP), which results in local relaxation of the penile smooth muscle. Some sympathetic post-ganglionic fibers also release nitric oxide in the penis[11,12,16–18,20,101]. The use of type 5 phosphodiesterase inhibitors such as sildenafil to block the degradation of cGMP is the most effective treatment for erectile dysfunction[22]. Parasympathetic nerves also release acetylcholine and vasoactive intestinal polypeptide, which aid in the erectile process. Noradrenaline and neuropeptide Y are released from sympathetic nerves and limit blood flow into the cavernous spaces. The molecular and physiological mechanisms of smooth muscle contraction and relaxation of the penis have been extensively reviewed[3,22].

Several studies have examined the brain regions activated during penile erection or have traced projections to the penis using transneuronal tracers. These studies have identified potential brain sites that regulate penile erection. Stimulation or lesions of the medial preoptic area, lateral hypothalamus, dorsomedial nucleus of the hypothalamus, medial amygdala, and PVN can evoke or block erections. Many studies have shown that the medial preoptic area is essential for male sexual behavior[80,105]. However, medial preoptic lesions do not abolish erections evoked by masturbation and do not decrease sexual motivation[33,108]. Therefore, other brain nuclei can also activate penile erection. Growing evidence suggests that the PVN is important for penile erection. Stimulation of the PVN evokes erections in awake or anesthetized male rats, and lesions of the PVN decrease the pro-erectile effects of apomorphine and oxytocin[81–83]. Experimental evidence supports the hypothesis that one mechanism of PVN-mediated erections is activation of oxytocin neurons that project directly to the lumbosacral spinal cord[6]. Alternatively, pathways that either activate spinal circuits indirectly or act to disinhibit brain nuclei that tonically inhibit spinal circuits may be involved. Different brain pathways may contribute to the regulation of the different components of sexual behavior. For example, lesions of parvocellular PVN neurons do not affect mounting behavior, which may be primarily controlled by the medial preoptic area[1].

## Emission

Emission is an involuntary process that involves sympathetic and parasympathetic innervation of multiple organs that produce, store, and move sperm and seminal fluids within the accessory sex glands (testes), vas deferens, seminal vesicle, prostatic urethra, and prostate. The vas deferens and the prostate have received the most attention. The vas deferens is primarily controlled by sympathetic nerves that evoke contractions of the muscle to facilitate the transport of sperm and the absorption and secretion of fluids that support sperm function[59]. The prostate produces secretions that accompany ejaculation of the sperm and is sensitive to levels of circulating testosterone.

An enlarged prostate (benign prostatic hyperplasia) is common in older men and is thought to be due to hormonal changes that occur with aging[95]. Seminal and prostatic fluids remain in the proximal urethra until ejaculation occurs, due to occlusion of the bladder neck and urethral sphincter (Figure 20–4). There is little research on the CNS control of emission, although there is evidence that the PVN may be involved in emission in rats[6].

## Ejaculation

Ejaculation is the expulsion of fluids from the urethra that is facilitated by rhythmic contractions of the perineal muscle[8,37,63]. Closure of the bladder neck and urethral sphincter by sympathetic and somatic pathways prohibits retrograde ejaculation to the prostate, seminal vesicles, and bladder as well as preventing urine flow during ejaculation. Stimulation of the sensory pudendal nerve or dorsal penile nerve can evoke ejaculation[77] (Figure 20–4). Interestingly, the rhythmic firing of the perineal muscles is accompanied by rhythmic firing of the cavernous, hypogastric, and pelvic nerves[77].

Neurophysiological recordings in humans have shown concomitant rhythmic contractions of the perineal muscles together with ejaculation and the sensation of orgasm/climax[14,37,97]. Recordings from ischiocavernosus and bulbospongiosus muscles during copulation in male rats have confirmed that these muscles fire in synchrony during mounting and intromission, and sometimes during ejaculation[48].

An animal model mimicking the physiological reflexes that occur during ejaculation was developed

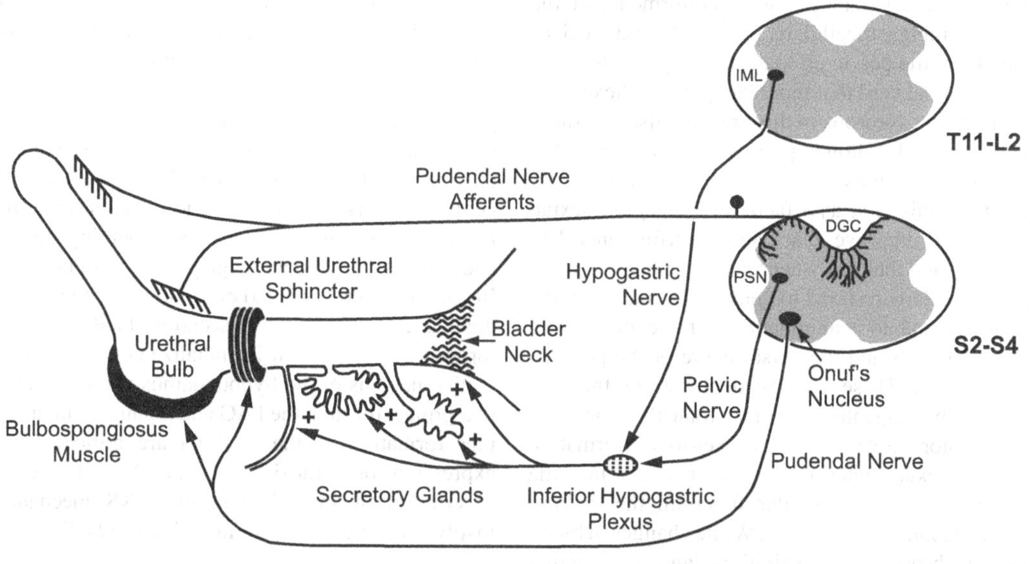


Figure 20–4 Diagram illustrating the major peripheral and spinal pathways mediating emission and ejaculatory responses in men. Sexual reflexes require coordination of the hypogastric, pelvic, and pudendal nerves. Pudendal nerve afferents, including those from the glans penis, terminate in the dorsal horn and dorsal gray commissure of the sacral spinal cord. Erection, emission, and ejaculation are mediated by the hypogastric (sympathetic), pelvic (parasympathetic), and pudendal (somatic) nerves that innervate the internal and external genital organs. Emission involves secretion of seminal fluids into the urethra via the secretary glands where it remains until ejected along with sperm, which is deposited in the urethra by contractions of the vas deferens. Ejaculation involves rhythmic contractions of the ischiocavernosus (not shown) and bulbospongiosus muscles and occlusion of the bladder neck. DGC, dorsal gray commissure; IML, intermediolateral cell column, PSN, sacral parasympathetic nucleus.

by McKenna and colleagues[77]. This model has been invaluable in furthering our understanding of the CNS control of ejaculation[71,73]. The urethrogenital reflex comprises rhythmic contractions of the perineal muscles (ischiocavernosus and bulbocavernosus muscles), penile erections, and expulsion of the urethral contents (ejaculation). The peripheral activity seen during the urethrogenital reflex strongly resembles that seen during sexual climax in humans, especially the clonic contractions of the perineal muscles and expulsion of fluid from the urethra. Stimulation of the pudendal sensory nerve triggers the urethrogenital reflex in the spinally transected, anesthetized rat as long as the lumbosacral spinal circuits are preserved. The responses cannot be evoked in the intact, anesthetized animal, suggesting supraspinal inhibition. The urethrogenital reflex is centrally generated by a spinal pattern generator, which involves multiple spinal segments that coordinate somatic, sympathetic, and parasympathetic efferents innervating the sexual organs. This spinal pattern generator may involve cells located in the medial gray matter in lumbar spinal segments 3 and 4.

Bilateral destruction of cell bodies in the nucleus paragigantocellularis in the rostral ventrolateral medulla (RVLM) allowed the urethrogenital reflex to be exposed in spinally intact, anesthetized animals. Neuroanatomical tracing studies confirmed that the nucleus paragigantocellularis projects to and receives inputs from the pelvic efferent pathways in the lumbosacral spinal cord that modulate pelvic reflexes[4,50,72] (Figure 20–5). Neurons in this area are also transneuronally labeled following virus injection into the penis, perineal muscles, uterus, and clitoris[67,74,92]. Lesions of this area also facilitate *ex copula* sexual reflexes and improve ejaculatory performance[70,115]. Excitatory and inhibitory neurons in the nucleus paragigantocellularis respond to genital stimulation in the female rat and to manipulations of the pelvic and pudendal nerves and the dorsal nerve of the penis in the male[52,104]. These studies demonstrate that the nucleus paragigantocellularis tonically inhibits somatomotor output and receives sensory information related to sexual function. The ventrolateral medulla also regulates cardiovascular function, the defense reaction, respiration, and pain. While changes in blood pressure, heart rate, respiration, and nociception accompany sexual function, the RVLM may coordinate the homeostatic responses to behavioral activation of many types.

The medial preoptic area has been implicated in several aspects of sexual behavior in males. Stimulation of this area induced sexual behavior, rhythmic firing of the pudendal motor nerve, and penile erection[44,73]. The medial preoptic area contains a high density of neurons that have receptors for gonadal androgens and is extensively interconnected with many other brain regions, including the limbic system and lower autonomic brainstem nuclei[75,106]. Therefore, the medial preoptic area is capable of integrating sensory and hormonal signals that regulate sexual reflexes.

## REFLEX MECHANISMS MEDIATING FEMALE SEXUAL FUNCTION

Understanding female sexual responses has lagged behind the understanding of male responses, primary due to the lack of suitable animal models and the lack of recognition that females suffer from physiologically based sexual dysfunction. Female sexual behavior is largely dependent on the level of the gonadal steroid hormones, estrogen, and progesterone. However, sexual behavior can occur in conditions of suboptimal or very low levels of these hormones, suggesting that sexual behavior can be triggered with adequate sensory inputs from the genitals or from the brain.

### Lordosis

Lordosis in the rat is the most thoroughly studied female reproductive behavior and has provided a great deal of knowledge about hormone-dependent reproductive behavior[66,98]. Male mounting or vaginocervical stimulation activates pudendal afferents that elicit a polysynaptic, multisegmental reflex in the axial motoneurons. This results in dorsiflexion (arching) of the back that facilitates vaginal penetration of the penis. Lordosis is greatly enhanced by sensory stimulation that is generated by male mounting behavior and is highly dependent on gonadal steroid hormones. In contrast to erection and ejaculation in the male, lordosis is controlled by a descending facilitation since lordosis does not occur in spinalized rats. The ventromedial nucleus of the hypothalamus and its pathways that project through the PAG and gigantocellular reticular formation in the medulla are critical for the expression of lordosis behavior. A more detailed description of lordosis and the CNS mechanisms involved can be found in Pfaff et al. (1994)[99].

### Genital Arousal

Genital arousal in females is associated with increased blood flow to the vagina and clitoris, which results in clitoral erection, vaginal engorgement, and vaginal lubrication[43,85]. There is some evidence that clitoral erection is mediated by local mechanisms similar to those involved in penile erection. Stimulation of the pelvic or pudendal nerve can elicit genital arousal

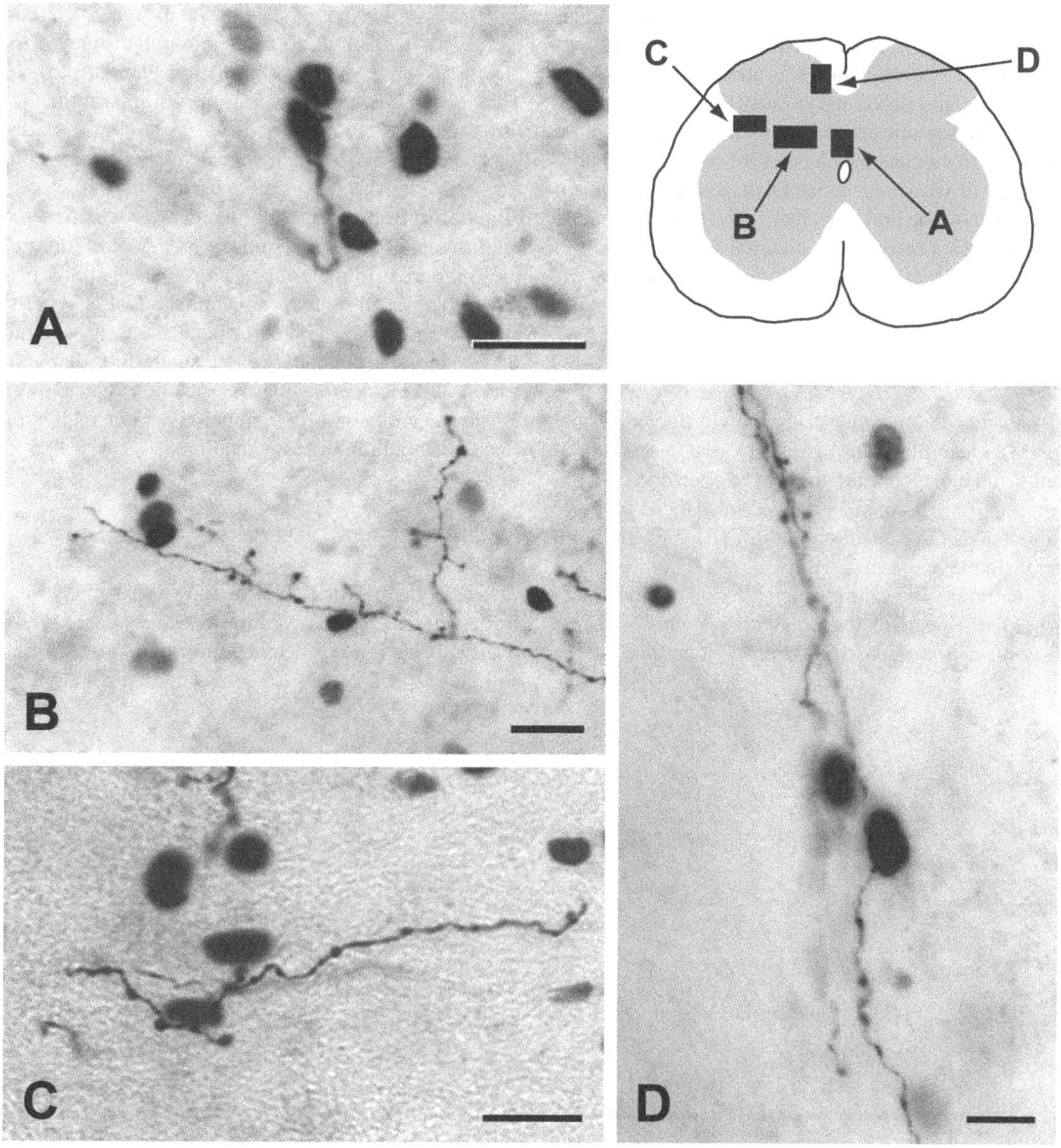


Figure 20–5 Descending inputs from the nucleus paragigantocellularis make multiple connections with spinal interneurons that are activated with sexual reflexes. Axons anterogradely labeled by injection of biotin dextran amine into the nucleus paragigantocellularis on Fos-immunoreactive nuclei. Dextran-containing axons enter the dorsal gray commissure from the lateral gray matter and dorsal horn and travel to other spinal regions. The *top* of each photograph is dorsal and the *left side* is lateral. *A:* In the dorsal gray commissure of lumbar spinal segment 6, labeled axons appear to closely appose nuclei that are immunoreactive for Fos. *B:* In the intermediate gray matter of sacral spinal segment 1, axons coursing horizontally from the sacral parasympathetic nucleus appear to make contact with Fos-positive neurons while traveling towards the medial gray matter. *C:* In the lateral gray matter of lumbar segment 6, labeled axons enter the sacral parasympathetic nucleus and appear to contact Fos-immunoreactive neurons there. *D:* A few axons run along the medial dorsal horn of lumbar segment 6 and occasionally make contacts with Fos-immunoreactive neurons. *Insert,* diagram of a transverse section through lumbar segment 6 showing the location of A–D. Scale bars in A-C, 20 μm; scale bar in *D:* 10 μm. Reproduced from Marson et al. (2003)[68] with permission.

responses[23,85]. In recent studies, we demonstrated that the increase in vaginal blood flow in response to pudendal nerve stimulation was abolished by bilateral hypogastric and pelvic nerve cuts (Figure 20–6), suggesting that somatic afferents activate automatic spinal pathways to mediate the changes in vaginal blood flow that lead to vasocongestion. Little research has been conducted on the brain mechanisms regulating female genital arousal responses, although one study demonstrated an increase in vaginal blood flow upon electrical stimulation of the medial preoptic area[40].

### Orgasm-Like Responses

In females, contractions of the pelvic floor and anal sphincter take place during orgasm, and these components of the response are thought to equate to ejaculation/orgasm in men. In women, these muscle contractions have been reported to be associated with the feeling of orgasm and climax[15,103]. Examination of the urethrogenital reflex in female rats demonstrated similar responses to those associated with orgasmic responses in women. Rhythmic contractions of the pudendal motor nerve, vagina, anal sphincter, and uterus were elicited by brief urethral distension or pudendal sensory nerve stimulation[78] (Figure 20–7). This response is neurologically very similar tothe urethrogenital reflex seen in male rats. A strong similarity between men and women was also noted in the contractions of the perineal muscles during sexual climax[13,15]. Brain and spinal pathways regulating the urethrogenital reflex in female rats appear similar to those reported in male rats. The proposed spinal pattern generator in lumbar segments 3 and 4 (Lst cells) appears not to be activated in females during copulation or the urethrogenital reflex, suggesting that activation of these neurons may be specific to ejaculation. Further elucidation of the spinal generator mediating female genital responses is required.

## NEUROTRANSMITTERS

Pharmacological studies have shown that many neurotransmitters are involved in male and female reproductive behavior. For detailed information on specific

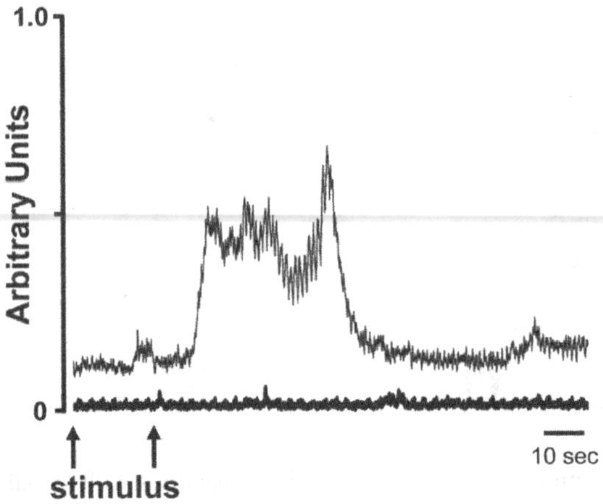


Figure 20–6 Vaginal blood flow before and after cutting autonomic nerves. Recording of vaginal blood flow using a Doppler laser probe in a urethane-anesthetized female rat with a spinal cord transection at T10. *Top trace,* Stimulation of the pudendal sensory nerve (10 μA, 0.2 msec, 40 Hz, 1 sec on/off, for 10 sec) evoked an increase in vaginal blood flow. *Bottom trace,* after cutting the hypogastric and pelvic nerves bilaterally, the increase in vaginal blood flow to pudendal sensory nerve stimulation is blocked. Vaginal blood flow responses are shown in arbitrary units.

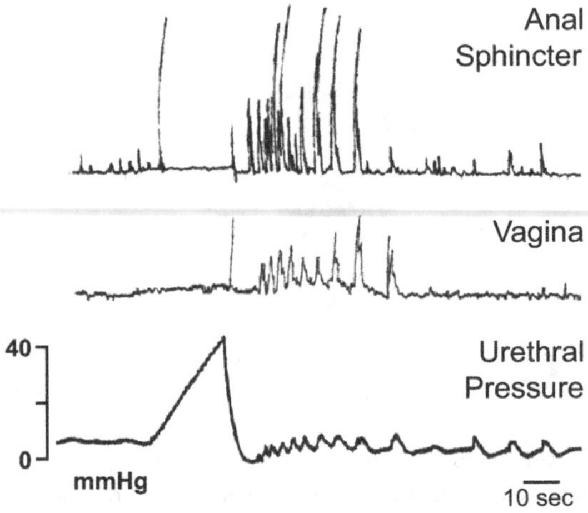


Figure 20–7 The urethrogenital reflexes in the female rat. The urethrogenital reflex was elicited by infusing saline and briefly occluding the urethral meatus in a urethane-anesthetized female rat with a spinal cord transection at T10. The rise in pressure produced by this procedure is shown in the *bottom trace.* Immediately after occlusion, rhythmic contractions of the anal sphincter and vagina were seen. Anal sphincter and vaginal EMG activity were rectified and integrated with a 100 msec time constant.

neurotransmitters and neuroendocrine mechanisms, the reader should examine reviews on the specific chemical of interest[5,7,28–30,39,41–43,46,53,94,109,110].

## Monoamines

Serotonin (5-hydroxytryptamine: 5-HT) acts through a large number of receptor subtypes and has many potential peripheral, spinal, and brain sites of action. Both facilitatory and inhibitory effects on sexual function have been reported. Increased levels of serotonin resulting from chronic administration of serotonin reuptake inhibitors are thought to mediate the high incidence of orgasmic dysfunction seen with antidepressant therapy in humans[84]. Chronic administration of serotonin reuptake inhibitors in rats delays ejaculation, increases the post ejaculatory interval, and decreases copulatory efficiency[21,27]. Other studies in rodents have shown that administration of $5\text{-HT}_{1A}$ agonists facilitates ejaculation, while administration of $5\text{-HT}_{1B}$ and $5\text{-HT}_{2C}$ receptor analogues inhibits ejaculation. $5\text{-HT}_{2C}$ receptors have been demonstrated to activate penile erection, whereas $5\text{-HT}_{2A}$ receptors may regulate initiation of copulation. Central 5-HT mechanisms (e.g., in the lateral hypothalamus) may be involved in inhibition of sexual behaviour, especially immediately after ejaculation[30].

Dopamine has a facilitatory effect on sexual behavior and sexual motivation, which is associated with reward in both males and females via its action on brain reward pathways, such as the amygdala, nucleus accumbens, hypothalamus, and ventral tegmental area[30]. Much of the basic research on dopamine began after reports appeared of increased libido and sexual potency from men treated with L-dopa (3, 4-dihydroxy-L-phenylalanine, the precursor of dopamine) for Parkinson's disease, and most of the research on dopamine has been conducted in male rats. The medial preoptic area is the major brain site for dopamine's regulation of sexual behavior (via $D_1$ and $D_2$ receptors), where it acts to facilitate copulation, genital reflexes, and sexual motivation. Dopamine pathways also act through the PVN to facilitate sexual behavior. Many neurotransmitters, including glutamate, 5-HT, nitric oxide, and oxytocin, have been shown to interact with dopamine pathways that regulate sexual function[30].

Noradrenergic fibers are abundant in spinal regions that regulate pelvic function, and electrophysiological studies have shown that drugs that act on adrenoceptors alter the activity of the hypogastric, pelvic, and pudendal nerves[26,31]. Administration of clonidine, an agonist at $\alpha_2$-adrenoceptors, inhibits erections and penile reflexes. Intrathecal infusion of noradrenaline accelerates pelvic thrusting, suggesting a facilitatory effect of the exogenous drug on the activity of lumbosacral motoneurons[47]. However, further studies are required to understand the central role of adrenergic pathways on sexual function.

## Neuropeptides

Oxytocin is one of the most important neuropeptides mediating sexual behavior in both males and females. Oxytocin is released during sexual behavior; and administration of oxytocin, either systemically or into the medial preoptic area or ventromedial nucleus of the hypothalamus, facilitates female receptive behavior and elicits penile erections[6,93]. While it is evident that central oxytocin pathways are engaged during sexual behavior, circulating oxytocin may also mediate contractions of peripheral smooth muscle (e.g., corpus cavernosus, uterus) that occur during erection and climax.

Melanocortin acts via the CNS to stimulate solicitation (arousal) behaviors and penile erections[100,113,114]. Activation of central melanocortin 3 and melanocortin 4 receptors in the ventromedial hypothalamic nucleus, PVN, and spinal cord and of peripheral receptors have all been implicated in the CNS-mediated facilitatory actions of melanocortin.

Several studies have focused on the role of peptide-containing afferent and efferent axons in the innervation of the pelvic organs[86,89,91]. The functional significance of this innervation is not yet clear, but it is likely that peptides act to both increase the sensitivity of sensory afferents to natural stimuli and may increase the responsiveness to glutamate and GABA of central pathways that control visceral tissues. Although the distribution of sensory afferents and many types of peptide-containing axons in sympathetic and parasympathetic spinal regions involved in regulating sexual function have been described (see Chapters 6 and 7), the role of peptides in the CNS control of sexual function requires further research at both spinal and supraspinal levels.

## SUMMARY

This chapter summarizes what is presently known about the CNS regions that regulate sexual responses. Over the past 50 years, there has been an increasing volume of research on the neural control of sexual function, using anatomical, physiological, pharmacological, and behavioral approaches. This has resulted in the identification of several specific brain nuclei and pathways that regulate sexual behavior in males and females. New functional neuroanatomical techniques—for example, induction of Fos expression and transneuronal tracing—have allowed visualization of

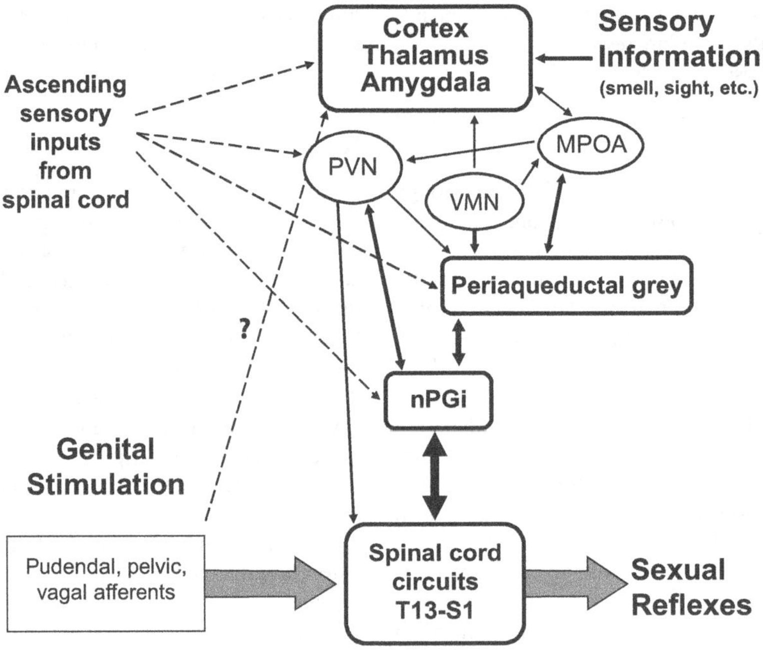


Figure 20–8 CNS regions that regulate sexual function. Diagram showing the regions within the central nervous system that are currently thought to regulate sexual responses in males and females.

the neurons activated with specific components of sexual function in males and females. The location of a spinal pattern generator involved in ejaculation has been identified. Brain-imaging techniques in humans have also provided important information allowing correlation with animal studies. The discovery of nitric oxide and its role in penile erection led to the development of drug treatments for erectile dysfunction and brought the field of sex research to the forefront.

Sexual reflexes are regulated by highly integrated autonomic and somatic pathways in the spinal cord and brain (Figure 20–8). The forebrain regions identified to date appear to regulate the initiation and execution of sexual function. The medial preoptic area is important for the integration of sensory and hormonal signals related to sexual function. Other forebrain regions, such as the amygdala, bed nucleus of the stria terminalis, and thalamic areas, appear to play a role in the execution and reward aspects of sexual function. The PVN and ventromedial nucleus of the hypothalamus play an important role in penile erection and lordosis, respectively. Many of these brain nuclei project to and relay through the PAG and medullary reticular formation, although there is direct innervation of the lumbosacral cord from the PVN. The spinal cord pathways, especially those mediating the physiological changes associated with the urethrogenital reflex, are tonically inhibited by neurons in the ventrolateral medulla. Brain nuclei may activate sexual reflexes either by direct action on spinal cord circuits or indirectly via excitatory mechanisms or disinhibition. Many of these brain regions also receive ascending sensory inputs from the pelvic, pudendal, and hypogastric nerves that mediate sexual reflexes (Figure 20–8).

Many neurotransmitters and receptor subtypes have been shown to modulate various aspects of sexual function at various sites in the brain and spinal cord. In addition, recent advances in behavioral pharmacology using *in situ* microdialysis have demonstrated that any individual neurotransmitter is unlikely to function on its own. Rather individual neurotransmitters act in coordination with other transmitters (for example, 5HT and dopamine; dopamine and nitric oxide; dopamine and prolactin, oxytocin, and vasopressin) to regulate sexual function.

ACKNOWLEDGEMENTS We would like to thank our colleagues who assisted in some of the studies described in this chapter: Rong S. Cai, Karla Gravitt, Karen Foley, Rosemary Orr, and Anne Z. Murphy. Thanks to Kevin McKenna, who introduced me to this line of research. The research was supported in part by National Institutes of Health grants #NS39166 and #HD30149.

## References

1. Ackerman, A. E., Lange, G. M., and Clemens, L. G. (1998). Effects of paraventricular lesions on sex behavior and seminal emission in male rats. *Physiology and Behavior* 63, 49–53.
2. Adler, N. T., Davis, P. G., and Komisaruk, B. R. (1977). Variation in the size and sensitivity of a genital sensory field in relation to the estrous cycle in rats. *Hormones and Behavior* 9, 334–344.
3. Andersson, K. E. (2003). Erectile physiological and pathophysiological pathways involved in erectile dysfunction. *Journal of Urology* 170, S6–S13; discussion S13–S14.
4. Andrezik, J. A., Chan-Palay, V., and Palay, S. L. (1981). The nucleus paragigantocellularis lateralis in the rat. Demonstration of afferents by the retrograde transport of horseradish peroxidase. *Anatomy and Embryology* 161, 373–390.
5. Argiolas, A., and Melis, M. R. (2004). The role of oxytocin and the paraventricular nucleus in the sexual behavior of male mammals. *Physiology and Behavior* 83, 309–317.
6. Argiolas, A., and Melis, M. R. (2005). Central control of penile erection: Role of the paraventricular nucleus of the hypothalamus. *Progress in Neurobiology* 76, 1–21.
7. Baskerville, T. A., and Douglas, A. J. (2008). Interactions between dopamine and oxytocin in the control of sexual behaviour. *Progress in Brain Research* 170, 277–290.
8. Beckett, S. D., Purohit, R. C., and Reynolds, T. M. (1975). The corpus spongiosum penis pressure and external penile muscle activity in the goat during coitus. *Biology Reproduction* 12, 289–292.
9. Berkley, K., Robbins, A., and Sato, Y. (1987). Uterine afferent fibers in the rat. In R. Schmidt, H. Schaible, and C. Vahle-Hinz (Eds.), *Fine Afferent Nerve Fibers and Pain*, pp. 129–136. Weinheim, Germany: VCH Verlage.
10. Bernabe, J., Rampin, O., Giuliano, F., and Benoit, G. (1995). Intracavernous pressure changes during reflexive penile erections in the rat. *Physiology and Behavior* 57, 837–841.
11. Bivalacqua, T. J., Liu, T., Musicki, B., Champion, H. C., and Burnett, A. L. (2007). Endothelial nitric oxide synthase keeps erection regulatory function balance in the penis. *European Urology* 51, 1732–1740.
12. Bivalacqua, T. J, Musicki, B., Usta, M. F., Champion, H. C., Kadowitz, P. J., Burnett, A. L., and Hellstrom, W. J. (2005). Endothelial nitric oxide synthase gene therapy for erectile dysfunction. *Current Pharmaceutical Design* 11, 4059–4067.
13. Bohlen, J., Held, J., and Anderson, M. (1982). Response of the circumvaginal musculature during masturbation. In B. Graber (Ed.), *Circumvaginal Musculature and Sexual Function*, pp. 43–60. Basel, Switzerland: Krager.
14. Bohlen, J. G., Held, J. P., and Sanderson, M. O. (1980). The male orgasm: Pelvic contractions measured by anal probe. *Archives of Sexual Behavior* 9, 503–521.
15. Bohlen, J. G., Held, J. P., Sanderson, M. O., and Ahlgren, A. (1982). The female orgasm: Pelvic contractions. *Archives of Sexual Behavior* 11, 367–386.
16. Burnett, A. L. (2002). Nitric oxide regulation of penile erection: Biology and therapeutic implications. *Journal of Andrology* 23, S20–S26.
17. Burnett, A. L. (2004). Novel nitric oxide signaling mechanisms regulate the erectile response. *International Journal of Impotence Research* 16 Suppl 1, S15–S19.
18. Burnett, A. L. (2008). Molecular pharmacotherapeutic targeting of PDE5 for preservation of penile health. *Journal of Andrology* 29, 3–14.
19. Burnett, A. L., Lowenstein, C. J., Bredt, D. S., Chang, T. S., and Snyder, S. H. (1992). Nitric oxide: A physiologic mediator of penile erection. *Science* 257, 401–403.
20. Burnett, A. L., and Musicki, B. (2005). The nitric oxide signaling pathway in the penis. *Current Pharmaceutical Design* 11, 3987–3994.
21. Cantor, J. M., Binik, Y. M., and Pfaus, J. G. (1999). Chronic fluoxetine inhibits sexual behavior in the male rat: Reversal with oxytocin. *Psychopharmacology* 144, 355–362.
22. Carson, C. C., and Lue, T. F. (2005). Phosphodiesterase type 5 inhibitors for erectile dysfunction. *British Journal of Urology International* 96, 257–280.
23. Cellek, S., and Moncada, S. (1998). Nitrergic neurotransmission mediates the non-adrenergic non-cholinergic responses in the clitoral corpus cavernosum of the rabbit. *British Journal of Pharmacology* 125, 1627–1629.
24. Collins, J. J., Lin, C. E., Berthoud, H. R., and Papka, R. E. (1999). Vagal afferents from the uterus and cervix provide direct connections to the brainstem. *Cell and Tissue Research* 295, 43–54.
25. Coolen, L. M., Allard, J., Truitt, W. A., and McKenna, K. E. (2004). Central regulation of ejaculation. *Physiology and Behavior* 83, 203–215.

26. Danuser, H., and Thor, K. B. (1995). Inhibition of central sympathetic and somatic outflow to the lower urinary tract of the cat by the alpha 1 adrenergic receptor antagonist prazosin. *Journal of Urology* 153, 1308–1312.
27. de Jong, T. R., Pattij, T., Veening, J. G., Waldinger, M. D., Cools, A. R., and Olivier, B. (2005). Effects of chronic selective serotonin reuptake inhibitors on 8-OH-DPAT-induced facilitation of ejaculation in rats: Comparison of fluvoxamine and paroxetine. *Psychopharmacology* 179, 509–515.
28. de Jong, T. R., Veening, J. G., Olivier, B., and Waldinger, M. D. (2007). Oxytocin involvement in SSRI-induced delayed ejaculation: A review of animal studies. *Journal of Sexual Medicine* 4, 14–28.
29. Dominguez, J. M, Gil, M., and Hull, E. M. (2006). Preoptic glutamate facilitates male sexual behavior. *Journal of Neuroscience* 26, 1699–1703.
30. Dominguez, J. M and Hull, E. M. (2005). Dopamine, the medial preoptic area, and male sexual behavior. *Physiology and Behavior* 86, 356–368.
31. Downie, J. W and Bialik, G. J. (1988). Evidence for a spinal site of action of clonidine on somatic and viscerosomatic reflex activity evoked on the pudendal nerve in cats. *Journal of Pharmacology and Experimental Therapeutics* 246, 352–358.
32. Erskine, M. S., Lehmann, M. L., Cameron, N. M., and Polston, E. K. (2004). Co-regulation of female sexual behavior and pregnancy induction: An exploratory synthesis. *Behavioral Brain Research* 153, 295–315.
33. Everitt, B. J., and Stacey, P. (1987). Studies of instrumental behavior with sexual reinforcement in male rats (Rattus norvegicus): II. Effects of preoptic area lesions, castration, and testosterone. *Journal of Comparative Psychology* 101, 407–419.
34. Fedirchuk, B., Song, L., Downie, J. W., and Shefchyk, S. J. (1992). Spinal distribution of extracellular field potentials generated by electrical stimulation of pudendal and perineal afferents in the cat. *Experimental Brain Research* 89, 517–520.
35. Ferretti, A., Caulo, M., Del Gratta, C., Di Matteo, R., Merla, A., Montorsi, F., Pizzella, V., Pompa, P., Rigatti, P., Rossini, P. M., Salonia, A., Tartaro, A., and Romani, G. L. (2005). Dynamics of male sexual arousal: Distinct components of brain activation revealed by fMRI. *Neuroimage* 26, 1086–1096.
36. Galindo, R., Barba, V., and Dail, W. G. (1997). The sensory branch of the pudendal nerve is the major route for adrenergic innervation of the penis in the rat. *The Anatomical Record* 247, 479–485.
37. Gerstenberg, T. C., Levin, R. J., and Wagner, G. (1990). Erection and ejaculation in man. Assessment of the electromyographic activity of the bulbocavernosus and ischiocavernosus muscles. *British Journal of Urology* 65, 395–402.
38. Gerstenberg, T. C., Nordling, J., and Hald, T. (1991). Evoked potentials from the lower urinary tract. II. The spino-cortical neuraxis. A methodological study. *Scandinavian Journal of Urology and Nephrology* Suppl 138, 41–46.
39. Giraldi, A., Marson, L., Nappi, R., Pfaus, J., Traish, A. M., Vardi, Y., Goldstein, I. (2004). Physiology of female sexual function: Animal models. *Journal of Sexual Medicine* 1, 237–253.
40. Giuliano, F., Allard, J., Compagnie, S., Alexandre, L., Droupy, S., Bernabe, J. (2001). Vaginal physiological changes in a model of sexual arousal in anesthetized rats. *American Journal of Physiology. Regulatory, Comparative and Integrative Physiology* 281, R140–R149.
41. Giuliano, F, Clement, P. (2005). Physiology of ejaculation: Emphasis on serotonergic control. *European Urology* 48, 408–417.
42. Giuliano, F., and Rampin, O. (2000). Central neural regulation of penile erection. *Neuroscience and Biobehavioral Reviews* 24, 517–533.
43. Giuliano, F., Rampin, O., and Allard, J. (2002). Neurophysiology and pharmacology of female genital sexual response. *Journal of Sexual Marital Therapy* 28 Suppl 1, 101–121.
44. Giuliano, F., Rampin, O., Brown, K., Courtois, F., Benoit, G., and Jardin, A. (1996). Stimulation of the medial preoptic area of the hypothalamus in the rat elicits increases in intracavernous pressure. *Neuroscience Letters* 209, 1–4.1
45. Guerit, J. M., and Opsomer, R. J. (1991). Bit-mapped imaging of somatosensory evoked potentials after stimulation of the posterior tibial nerves and dorsal nerve of the penis/clitoris. *Electroencephalography and Clinical Neurophysiology* 80, 228–237.
46. Hadley, M. E. (2005). Discovery that a melanocortin regulates sexual functions in male and female humans. *Peptides* 26, 1687–1689.
47. Hernandez Gonzalez, M., Oropeza, M. V., Guevara, M. A., Cervantes, M., Moralí, G. (1994). Effects of intrathecal administration of adrenergic agonists on the frequency of copulatory pelvic thrusting of the male rat. *Archives of Medical Research* 25, 419–425.
48. Holmes, G. M., Chapple, W. D., Leipheimer, R. E., and Sachs, B. D. (1991). Electromyographic analysis of male rat perineal muscles during copulation and reflexive erections. *Physiology and Behavior* 49, 1235–1246.

49. Holstege, G., Georgiadis, J. R., Paans, A. M., Meiners, L. C., van der Graaf, F. H., and Reinders, A. A. (2003). Brain activation during human male ejaculation. *Journal of Neuroscience* 23, 9185–9193.
50. Holstege, G., and Tan, J. (1987). Supraspinal control of motoneurons innervating the striated muscles of the pelvic floor including urethral and anal sphincters in the cat. *Brain* 110, 1323–1344.
51. Honda, C. N. (1985). Visceral and somatic afferent convergence onto neurons near the central canal in the sacral spinal cord of the cat. *Journal of Neurophysiology* 53, 1059–1078.
52. Hubscher, C. H., and Johnson, R. D. (1996). Responses of medullary reticular formation neurons to input from the male genitalia. *Journal of Neurophysiology* 76, 2474–2482.
53. Hull, E. M., Muschamp, J. W., and Sato, S. (2004). Dopamine and serotonin: Influences on male sexual behavior. *Physiology and Behavior* 83, 291–307.
54. Janig, W., and McLachlan, E. M. (1987). Organization of lumbar spinal outflow to distal colon and pelvic organs. *Physiological Reviews* 67, 1332–1404.
55. Keast, J. R. (1999). The autonomic nerve supply of male sex organs—an important target of circulating androgens. *Behavioral Brain Research* 105, 81–92.
56. Keast, J. R. (2004). Remodelling of connections in pelvic ganglia after hypogastric nerve crush. *Neuroscience* 126, 405–414.
57. Keast, J. R. (2006). Plasticity of pelvic autonomic ganglia and urogenital innervation. *International Review of Cytology* 248, 141–208.
58. Kepper, M., and Keast, J. (1995). Immunohistochemical properties and spinal connections of pelvic autonomic neurons that innervate the rat prostate gland. *Cell and Tissue Research* 281, 533–542.
59. Kihara, K., Sato, K., and Oshima, H. (1998). Sympathetic efferent pathways projecting to the vas deferens. *Microscopy Research and Technique* 42, 398–408.
60. Komisaruk, B. R., Whipple, B., Crawford, A., Liu, W. C., Kalnin, A., and Mosier, K. (2004). Brain activation during vaginocervical self-stimulation and orgasm in women with complete spinal cord injury: FMRI evidence of mediation by the vagus nerves. *Brain Research* 1024, 77–88.
61. Kow, L. M., and Pfaff, D. W. (1973). Effects of estrogen treatment on the size of receptive field and response threshold of pudendal nerve in the female rat. *Neuroendocrinology* 13, 299–313.
62. Langworthy, O. R. (1965). Innervation of the pelvic organs of the rat. *Investigative Urology* 15, 491–511.
63. Lavoisier, P., Courtois, F., Barres, D., and Blanchard, M. (1986). Correlation between intracavernous pressure and contraction of the ischiocavernosus muscle in man. *Journal of Urology* 136, 936–939.
64. Lee, J. W., and Erskine, M. S. (1996). Vaginocervical stimulation suppresses the expression of c-Fos induced by mating in thoracic, lumbar and sacral segments of the female rat. *Neuroscience* 74, 237–249.
65. Llewellyn-Smith, I. J., Weaver, L. C., and Keast, J. R. (2006). Effects of spinal cord injury on synaptic inputs to sympathetic preganglionic neurons. *Progress in Brain Research* 152, 11–26.
66. Mani, S. (2003). Emerging concepts in the regulation of female sexual behavior. *Scandinavian Journal Psychology* 44, 231–239.
67. Marson, L. (1995). Central nervous system neurons identified after injection of pseudorabies virus into the rat clitoris. *Neuroscience Letters* 190, 41–44.
68. Marson, L., Cai, R., and Makhanova, N. (2003). Identification of spinal neurons involved in the urethrogenital reflex in the female rat. *Journal of Comparative Neurology* 462, 355–370.
69. Marson, L., and Gravitt, K. (2004). Spinal neurons activated with the urethrogenital reflex in the male rat. *Brain Research* 1026, 108–115.
70. Marson, L., List, M. S., and McKenna, K. E. (1992). Lesions of the nucleus paragigantocellularis alter *ex copula* penile reflexes. *Brain Research* 592, 187–192.
71. Marson, L., and McKenna, K. E. (1990). The identification of a brainstem site controlling spinal sexual reflexes in male rats. *Brain Research* 515, 303–308.
72. Marson, L., and McKenna, K. E. (1992). A role for 5-hydroxytryptamine in descending inhibition of spinal sexual reflexes. *Experimental Brain Research* 88, 313–320.
73. Marson, L., and McKenna, K. E. (1994). Stimulation of the hypothalamus initiates the urethrogenital reflex in male rats. *Brain Research* 638, 103–108.
74. Marson, L., and McKenna, K. E. (1996). CNS cell groups involved in the control of the ischiocavernosus and bulbospongiosus muscles: A transneuronal tracing study using pseudorabies virus. *Journal of Comparative Neurology* 374, 161–179.
75. Marson, L., and Murphy, A. Z. (2006). Identification of neural circuits involved in female genital responses in the rat: A dual virus and anterograde tracing study. *American Journal of Physiology. Regulatory, Comparative and Integrative Physiology* 291, R419–R428.

76. McCarthy, M. M., Besmer, H. R., Jacobs, S. C., Keidan, G. M., and Gibbs, R. B. (1997). Influence of maternal grooming, sex and age on Fos immunoreactivity in the preoptic area of neonatal rats: Implications for sexual differentiation. *Developmental Neuroscience* 19, 488–496.
77. McKenna, K. E., Chung, S. K., and McVary, K. T. (1991). A model for the study of sexual function in anesthetized male and female rats. *American Journal of Physiology* 261, R1276–R1285.
78. McKenna, K. E., Knight, K. C., and Mayers, R. (1991). Modulation by peripheral serotonin of the threshold for sexual reflexes in female rats. *Pharmacology Biochemistry and Behavior* 40, 151–156.
79. McKenna, K. E., and Marson, L. (1997). Spinal and brainstem control of sexual function. In D. Jordan (Ed.), *Central Control of Autonomic Function*, pp. 151–187. London, U.K.: Hardwood Academic Publishers.
80. Meisel, R., and Sachs, B. (1994). The physiology of male sexual behavior. In E. Knobil and, J. Neill (Eds.), *The Physiology of Reproduction*, pp. 3–105. New York: Raven Press.
81. Melis, M. R., Stancampiano, R., and Argiolas, A. (1994). Penile erection and yawning induced by paraventricular NMDA injection in male rats are mediated by oxytocin. *Pharmacology Biochemistry and Behavior* 48, 203–207.
82. Melis, M. R., Succu, S., Spano, M. S., and Argiolas, A. (1999). Morphine injected into the paraventricular nucleus of the hypothalamus prevents noncontact penile erections and impairs copulation: Involvement of nitric oxide. *European Journal of Neuroscience* 11, 1857–1864.
83. Melis, M. R., Succu, S., Spano, M. S., and Argiolas, A. (2000). Effect of excitatory amino acid, dopamine, and oxytocin receptor antagonists on noncontact penile erections and paraventricular nitric oxide production in male rats. *Behavioral Neuroscience* 114, 849–857.
84. Modell, J. G., Katholi, C. R., Modell, J. D., and DePalma, R. L. (1997). Comparative sexual side effects of bupropion, fluoxetine, paroxetine, and sertraline. *Clinical Pharmacology and Therapeutics* 61, 476–487.
85. Munarriz, R., Kim, S. W., Kim, N. N., Traish, A., and Goldstein, I. (2003). A review of the physiology and pharmacology of peripheral (vaginal and clitoral) female genital arousal in the animal model. *Journal of Urology* 170, S40–S44; discussion, S44–S45.
86. Nance, D. M., Burns, J., Klein, C. M., and Burden, H. W. (1988). Afferent fibers in the reproductive system and pelvic viscera of female rats: Anterograde tracing and immunocytochemical studies. *Brain Research Bulletin* 21, 701–709.
87. Newton, B. W. (1993). Galanin immunoreactivity in rat spinal lamina IX: Emphasis on sexually dimorphic regions. *Peptides* 14, 955–969.
88. Niel, L., Willemsen, K. R., Volante, S. N., and Monks, D. A. (2008). Sexual dimorphism and androgen regulation of satellite cell population in differentiating rat levator ani muscle. *Developmental Neurobiology* 68, 115–122.
89. Ottesen, B., Wagner, G., and Fahrenkrug, J. (1988). *Peptidergic Innervation of the Sexual Organs*, vol. 6, pp. 66–97. Amsterdam, Netherlands: Elsevier Science Publishers.
90. Paick, J. S., and Lee, S. W. (1994). The neural mechanism of apomorphine-induced erection: An experimental study by comparison with electrostimulation-induced erection in the rat model. *Journal of Urology* 152, 2125–2128.
91. Papka, R. E., Newton, B. W., and McNeill, D. L. (1991). Origin of galanin-immunoreactive nerve fibers in the rat paracervical autonomic ganglia and uterine cervix. *Journal of the Autonomic Nervous System* 33, 25–33.
92. Papka, R. E., Williams, S., Miller, K. E., Copelin, T., and Puri, P. (1998). CNS location of uterine-related neurons revealed by trans-synaptic tracing with pseudorabies virus and their relation to estrogen receptor-immunoreactive neurons. *Neuroscience* 84, 935–952.
93. Pedersen, C. A., and Boccia, M. L. (2006). Vasopressin interactions with oxytocin in the control of female sexual behavior. *Neuroscience* 139, 843–851.
94. Peeters, M., and Giuliano, F. (2008). Central neurophysiology and dopaminergic control of ejaculation. *Neuroscience and Biobehavioral Reviews* 32, 438–453.
95. Pennefather, J. N., Lau, W. A., Mitchelson, F., and Ventura, S. (2000). The autonomic and sensory innervation of the smooth muscle of the prostate gland: A review of pharmacological and histological studies. *Journal of Autonomic Pharmacology* 20, 193–206.
96. Peters, L. C., Kristal, M. B., and Komisaruk, B. R. (1987). Sensory innervation of the external and internal genitalia of the female rat. *Brain Research* 408, 199–204.
97. Petersen, I., and Stener, I. (1970). An electromyographical study of the striated urethreal sphincter, the striated anal sphincter, and the levator ani muscle during ejaculation. *Electromyography* 10, 23–44.
98. Pfaff, D., Westberg, L., and Kow, L. M. (2005). Generalized arousal of mammalian central

nervous system. *Journal of Comparative Neurology* 493, 86–91.
99. Pfaff, D. W., Schwartz-Giblin, S., McCarthy, M. M., and Kow, L. M. (1994). Cellular and molecular mechanisms of female reproductive behavior. In E. Knobil, J. D. Neill, G. S. Greenwald, C. L. Markert, and, D. W. Pfaff (Eds.), *The Physiology of Reproduction*, vol. 2, pp. 107–220, New York: Raven Press, Ltd.
100. Pfaus, J. G., Shadiack, A., Van Soest, T., Tse, M., and Molinoff, P. (2004). Selective facilitation of sexual solicitation in the female rat by a melanocortin receptor agonist. *Proceedings of the National Academy Sciences, USA* 101, 10201–10204.
101. Prieto, D. (2008). Physiological regulation of penile arteries and veins. *International Journal of Impotence Research* 20, 17–29.
102. Rasia-Filho, A. A., Fabian, C., Rigoti, K. M., and Achaval, M. (2004). Influence of sex, estrous cycle and motherhood on dendritic spine density in the rat medial amygdala revealed by the Golgi method. *Neuroscience* 126, 839–847.
103. Rellini, A. H., McCall, K. M., Randall, P. K., and Meston, C. M. (2005). The relationship between women's subjective and physiological sexual arousal. *Psychophysiology* 42, 116–124.
104. Rose, J. (1990). Brainstem influences on sexual behavior. In W. Klemm and, R. Vertes (Eds.), *Brainstem Influences on Sexual Behavior*, pp. 407–463, New York: John Wiley and Sons.
105. Shimura, T., Yamamoto, T., and Shimokochi, M. (1994). The medial preoptic area is involved in both sexual arousal and performance in male rats: Re-evaluation of neuron activity in freely moving animals. *Brain Research* 640, 215–222.
106. Simerly, R. B., and Swanson, L. W. (1986). The organization of neural inputs to the medial preoptic nucleus of the rat. *Journal of Comparative Neurology* 246, 312–342.
107. Sipski, M., Alexander, C., Gomez-Marin, O., and Spalding, J. (2007). The effects of spinal cord injury on psychogenic sexual arousal in males. *Journal of Urology* 177, 247–251.
108. Slimp, J. C., Hart, B. L., and Goy, R. W. (1975). Heterosexual, autosexual, and social behavior of adult male rhesus monkeys with medial pre-optic anterior hypothalamic lesions. *Brain Research* 142, 105–122.
109. Succu, S., Mascia, M. S., Melis, T., Sanna, F., Melis, M. R., Possenti, R., and Argiolas, A. (2005). Pro-VGF-derived peptides induce penile erection in male rats: Involvement of paraventricular nitric oxide. *Neuropharmacology* 49, 1017–1025.
110. Succu, S., Sanna, F., Melis, T., Boi, A., Argiolas, A., and Melis, M. R. (2007). Stimulation of dopamine receptors in the paraventricular nucleus of the hypothalamus of male rats induces penile erection and increases extra-cellular dopamine in the nucleus accumbens: Involvement of central oxytocin. *Neuropharmacology* 52, 1034–1043.
111. Truitt, W. A., and Coolen, L. M. (2002). Identification of a potential ejaculation generator in the spinal cord. *Science* 297, 1566–1569.
112. Uhl-Bronner, S., Waltisperger, E., Martinez-Lorenzana, G., Condes Lara, M., and Freund-Mercier, M. J. (2005). Sexually dimorphic expression of oxytocin binding sites in forebrain and spinal cord of the rat. *Neuroscience* 135, 147–154.
113. Van der Ploeg, L. H., Martin, W. J., Howard, A. D., Nargund, RP, Austin, C. P., Guan, X., Drisko, J., Cashen, D., Sebhat, I., Patchett, A. A., Figueroa, D. J., DiLella, A. G., Connolly, B. M., Weinberg, D. H., Tan, C. P., Palyha, O. C., Pong, S. S., MacNeil, T., Rosenblum, C., Vongs, A, Tang, R., Yu, H., Sailer, A. W., Fong, T. M., Huang, C., Tota, M. R., Chang, R. S., Stearns, R., Tamvakopoulos, C., Christ, G., Drazen, D. L., Spar, B. D., Nelson, R. J., and MacIntyre, D. E. (2002). A role for the melanocortin 4 receptor in sexual function. *Proceedings of the National Academy Sciences, USA* 99, 11381–11386.
114. Wessells, H., Blevins, J. E., and Vanderah, T. W. (2005). Melanocortinergic control of penile erection. *Peptides* 26, 1972–1977.
115. Yells, D. P., Hendricks, S. E., and Prendergast, M. A. (1992). Lesions of the nucleus paragigantocellularis: Effects on mating behavior in male rats. *Brain Research* 596, 73–79.

# Index

**NOTE: Numbers in italics indicate that the indexing term occurs in a Figure.**

The manufacturer's authorised representative in the EU for product safety is Oxford University Press España S.A. of El Parque Empresarial San Fernando de Henares, Avenida de Castilla, 2 – 28830 Madrid (www.oup.es/en or product.safety@oup.com). OUP España S.A. also acts as importer into Spain of products made by the manufacturer.

Printed in the USA/Agawam, MA
May 14, 2026

905056.149